MEDICAL TERMINOLOGY
A Programmed Learning Approach
to the Language of Health Care

MEDICAL TERMINOLOGY

A Programmed Learning Approach to the Language of Health Care

MARJORIE CANFIELD WILLIS, CMA-AC
Program Director
Medical Assisting/Medical Transcription Programs
Orange Coast College
Costa Mesa, California

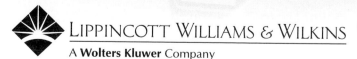

LIPPINCOTT WILLIAMS & WILKINS
A **Wolters Kluwer** Company

Philadelphia · Baltimore · New York · London
Buenos Aires · Hong Kong · Sydney · Tokyo

Editor: John Goucher
Managing Editor: Jacquelyn Merrell
Marketing Manager: Christen DeMarco
Production Editor: Jennifer Ajello
Designer: Risa Clow
Compositor: Graphic World
Printer: Quebecor World-Dubuque

351 West Camden Street
Baltimore, MD 21201

530 Walnut St.
Philadelphia, PA 19106

The publisher is not responsible (as a matter of product liability, negligence, or otherwise) for any injury resulting from any material contained herein. This publication contains information relating to general principles of medical care that should not be construed as specific instructions for individual patients. Manufacturers' product information and package inserts should be reviewed for current information, including contraindications, dosages, and precautions.

Printed in the United States of America

Library of Congress Cataloging-in-Publication Data

Willis, Marjorie Canfield.
    Medical terminology : a programmed learning approach to the language of health care /
Marjorie Canfield Willis.
        p. cm.
    Includes index.
    ISBN 0-7817-3394-4
        1. Medicine—Terminology. I. Title.

R123 . W4758 2002
610'.1'4—dc21

2002066081

The publishers have made every effort to trace the copyright holders for borrowed material. If they have inadvertently overlooked any, they will be pleased to make the necessary arrangements at the first opportunity.

To purchase additional copies of this book, call our customer service department at **(800) 638-3030** or fax orders to **(301) 824-7390**. International customers should call **(301) 714-2324**.

Visit Lippincott Williams & Wilkins on the Internet: *http://www.LWW.com.* Lippincott Williams & Wilkins customer service representatives are available from 8:30 am to 6:00 pm, EST.

02 03 04 05
1 2 3 4 5 6 7 8 9 10

Dedicated to the memory of

Dell A. Canfield,

my father, my inspiration

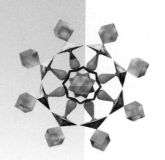

Preface to the Students

Summary of Objectives

Upon completion of this text, you will be able to:

* Describe the origin of medical language.

* Analyze the component parts of a medical term and use basic prefixes, suffixes, and combining forms to build medical terms.

* Explain the common rules for proper medical term formation, pronunciation, and spelling of medical terms.

* Define basic terms and abbreviations used in documenting health records.

* Identify common pharmaceutical terms and abbreviations used in documenting medical records.

* Identify the common forms used in documenting the care of a patient.

* Identify common anatomic terms related to the major systems of the body.

* Identify common terms related to symptoms, diagnosis, surgeries, therapies, and diagnostic tests related to the major systems of the body.

* Explain common terms and abbreviations used in documenting medical records related to the major systems of the body.

Getting Started

GOALS AND PLANNING

To reach the goal of learning the language of health care, you'll need a reasonable plan for completion. Follow the study path that this text or your instructor provides, and work the necessary study time into your personal schedule.

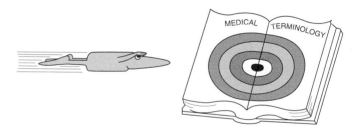

ORGANIZING THE STARTER SET OF FLASH CARDS

A "starter set" of common prefixes, suffixes, and a selected number of combining forms are provided on flash cards at the back of the text. These cards are a base on which to build, and you should review them often. Each component in the starter set is numbered and color coded according to division: **prefixes** are printed on **peach** cards, **combining forms** on **purple** cards, and **suffixes** on **green** cards. The term component is printed on the front of the card, and its meaning, including a term example, is on the back. Reinforce your learning by drawing lines to separate the components in each of the term examples, and write definitions for each in the margins.

Using a punch, put a hole in the top of each flash card. Loop each card through a key chain or ring holder to make a "rotary file." This method keeps groups of cards together and prevents them from becoming lost or scattered. Within this file, group together associated cards for components related to color, size, position, direction, and so on.

MAKING ADDITIONAL FLASH CARDS

It is highly recommended that you make flash cards for all of the additional term components introduced in each body system chapter. You can follow the example of the cards provided in the starter set, or you can see the space-saving **frugal flash card** method illustrated below. The extra benefit of handwriting them yourself is a memory boost.

You can also extend the use of flash cards to include abbreviations, symbols, and terms found throughout the text. If your stack of flash cards becomes large and cumbersome, you may want to use the following method that consolidates paper and is inexpensive, known as the frugal flash card:

1. Divide a piece of 8 1/2 × 11" lined paper in half lengthwise by making a fold down the center, creating two columns. Write the word component, symbol, or term on the first line of the first column, and its definition on the **same** line in the second column.

2. Skip down a line, then write the next word component, symbol, or term with its definition on the **same** line in the second column.

3. Continue listing any desired series of terms with corresponding definitions on the paper in this fashion until you reach the bottom of the paper. The next step is to fold the paper at the lengthwise crease, dividing the columns so that the word component, symbol, or term is listed on one side of the paper, and the definition appears on the same line on the other side of the paper. This allows you to flip from one side to the other, "flashing" and reinforcing the meanings of the terms with corresponding definitions. Use the other side of the paper in the same way.

SNATCHING MOMENTS!

Carry your flash cards with you at all times. During most days there are times when you can snatch a moment to flash your cards. You will feel less stress when waiting in a line or waiting room for an appointment if you know that you can make good use of those moments for study time.

Study Tips

USING YOUR SENSES

An effective memory depends on intricate processes that recall mental images of sights, sounds, feelings, tastes, and smells. For this reason, try to include as many senses as possible in the process of reinforcing learning.

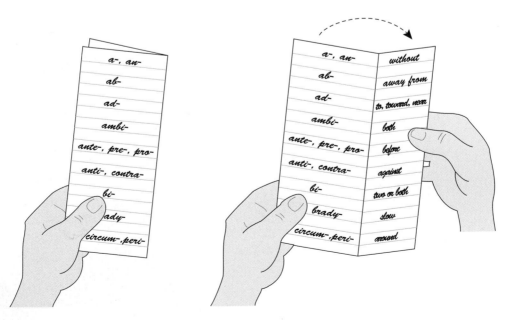

SEE IT	Employ your visual (seeing) sense by making and repeatedly reviewing your flash cards.
SAY IT	Pronounce each component out loud three times as you flash each card to reinforce your auditory (hearing) sense.
WRITE IT	Write and rewrite responses to programmed inquiries before highlighting the correct answers. Make flash cards by hand using pleasant colored paper and ink to satisfy your kinesthetic (feeling) sense.

MNEMONICS CAN HELP

Mnemonics, referring to any device for aiding memory, is named for the goddess of memory in Greek mythology. Mnemonic techniques link things to be remembered with clues for their recall using the stimulus of images, sounds, smell, and touch. Consider the following applications:

- Make up rhymes or stories that help to differentiate between meanings. For example: peri-, the prefix meaning *around*, is often confused with para-, the prefix meaning *along side of*. Use the two components in a sentence to compare their meanings; for example, I sat "para" (**alongside of**) Sarah on the merry-"peri"-go-**around.** Often the most absurd associations can help you to remember. It doesn't matter if they don't make sense to anyone but you!

- Make up songs and rhythms to help remember facts. Take a song you are familiar with like "Row, row, row, your boat . . . " and insert words with definitions that are in tune with the song.

- Draw pictures depicting term components for reinforcement.

MEMORY DRILL

Give yourself a memory drill by listing word components, symbols, or terms on one side of a piece of paper, and then filling in with the definitions from memory. Correct your paper by writing out the correct answer over the incorrect one in red ink. Make a list of incorrectly defined components on a separate piece of paper, and repeat the drill. Repeat this process until you have identified a list of the most continually found incorrect. Spend additional time on those most troublesome terms.

Additional Resources

The CD-ROM has additional fun activities to help remember medical terminology. Use this

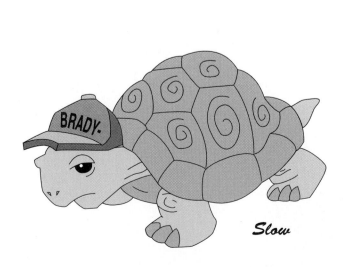

Slow

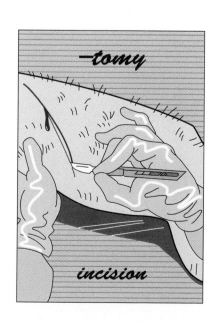

-tomy

incision

CD to reinforce what you've learned in the text. Activities on the CD include:

- Spelling bees to help you recognize and correctly spell medical terms

- A pronunciation glossary with audio pronunciations

- Interactive medical record exercises

- Labeling exercises to reinforce your knowledge of both medical terms and basic anatomy

- Concentration games, in which you match combining forms or word list with definitions

- Answers to the questions in Medical Records For Additional Study

- Scored and unscored chapter quizzes to test your knowledge

Ready, Set, Go!

Everything is laid out for you to proceed with your study. The techniques employed here have proven beneficial in learning and are geared toward efficient memorization. Be creative and enjoy the learning process!

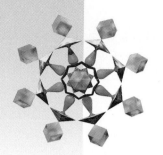

Preface to the Instructor

This text provides a sequential, programmed process for learning the language of health care that is intended to meet the needs of students working independently or within a classroom. The approach is self-directed. Learning segments are presented in self-study increments followed by programmed review frames for immediate feedback and reinforcement. Diagrams, illustrations, and term tips support learning segments, and practice exercises at the end of each chapter provide additional reinforcement. Learning builds from an understanding of the origin of medical terms and basic term construction, to the comprehension of more difficult terms and concepts encountered in relation to the body systems and medical specialty areas. The process culminates in applying the knowledge to understanding selected medical records.

The first two chapters give the basics for understanding the language of health care. Chapter 1 introduces basic term components (prefixes, suffixes, and a selected number of combining forms) and shows how these structures are combined to form medical terms. Rules of pronunciation, spelling, and formation of singular and plural froms are included. Medical word components introduced in this chapter are used repeatedly throughout the text. They are included in the starter set of flash cards for medical term components in the back of the text. Chapter 2 explains how medical terms will be learned and reinforced throughout the text using health records. Common forms, formats, abbreviations, symbols, and methods of documenting patient care are introduced. This helps students understand basic communication between professionals, including physician/provider orders and prescriptions. This chapter prepares students for medical record analyses in succeeding chapters.

Chapters 3 through 15 cover terms related to body systems. Additional combining forms are introduced along with terms related to symptoms, diagnoses, tests, procedures, surgeries, and therapies. After mastering the programmed portions and review exercises, completion of medical record analyses provides further reinforcement of learning through application of knowledge.

The CD-ROM contains additional exercises to reinforce learning. Among these exercises are scored and uscored chapter quizzes, a pronunciation glossary with 2,700 terms (organized both alphabetically and by chapter), interactive medical record exercises, labeling exercises based on the figures in the text, spelling bees, and concentration matching games.

Special Features:

- A CD-ROM with learning activities to reinforce understanding

- A connection web site specially created for instructors with PowerPoint images, a testbank, and additional activities

- A starter set of common medical term components on flash cards

- Self-study instructional increments followed by programmed reinforcement

- Unique health record orientation in Chapter 2

- Medical record analyses at the end of each body system chapter

- Pertinent color illustrations

- Chapter Review exercises to meet all learning needs

- Anatomy review with labeling exercises

- Term Tips related to spelling, pitfalls to avoid, and more

- Three appendices, including a glossary of abbreviations and symbols, term components, and commonly prescribed drugs

User's Guide

Medical Terminology: A Programmed Learning Approach to the Language of Health Care gives you a complete system for learning and using medical terminology. This User's Guide shows you how to put the book's features to work for you!

CHAPTER 3

Integumentary System

Integumentary System Overview

Tissues of the integumentary system (Fig. 3-1):
* Skin (also called the *integument*)
* Hair
* Nails
* Sweat glands
* Sebaceous glands

Functions of the integumentary system:

* Protects the body from injury
* Protects the body from intrusion of microorganisms
* Helps regulate body temperature
* Houses receptors for sense of touch, including pain a[...]

The skin has three layers:

* The **epidermis** consists of several layers of stratif[...]
  1. Cells are produced in the innermost (basal) la[...]
     face.
  2. Cells that are pushed up flatten, fill with a [...]
  3. Layers of packed dead cells accumulate in[...]
     sloughed off.
* The **dermis**, the connective tissue layer, co[...]
  (Fig. 3-1). Collagen fibers make the skin to[...]
* The **subcutaneous layer** below the derm[...]
  (fatty) tissue.

BODY SYSTEM OVERVIEW

Each chapter opens with a **body system overview**. This overview sets the stage for each chapter, introducing the body system, and laying the foundation for your work.

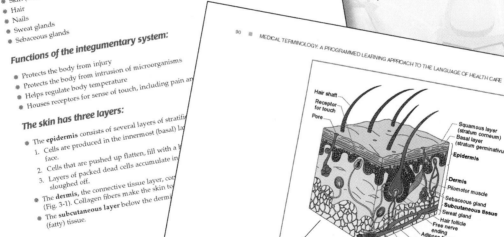

Hair shaft
Receptor for touch
Pore
Squamous layer (stratum corneum)
Basal layer (stratum germinativum)
Epidermis
Dermis
Pilomotor muscle
Sebaceous gland
Subcutaneous tissue
Sweat gland
Hair follicle
Free nerve ending
Adipose tissue
Receptor for pressure
Venule
Arteriole
Nerve

■ FIGURE 3-1. The skin.

SELF-INSTRUCTION: COMBINING FORMS

Study the following:

Combining Form	Meaning
adip/o	
lip/o	fat
steat/o	
	skin

A detailed illustration presents a visual overview of each body system being presented.

FRAMES

The book is broken into learning frames. Two types of frames are used:
Self-Instruction frames and Programmed Review frames.

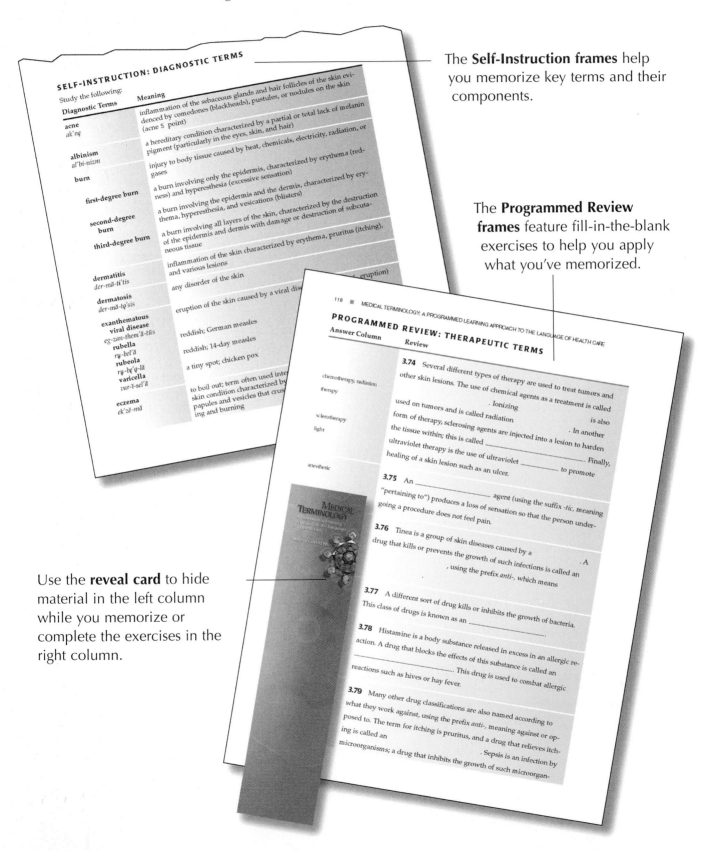

The **Self-Instruction frames** help you memorize key terms and their components.

The **Programmed Review frames** feature fill-in-the-blank exercises to help you apply what you've memorized.

Use the **reveal card** to hide material in the left column while you memorize or complete the exercises in the right column.

SELF-INSTRUCTION: DIAGNOSTIC TERMS

Study the following:

Diagnostic Terms	Meaning
acne ak'nē	inflammation of the sebaceous glands and hair follicles of the skin evidenced by comedones (blackheads), pustules, or nodules on the skin (acne 5 point)
albinism al'bi-nizm	a hereditary condition characterized by a partial or total lack of melanin pigment (particularly in the eyes, skin, and hair)
burn	injury to body tissue caused by heat, chemicals, electricity, radiation, or gases
first-degree burn	a burn involving only the epidermis, characterized by erythema (redness) and hyperesthesia (excessive sensation)
second-degree burn	a burn involving the epidermis and the dermis, characterized by erythema, hyperesthesia, and vesications (blisters)
third-degree burn	a burn involving all layers of the skin, characterized by the destruction of the epidermis and dermis with damage or destruction of subcutaneous tissue
dermatitis der-mă-tī'tis	inflammation of the skin characterized by erythema, pruritus (itching), and various lesions
dermatosis der-mă-tō'sis	any disorder of the skin
exanthematous viral disease eg-zan-them'ă-tŭs	eruption of the skin caused by a viral dise... ...eruption)
rubella ru-bel'ă	reddish; German measles
rubeola ru-bē'ŏ-lă	reddish; 14-day measles
varicella var-ĭ-sel'ă	a tiny spot; chicken pox
eczema ek'zĕ-mă	to boil out; term often used inter... skin condition characterized by... papules and vesicles that crus... ing and burning

PROGRAMMED REVIEW: THERAPEUTIC TERMS

Answer Column	Review
chemotherapy, radiation therapy	**3.74** Several different types of therapy are used to treat tumors and other skin lesions. The use of chemical agents as a treatment is called _____. Ionizing _____ is also used on tumors and is called radiation _____. In another
sclerotherapy	form of therapy, sclerosing agents are injected into a lesion to harden the tissue within; this is called _____. Finally,
light	ultraviolet therapy is the use of ultraviolet _____ to promote healing of a skin lesion such as an ulcer.
anesthetic	**3.75** An _____ agent (using the suffix -tic, meaning "pertaining to") produces a loss of sensation so that the person undergoing a procedure does not feel pain.
	3.76 Tinea is a group of skin diseases caused by a _____. A drug that kills or prevents the growth of such infections is called an _____, using the prefix anti-, which means _____
	3.77 A different sort of drug kills or inhibits the growth of bacteria. This class of drugs is known as an _____.
	3.78 Histamine is a body substance released in excess in an allergic reaction. A drug that blocks the effects of this substance is called an _____. This drug is used to combat allergic reactions such as hives or hay fever.
	3.79 Many other drug classifications are also named according to what they work against, using the prefix anti-, meaning against or opposed to. The term for itching is pruritus, and a drug that relieves itching is called an _____. Sepsis is an infection by microorganisms; a drug that inhibits the growth of such microorgan-

MEDICAL TERMINOLOGY

INTRODUCTORY CHAPTERS

The first two chapters set the stage for learning throughout the text. Chapter 1 provides analysis of **basic term components and rules** for forming, spelling, and pronouncing medical terms. Chapter 2 introduces the framework of **health care documents** so that real-life medical records can be used to reinforce the understanding of terms presented in the subsequent body system chapters.

COMMON SUFFIXES

Instructional Frame #6

Suffixes are endings that modify the root. They give the root essential meaning by forming a noun, verb, or adjective. The two basic types of suffixes are simple and compound. Simple suffixes form basic terms. For example, -ic (pertaining to), a simple suffix combined with the root gastr (stomach), forms the term gastric (pertaining to the stomach). Compound suffixes are formed by a combination of basic term components. For example, the root tom (to cut) combined with the simple suffix -y (denoting a process of) forms the compound suffix -tomy (incision); the compound suffix -ectomy (excision or removal) is formed by a combination of the prefix ec- (out) with the root tom (to cut) and the simple suffix -y (a process of).

Compound suffixes are added to roots to provide a specific meaning. For example, hyster (a root meaning uterus) combined with -ectomy forms hysterectomy (excision of the uterus). Noting the differences between simple and compound suffixes will help you analyze medical terms.

Suffixes in this text are divided into four categories:

1. Symptomatic suffixes, which describe the evidence of illness
2. Diagnostic suffixes, which provide the name of a medical condition
3. Surgical (operative) suffixes, which describe a surgical treatment
4. General suffixes, which have general application

A listing of commonly used suffixes follows. Each suffix is included on a flash card in the starter set. Organize the cards into the four categories of suffixes. Draw lines to separate the components in each of the term examples, and write definitions in the margins to prepare for review exercises. Appendix A contains a summary of suffixes.

SELF-INSTRUCTION: COMMON SUFFIXES

Study the following:

Suffix	Meaning	Flash Card ID#

SYMPTOMATIC SUFFIXES (WORD ENDINGS THAT DESCRIBE A CONDITION OR DISEASE)

Suffix	Meaning	Flash Card ID#
-algia, -dynia	pain	
-genesis	origin or production	S-2
-lysis	breaking down or dissolution	S-11
	enlargement	S-20
	trembling	S-22
	mal reduction	S-24
	age	S-27
	ary contraction	S-35
		S-38

...THAT DESCRIBE A CONDITION OR DISEASE)

	hernia	S-4
	dilation	S-8
	ence of	S-10
		S-15

PROGRESS NOTE

Merrell, Ellen
June 9, 20xx

Subjective **S:** The patient returns for lab results. She still feels "fatigue" but admits to very heavy and irregular menstrual periods for the past 6 months or so.

Objective **O:** Thyroid panel is *within normal limits*. The CBC reveals a Hgb of 8.0 and Hct of 23. **WNL**

A:
1. Anemia, probably due to iron deficiency
2. Menorrhagia
3. R/O obesity related diabetes **Rule out**

Assessment (Impression, Diagnosis)

P:
1. Rx: Feosol 1 po tid with meals
2. Repeat CBC and include serum iron
3. Schedule glucose tolerance test
4. Refer to Dr. Chang for gynecological followup

Plan (Disposition, Recommendation)

Reyna James
Reyna James, M.D.

RJ:bst
D: 6/9/20xx
T: 6/10/20xx

FIGURE 2-2. SOAP note.

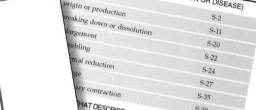

H & P	history and physical
Hx	history
HPI, PI	history of present illness, present illness
IMP	impression

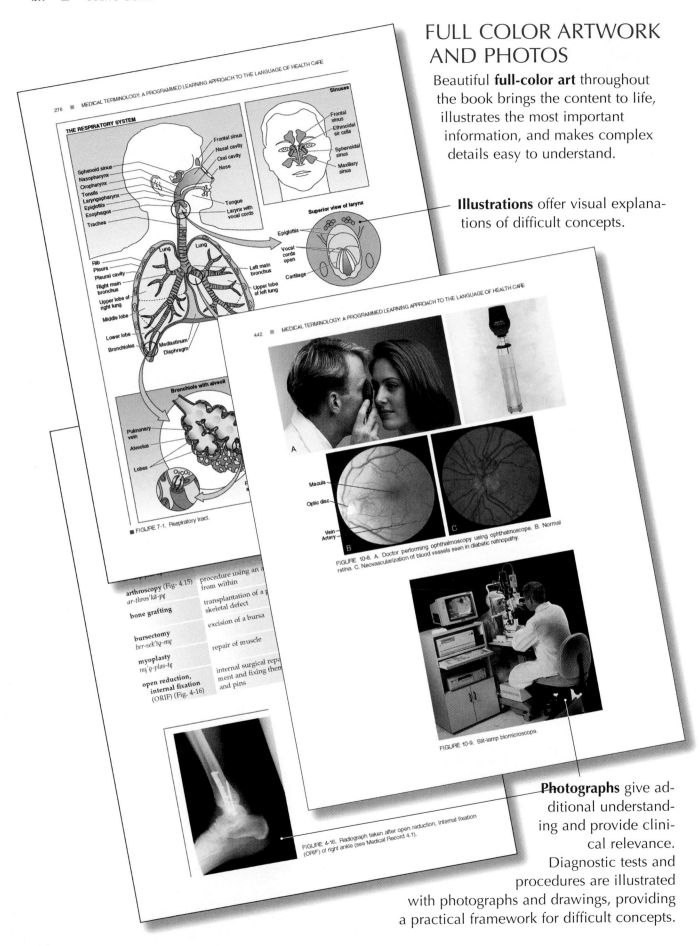

FULL COLOR ARTWORK AND PHOTOS

Beautiful **full-color art** throughout the book brings the content to life, illustrates the most important information, and makes complex details easy to understand.

Illustrations offer visual explanations of difficult concepts.

Photographs give additional understanding and provide clinical relevance. Diagnostic tests and procedures are illustrated with photographs and drawings, providing a practical framework for difficult concepts.

PRACTICE EXERCISES

Exercises are included throughout the book to help you completely understand the content, assess your progress, and review and prepare for quizzes
and tests. Put your knowledge to the test with
word part exercises, labeling diagrams, fill-in-
the-blanks, spelling bees, and medical record
exercises found throughout each chapter.

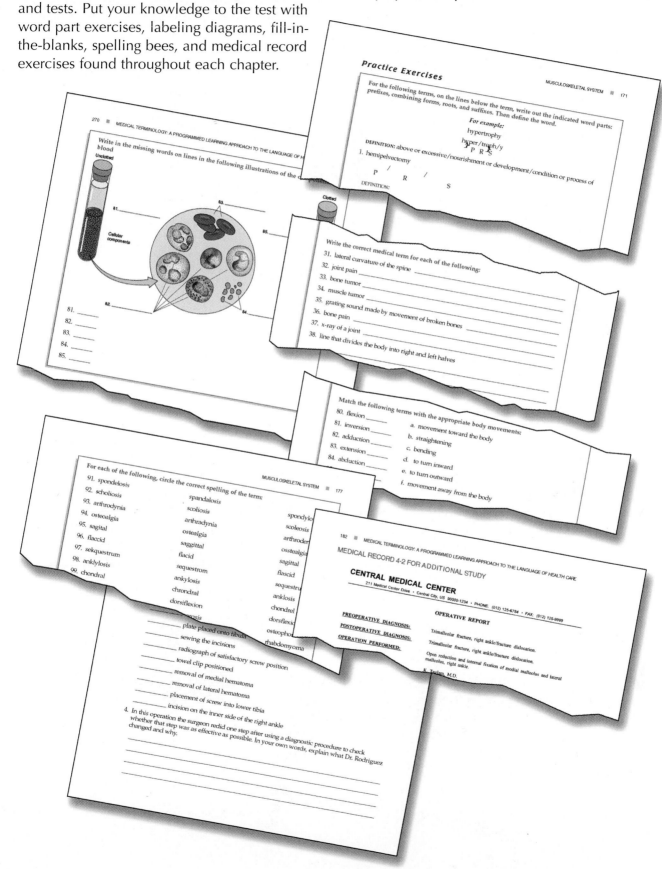

FLASHCARDS

A set of **flashcards** is included to help you maximize your study time. Use this system to make additional flash cards as you work through the text.

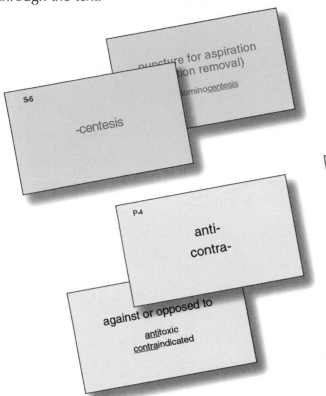

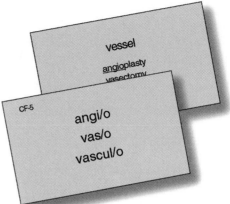

CD-ROM

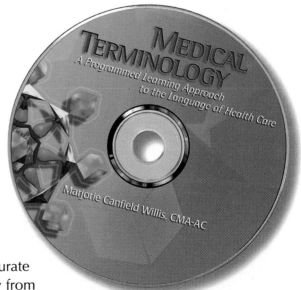

The free **CD-ROM** is your ace-in-the-hole! Use these additional exercises to test your knowledge, assess your progress, and study and review for quizzes and tests. Have FUN while you learn.

- The Concentration/matching games help you remember the links between word parts and their meanings.

- Interactive Labeling activities help you reinforce your understanding of anatomy.

- The pronunciation glossary allows you to hear accurate pronunciations of over 1,500 terms, pulled directly from Stedman's Medical Dictionary.

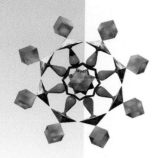

Acknowledgments

There are many dedicated professionals to thank . . .

I consider myself most fortunate to have the publishing industry's best at my side through the development and production of this text. I'm forever grateful to John Butler, my very first editor, for his belief in this book and dedication to ensuring that it would become a reality. I thank my current editor, John Goucher, for his commitment to see it through to fruition. Tom Lochhaas, developmental editor, has also been steadfast in his support and has skillfully guided me through each of my authoring endeavors. Jacqui Merrell, managing editor, did an exemplary job of organizing this project and was always available with encouragement and support and a very special thanks goes to Jennifer Ajello and the production team for all their efforts.

I'd also like to express appreciation to the faculty of Orange Coast College, School of Allied Health Professions, for their ongoing support. I owe a special debt of gratitude to my boss, Kevin Ballinger, Dean of the Consumer and Health Sciences Division.

The following reviewers were extraordinarily helpful, and I thank them for their careful atention and valuable comments:

Sandra Cutler, MEd, RRT
Springfield Technical College
Springfield, MA

Thomas Falen, MA
Health Services Administration
University of Central Florida
Orlando, FL

Connie Morgan, Division Chair
Ivy Tech State College
Kokomo, IN

Alice Slusher, Masters in Health and Human Services
Youngstown State University
Youngstown, OH

Mary Teslow, Master of Arts Library & Information Studies RHIA
Broward Community College
Ft. Lauderdale, FL

M.C.W.

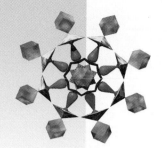

Contents

CHAPTER 1

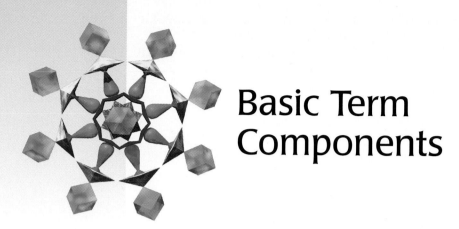

Basic Term Components

Introduction

Most medical terms have Greek or Latin origins. These terms date back to the founding of modern medicine by the Greeks and by the influence of Latin when it was the universal language in the Western world. Other languages, such as German and French, have also influenced medical terms. Today, many new terms are derived from English, which is considered the universal language. Most of the terms related to diagnosis and surgery have Greek origin, and most anatomic terms come from Latin.

Once you understand the basic medical term structure and know the commonly used prefixes, suffixes, and combining forms, you can learn the meaning of most medical terms by analyzing their component parts. Those mysterious words, which are almost frightening at first glance, will soon seem commonplace. You will learn to analyze each term you encounter with your newfound knowledge and the help of a good medical dictionary.

This chapter includes the most common prefixes and suffixes and a selection of common combining forms. More combining forms and other pertinent prefixes and suffixes are added in following chapters as you learn terms related to the body systems. This chapter also provides basic rules for proper medical term formation, pronunciation, and spelling.

Start Now

Remove the starter set of flash cards at the back of the text and organize them as recommended in the Getting Started section. Make the most of each moment of study time available to you. The key to success in building a medical vocabulary is memorizing the basic structures in this chapter.

HOW TO USE PROGRAMMED LEARNING SEGMENTS

Take time to study the material in each instructional frame before starting on a review segment. Key term components included in the flash card starter set are identified by letter and number. Locate and use them for additional reinforcement.

Remove the Reveal Card from the back cover of the text. Place the card over the shaded portion of the left column of the page to hide the appropriate responses to the questions in the learning material in the right column. Slide the card down the page to reveal the answer only after you have written your response in the fill-in space on the right. Note: Use a pencil so that you can quickly erase any inappropriate response and replace it with the correct one. Go over all the correct responses with a highlighter pen for additional reinforcement.

You can move at your own pace given the time allotted. Between study periods, use the reveal card as a bookmark.

TERM COMPONENTS

Instructional Frame #1
Study the flash cards for the word structures listed below in preparation for the programmed review that follows.

SELF-INSTRUCTION: TERM COMPONENTS

Study the following:

Term Component	Category	Meaning	Flash Card ID#
lip	root	fat	
lip/o	combining form	fat	CF-28
-emia	suffix	blood condition	S-10
hyper-	prefix	excessive	P-19
protein	root	protein	

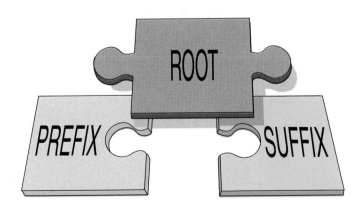

Most medical terms have three basic component parts: the root, the suffix, and the prefix. Each term is formed by combining at least one root, the foundation or subject of the word, and a suffix, the word ending that modifies and gives essential meaning to the root. A prefix is placed at the beginning of a term only when needed, to further modify the root or roots.

PROGRAMMED REVIEW: THE ROOT AND SUFFIX

Answer Column	Review
fat foundation or subject blood condition	**1.1** In the word lipemia, *lip* (meaning _____) is the *root* and _____ of the term. It is modified and given essential meaning by the link to the suffix *-emia*, meaning _blood_ _Condition_.
root, fat, suffix blood condition fat, blood	**1.2** Breaking down and defining the key components in a term often defines the term or gives clues to its meaning. In the term *lipemia*, *lip* is the _____ that means _____, and *-emia* is the _____ that means _____ _____. Memorizing key medical term components makes it possible to decipher that the term refers to the condition of _fat_ in the _blood_. Note: Lipemia is synonymous with lipidemia (formed from *lip, -oid,* and *-emia*)

PROGRAMMED REVIEW: THE PREFIX

Answer Column	Review
prefix beginning, modify excessive	**1.3** The prefix is a word structure at the beginning of a term used when needed to further modify the root or roots. For example, in the term hyperlipemia, *hyper-* is a _____ placed at the _____ of the term to further _____ the meaning of the term to denote _____ fat in the blood.

PROGRAMMED REVIEW: ADDITIONAL ROOTS

Answer Column	Review
root protein	**1.4** Often, a medical term is formed from two or more roots. For example, in the term hyperlipo*protein*emia, the addition of the _____ *protein* further defines the word to indicate an excessive amount of fat and _____ in the blood.

COMBINING FORMS AND COMBINING VOWELS

When a medical term has more than one root, the roots are joined together by a vowel, usually an "o." As shown in hyper/lip/o/protein/emia, the "o" is used to link the two roots, and it provides easier pronunciation. This vowel is known as a combining vowel. "O" is the most common combining vowel (i is the second most common) and is used so frequently to join root to root or root to suffix that it is routinely attached to the root and presented as a combining form.

PROGRAMMED REVIEW: COMBINING FORMS AND COMBINING VOWELS

Answer Column	Review
root, combining form o, combining vowel i	**1.5**　In *lip/o, lip* is the _____, and *lip/o* is the _____ _____ (root with combining vowel attached). The vowel ___ is the most common _____ _____ and ___ is the second most common.

This text uses combining forms rather than roots for easier term analysis. Each is presented with a slash between the root and the combining vowel. Hyphens are placed after prefixes to indicate their placement in the beginning of a medical term, and hyphens are placed before suffixes to indicate their link at the end of a term.

PROGRAMMED REVIEW

Answer Column	Review
root, suffix, prefix	**1.6**　Most medical terms have three basic component parts: the _____, _____, and _____.
foundation or subject	**1.7**　The root is the _____ of the term.
suffix	**1.8**　The _suffix_ is the word ending that modifies and gives essential meaning to the root.
prefix	**1.9**　The _prefix_ is a word structure at the beginning of a term that is used when needed to further modify the root.
two	**1.10**　Often a medical term is formed of _____ or more roots.
combining vowel, o	**1.11**　When a medical term has more than one root, it is joined together by a _____ _____, usually an ___.
root, vowel	**1.12**　A combining form is a _____ with a _____ attached.

Note that each component depends on the other to express the meaning of the term. Few components can stand alone.

A Few Exceptions

Most medical terms are formed by combining a root or roots and modified by suffixes and prefixes. (See examples in Instructional Frame #3.) Occasionally, terms are formed by a root alone or a combination of roots.

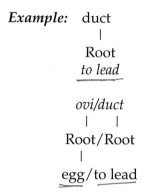

Example: duct
|
Root
to lead

ovi/duct
| |
Root/Root
|
egg/to lead

Oviduct refers to the uterine tube.

Sometimes, a term is formed from the combination of a prefix and suffix.

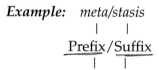

Example: *meta/stasis*
| |
Prefix/Suffix
| |
beyond, after, or change/stop or stand

Metastasis refers to the spread of a disease, such as cancer, from one location to another.

DEFINING MEDICAL TERMS THROUGH WORD STRUCTURE ANALYSIS

You can usually define a term by interpreting the suffix first, then the prefix (if present), then the root or roots.

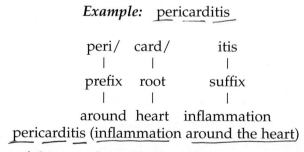

Example: pericarditis

peri/   card/   itis
| | |
prefix   root   suffix
| | |
around   heart   inflammation
pericarditis (inflammation around the heart)

You sense the basic meaning of this term by understanding its components; however, the dictionary clarifies that the term refers to inflammation of the pericardium, the sac that encloses the heart.

Beginning students often have difficulty differentiating between prefixes and roots (or combining forms) because the root appears first in a medical term when a prefix is not used. It is important to memorize the most common prefixes (those in your starter flash card set) so that you can tell the difference. Also, keep in mind that a prefix is used only as needed to further modify the root or roots.

RULES FOR FORMING AND SPELLING MEDICAL TERMS

Instructional Frame #2

Study the flash cards for the word structures listed below in preparation for the instruction and review that follows.

SELF-INSTRUCTION: RULES FOR FORMING AND SPELLING MEDICAL TERMS

Study the following:

Combining Form	Meaning	Flash Card ID#
angi/o, vas/o, vascul/o	vessel	CF-5
cardi/o	heart	CF-8
enter/o	small intestine	CF-15
esophag/o	esophagus	CF-17
gastr/o	stomach	CF-20
hem/o, hemat/o	blood	CF-23
hepat/o	liver	CF-24
oste/o	bone	CF-39
ur/o, urin/o	urine	CF-54

Suffixes	Meaning	Flash Card ID#
-al, -eal	pertaining to	S-1
-ectasis	expansion or dilation	S-8
-ectomy	excision (removal)	S-9
-ia	condition of	S-13
-itis	inflammation	S-17
-logy	study of	S-19
-megaly	enlargement	S-22
-stomy	creation of an opening	S-40
-tomy	incision	S-41

Prefixes	Meaning	Flash Card ID#
oligo-	few or deficient	P-28
para-	alongside of, or abnormal	P-30
peri-	around	P-8

Once you understand the basics of medical word building, the next steps are to memorize common term components and learn the rules for correctly spelling medical terms. Study the following five basic rules, and use them to construct words using the components provided in frame #2.

SELF-INSTRUCTION: FIVE BASIC RULES FOR FORMING AND SPELLING MEDICAL TERMS

Answer Column	Instruction
enlargement of liver	**1.13** If the root ends in a consonant (any letter *except* a, e, i, o, u) and the suffix begins with a consonant, insert a combining vowel (usually an "o") between the component parts: hepato/o + -megaly is spelled hepatomegaly and is defined as _____.
excision (removal) of a vessel	**1.14** A combining vowel is *not* used before a suffix that begins with a vowel: vas/o + -ectomy is spelled vasectomy and is defined as _____ *removal of vessel* _____.
inflammation of the heart	**1.15** If the root ends in a vowel and the suffix begins with the *same vowel*, drop the final vowel from the root and do *not* use a combining vowel: cardi/o + -itis is spelled carditis and is defined as _____.
pertaining to the heart and esophagus	**1.16** Most often, a combining vowel is inserted between two roots even when the second root begins with a vowel: cardi/o + esophag/o + -eal is spelled cardioesophageal and is defined as _____.
pertaining to alongside of the small intestine	**1.17** Occasionally, when a prefix ends in a vowel, and the root begins with a vowel, the final vowel is dropped from the prefix: para- + enter/o + -al is spelled parenteral and is defined as _____.

Note: All these rules have exceptions. Follow the basic guidelines set forth in this text, but be prepared to accept exceptions as you encounter them. Rely on your medical dictionary for additional guidance.

In the following review, construct the following words using the rules previously provided, and give the meaning for each.

PROGRAMMED REVIEW: RULES FOR FORMING AND SPELLING MEDICAL TERMS

Answer Column	Review
angiectasis expansion or dilation of a vessel	**1.18** angi/o + -ectasis is spelled _____ and means _____
gastrotomy incision in stomach	**1.19** gastr/o + -tomy is spelled _____ and means _____
hematology study of blood	**1.20** hemat/o + -logy is spelled _____ and means _____
gastroenterostomy creation of an opening (between) stomach and small intestine	**1.21** gastr/o + enter/o + -stomy is spelled _____ and means _____
oliguria condition of deficient urine	**1.22** oligo- + ur/o + -ia is spelled _____ and means _____
ostectomy excision (removal) of bone	**1.23** oste/o + -ectomy is spelled _____ and means _____
pericarditis inflammation around the heart	**1.24** peri- + cardi/o + -itis is spelled _____ and means _____

THE FORMATION OF MEDICAL TERMS

Instructional Frame #3

Study the flash cards for the word structures listed below to prepare for the review that follows.

SELF-INSTRUCTION: PATTERNS OF TERM FORMATION

Study the following:

Combining Form	Meaning	Flash Card ID#
cardi/o	heart	CF-8
vascul/o	vessel	CF-5

Suffixes	Meaning	Flash Card ID#
-ac, -al, -ar	pertaining to	S-1
-dynia	pain	S-2
-ium	structure or tissue	S-18
-logy	study of	S-19
-rrhaphy	suture	S-34
-rrhexis	rupture	S-36

Prefixes	Meaning	Flash Card ID#
endo-	within	P-15
epi-	upon	P-16
sub-	below or under	P-36

All medical terms build from the root. Prefixes and suffixes are attached to the root to modify its meaning. Two or more roots are often linked together before being modified.

The following examples show the common patterns of medical term formation using the root cardi (heart) as a base. Using the term components listed earlier, define the term as you examine each pattern. Also, note the rules used for forming each term.

PROGRAMMED REVIEW: PATTERNS OF TERM FORMATION

Answer Column	Review
	1.25 Root/Suffix
pertaining to the heart	cardi/ac means _____

1.26 Prefix/Root/Suffix

structure or tissue upon the heart

epi/card/ium means _____

1.27 Prefix/Prefix/Root/Suffix

pertaining to below or under and within the heart

sub/endo/cardi/al means _____

_____

1.28 Root/Combining Vowel/Root/Suffix

pertaining to the heart and vessels

cardi/o/vascul/ar means _____

_____

1.29 Root/Combining Vowel/Suffix

study of the heart

cardi/o/logy means _____

1.30 Root/Combining Vowel/Suffix (Symptomatic) [page 17]

pain in the heart

cardi/o/dynia means _____

1.31 Root/Combining Vowel/Suffix (Diagnostic) [page 17]

rupture of the heart

cardi/o/rrhexis means _____

1.32 Root/Combining Vowel/Suffix (Operative) [page 17]

suture of the heart

cardi/o/rrhaphy means _____

SPELLING MEDICAL TERMS

Correct spelling of medical terms is crucial for communication among health care professionals. Careless spelling causes misunderstandings that can have serious consequences. The following list shows some of the pitfalls to avoid.

1. Some words sound the same but are spelled differently and have different meanings. Context is the clue to spelling. For example,

ileum (part of the intestine)   ilium (part of the hip bone)
sitology (study of food)   cytology (study of cells)

2. Other words sound similar but are spelled differently and have different meanings. For example,

abduction (to draw away from)   adduction (to draw toward)
hepatoma (liver tumor)   hematoma (blood tumor)
aphagia (inability to swallow)   aphasia (inability to speak)

3. When letters are silent in a term, they risk being omitted when spelling the word. For example,

> pt has a "t" sound if found at the beginning of a term, e.g., pterygium, but both the "p" and "t" are pronounced when found within a term, e.g., nephroptosis   (nef-rop-tō'sis)
> ph has an "f" sound, e.g., diaphragm
> ps has an "s" sound, e.g., psychology

4. Some words have more than one accepted spelling. For example,

> orthopedic   orthopaedic
> leukocyte   leucocyte

5. Some combining forms have the same meaning but different origins that compete for usage. For example, three combining forms mean uterus:

> hyster/o (Greek)
> metr/o (Greek)
> uter/o (Latin)

ACCEPTABLE TERM FORMATIONS

As you learn medical terms, you can have fun experimenting with creating words, such as glyco (sweet) + cardio (heart) = sweetheart! However, in the real medical world, the word is formed when the term itself is coined. Often there seems to be no reason why a particular word form became acceptable. That is why you should check your medical dictionary when the spelling, formation, or precise meaning is in doubt.

RULES OF PRONUNCIATION

When you first learn to pronounce medical terms, the task can seem insurmountable. The first time you open your mouth to say a term is a tense moment for those who want to get it right! The best preparation is to study the basic rules of pronunciation; to repeat the words after hearing them pronounced on the CD-ROM accompanying this text or after your instructor has said them; and to try to keep the company of others who use medical language. There is nothing like the validation you get from the fact that no one laughed or snarled at you when you said something "medical" for the very first time! Your confidence will build with every word you use.

Following are some helpful shortcuts:

SHORTCUTS TO PRONUNCIATION

Consonant	Example
1. c (before a, o, u) = k	cavity, colon, cure
2. c (before e, i) = s	cephalic, cirrhosis
3. ch = k	cholesterol
4. g (before a, o, u) = g	gallstone, gonad, gurney
5. g (before e, i) = j	generic, giant
6. ph = f	phase
7. pn = n	pneumonia
8. ps = s	psychology
9. pt = t	ptosis, pterygium
10. rh, rrh = r	rhythm, hemorrhoid
11. x = z (as first letter)	xerosis

Phonetic spelling for the pronunciation of most medical terms in this text is provided in parentheses below the term. The phonetic system used here is basic and has only a few standard rules. The macron and breve are the two diacritical marks used. The macron (¯) is placed over vowels that have a long sound:

ā in day
ē in bee
ī in pie
ō in no
ū in unit

The breve (˘) is placed over vowels that have a short sound:

ă in alone
ĕ in ever
ĭ in pit
ŏ in ton
ŭ in sun

The primary accent (´) is placed after the syllable that is stressed when saying the word. Monosyllables do not have a stress mark. Other syllables are separated by hyphens.

SINGULAR AND PLURAL FORMS

Instructional Frame #4
Plurals are usually formed by adding "s" or "es" to the end of a singular form. The following are common exceptions for forming plurals of Latin and Greek derivatives. Study the exceptions to prepare for the review that follows.

SELF-INSTRUCTION: SINGULAR AND PLURAL FORMS

Singular Ending In	Example	Plural Ending	Example
-a	vertebra	-ae	vertebrae
-is	diagnosis	-es	diagnoses
-ma	condyloma	-mata	condylomata
-on	phenomenon	-a	phenomena
-um	bacterium	-a	bacteria
*-us	fungus	-i	fungi
-ax	thorax	-aces	thoraces
-ex	apex	-ices	apices
-ix	appendix	-ices	appendices
-y	myopathy	-ies	myopathies

*Exceptions to this rule: viruses and sinuses.

PROGRAMMED REVIEW: SINGULAR AND PLURAL FORMS

Answer Column	Review
t	**1.33** The *pt* in *pterygium* has a/an __ sound.
ovaries, ova	**1.34** An ov<u>um</u> is an egg produced by an ovary. There are two _____ in the female that produce eggs or _____.
k	**1.35** The *ch* in the word *chronic* has a/an __ sound.
metastases	**1.36** The spread of cancer to a distant organ is called metastasis. The spread of cancer to more than one organ is _____.
s	**1.37** The *c* in the word *cirrhosis* has a/an __ sound.
verrucae	**1.38** A verruca is a wart. The term for several warts is _____.
z	**1.39** The *x* in *xerosis* has a/an __ sound.
condyloma	**1.40** Condylomata are genital warts. One genital wart is a _____.
j	**1.41** The *g* in *genital* has a/an __ sound.
index	**1.42** Indices is a plural form of _____.
thrombi	**1.43** A thrombus is a clot. Several clots are termed _____.
n	**1.44** The *pn* in *pneumatic* has a/an __ sound.

COMMON PREFIXES

Instructional Frame #5

Prefixes are word structures found at the beginning of a term when needed to further modify the root or roots. A list of commonly used prefixes organized within categories follows. Each is included on a flash card in the starter set. Organize the cards into the categories listed here. Draw lines to separate the components in each of the term examples, and write definitions in the margins in preparation for review exercises.

Appendix A contains a summary list of prefixes.

SELF-INSTRUCTION: COMMON PREFIXES

Study the following:

Prefix	Meaning	Flash Card ID#
Negation		
a-, an-	without	P-1
anti-, contra-	against or opposed to	P-5
de-	from, down, or not	P-10
Position/Direction		
ab-	away from	P-2
ad-	to, toward, or near	P-3
circum-, peri-	around	P-8
dia-, trans-	across or through	P-11
e-, ec-, ex-	out or away	P-13
ecto-, exo-, extra-	outside	P-14
en-, endo-, intra-	within	P-15
epi-	upon	P-16
inter-	between	P-21
meso-	middle	P-23
meta-	beyond, after, or change	P-24
para-*	*alongside of, or abnormal	P-30
retro-	backward or behind	P-35
Quantity of Measurement		
bi-	two, or both	P-6
hemi-, semi-	half	P-18
hyper-	above or excessive	P-19
hypo-	below or deficient	P-20
macro-	large or long	P-22

micro-	small	P-25
mono-, uni-	one	P-26
oligo-	few or deficient	P-28
pan-	all	P-29
poly-, multi-	many	P-31
quadri-	four	P-33
sub-, infra-	below or under	P-36
super-, supra-	above or excessive	P-37
tri-	three	P-39
ultra-	beyond or excessive	P-40

Time

ante-, pre-, pro-	before	P-4
brady-	slow	P-7
tachy-	fast	P-38
post-	after, or behind	P-32
re-	again or back	P-34

General

con-, syn-, sym-	together or with	P-9
dys-	painful, difficult, or faulty	P-12
eu-	good or normal	P-17
neo-	new	P-27

Study the flash cards for the prefixes listed above in preparation for the following review.

PROGRAMMED REVIEW: PREFIXES

Answer Column	Review
	1.45 Several prefixes modify direction when used in a term. _Abduction_
away	is used to describe movement _____ from the body, and _adduction_
to, toward, or near	describes movement _____ the body.

around

across or through

out or away

one, bi

Circumduction is movement that is _____. A diagonal is an angle that moves _____. *Inversion* refers to turning in and eversion means to turn _____. *Unilateral* refers to _____ side, whereas _____ lateral means both sides.

exo

endo

within

1.46 Glands that secrete within the body are the endocrine glands, and those that secrete outside are the _____ crine glands. An instrument to examine within the body is an _____scope. When something is encapsulated, it is held _____.

upon

across or through

within

1.47 Epidermal refers to something _____ the skin. *Transdermal* pertains to _____ the skin, and *intradermal* means _____ the skin.

again

from, down, or not

before

backward or behind

1.48 When something is reactivated, it is made active _____. *Deactivate* refers to something that is _____ active. *Proactive* refers to an action made _____. *Retroposition* refers to a structure that is _____.

before

pre

around, after

Neo

1.49 Natal pertains to birth. Antenatal is the time _____ birth, also known as the _____natal period. *Perinatal* is the time _around_____ birth, and *postnatal* is the time _____ birth. _____natal pertains to newborn.

good or normal

difficult

1.50 Toc/o is a combining form meaning labor. *Eutocia* is a condition of _____ labor, and *dystocia* is a condition of _____ labor.

a

dys

a

1.51 Dysphasia is a condition of difficult speech. A patient without the ability to speak has a condition called ___phasia. A condition of difficulty swallowing is termed _____phagia. The patient without the ability to swallow has ___phagia.

An

1.52 Aerobic pertains to air. _____aerobic pertains to without air.

COMMON SUFFIXES

Instructional Frame #6

Suffixes are endings that modify the root. They give the root essential meaning by forming a noun, verb, or adjective. The two basic types of suffixes are simple and compound. Simple suffixes form basic terms. For example, -ic (pertaining to), a simple suffix combined with the root gastr (stomach), forms the term gastric (pertaining to the stomach). Compound suffixes are formed by a combination of basic term components. For example, the root tom (to cut) combined with the simple suffix -y (denoting a process of) forms the compound suffix -tomy (incision); the compound suffix -ectomy (excision or removal) is formed by a combination of the prefix ec- (out) with the root tom (to cut) and the simple suffix -y (a process of).

Compound suffixes are added to roots to provide a specific meaning. For example, hyster (a root meaning uterus) combined with -ectomy forms hysterectomy (excision of the uterus). Noting the differences between simple and compound suffixes will help you analyze medical terms.

Suffixes in this text are divided into four categories:

1. Symptomatic suffixes, which describe the evidence of illness
2. Diagnostic suffixes, which provide the name of a medical condition
3. Surgical (operative) suffixes, which describe a surgical treatment
4. General suffixes, which have general application

A listing of commonly used suffixes follows. Each suffix is included on a flash card in the starter set. Organize the cards into the four categories of suffixes. Draw lines to separate the components in each of the term examples, and write definitions in the margins to prepare for review exercises. Appendix A contains a summary of suffixes.

SELF-INSTRUCTION: COMMON SUFFIXES

Study the following:

Suffix	Meaning	Flash Card ID#
SYMPTOMATIC SUFFIXES (WORD ENDINGS THAT DESCRIBE A CONDITION OR DISEASE)		
-algia, -dynia	pain	S-2
-genesis	origin or production	S-11
-lysis	breaking down or dissolution	S-20
-megaly	enlargement	S-22
-oid	resembling	S-24
-penia	abnormal reduction	S-27
-rrhea	discharge	S-35
-spasm	involuntary contraction	S-38
DIAGNOSTIC SUFFIXES (WORD ENDINGS THAT DESCRIBE A CONDITION OR DISEASE)		
-cele	pouching or hernia	S-4
-ectasis	expansion or dilation	S-8
-emia	blood condition	S-10
-iasis	formation or presence of	S-15

-itis	inflammation	S-17
-malacia	softening	S-21
-oma	tumor	S-25
-osis	condition or increase	S-26
-phil, -philia	attraction for	S-29
(-ptosis)	falling or downward displacement	S-32
-rrhage, -rrhagia	to burst forth (usually blood)	S-33
-rrhexis	rupture	S-36

SURGICAL (OPERATIVE) SUFFIXES (WORD ENDINGS THAT DESCRIBE A SURGICAL (OPERATIVE) TREATMENT)

-centesis	puncture for aspiration	S-5
-desis	binding	S-6
-ectomy	excision (removal)	S-9
-pexy	suspension or fixation	S-28
-plasty	surgical repair or reconstruction	S-30
-rrhaphy	suture	S-34
-tomy	incision	S-41
-stomy	creation of an opening	S-40

GENERAL SUFFIXES (SIMPLE OR COMPOUND SUFFIXES THAT HAVE GENERAL APPLICATION)

Noun Endings (suffixes that form a noun when combined with a root)

-ation	process	S-3
-e	noun marker	S-7
-ia, -ism	condition of	S-13
-y	condition or process of	S-42
-ium	structure or tissue	S-18

Adjective Endings (suffixes that form an adjective when combined with a root)

-ac, -al, -ar, -ary, -eal, -ic, -ous, -tic	pertaining to	S-1

Diminutive Endings (suffixes meaning small)

-icle, -ole, -ula, -ule		S-16

Other General Suffixes

-gram	record	S-12
-graph	instrument for recording	S-12
-graphy	process of recording	S-12
-iatrics, -iatry	treatment	S-14
-logy	study	S-19
-logist	one who specializes in the study or treatment of	S-19
-ist	one who specializes in	S-19
-meter	instrument for measuring	S-23
-metry	process of measuring	S-23
-poiesis	formation	S-31
-scope	instrument for examination	S-37
-scopy	process of examination	S-37
-stasis	stop or stand	S-39

Don't be rolled over by the

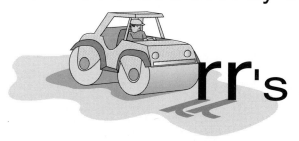

rr's

We have the Greeks to thank for the suffixes with **double rr's.** Take a careful look at each so that you will spell them correctly in a term!

Suffix	Meaning	Example
-rrhea	discharge	pyorrhea—a discharge of pus
-rrhage or -rrhagia	to burst forth (usually blood)	hemorrage—a burst forth of blood
		menorrhagia—a burst forth of blood during menstruation
-rrhexis	rupture	angiorrhexis—a rupture of a vessel
-rrhaphy	suture	nephorrhaphy—a suture of the kidney

Each component also has an h and -rrhaphy has two!

Study the flash cards for the suffixes listed above in preparation for the following review.

PROGRAMMED REVIEW: SUFFIXES

Answer Column	Review

1.53 *Gastr/o* is a combining form meaning _____.

stomach

In *epigastrium*, epi- is the _____ meaning _____, and

prefix, upon

_____ is the noun ending meaning _____ or

-ium, structure

_____.

tissue

1.54 In *epigastric*, use of the suffix _____ forms an adjective denoting

-ic

_____ _____ the stomach—specifically referring to

pertaining to

the tissue region _____ the stomach known as the

upon

_____. In *gastroesophageal*, _____ is the adjective

epigastrium, -eal

ending that modifies the term to mean _____ _____

pertaining to

the stomach and _____.

esophagus

1.55 A symptomatic suffix is a term _____ used to describe

ending

evidence of illness. *-Algia* or *-dynia* meaning _____, *-megaly* meaning

pain

_____, *-rrhea* meaning ~~discharge~~, and

enlargement, discharge

-spasm meaning _____ _____

involuntary contraction

are examples of suffixes used to form_____ terms

symptomatic

that describe evidence of _____.

illness

1.56 The symptomatic term that describes stomach pain is

_____. Pain located in the tissue upon the stomach is

gastralgia or gastrodynia

termed _____. Involuntary contraction of the

epigastralgia

stomach is called _____, and the term to describe

gastrospasm

the discharge of gastric juice from the stomach is *gastro*_____.

rrhea

The term to describe an enlargement of the stomach is

_____.

gastromegaly

1.57 Physical examination and test procedures are key to identifying

the cause of symptoms in order to make a diagnosis (the name of a con-

dition or disease).

In evaluating the cause of a symptom such as gastrodynia, or _____

pain

examination	in the stomach, a gastroscopy or _____ of the
stomach	_____ may be performed . The specific endoscope (instru-
within	ment to examine _____) used in gastroscopy is called a
gastroscope	_____ .

1.58 Diagnostic suffixes are word _____ used to describe a

endings	condition or name of a disease called a _~diagnosis~_ . If, on
diagnosis	gastroscopic examination, the physician notes an inflammation of the
	stomach, a diagnosis of _____ is made. The presence of
gastritis	a stone in the stomach is termed gastrolith_____ , and a finding
iasis	of softening of the stomach wall is called _____ .
gastromalacia	

1.59 Once a diagnosis is made, treatment follows. Some treatments require surgery. Operative suffixes are term _____ that de-

endings	scribe a surgical or _____ treatment. Given a diagnosis
operative	of stomach tumor, termed _____ , a surgical remedy might
gastroma	involve a partial or complete removal of the stomach called a
gastrectomy	_____ . Gastroptosis, defined as a falling or
downward displacement	_____ _____ of the
stomach	_____ , may necessitate a surgical suspension or fixation
pexy	called a gastro _pexy_ . The operative term describing a surgical re-
gastroplasty	pair of the stomach is _____ .

COMMON COMBINING FORMS

Instructional Frame #7

The following table shows selected combining forms (roots with vowels attached) to give you a start toward building medical terms. Each is included on a flash card in the starter set. Organize them in categories such as on the following list. Review them by drawing lines to separate the components in each term example, and write definitions in the margins in preparation for review exercises. Additional combining forms are introduced at the beginning of Chapters 3 through 15 on body systems. Appendix A contains a summary of combining forms.

Study the entire starter set of flash cards in preparation for the following review

SELF-INSTRUCTION: COMMON COMBINING FORMS

Study the following:

Combining Form	Meaning	Flash Card ID#
COLORS		
cyan/o	blue	CF-12
erythr/o	red	CF-16
leuk/o	white	CF-27
melan/o	black	CF-30
SUBSTANCES		
aer/o	air, gas	CF-4
hem/o, hemat/o	blood	CF-23
hydr/o	water	CF-26
lip/o	fat	CF-28
py/o	pus	CF-48
ur/o, urin/o	urine	CF-54
ORGANS/STRUCTURES		
abdomin/o, lapar/o	abdomen	CF-1
✓ acr/o	extremity or topmost	CF-2
✓ aden/o	gland	CF-3
angi/o, vas/o, vascul/o	vessel	CF-5
✓ arthr/o	joint	CF-6
cardi/o	heart	CF-8
cephal/o	head	CF-9
col/o, colon/o	colon	CF-10
cyt/o	cell	CF-13
derm/o, dermat/o, cutane/o	skin	CF-14
enter/o	small intestine	CF-15
esophag/o	esophagus	CF-17
gastr/o	stomach	CF-20
hepat/o	liver	CF-24
✓ hist/o	tissue	CF-25

nas/o, rhin/o	nose	CF-32
nephr/o, ren/o	kidney	CF-34
neur/o	nerve	CF-35
or/o	mouth	CF-37
oste/o	bone	CF-39
pneumon/o	air or lung	CF-46

GENERAL

carcin/o	cancer	CF-7
crin/o	to secrete	CF-11
esthesi/o	sensation	CF-18
fibr/o	fiber	CF-19
gen/o	origin or production	CF-21
gynec/o	woman	CF-22
lith/o	stone	CF-29
morph/o	form	CF-31
necr/o	death	CF-33
onc/o	tumor, mass	CF-36
orth/o	straight, normal, correct	CF-38
path/o	disease	CF-40
ped/o	child or foot	CF-41
phag/o	eat or swallow	CF-42
phas/o	speech	CF-43
plas/o	formation	CF-45
phob/o	exaggerated fear or sensitivity	CF-44
psych/o	mind	CF-47
scler/o	hard	CF-49
son/o	sound	CF-50
sten/o	narrow	CF-51
tox/o, toxic/o	poison	CF-52
troph/o	nourishment or development	CF-53

PROGRAMMED REVIEW: COMBINING FORMS

Answer Column	Review

kidney	**1.60** *Neph* is a Greek root meaning _____ . Combined with an
combining form	o, it becomes *nephr/o*, a _____ _____ . *Nephr/o* can-
suffix	not stand alone as a term. At the least, it needs a _____ to give
	it essential meaning. In the term *nephrology,* the addition of the suffix
study	*-logy* forms a term with a specific meaning: _____ of the
kidney	_____ .

	1.61 In nephrolithiasis, the link of *nephr/o* to *lith,* a root meaning
stone, -iasis	_____ , and the suffix _____ forms the term referring to
presence or formation of	the _presence or formation of_____ . The combining
kidney stones	
o	vowel for *lith* is _o_ . Notice that the vowel was not used when linked to
suffix	*-iasis* because the _suffix_____ began with a vowel. Nephrolithiasis is
ren/o	a renal disease. Renal is a term formed using _____ , the Latin
	combining form meaning kidney.

combining form	**1.62** *Abdomin/o* is a _____ _____ meaning
abdomen	_abdomen_____ , the central part of the body trunk. Note that the
	spelling of *abdomin/o* is different from the anatomic part it represents.
lapar/o	Another combining form meaning abdomen is _lapar_____ . A la-
abdomen	paroscope is an instrument used to examine the _____ .

blood	**1.63** *Hem/o* and *hemat/o* are combining forms meaning _blood_____ .
hematology	The study of blood is called _hematology_____ . It includes analy-
cell	sis of blood and its cellular components. *Cyt/o* means _____ . Cells
red	of the blood include erythrocytes, or _____ cells, and
leukocytes	_____ , or white cells. *Hemopoiesis* is a term referring
blood, suffix	to the formation of _blood____ . *-Emia* is the _____ that means
poison	blood. Toxemia is a condition of blood _____ .

water head	**1.64** *Hydr/o* is a combining form meaning _____. A person with hydrocephaly has a condition of water (fluid) within the _____.
(acro) topmost, acro	**1.65** An enlarged extremity is called _acro_ megaly. *Acr/o* also means _topmost_. A person with _acro_ *phobia* has a fear of high places.
gen/o origin or production cancer	**1.66** The suffix meaning origin or production is *-genesis*. The combining form meaning origin or production is _____. The suffix *-genic* pertains to _____. *Carcinogenic* pertains to the origin or production of _cancer_.
white red melan/o, blue cyan black skin	**1.67** Besides *leuk/o* meaning _____ and *erythr/o* meaning _____, other combining forms are listed in the starter set related to color: _melan_ is black, and *cyan/o* is _____. When the skin turns blue from lack of oxygen, the term for it is _cyan_ osis. *Melanoma*, referring to a _black_ tumor, is a common cutaneous cancer, or _skin_ cancer.

CELLS/TISSUES/ORGANS/SYSTEMS (FIG. 1-1)

Study the entire starter set of flash cards to prepare for the review that follows.

PROGRAMMED REVIEW: CELLS/TISSUES/ORGANS/SYSTEMS

Answer Column	Review
   small cyto histology	**1.68** The term *cell,* meaning small room, was used to describe the structures first observed in 1665 by Robert Hooke as he examined cork using a microscope, an instrument to examine something _____. He noted that the small cells were part of a larger web of woven tissue. The study of cells that comprise the human body became known as _cyto_ logy and the study of tissue became known as _histology_.

Levels of organization

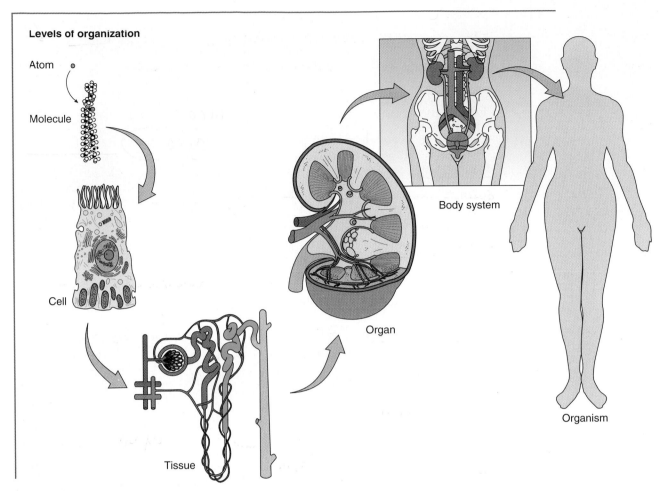

■ **FIGURE 1-1.** Levels of organization in the body.

larger

organs

urine

pertaining to

1.69 Body cells combine to form tissues and combinations of tissues compose the organs necessary for body functions. Organs act together as part of the _____ body systems. For example, the kidneys are _____ that function to filter blood as part of the urinary system (*urin/o* means _____, and -ary means _____).

ren/o

urology

nephro

1.70 The Greek combining form for kidney is *nephr/o,* and the Latin is _____. The medical specialty concerned with the study and treatment of the urinary tract is called _____. The physician who particularly specializes in the study and treatment of the kidneys is known as a _____logist.

patho

pathologist

1.71 Examination of body cells and tissues is part of the medical specialty concerned with the study of *disease*, known as _____logy. The physician who is a specialist in the study of disease is called a _____.

formation

faulty

new

-oma

carcinoma

oncology

1.72 *Plas/o* is a combining form meaning _____, and *dys-* is a prefix meaning bad, difficult, or _____. Dysplasia is the term used to describe abnormal cell and tissue development, and neoplasia, referring to a condition of _____ formation, is the term used to describe the formation of cells and tissue into tumor. The suffix for tumor is __oma__. A cancerous tumor is called a ___carcinoma___. The specialty concerned with the study of tumors and cancers is ___oncology___.

skin

dermatology

dermatologist

1.73 The largest organ of the body, the skin, is part of the integumentary system. Integument is Latin for skin, and *dermat/o* is Greek meaning _____. The specialty field involved with the study and treatment of skin diseases is called _____. The specialist is called a _____.

Oste/o

joint

1.74 The musculoskeletal system provides support and gives shape to the body. Bones, which form the skeleton, are covered with muscle to supply the forces that make movement possible. ___oste/o___ is the combining form for bone, and *arthr/o* is the combining form meaning ___joint___, the hinge between bones.

heart

vessels

hematology

1.75 The cardiovascular system consists of the ___heart___ and ___vessels___ that transport blood throughout the body. Blood provides transport for oxygen, nutrients, and wastes. The study of blood is called ___hematology___.

air or lung

1.76 *Pneum/o*, meaning ___lung___, is the key combining form of the respiratory system, which is responsible for the exchange of gases (oxygen and carbon dioxide) within the body. The nose is the first structure to receive oxygen.

nose

nas/o

Rhin/o is the Greek combining form meaning _____. The Latin combining form with the same meaning is _____.

Neur/o

1.77 The nervous system is a complicated network of nerves and fibers that control all functions of the body. _Neur/o_ is the combining form for nerve.

within

to secrete

1.78 The ductless glands of the endocrine system affect the function of organs by the secreting hormones. *Endo* means _within_, and *crin/o* means _to secrete_.

mouth

esophagus, stomach

small, large

liver

1.79 The gastrointestinal system provides for digestion and elimination. Combining forms related to key structures of the tubular digestive tract are: *or/o* meaning _mouth_, *esophag/o* meaning _esophagus_, *gastr/o* meaning _stomach_, *enter/o* meaning _small_ intestine, and *col/o* or *colon/o* meaning _large_ intestine. *Hepat/o* is the combining form for _liver_, the organ that produces bile necessary for digestion.

logist

gynecology

1.80 The male and female reproductive systems produce the sex cells and maintain the organs necessary for production of human offspring. The physician who specializes in the treatment of the male and female urinary system, as well as the male reproductive system, is called a uro _logist_. Treatment of the female reproductive system involves two medical specialties: obstetrics and _gynecology_ (study of woman).

Practice Exercises

Circle the correct meaning for the following term components:

1. inter-

   a. difficult   b. between   c. within   d. out, away   e. behind

2. ultra-

   a. across   b. excessive   c. against   d. around   e. without

3. anti-

   a. beside   b. outside   c. against   d. around   e. away from

4. a-

   a. double   b. both   c. two   d. without   e. against

5. bi-

   a. without   b. upon   c. excessive   d. two   e. back, again

6. pre-

   a. against   b. out   c. toward   d. before   e. after

7. poly-

   a. many   b. few   c. above   d. before   e. after

8. neo-

   a. birth   b. death   c. origin   d. new   e. disease

9. peri-

   a. many   b. all   c. alongside of   d. attraction for   e. around

10. hyper-

   a. below   b. after   c. beyond   d. excessive   e. deficient

11. -plasty

   a. surgical repair   b. cancer   c. tumor   d. excision   e. incision

12. -megaly

   a. development   b. tumor   c. fixation   d. enlargement   e. softening

13. -itis

   a. excision   b. condition   c. abnormal reduction   d. formation   e. inflammation

14. -rrhagia

   a. discharge   b. suture   c. rupture   d. burst forth   e. repair

15. -penia

    a. discharge   b. fixation   c. rupture   d. reduction e. suspension

16. necr/o

    a. fear   b. death   c. black   d. tumor   e. large

17. toxic/o

    a. poisen   b. poison   c. poieson   d. poissen   e. poeson

18. acr/o

    a. gland   b. blue   c. air   d. extremity   e. red

19. angi/o

    a. artery   b. heart   c. vessel   d. red   e. gland

20. cyt/o

    a. color   b. sac   c. blue   d. colon   e. cell

21. melan/o

    a. death   b. disease   c. black   d. dissolution   e. large

Circle the term component for the following:

22. kidney

    a. enter/o   b. gastr/o   c. ren/o   d. hepat/o   e. necr/o

23. large

    a. poly-   b. -malacia   c. -oma   d. hyper-   e. macro-

24. record

    a. -meter   b. -metry   c. -gram   d. -graph   e. graphy

25. surgical fixation

    a. -ptosis   b. -plasia   c. -penia   d. -pexy   e. -plasty

26. condition or increase

    a. -itis   b. -iasis   c. -osis   d. -ium   e. -ous

27. excision

    a. -tomy   b. stomy   c. ectomy   d. -centesis   e. -cele

Circle the correct plural for the following:

28. vertebra

    a. vertebray   b. vertebras   c. vertebrae   d. vertebrus   e. vertebraes

29. bulla

    a. bulli   b. bullia   c. bullae   d. bullas   e. bullata

30. speculum

    a. speculata   b. speculumes   c. specula   d. speculae   e. speculuma

31. fungus

    a. fungi   b. fungae   c. funges   d. funguses   e. fungea

32. stoma

    a. stomata   b. stomatae   c. stomes   d. stomatus   e. stomatum

33. macula

    a. maculus   b. maculas   c. maculi   d. maculae   e. maculies

34. radius

    a. radii   b. radiusos   c. radiuses   d. radia   e. radiis

35. diagnosis

    a. diagnosa   b. diagnoses   c. diagnosses   d. diagnosi   e. diagnosae

Circle the operative term in each of the following:

36. a. nephroptosis   b. hemolysis   c. angiectasis   d. colostomy   e. necrosis

37. a. vasorrhaphy   b. hematoma   c. gastrocele   d. endoscope   e. cardiorrhexis

38. a. morphologic b. adenolysis c. abdominocentesis d. osteomalacia e. polyrrhea

Circle the correct spelling:

39. a. nephoraphy   b. nephorrapy   c. nephrorrhaphy   d. nephorrhapy

40. a. abdominoscopy   b. abdemenoscopi   c. abdomenscopy   d. abdominoschope

41. a. perrycardium b. pericardium c. periocardium d. parcardium e. paracardium

For the following words, draw a line or lines to separate prefixes, combining forms (roots), and suffixes. Then define the word according to the meaning of its components. Note: P = prefix; R = root; S = suffix.

For example:
hyperlipemia

<u>hyper / lip / emia</u>
  P   R   S

DEFINITION: above or excessive/fat/blood condition

42. microlithiasis

<u>Small</u> / <u>lith</u> / <u>iasis.</u>
  P   R   S

DEFINITION: Small / Stone / presence of

43. sympathy

    <u>sym</u> / <u>path</u> / <u>y</u>
      P   R   S

    DEFINITION: _____

44. toxoid

    <u>tox</u> / <u>oid</u>
      R   S

    DEFINITION: poisong resonbea _____

45. mesomorphic

    _____ / _____ / _____
      P   R   S

    DEFINITION: _____

46. pancytopenia

    <u>pan</u> / <u>cyto</u> / <u>penia</u>
      P   CF   S

    DEFINITION: all   cell   abnormal reduction _____

47. metastasis

    <u>meta</u> / <u>stasis</u>
      P   S

    DEFINITION: beyond / stop or stand _____

48. acrodynia

    <u>acro</u> / <u>dynia</u>
      CF   S

    DEFINITION: peripheral: pain _____

49. tachycardia

    <u>tach</u> / <u>card</u> / <u>ia</u>
      P   R   S

    DEFINITION: rapid fast   heart   condition of _____

50. pyogenesis

    <u>pyo</u> / <u>genesis</u>
      CF   S

    DEFINITION: pus   origin or prod'n _____

51. adenitis

aden / _itis_
R   S

DEFINITION: _gland inflamm_

52. macrocephalous

large / _head_ / _ous_
P   R   S

DEFINITION: _large head pertaing to_

53. paracentesis

para / _centesis_
P   S

DEFINITION: _alongside of puncture for aspiration_

54. ultrasonography

ultra / _Sono_ / _graphy_
P   CF   S

DEFINITION: _beyond_

55. orthopedic

ortho / _____ / _ic_
CF   R   S

DEFINITION: _Straight / normal per_

56. angiomegaly

_____ / _____
CF   S

DEFINITION: _____

57. psychiatry

_____ / _____
R   S

DEFINITION: _____

58. carcinophobia

_____ / _____ / _____
CF   R   S

DEFINITION: _____

59. endocrinologist

within / _crino_ / _____
   P   CF   S

DEFINITION: _____

60. rhinostenosis

_____ / _____ / _osis_
   CF   R   S

DEFINITION: _____

61. hypoesthesia

_____ / _____ / _____
   P   R   S

DEFINITION: _____

62. aerophagia

_____ / _eat or swallow_ / _____
   CF   R   S

DEFINITION: _____

63. fibroma

fiber / _tumor_
   R   S

DEFINITION: _____

64. pneumophilia

_____ / _____
   CF   S

DEFINITION: _lung_ / _attract_

65. sclerosis

harden / _osis_
   R   S

DEFINITION: _____ / condition or increase.

66. hemolysis

hemo / _lysis_
   CF   S

DEFINITION: blood / breaking down

67. hydrocephaly

_____ / _____ / __y__
   CF   R   S

DEFINITION: _____ condition _____

68. cytometer

_____ / _____
   CF   S

DEFINITION: _____

69. cyanotic

__cyano__ / __tic__
   CF   S

DEFINITION: __blue, pertaining to_____

70. extravasation

__extra__ / __vas__ / __ation__
   P   R   S

DEFINITION: __outside vessel process_____

71. hypertrophy

__hyper__ / __troph__ / __y__
   P   R   S

DEFINITION: __above / nourishment / condition · pwcim of__

Circle the appropriate prefix to complete the following terms:

72. _____nasal = <u>above</u> the nose

   a. para   b. peri   c. supra   d. infra   e. sub

73. _____activate = make active <u>again</u>

   a. de   b. retro   c. pro   d. re   e. hyper

74. _____ operative = <u>before</u> surgery

   a. intra   b. post   c. pre   d. peri   e. circum

75. _____partum = <u>after</u> labor

   a. ante   b. anti   c. post   d. pro   e. retro

76. _____hydrated = <u>not</u> watered

   a. anti   b. de   c. ec   d. dys   e. contra

77. _____morphic = pertaining to <u>one</u> form

   a. bi   b. micro   c. mono   d. tri   e. meta

78. _____dermal = <u>across or through</u> the skin

    a. ecto   b. endo   c. intra   d. epi   e. trans

79. _____acute = <u>excessively</u> severe

    a. sub   b. hypo   c. super   d. oligo   e. pan

80. _____umbilical = <u>below or under</u> the navel

    a. hyper   b. infra   c. peri   d. para   e. pre

81. _____cardia = <u>outside</u> the heart

    a. exo   b. endo   c. retro   d. para   e. peri

82. _____flexion = bend <u>before</u>

    a. retro   b. de   c. ante   d. anti   e. re

83. _____phasia = <u>difficult</u> speech

    a. ab   b. dys   c. a   d. eu   e. para

84. _____duction = to turn <u>away from</u>

    a. ad   b. ab   c. ecto   d. pro   e. ante

85. _____phylaxis = to guard <u>before</u>

    a. retro   b. pro   c. post   d. peri   e. anti

86. _____arthritis = inflammation of <u>many</u> joints

    a. meta   b. poly   c. macro   d. pan   e. ultra

87. _____cardia = <u>slow</u> heart

    a. hypo   b. tachy   c. brady   d. hyper   e. dys

88. _____vascular = <u>around</u> a blood vessel

    a. intra   b. inter   c. para   d. circum   e. endo

89. _____aerobic = pertaining to life <u>without</u> air

    a. an   b. a   c. hypo   d. hyper   e. dys

90. _____sexual = pertaining to <u>both</u> sexes

    a. uni   b. bi   c. tri   d. quadri   e. poly

91. _____plegia = <u>half</u> paralysis

    a. quadri   b. peri   c. hemi   d. bi   e. mono

Match the following:

92. black ___f___   a. tri-

93. three ___a___   b. leuk/o

94. red ___h___   c. cyan/o

95. four ___g___   d. bi-

96. white ___b___   e. uni-

97. one ___e___   f. melan/o

98. blue ___c___   g. quadri-

99. two ___d___   h. erythr/o

100. few ___i___   i. oligo-

Answers to Practice Exercises

1. b. between
2. b. excessive
3. c. against
4. d. without
5. d. two
6. d. before
7. a. many
8. d. new
9. e. around
10. d. excessive
11. a. surgical repair
12. d. enlargement
13. e. inflammation
14. d. burst forth
15. d. reduction
16. b. death
17. b. poison
18. d. extremity
19. c. vessel
20. e. cell
21. c. black
22. c. ren/o
23. e. macro-
24. c. -gram
25. d. -pexy
26. c. -osis
27. c. -ectomy
28. c. vertebrae
29. c. bullae
30. c. specula

31. a. fungi
32. a. stomata
33. d. maculae
34. a. radii
35. b. diagnoses
36. d. colostomy
37. a. vasorrhaphy
38. c. abdominocentesis
39. c. nephrorrhaphy
40. a. abdominoscopy
41. b. pericardium
42. micro / lith / iasis
    P   R   S
    Small/stone/presence or
    formation of
43. sym / path / y
    P   R   S
    together or with/disease/
    condition or process of
44. tox / oid
    R   S
    poison/resembling
45. meso / morph / ic
    P   R   S
    middle/form/pertaining to
46. pan / cyto / penia
    P   CF   S
    all/cell/abnormal reduction
47. meta / stasis
    P   S
    beyond, after, or change/
    stop or stand
48. acro / dynia
    CF   S
    extremity/pain

49. tachy / card / ia
    P   R   S
    fast/heart/condition of
50. pyo / genesis
    CF   S
    pus/origin or production
51. aden / itis
    R   S
    gland/inflammation
52. macro / cephal / ous
    P   R   S
    large or long/head/
    pertaining to
53. para / centesis
    P   S
    alongside of/puncture for
    aspiration
54. ultra / sono / graphy
    P   CF   S
    beyond or excessive/sound/
    process of recording
55. ortho /ped / ic
    CF   R   S
    straight, normal, or
    correct/foot/ pertaining to
56. angio / megaly
    CF   S
    vessel/enlargement
57. psych / iatry
    R   S
    mind/treatment
58. carcino / phob / ia
    CF   R   S
    cancer/fear or sensitivity/
    condition of

59. endo / crino / logist
    P   CF   S
    within/to secrete/one who
      specializes in the study or
      treatment of
60. rhino / sten / osis
    CF   R   S
    nose/narrow/condition or
      increase
61. hypo / esthes / ia
    P   R   S
    below or deficient/
      sensation/condition of
62. aero / phag / ia
    CF   R   S
    air or gas/eat or swallow/
      condition of
63. fibr / oma
    R   S
    fiber/tumor
64. pneumo / philia
    CF   S
    air or lung/attraction for
65. scler / osis
    R   S
    hard/condition or increase

66. hemo / lysis
    CF   S
    blood/breaking down
      or dissolution
67. hydro / cephal / y
    CF   R   S
    water/head/condition or
      process of
68. cyto / meter
    CF   S
    cell/instrument for
      measuring
69. cyano / tic
    CF   S
    blue/pertaining to
70. extra / vas / ation
    P   R   S
    outside/vessel/process
71. hyper / troph / y
    P   R   S
    above or excessive/
      nourishment or
      development/condition
      or process of
72.   c. supra
73.   d. re
74.   c. pre

75.   c. post
76.   b. de
77.   c. mono
78.   e. trans
79.   c. super
80.   b. infra
81.   a. exo
82.   c. ante
83.   b. dys
84.   b. ab
85.   b. pro
86.   b. poly
87.   c. brady
88.   d. circum
89.   a. an
90.   b. bi
91.   c. hemi
92.   f. melan/o
93.   a. tri
94.   h. erythr/o
95.   g. quadri-
96.   b. leuk/o
97.   e. uni-
98.   c. cyan/o
99.   d. bi-
100.   i. oligo-

CHAPTER 2

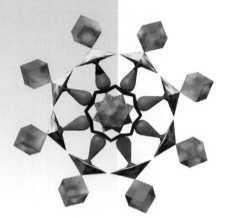

Health Care Records

Common Records Used in Documenting the Care of a Patient

To actually use your knowledge of medical terminology, you need to see how this language is used in everyday communications about patients. Learning the common abbreviations, symbols, forms, and formats used in recording patient care will help you comprehend medical record documentation.

THE HISTORY AND PHYSICAL

The cornerstone for patient care is the **history and physical (H & P)** record (Fig. 2-1). It documents the patient's medical history and findings from the physical examination. It is usually the first document generated when a patient **presents** for care. It is usually recorded at a new patient visit or as part of a consultation.

The first portion of the **H & P,** the **history (Hx),** provides **subjective information (S)** obtained from the patient about his or her personal perceptions. It is the patient's personal statement about their medical history. Information regarding past injuries, illnesses, operations, defects, and habits is included here. It begins with the **chief complaint (CC),** the patient's reason for seeking medical care. It is usually brief and is often documented in the patient's own words, which are indicated within quotes (e.g., CC: "flu"). Often, especially in handwritten notes, the abbreviation **c/o (complains of)** is also used. Next, the complaint is amplified in the **present illness (PI)** or **history of present illness (HPI)** to note the duration and severity of the complaint (how long the patient has had the complaint and how bad it is). Notations about the patient's **symptoms (sx),** which are subjective evidences of illness, indicate what the patient is experiencing.

Information about the patient's **past history (PH) or past medical history (PMH)** is recorded next. It includes a record of information about the patient's past illnesses starting with childhood, and it includes surgical operations, injuries, physical defects, medications, and allergies. **UCHD (usual childhood diseases)** is the abbreviation used here to record that the patient had all the "usual" or commonly contracted illnesses during childhood. **NKA (no known allergies)** or **NKDA (no known drug allergies)** indicates that the patient has had no known allergic reaction to a previously administered drug. The **family history (FH)** includes the state of health of immediate family members (mother, father, siblings), and the **social history (SH)** notes the patient's recreational interests, hobbies, and use of tobacco and drugs, including alcohol. A record of work habits that may involve health risks is included in the **occupational history (OH).** The history is complete after doc-

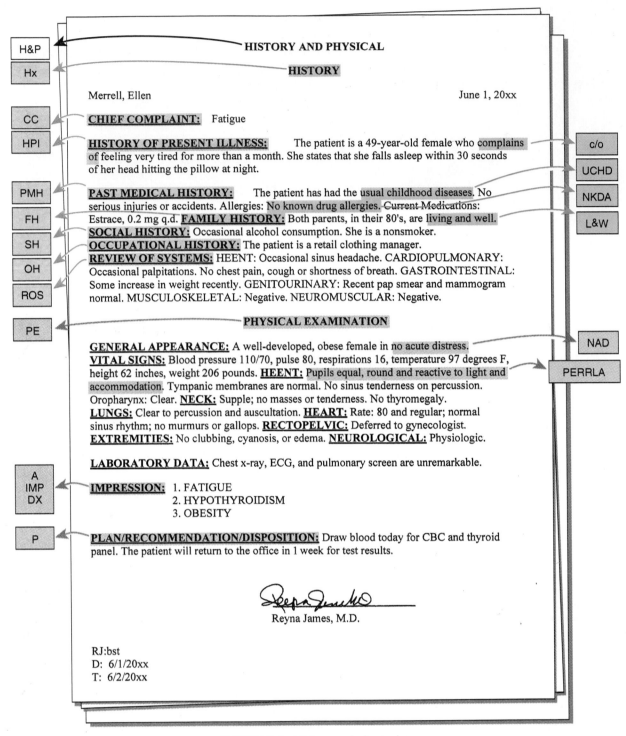

FIGURE 2-1. History and physical.

umenting the patient's answers to questions related to the **review of systems,** a head-to-toe review of the function of all body systems. This review makes it possible to evaluate other symptoms that may not have been previously mentioned.

After the subjective data are recorded, the provider begins a **physical examination** to obtain **objective information,** facts that can be seen or detected by testing. **Signs,** or objective evidences of disease, are documented, and selected diagnostic tests are performed or ordered when further evaluation is necessary. Several abbreviations are used to document the findings of physical examination; for example, **HEENT (head, eyes, ears, nose, throat), PERRLA (pupils equal, round, and reactive to light and accommodation), NAD (no acute distress),** and **WNL (within normal limits).**

The identification of a disease or condition is recorded in the **impression, diagnosis, or assessment,** which is made after the evaluation of all subjective and objective data. Often, when one or more diagnoses are in question, a **differential diagnosis** is made using the abbreviation **R/O (rule out).** The possible conditions are identified, and further investigation, often involving diagnostic tests and procedures, is done to **rule out** or eliminate each suspect and verify the final diagnosis.

Final notations include the provider's **plan,** also called a **recommendation,** or **disposition.** Here, the provider outlines strategies designed to remedy the patient's condition, including instructions to the patient, orders for medications, diagnostic tests, or therapies.

Often, physicians are required to dictate a current history and physical report before admitting a patient to the hospital, e.g., for elective surgery. When the patient is to have surgery, the report is often called a "preoperative" history and physical.

SOAP Notes

After the initial history and physical is recorded, further documentations in the form of **progress notes** are made as care continues. The SOAP method of documenting a patient's progress is most common. The letters represent the order in which progress is noted as each complaint or problem is addressed (Fig. 2-2).

S – <u>Subjective</u>   That which the patient describes

O – <u>Objective</u>   Observable information (e.g., test results and blood pressure readings)

A – <u>Assessment</u>
or Dx, IMP   Patient's progress and evaluation of the plan's effectiveness—any new-found problem or diagnosis is also noted here

P – <u>Plan</u>   Decision to proceed or alter the plan strategy

Make flash cards, and memorize the following abbreviations used in documenting a history and physical examination and progress notes so that you will recognize them in the health records found throughout this book.

SELF-INSTRUCTION: MEDICAL RECORD ABBREVIATIONS

Study the following:

Combining Form	Meaning
A	assessment
A & W	alive and well
CC	chief complaint
c/o	complains of
Dx	diagnosis
FH	family history
HEENT	head, eyes, ears, nose, throat

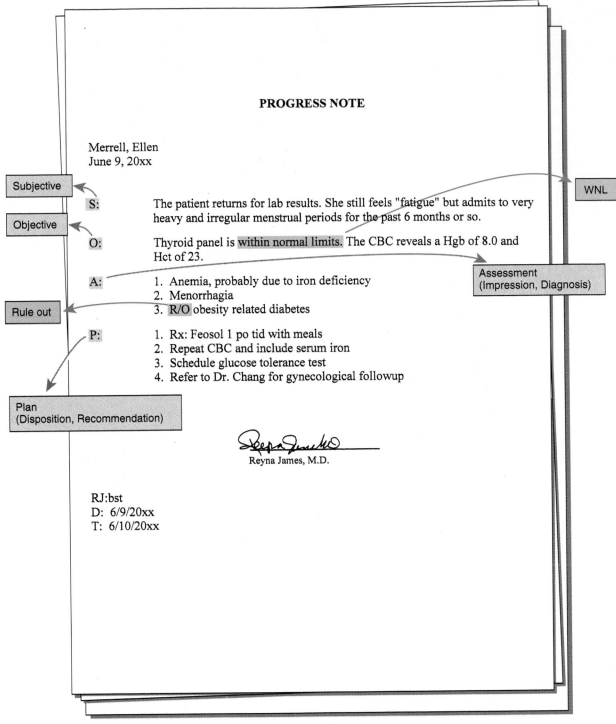

FIGURE 2-2. SOAP note.

H & P	history and physical
Hx	history
HPI, PI	history of present illness, present illness
IMP	impression

L & W	living and well
NAD	no acute distress
NKA, NKDA	no known allergies, no known drug allergies
O	objective information
OH	occupational history
P	plan (recommendation, disposition)
PE, Px	physical examination
PERRLA	pupils equal, round, and reactive to light and accommodation
PH, PMH	past history, past medical history
ROS, SR	review of systems, systems review
R/O	rule out
S	subjective information
SH	social history
Sx	symptom
UCHD	usual childhood diseases
WNL	within normal limits

PROGRAMMED REVIEW: MEDICAL RECORD ABBREVIATIONS

Study the following:

Answer Column	Review

history and physical

2.1 The H & P, or _____ _____ _____, is the first document generated in the care of a patient. It is divided into

history two categories: the Hx, or _____, that provides all

subjective _____ information obtained from the patient, includ-

physical ing his or her own perceptions, and the Px, or _____, or

physical examination PE, or _____ _____, that records

objective all _____ information that can be seen or verified by the examiner.

2.2 The first thing that is noted in the history is the CC, or

chief complaint _____ _____, or what the patient c/o, or complains of

present illness

history, present illness

symptoms

_____ ____. It is a brief explanation of what brought the patient to seek medical care. Next, an amplification of the complaint is made in the PI, or _____ _____, or HPI, or _____ of _____ _____ to report how long the patient has had the complaint and how bad it is. All subjective evidences of disease that the patient reports are noted as Sx, or _____.

past history, past

medical history

usual childhood diseases

no

known allergies, no known

drug allergies

2.3 The history continues by gathering information regarding past injuries, illnesses, operations, physical defects, medications, and allergies in the PH, or _____ _____, or PMH, or _____ _____ _____. UCHD means that the patient had the _____ _____ _____, or commonly contracted illnesses during childhood. NKA, or _____ _____ _____, or NKDA, ____ _____ _____ _____, indicates that the patient has had no known allergic reaction to a previously administered drug.

family history

social history

occupational history

review of

systems, systems review

2.4 "Father, age 58, mother, age 54, brother, age 32, all L&W" is an example of a FH, or _____ _____. Notes about recreational interests, hobbies, and use of tobacco and drugs such as alcohol are noted in the SH, or _____ _____. Work habits that may involve health risks are included in the OH, or _____ _____. The history is complete after the patient answers questions related to a review of the functions of the body systems in the ROS, or _____ ____ _____, or SR: *Systems Review*.

physical

physical examination

signs

2.5 The second portion of the H & P is the Px, or _____, or PE, _____ _____. Objective evidences of disease called _____ are documented, selected tests are ordered, and findings are recorded. Common abbreviations: HEENT

head, eyes, ears, nose, throat	means _____, _____, _____, _____ and _____;
pupils equal, round,	PERRLA means _____ _____, _____ and
reactive, light,	_____ to _____ and
accommodation, within	_____; WNL means _____
normal limits, no acute	_____ _____. NAD indicates _____ _____
distress	_____.

2.6 The identification of a disease or condition is recorded in the IMP,

impression, diagnosis	or _____ , Dx, or _____ , or A, or
assessment	_____, which is made after all subjective and objec-
	tive data are evaluated. When one or more diagnoses are in question, a
rule	differential diagnosis is made using the abbreviation R/O, or _____
out	_____.

2.7 An outline of strategies designed to remedy the patient's condition

plan	is noted in the provider's P, or _____, also called a
recommendation, disposition	_____ or _____,
	which includes instructions to the patient, orders for medications, diag-
	nostic tests, or therapies.

2.8 *SOAP Notes:* After the initial history and physical is recorded, fur-

progress	ther documentations in the form of _____ notes are made
	as care continues. The letters represent the order in which progress is
	noted:
subjective	S – _____ ; that which the patient describes
objective	O – _____ ; observable information (e.g., test results or
	blood pressure readings)
assessment	A – _____ ; patient's progress and evaluation of the
	effectiveness of the plan
plan	P – _____ ; decision to proceed or alter the plan strategy

Hospital Records

The **history and physical** (Fig. 2-3) is often the first document entered into the patient's hospital record and is commonly required before elective admission for surgery. **Physician's Orders** (Fig. 2-4) list the directives for care prescribed by the doctor attending the patient. The **Nurse's Notes** (Fig. 2-5) and **Physician's Progress Notes** (Fig. 2-6) chronicle the care throughout the patient's stay. In a difficult case, a specialist may be called in by the attending physician, and a **Consultation Report** is filed. If a surgical remedy is indicated, a narrative **Operative Report** (Fig. 2-7) is required of the primary surgeon. In this report, a detailed account of the operation is given, including the method of incision, technique, instruments used, types of suture, method of closure, and the patient's responses during the procedure and at the time of transfer to recovery. The anesthesiologist, who is in charge of life support during surgery, must file the **Anesthesiologist's Report,** which includes details of anesthesia during surgery, including the drugs used, the dose and time given, and the patient's vital status throughout the procedure. When a surgery or procedure involves a reasonable risk to the patient, an **Informed Consent** form signed by the patient is required to advise the patient of the risks and benefits of the proposed treatment as well as alternatives. **Ancillary Reports** note the various procedures and therapies, including **Diagnostic Tests** and **Pathology Reports** (Fig. 2-8).

The final hospital document that is recorded at the time of discharge is the **Discharge Summary** (also termed **Clinical Resume, Clinical Summary,** or **Discharge Abstract).** It is a summary of the patient's hospital care, including date of admission, diagnosis, course of treatment, final diagnosis, and date of discharge (Fig 2-9).

The sample medical records in Figures 2-3 through 2-9 chronicle the medical care of Carleen Perron, a 28-year-old woman who was seen in consultation by Dr. Patrick Rodden, an ears, nose, and throat (ENT) specialist, who recommended a surgical remedy for the repeated infections she has had over the past 6 months.

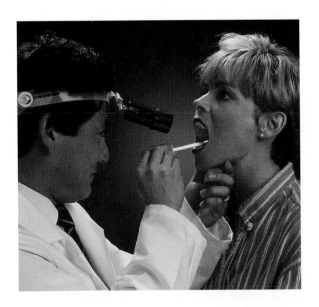

Common Diagnostic Tests and Procedures

Diagnostic tests and procedures are an integral part of patient care. Analyses of urine, stool, and blood specimens are recorded among the earliest efforts to understand conditions of disease. The advance of technology has led to the development of a whole myriad of highly sophisticated laboratory testing, examples of which will be featured in this text as they pertain to a specific body system. The two most common laboratory tests performed as part of a general health inquiry or

CENTRAL MEDICAL CENTER

211 Medical Center Drive • Central City, US 90000-1234 • PHONE: (012) 125-6784 • FAX: (012) 125-9999

PREOPERATIVE HISTORY AND PHYSICAL

HISTORY

DATE OF ADMISSION: June 3, 20xx

HISTORY OF PRESENT ILLNESS:
The patient is a 28-year-old white female with a chief complaint of frequent, recurrent, suppurative tonsillitis. She has had some eight infections over the last 6 months and is admitted at this time for elective tonsillectomy. The surgery has been discussed with the patient and family, including risks and complications. The patient's internist is C. Camarillo, M.D.

MEDICATIONS: None.

ALLERGIES: None known.

PAST SURGICAL HISTORY: None.

PAST MEDICAL HISTORY: UCHD (usual childhood diseases).

REVIEW OF SYSTEMS: CARDIOVASCULAR: No high blood pressure, heart murmurs, or shortness of breath. PULMONARY: No chronic lung disease; no asthma. GASTRO-INTESTINAL: No hepatitis. RENAL HISTORY: Negative for infections. ENDOCRINE: No diabetes or thyroid disease. MUSCULOSKELETAL: Negative for arthritis. HEMATOLOGIC: No history of anemia or bleeding tendencies.

FAMILY HISTORY: Grandmother has history of diabetes.

GYNECOLOGICAL HISTORY: Regular menses.

SOCIAL HISTORY: The patient is a nonsmoker. Alcohol use was denied, and drug use was denied.

(continued)

P. Rodden MD
PATRICK RODDEN, M.D.

JR:bst

D: 6/1/20xx
T: 6/2/20xx

HISTORY AND PHYSICAL Page 1	PT. NAME: PERRON, CARLEEN ID NO: 672894017 ROOM NO: ATT. PHYS: PATRICK RODDEN, M.D.

FIGURE 2-3. Preoperative history and physical submitted to the hospital before surgical admission.

CENTRAL MEDICAL CENTER

211 Medical Center Drive • Central City, US 90000-1234 • PHONE: (012) 125-6784 • FAX: (012) 125-9999

PREOPERATIVE HISTORY AND PHYSICAL

PHYSICAL EXAMINATION

VITAL SIGNS: Afebrile, alert, oriented, normotensive. Blood Pressure: 124/80. Pulse: 84. Respirations: 18.

HEENT: PERRLA (pupils equal, round, and reactive to light and accommodation). Tympanic membranes are clear. Light reflex is present. No sinus tenderness on percussion. Oropharynx: Clear. Hypertrophic tonsils. No exudates. Nasopharynx: No masses. Larynx: Clear.

NECK: Supple; no masses or tenderness. No cervical adenopathy.

LUNGS: Clear to percussion and auscultation.

HEART: Rate: 84 and regular; normal sinus rhythm; no murmurs or gallops.

RECTOPELVIC: Deferred.

EXTREMITIES: No peripheral edema. No ecchymoses.

NEUROLOGICAL: Physiologically intact.

IMPRESSION: Chronic, recurrent tonsillitis. The patient is admitted for an elective tonsillectomy.

P. Rodden MD
PATRICK RODDEN, M.D.

JR:bst
D: 6/1/20xx
T: 6/2/20xx

HISTORY AND PHYSICAL PAGE 2	PT. NAME: PERRON, CARLEEN
	ID NO: 672894017
	ROOM NO:
	ATT. PHYS: PATRICK RODDEN, M.D.

FIGURE 2-3. (CONTINUED)

CENTRAL MEDICAL CENTER

211 Medical Center Drive • Central City, US 90000-1234 • PHONE: (012) 125-6784 • FAX: (012) 125-9999

DOCTOR: PLEASE STATE PERTINENT CLINICAL INFORMATION WHEN ORDERING RADIOLOGY PROCEDURES

WRITE WITH BALLPOINT INK PEN; PRESS HARD

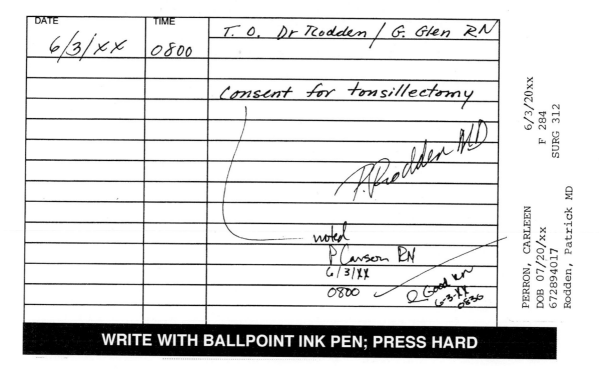

DATE	TIME	
6/3/XX	0800	T. O. Dr Rodden / G. Glen RN
		Consent for tonsillectomy
		P. Rodden MD
		noted
		P Carson RN
		6/3/XX
		0800 Q Gooder 6-3-XX 0830

(right margin:) 6/3/20xx F 284 SURG 312 PERRON, CARLEEN DOB 07/20/xx 672894017 Rodden, Patrick MD

WRITE WITH BALLPOINT INK PEN; PRESS HARD

DATE	TIME	
6/3/XX	10⁰⁰	Anesthesia post-op care
		1) mask O2 8 L/min
		2) VS per PAR routine
		3) Demerol 20-40 mg IV q 5-15 min prn
		4) Droperidol 0.6 - 1.2 mg IV
		q 15-30 min prn
		5) maybe DC'd when awake & VS
		stable X 1 h
		noted 6-3-XX Robert Jung, MD
		P Carson RN
		10¹⁰

(right margin:) 6/3/20xx F 284 SURG 312 PERRON, CARLEEN DOB 07/20/xx 672894017 Rodden, Patrick MD

PHYSICIAN'S ORDERS

FIGURE 2-4. Physician's orders: orders written by the anesthesiologist and surgeon and noted by the nursing staff during the patient's surgical care.

CENTRAL MEDICAL CENTER

211 Medical Center Drive • Central City, US 90000-1234 • PHONE: (012) 125-6784 • FAX: (012) 125-9999

DOCTOR: PLEASE STATE PERTINENT CLINICAL INFORMATION WHEN ORDERING RADIOLOGY PROCEDURES

WRITE WITH BALLPOINT INK PEN; PRESS HARD

DATE	TIME	
6-3-XX	10⁰⁰	POST-OP

POST-OP
1) V.S. q ½ h x 4 then q 2h x 4, then q 4h
2) bed rest c̄ BRP when alert
3) Continue IV's 80cc/hr 5% D/.2 NS until taking fluids well
4) tylenol elixir c̄ cod ΙΙΙ tsp q 4h po prn pain)
5) Demerol 50mg IM q 4h Vistaril 50mg prn severe pain
6) Ice & liquids at bedside & encourage   P Rodden MD

noted W. Cliff, R.N. 6-3-xx 1130

M 6/3/xx 11⁴⁵

PERRON, CARLEEN
DOB 07/20/xx
67289401 7
Rodden, Patrick MD

6/3/20xx
F 284
SURG 312

WRITE WITH BALLPOINT INK PEN; PRESS HARD

DATE	TIME	
6-3-XX	12³⁰	

1) full liquids requiring soft diet
2) admit
3) Dalmane 15 mg po q hs prn sleep MRX1 prn   P Rodden M

noted W. Cliff R.N. 12:30

M 6/3/xx 12³⁰

PERRON, CARLEEN
DOB 07/20/xx
67289401 7
Rodden, Patrick MD

6/3/20xx
F 284
SURG 312

PHYSICIAN'S ORDERS

FIGURE 2-4. (CONTINUED)

DATE	TIME	REMARKS
6/3/xx	0615	admitted & oriented to room 312. In no acute distress. VS stable. Afebrile NPO maintained. Condition stable. K. Brown RN
6/3/xx	0800	To OR via gurney - awake & oriented accompanied by her mother - condition stable K. Brown RN
6/3/xx	1110	Returned from PAR drowsy but arouses easily skin warm & dry. Color pink - VS stable - Throat dry unable to take sips of water very well - no nausea - c/o severe sore throat medicated x̄ with IM pain medication with desired effect - mother very supportive & remains @ bedside - Using a bedpan but unable to urinate - IV infusing well K. Brown RN

CENTRAL MEDICAL CENTER **PATIENT'S PROGRESS NOTES** **GENERAL CARE & TREATMENT**	PT. NAME: PERRON, CARLEEN ID NO: 672894017 ROOM NO: 312 ATT. PHYS: PATRICK RODDEN, M.D.

FIGURE 2-5. Nurse's notes: a recording by the nursing staff of the patient's progress made during general care and treatment.

DATE	TIME	REMARKS
6/3/xx	10⁰⁵	*op note*
		Chronic, recurrent tonsillitis
		Procedure: tonsillectomy
		Surgeon: P. Rodden MD
		Anesthesiologist: Robert Jung MD
		Procedure tolerated well
		P Rodden MD
6/3/xx	12²⁰	*post op check*
		VS stable
		C/o pain & poor p o fluid intake
		Will keep pt overnight for observation
		Plan to DC in am
		P Rodden MD
6/4/xx	08⁰⁰	*Doing much better – no bleeding*
		taking liquids freely
		DC'd on fluids
		Given RX for Tylenol.
		RTO in 48h
		P. Rodden MD

CENTRAL MEDICAL CENTER **PHYSICIAN'S PROGRESS NOTES**	**PT. NAME:** PERRON, CARLEEN **ID NO:** 672894017 **ROOM NO:** 312 **ATT. PHYS:** PATRICK RODDEN, M.D.

FIGURE 2-6. Physician's progress notes: physician's notations of the patient's progress throughout care.

CENTRAL MEDICAL CENTER

211 Medical Center Drive • Central City, US 90000-1234 • PHONE: (012) 125-6784 • FAX: (012) 125-9999

OPERATIVE REPORT

DATE OF OPERATION: June 3, 20xx.

PREOPERATIVE DIAGNOSIS: Chronic tonsillitis.

POSTOPERATIVE DIAGNOSIS: Frequent, recurrent tonsillitis.

SURGEON: Patrick Rodden, M.D.

ASSISTANT SURGEON: None

ANESTHESIOLOGIST: Robert Jung, M.D.

ANESTHESIA: General.

SURGERY PERFORMED: Tonsillectomy.

DESCRIPTION OF OPERATION: After general anesthesia induction, with intubation, the McGivor mouth gag and tongue retractor were utilized for exposure of the oropharynx. Local anesthetic consisting of 6 cc of 0.5% Xylocaine with 1:100,000 epinephrine was utilized. Tonsillectomy was carried out using dissection and air technique. The right tonsillectomy electrocoagulation Bovie suction was utilized for hemostasis. Examination of the nasopharynx was normal.

The patient tolerated the procedure well and went to the recovery room in good condition.

P. Rodden MD

PATRICK RODDEN, M.D.

JR:as
D: 6/3/20xx
T: 6/4/20xx

OPERATIVE REPORT	PT. NAME:	PERRON, CARLEEN
	ID NO:	672894017
	ROOM NO:	312
	ATT. PHYS:	PATRICK RODDEN, M.D.

FIGURE 2-7. Operative report: surgeon's account of surgical procedure.

CENTRAL MEDICAL CENTER

211 Medical Center Drive • Central City, US 90000-1234 • PHONE: (012) 125-6784 • FAX: (012) 125-9999

PATHOLOGY REPORT

PATIENT: PERRON, CARLEEN
28 Y (FEMALE)

DATE RECEIVED: June 3, 20xx. DATE REPORTED: June 4, 20xx

GROSS:

Received are two tonsils each 2.5 cm in greatest diameter.

MICROSCOPIC:

The sections show deep tonsilar crypts associated with follicular lymphoid hyperplasia. No bacterial granules are seen.

DIAGNOSIS:

CHRONIC LYMPHOID HYPERPLASIA OF RIGHT AND LEFT TONSILS.

Mary Needham MD
MARY NEEDHAM, M.D.

MN:gds

D: 6/4/20xx
T: 6/5/20xx

FIGURE 2-8. Pathology report.

	MEDICAL RECORDS USE
THAT CONDITION WHICH AFTER STUDY IS DETERMINED TO BE THE REASON FOR ADMISSION TO THE HOSPITAL PRINCIPAL DIAGNOSIS - *Chronic tonsillitis*	
	474.00
FINAL DIAGNOSIS - NO ABBREVIATIONS	474.00
Same	
SECONDARY DIAGNOSIS:	
—	
COMPLICATIONS AND/OR COMORBIDITY:	
—	
PRINCIPAL OPERATION/PROCEDURES(S)/TREATMENT RENDERED:	
Tonsillectomy	
SECONDARY OPERATIONS/PROCEDURES:	

CONDITION ON DISCHARGE *Stable*

☐ DISCHARGE INSTRUCTIONS   ☐ PRE-PRINTED INSTRUCTIONS GIVEN

MEDICATIONS	*Tylenol*
PHYSICAL ACTIVITY	*Bed rest*
DIET	*full liquid*
FOLLOW-UP	*office in 48 h*

DATE OF SUMMARY IF DICTATED:

DATE ADMITTED: 6/3/XX	DATE DISCHARGED: 6/4/XX	ATTENDING PHYSICIAN *P. Rodden*	M.D.

FOR MED. RECORDS USE ONLY	ASSEMBLY	ANALYSIS	CODED	KEYED	FINAL CHECK		06/03/20XX
	SL	*MC/37*	*MZ*	*LY*	*S*		
CONSULTANTS:				AA	1		
				DP	R48		
				SC	1211		

CENTRAL MEDICAL CENTER

DIAGNOSIS RECORD/
DISCHARGE SUMMARY

FIGURE 2-9. Discharge summary (abstract). Final report documented at time of discharge. This abstract is more commonly seen in outpatient surgery.

to rule out a particular condition are the complete blood count (CBC) (See Fig. 6-9 in Chapter 6) and urinalysis (UA) (See Fig. 13-8 in Chapter 13).

It is valuable for health care professionals to recognize common diagnostic tests and procedures, and the types of technology used to produce them.

DIAGNOSTIC IMAGING MODALITIES

Methods of diagnostic imaging have rapidly expanded in the years since the discovery of x-ray by Wilhelm Roentgen in 1885. Radiation from x-rays, that could see through the body to produce images of the skeleton and other body structures, was found to be <u>ionizing, a process that changes the electrical charge of atoms with a possible effect on body cells</u>. Overexposure to ionizing radiation can have harmful side effects, e.g. cancer; however, technological advances have produced images requiring significantly lower doses of radiation to minimize risk.

Further advancement has led to the discovery and use of other imaging modalities (techniques) under the umbrella of the medical specialty known as radiology. Common ionizing modalities include: radiography (x-ray), computed tomography (CT) , and nuclear medicine. Common non-ionizing modalities that present no apparent risk include magnetic resonance imaging and sonography.

IONIZING IMAGING

RADIOGRAPHY (X-RAY)

Radiography is a modality using x-rays (ionizing radiation) to provide images of the body's anatomy to diagnose a condition or impairment. An image is produced when a small amount of radiation is passed through the body to expose a sensitive film. The image is called a radiograph. (There is an exception to the rule: graph is the preferred suffix used in radiology to refer to an x-ray record. It is taken by a radiologic technologist [also known as a radiographer] and interpreted or read by a radiologist, a physician specializing in the study of radiology.) (Fig. 2-10).

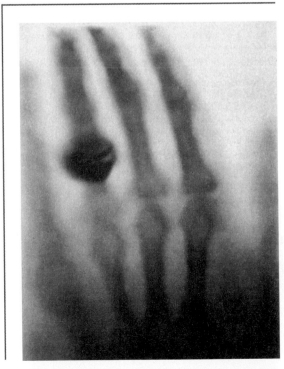

■ **FIGURE 2-10.** First published radiograph of the hand and signet ring of Professor Roentgen's wife; produced on December 22, 1895.

COMPUTED TOMOGRAPHY OR COMPUTED AXIAL TOMOGRAPHY

Computed tomography (CT), also known as computed axial tomography (CAT), is a radiologic procedure that uses a machine (called a scanner) to examine a body site by taking a series of cross-sectional (tomographic) x-ray films in a full circle rotation. A computer then calculates and converts the rates of absorption and density of the x-rays into a three-dimensional picture on a screen (Fig. 2-11).

NUCLEAR MEDICINE IMAGING OR RADIONUCLIDE ORGAN IMAGING

This diagnostic imaging technique uses an injected or ingested radioactive isotope, also called radionuclide (a chemical that has been tagged with radioactive compounds that emit gamma rays). A gamma camera detects and produces an image of the distributed gamma rays in the body. This technique is useful in determining size, shape, location, and function of body organs such as the brain, lungs, bones, and heart (Fig. 2-12).

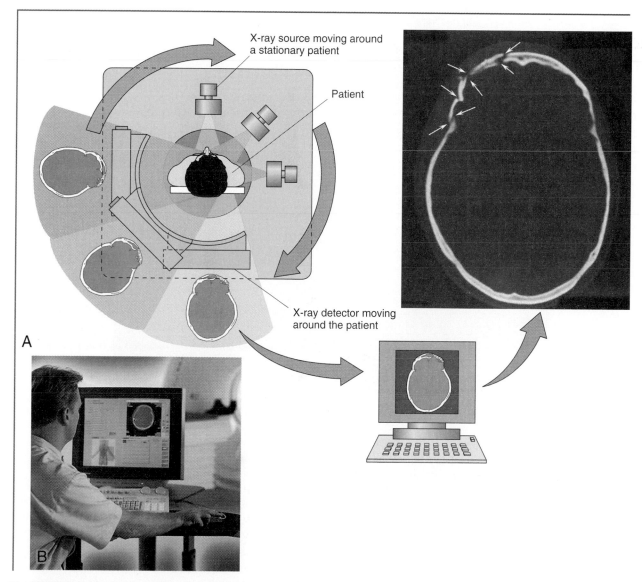

■ **FIGURE 2-11. A.** Principles of computed tomography (CT). Inset, CT showing multiple open fractures (*arrows*) of skull. **B.** CT imaging process.

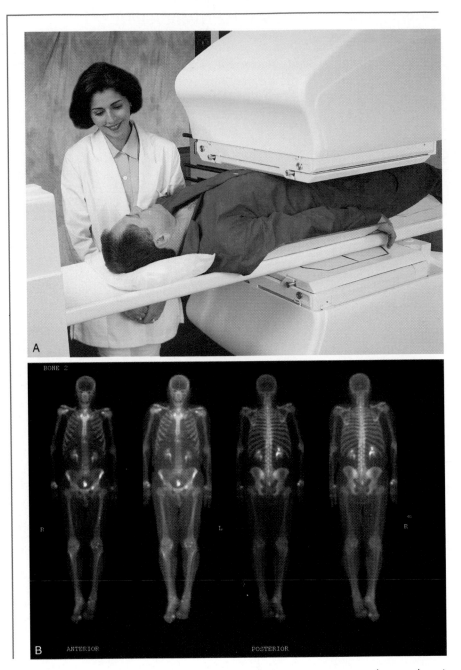

■ **FIGURE 2-12.** Nuclear medicine imaging. **A.** Gamma camera used to produce image **B.** Radionuclide whole body bone scan. (*See also* Figure 7-10.)

NON-IONIZING IMAGING

MAGNETIC RESONANCE IMAGING

Magnetic resonance imaging (MRI) is a non-ionizing imaging technique using magnetic fields and radio frequency waves to visualize anatomic structures within the body. A large magnet surrounds the patient as a scanner subjects the body to a radio signal that temporarily alters the alignment of the hydrogen atoms in the patient's tissue. As the radio wave signal is turned off, the atoms realign, and the energy produced is absorbed by detectors and interpreted using computers to provide detailed anatomic images of the body part. MRI is particularly useful in examining soft tissues, joints, and the brain and spinal cord (Fig. 2-13).

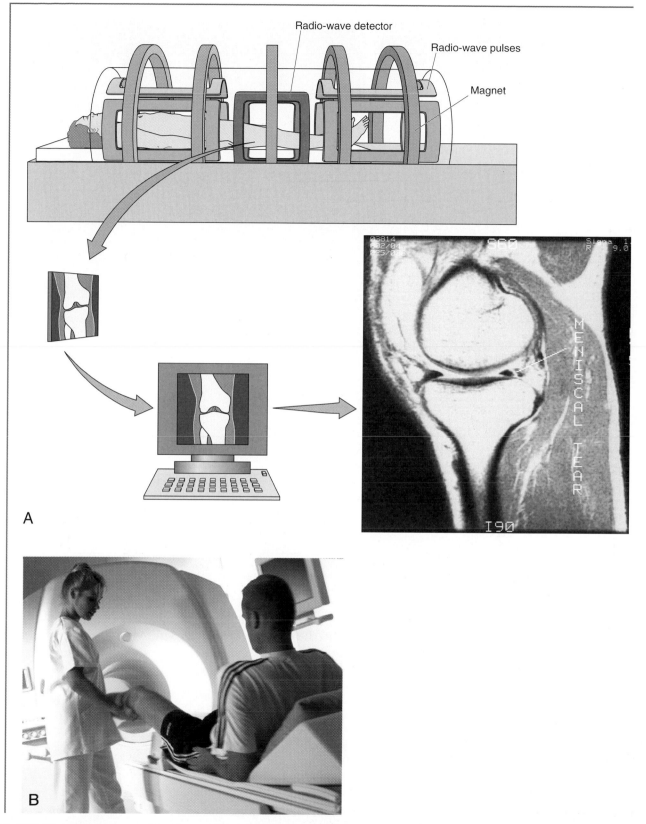

■ **FIGURE 2-13. A.** Principles of magnetic resonance imaging (MRI). Patient is positioned within a magnetic field as radiowave signals are conducted through selected body part. Energy is absorbed by tissues and then released. A computer processes the released energy and formulates the image. *Inset,* MRI of the knee (lateral view) identifying a torn meniscus. **B.** MRI unit.

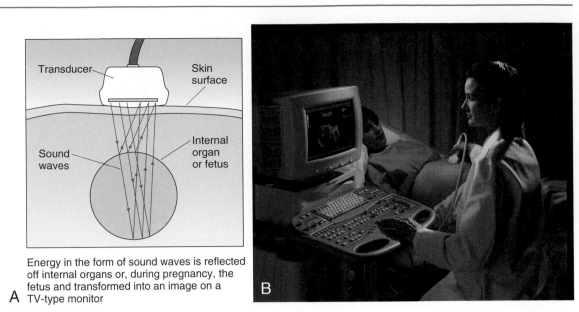

Energy in the form of sound waves is reflected off internal organs or, during pregnancy, the fetus and transformed into an image on a TV-type monitor

■ **FIGURE 2-14. A.** Principles of sonography. **B.** Obstetric sonography.

Magnetic resonance angiography (MRA) applies MR technology in the study of blood flow (see Diagnostic Tests and Procedures in Chapters 5 and 8.)

SONOGRAPHY

Sonography (diagnostic ultrasound) [U/S or US] is the use of high frequency sound waves (ultrasound) to visualize body tissues. Ultrasound waves sent through a scanning device, called a transducer, are reflected off structures within the body and analyzed by a computer to produce moving images on a monitor. Sonography is used to examine many parts of the body, including the abdomen, male and female reproductive organs, thyroid and parathyroid glands, and the cardiovascular system (Fig. 2-14).

USE OF CONTRAST

Some imaging procedures require the internal administration of a contrast medium to enhance the visualization of anatomic structures. There are many different kinds of contrast media, including barium, iodinated compounds, gasses (air, carbon dioxide), and other chemicals known to increase visual clarity. Depending on the medium, it may be injected, swallowed, or introduced through an enema or catheter. Compare Figures 13-5 and 13-7 (x-rays of the urinary tract) in Chapter 13, which show images taken with and without contrast.

PROGRAMMED REVIEW: DIAGNOSTIC IMAGING

Study the following:

Answer Column	Review
ionizing	**2.9** The diagnostic modality using _____ radiation in x-rays to produce images of the body's anatomy is called
radiology	_____, a term derived from the combining form *radi/o*

study of

radiograph

radiologic technologist

radiologist

cancer

meaning radiation and *-logy* meaning _____ ____. The x-ray image is called a _____. It is taken by a radiographer or _____ _____ and is interpreted by a physician who specializes in the study of radiology, called a _____. Ionizing radiation has an effect on body tissue, and overexposure can have harmful side effects such as _____.

CT

process of recording

tomo

computer

2.10 The application of computer technology to medical imaging was first applied by the x-ray development of computed tomography, abbreviated ____. *Tom/o*, a combining form meaning to cut, and *-graphy* meaning _____ ____ _____, give clues to how the CT scanner operates. The scanner is used to take a series of cross-sectional or _tomo_ graphic x-ray films that are converted by a _____ into a three-dimensional picture on a screen.

radionuclide

organ, ionizing

isotope

gamma

function

2.11 Nuclear medicine imaging, or _radio nuclide_ _organ_ imaging, is another modality using _ionizing_ radiation. The technique involves the injection or ingestion of a radioactive _isotope_ that emits gamma rays. An image is produced using a _gamma_ camera to detect the distribution of the gamma rays. Radionuclide organ images are useful in determining size, shape, location, and _function_ of body organs.

risk, magnetic

resonance imaging

sonography, magnet

radio

soft

sound

recording

2.12 There are two major non-ionizing imaging modalities that have shown no apparent _____ to patients: MRI, or _Magnetic_ _resonance_ _Imaging_, and ultrasound, or _Sonography_. MRI uses a large _magnet_ and _radio_ waves to visualize anatomic structures within the body, especially _soft_ tissues. Sonography, from the combining form *son/o* meaning _Sound_ and *-graph(y)* meaning a process of _recording_, uses high-frequency sound waves to produce body images.

Common Medical Record Terms Related to Disease

The following terms related to disease are common in medical records. Learn them as a foundation on which to build as your vocabulary expands.

SELF-INSTRUCTION: DISEASE TERMS

Study the following:

Term	Meaning
acute	sharp; having severe symptoms and a short course
chronic	a condition developing slowly and persisting over a period of time
benign	mild or noncancerous
malignant	harmful or cancerous
degeneration	gradual deterioration of normal cells and body functions
degenerative disease	any disease in which there is deterioration of structure or function of tissue
diagnosis	determination of the presence of a disease based on an evaluation of symptoms, signs, and test findings (results) (dia = through; gnosis = knowing)
etiology	study of the cause of a disease (etio = cause)
exacerbation	increase in severity of a disease with aggravation of symptoms (ex = out; acerbo = harsh)
remission	a period in which symptoms and signs stop or abáte
febrile	relating to a fever (elevated temperature)
idiopathic	a condition occurring without a clearly identified cause (idio = one's own)
localized	limited to a definite area or part
systemic	relating to the whole body rather than only a part
malaise	a feeling of unwellness, often the first indication of illness
marked	significant
morbidity	sick; a diseased state
mortality	the state of being subject to death
prognosis	foreknowledge; prediction of the likely outcome of a disease based on the general health status of the patient along with knowledge of the usual course of the disease—often noted in one word (e.g., Prognosis: good)

progressive	pertaining to the advance of a condition as signs and symptoms increase in severity
prophylaxis	a process or measure that prevents disease (pro = before; phylassein = guard)
recurrent	to occur again; describes a return of symptoms and signs after a period of quiescence (rest or inactivity)
sequela	a disorder or condition, usually resulting from a previous disease or injury
sign	a mark; objective evidence of disease that can be seen or verified by an examiner
syndrome	a running together; combination of symptoms and signs that give a distinct clinical picture indicating a particular condition or disease (e.g., menopausal syndrome)
noncontributory	not involved in bringing on the condition or result
unremarkable	not significant or worthy of noting

PROGRAMMED REVIEW: DISEASE TERMS

Answer Column	Review
Malaise	**2.13** There are many different signs and symptoms that manifest disease in the body. _____ is used to describe a patient who
febrile	feels unwell. A patient is considered _____ if he or she
a	has an increase in body temperature, and __ febrile if without a fever.
	Conditions limited to a definite area or part are considered
localized, systemic	_____, whereas those that are _____ affect the whole body.
acute	**2.14** Some conditions have a sudden, severe, or _____ onset,
chronic	whereas others that are _____ develop slowly and persist
progressive	over time. A condition is considered _progressive_ when
	the symptoms and signs advance with increased severity. A flare-up, or
exacerbation	_exacerbation_, occurs when the severity of symptoms
remission	are increased. A condition is said to be in _remission_ during
	the period in which signs and symptoms have stopped.

Recurrent	_recurrent_ describes a return of symptoms and signs after a period of inactivity.
etiology idiopathic malignant, benign marked	**2.15** The cause or _____ of a disease is often unknown. A condition is considered _____ when there is no clear identifying cause. If a condition is cancerous, it is _____, and is _____ if it is noncancerous. A patient with significant weakness can be said to have _____ weakness.
diagnosis prognosis	**2.16** The doctor makes a _____ when naming a disease and gives a _____ when predicting its likely outcome.
prophylaxis	**2.17** A _____ is a process or measure that prevents disease.

Medical Record Abbreviations

The following table lists common medical record abbreviations used in patient-care documentation. They represent the "acceptable" terms used extensively throughout this text. Remember that individual medical facilities provide their own list of acceptable terms and abbreviations that may not be used elsewhere. Memorize the terms and abbreviations from this list, and plan to adapt them to the variations you encounter.

SELF-INSTRUCTION: ABBREVIATIONS

Study the following:

Abbreviation	Meaning
MEDICAL CARE FACILITIES	
CCU	coronary (cardiac) care unit
ECU	emergency care unit
ER	emergency room
ICU	intensive care unit
IP	inpatient (a registered bed patient)

OP	outpatient
OR	operating room
PAR	post anesthetic recovery
post-op/postop	postoperative (after surgery)
pre-op/preop	preoperative (before surgery)
RTC	return to clinic
RTO	return to office

PATIENT CARE

BRP	bathroom privileges
CP	chest pain
DC, D/C	discharge, discontinue
ETOH	ethyl alcohol
L	left
R	right
pt	patient
RRR	regular rate and rhythm
SOB	shortness of breath
Tr	treatment
Tx	treatment or traction
VS	vital signs
T	temperature
P	pulse
R	respiration
BP	blood pressure
Ht	height
Wt	weight
WDWN	well-developed and well-nourished
y/o, y.o.	year old
#	number or pound: if before the numeral it means number (e.g., #2 = number 2); if after the numeral it means pound (e.g., 150# = 150 pounds)

♀	female
♂	male
°	degree, or hour
↑	increased
↓	decreased
∅	none or negative
♀	standing
♀	sitting
o—	lying

PROGRAMMED REVIEW: ABBREVIATIONS

Answer Column	**Review**

2.18 The patient seeking emergency care is often seen in the ECU or

emergency care unit _____ _____ _____, most commonly known as

ER the hospital ____. Depending on the circumstances of the accident or

outpatient illness, the patient is treated as an OP, or _____, or

inpatient admitted as an IP, or _____. Sometimes, in a critical

case, the patient is transferred directly to the ICU, or

intensive care unit _____ _____ _____. If surgery is necessary it is

operating room performed in the OR, or _____ _____, after which a

post period of recovery is made in PAR, or _____

anesthetic recovery _____ _____.

2.19 While hospitalized, the pt, or _____, is seen by the at-

patient tending physician and cared for by the nursing staff. The doctor writes

orders for all Tx, or _____, including how often the VS,

treatment or _____ _____ (T, or _____, P, or

vital signs, temperature _____, R, or _____, and BP, or _____

pulse, respiration, blood _____) are to be taken and whether the patient is to have

pressure

bathroom privileges BRP, or _____ _____. The nurses must

document the care and report any abnormal findings such as CP, or

chest pain, shortness of	_____ _____, SOB, or _____ ____
breath	_____. The doctor usually asks the patient to RTO, or
return to office	_____ ____ _____ within a few days of DC, or
discharge	_____ from the hospital.

Pharmaceutical Abbreviations and Symbols

Pharmaceutical abbreviations and symbols are frequently used in documenting patient care. They are found throughout the medical record. Efficient medical record keeping and effective communication among health care workers depends on knowledge of commonly used pharmaceutical abbreviations and symbols.

UNITS OF MEASURE

The following are common metric and apothecary units of measurement. Consult your medical dictionary for a complete listing of units of measurement and conversion formulas.

THE METRIC SYSTEM

Metric is the most commonly used system of measurement in health care. It is a decimal system based on the following units:

meter (m)	length (39.37 inches)
liter (L)	volume (1.0567 US quarts)
gram (g or gm)	weight (15.432 grains)

THE APOTHECARY SYSTEM

The apothecary system is an outdated method of liquid and weight measure used by the earliest chemists and pharmacists. The liquid measure was based on one drop. The weight measure was based on one grain of wheat. Although the small apothecary measures are rarely used, the larger ones (e.g., fluid ounces) are still common.

SELF-INSTRUCTION: UNITS OF MEASURE

Study the following:

Abbreviation	Meaning
METRIC	
cc	cubic centimeter (1 cc = 1 ml)
cm	centimeter (2.5 cm = 1 inch)
g or gm	gram
kg	kilogram [1,000 g (2.2 pounds)]

L	liter
mg	milligram [one-thousandth (0.001) of a gram]
ml or mL	milliliter [one-thousandth (0.001) of a liter]
mm	millimeter [one-thousandth (0.001) of a meter]
cu mm	cubic millimeter = mm^3

APOTHECARY

fl oz	fluid ounce
gr	grain
gt	drop (L. gutta = drop)
gtt	drops
dr	dram (1/8 ounce)
oz	ounce
lb or #	pound (16 ounces)
qt	quart (32 ounces)

Medication Administration

Prescribed medications can be administered to patients in a variety of ways, depending on the indication for the drug and on the patient's status. The following table gives an overview of forms of drugs and routes of administration including abbreviations and symbols:

SELF-INSTRUCTION: MEDICATION ADMINISTRATION

Study the following:

Drug Form	Route of Administration	
SOLID AND SEMISOLID FORMS		
tablet (tab)	oral	by mouth [per os (po)]
capsule (cap)	sublingual	under the tongue (SL)
	buccal	in the cheek
suppository	vaginal	inserted in the vagina [per vagina (PV)]
	rectal	inserted in the rectum [per rectum (PR)]

LIQUID FORMS

fluid	inhalation	inhaled through nose or mouth [e.g., aerosol (spray) or nebulizer (device used to produce a fine spray or mist, often in a metered dose)]
parenteral	by injection	
	intradermal (ID)	within the skin
	intramuscular (IM)	within the muscle
	intravenous (IV)	within the vein
	subcutaneous (SC or SQ)	under the skin
cream, lotion, ointment	topical	applied to surface of skin
other delivery systems	transdermal	absorption of drug through unbroken skin
implant	a drug reservoir imbedded in the body to provide continual infusion of a medication, e.g., insulin pump	

THE PRESCRIPTION

A prescription is a written direction by a physician for dispensing or administering a medication to a patient. It is an order to supply a named patient with a particular drug of a specific strength and quantity, along with specific instructions for administration. The prescription is a legal document that must be written in a specific format (Fig. 2-15).

DRUG NAMES

The **chemical name** is assigned to a drug in the laboratory at the time it is invented. It is the formula for the drug, which is written exactly according to its chemical structure. The **generic name** is

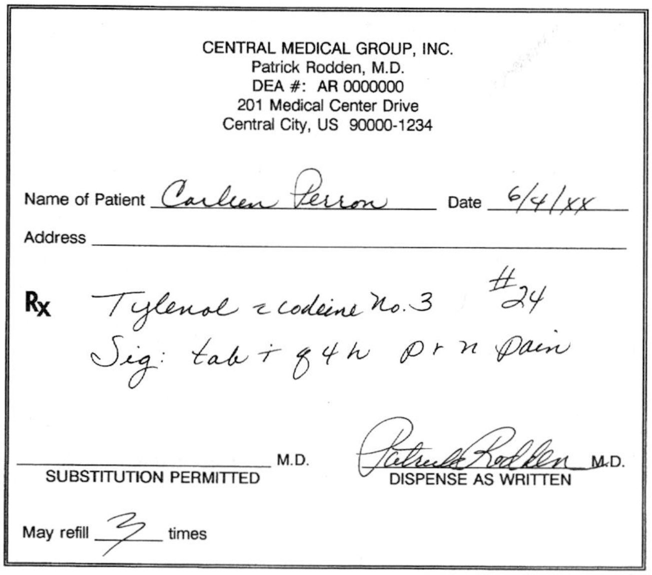
CENTRAL MEDICAL GROUP, INC.
Patrick Rodden, M.D.
DEA #: AR 0000000
201 Medical Center Drive
Central City, US 90000-1234

Name of Patient Carleen Perron Date 6/4/xx

Address

Rx Tylenol c̄ codeine No. 3 #24
Sig: tab i q4h prn pain

M.D.
SUBSTITUTION PERMITTED

Patrick Rodden M.D.
DISPENSE AS WRITTEN

May refill 3 times

FIGURE 2-15. Sample prescription.

the official, nonproprietary name given a drug. The **trade** or **brand** is the manufacturer's name for a drug. For example:

chemical name:	1-[[3-(6,7-dihydro-1-methyl-7-oxo-3-propyl-
	1H-pyrazolo[4,3-d]pyrimidin-5-yl)-4-ethoxyphenyl]sulfonyl]-4-methylpiperazine citrate
generic name:	sildenafil
brand or trade name:	Viagra (Pfizer Pharmaceutical Company)

Appendix C lists commonly prescribed drugs, including therapeutic categories.

PRESCRIPTION ABBREVIATIONS

Many Latin abbreviations and symbols are commonly used in prescription writing as well as in physician's orders. A familiarity with these symbols makes it possible to read a prescription or physician's order.

Historically, prescriptions were written in Latin. The words were abbreviated for convenience. For example, quater in die, Latin for four times a day, is abbreviated q.i.d. The dots were included to indicate the abbreviation of three words; however, if not carefully documented, the abbreviation can be interpreted with drastic implications. For example, the dot in q.d (meaning once a day) can be misinterpreted as q.i.d (4 times a day) when handwritten. Most pharmacy organizations today discourage the use of dots, especially in writing, because they can be misinterpreted.

In an effort to promote clarity, dots in abbreviations have been eliminated from the following tables. In practice, you will find variations, including the inclusion of dots and differing uses of uppercase instead of lowercase (e.g., QID versus qid).

Roman numerals were used exclusively in the early days and are still used today; however, most pharmacy organizations now promote the use of Arabic numerals only.

SELF-INSTRUCTION: COMMON ABBREVIATIONS AND SYMBOLS

Study the following:

Abbreviation	Meaning	Latin*
TIME AND FREQUENCY		
$\bar{a}$	before	ante
ac	before meals	ante cibum
am	before noon	ante meridiem
bid	twice a day	Bis in die
d	day	
h	hour	hora
hs	at hour of sleep (bedtime)	hora somni
noc	night	noctis
$\bar{p}$	after	post
pp	after meals	post prandial

*Original Latin given when deemed helpful.

pc	after meals	post cibum
pm	after noon	post meridiem
prn	as needed	Pro re nata
q	every	quaque
qd	every day	quaque die
qh	every hour	quaque hora
q2h	every 2 hours	
qid	four times a day	quarter in die
qod	every other day	quaque altera die
STAT	immediately	statium
tid	three times a day	ter in die
wk	week	
yr	year	

MISCELLANEOUS

AD	right ear	auris dextra
AS	left ear	auris sinstra
AU	both ears	auris unitas
ad lib	as desired	ad libitum
amt	amount	
aq	water	aqua
Ⓑ	bilateral	
C	Celsius, centigrade	
c̄	with	cum
F	Fahrenheit	
ⓜ	murmur	
NPO	nothing by mouth	non per os
OD	right eye	oculus dexter
OS	left eye	oculus sinister
OU	both eyes	oculi unitas

per	by or through	
po	per os (by mouth)	per os
PR	through rectum	per rectum
PV	through vagina	per vagina
qns	quantity not sufficient	
qs	quantity sufficient	
Rx	recipe; prescription	
Sig	label; instruction to the patient	signa
$\overline{s}$	without	sine
$\overline{ss}$	one-half	semis
wa	while awake	
x	Times or for [e.g., x 6 (six times), x 2 d (for 2 days)]	
>	greater than	
<	less than	
ī	one (modified lower-case Roman numeral i)	
īī	two (modified lower-case Roman numeral ii)	
īīī	three (modified lower-case Roman numeral iii)	
īv	four (modified lower-case Roman numeral iv)	
I, II, III, IV, V, VI, VII, VIII, IX, X	upper-case Roman numerals 1 through 10	

PROGRAMMED REVIEW: PHARMACEUTICAL ABBREVIATIONS AND SYMBOLS

Answer Column	Review
Metric	**2.20** _____ is the most commonly used system of measurement in health care.
gm kg, one	**2.21** Gram, abbreviated g or _____, is a weight measure. _Kilo-_ is a prefix meaning one thousand. A kilogram, or _____, contains _____ thousand grams (2.2 pounds). Body weight is often measured in kilograms

mg, gram	instead of pounds. *Milli-* is a prefix signifying one-thousandth. A milligram, or _____, is one-thousandth of a _____.
L quart, mL liter	**2.22** Liter, abbreviated __, is a volume measure. One liter is equal to 1.0567 US qt, or _____. An ml, or _____, is one-thousandth of a _____.
length mm, meter cm centimeters	**2.23** Meter is a measure of _____. There are 39.37 inches in a meter. A millimeter or _____ is one-thousandth of a _____. *Centi-* is a prefix meaning one hundred. A centimeter, or _____, is one-hundredth of a meter. There are 2.5 cm or _____ in an inch. The diameter of a lesion is commonly measured in cm.
cubic centimeter one, milliliter, 3 cu mm	**2.24** One cc, or _____ _____, is equal to _____ ml, or _____. A 3-cc syringe holds __ mL. Cubic millimeter is abbreviated _____ _____.
fluid ounce, drop, drops, pound quart	**2.25** Measures of the apothecary system, such as fl oz, or _____ _____, gt, or _____, gtt, or _____, #, or _____, and qt, or _____ are common.
tablet, by mouth, sublingual buccal through rectum, through vagina injection, intradermal intramuscular, intravenous subcutaneous through	**2.26** Drugs are administered in many ways. The most common drug form is the tab, or _____, which is usually taken po, or _____ _____, under the tongue, or _____, and sometimes in the cheek, or _____. Suppositories are inserted PR, or _____ _____, or PV, or _____ _____. The parenteral route of administration is by _____: ID, or _____, IM, or _____, IV, or _____, or SQ, or _____. Transdermal penetrates _____ the skin.
generic brand	**2.27** The _____ is the official, nonproprietary name for a drug, and the trade or _____ name is given to a drug by the

chemical	manufacturer. 8- Chloro-1-methyl-6-phenyl-4H-s-triazolo[4,3-a] [1,4]benzodiazepine is a _____ name.

before, $\bar{a}$	**2.28** Ante, meaning _____ , is abbreviated __. Post, meaning
after, $\bar{p}$, pm	_____ , is abbreviated __. After noon is abbreviated _____, and
after meals, d, noc	pc is _____ _____. Day is abbreviated __, night is _____,
hs, as	and bedtime is _____. If a medication is taken prn, it is taken _____
needed	_____. If the patient can have as much as desired, the abbreviation is ad _____. Every hour is abbreviated _____, every day is _____,
lib, qh, qd	
qod	and every other day is _____. Some drugs are taken twice a day, or
bid, tid, four	_____, three times a day, or _____, or qid, or _____ times a day.
immediately	STAT means _____.

✝	**2.29** The modified lower-case Roman numeral that means one is __,
$\bar{ss}$, $\bar{c}$, $\bar{s}$, OD	one- half is _____, with is __, and without is __. The right eye is _____,
AS	and left ear is _____. Sometimes the doctor wants the patient to take
NPO	nothing by mouth, or _____.

Recording Date and Time

The date and time are usually required in entries in a medical record. Always include the month, day of the month, and year (e.g., 2/25/xx); sometimes six digits are required (e.g., 01/08/xx). Military time is often used (Fig. 2-16).

Standard	Military	Standard	Military
1:00 AM	0100 zero one hundred hours	1:00 PM	1300 thirteen hundred hours
2:00 AM	0200 zero two hundred hours	2:00 PM	1400 fourteen hundred hours
2:15 AM	0215 zero two fifteen hours	3:00 PM	1500 fifteen hundred hours
3:00 AM	0300 zero three hundred hours	4:00 PM	1600 sixteen hundred hours
4:00 AM	0400 zero four hundred hours	5:00 PM	1700 seventeen hundred hours
4:30 AM	0430 zero four thirty hours	6:00 PM	1800 eighteen hundred hours
5:00 AM	0500 zero five hundred hours	7:00 PM	1900 nineteen hundred hours
6:00 AM	0600 zero six hundred hours	8:00 PM	2000 twenty hundred hours
7:00 AM	0700 zero seven hundred hours	9:00 PM	2100 twenty-one hundred hours
8:00 AM	0800 zero eight hundred hours	10:00 PM	2200 twenty-two hundred hours
9.00 AM	0900 zero nine hundred hours	11:00 PM	2300 twenty-three hundred hours
10:00 AM	1000 ten hundred hours	12:00 AM	2400 twenty-four hundred hours
11:00 AM	1100 eleven hundred hours	(midnight)	
12:00 PM	1200 twelve hundred hours		
(noon)			

Regulations and Legal Considerations

Medical record documentations are made by physicians caring for the patient and by other authorized health care professionals involved with care. State, federal, and private accrediting agencies

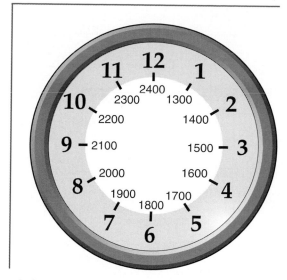

■ **FIGURE 2-16.** Military and standard time.

(e.g., the Joint Commission on Accreditation of Healthcare Organizations) provide specific guidelines that regulate how medical records are kept, including proper format for all forms; use of appropriate terminology and accepted abbreviations; protocol for personnel having access to records; and responsibilities for documentation.

Corrections

Sometimes mistakes are made when making an entry in a medical record. Careful clarification of the error is essential. The format may vary according to specific facility or organizational guideline. Generally, if a mistake is made in a handwritten entry, it should be identified by drawing a single line through it, and then writing the correction in the margin above or immediately after the mistake. Include the date and the initials of the person making the correction. The use of correction fluid is forbidden!

The medical record often becomes evidence in medical malpractice cases. Obliterations and signs of possible tampering can be construed as trying to withhold information or covering up negligent wrongdoing. Complete and accurate record keeping is your best defense against any possible legal action (Fig. 2-17).

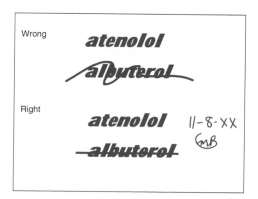

FIGURE 2-17. Proper correction of a handwritten chart entry.

Practice Exercises

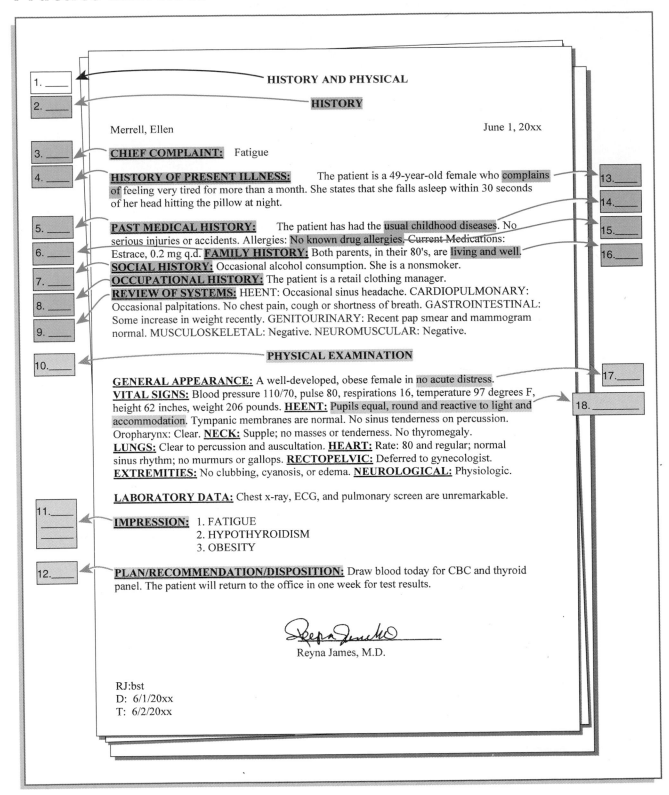

1. _____

2. _____

3. _____

4. _____

5. _____

6. _____

7. _____

8. _____

9. _____

10. _____

11. _____ _____

12. _____

13. _____

14. _____

15. _____

16. _____

17. _____

18. _____

HISTORY AND PHYSICAL

HISTORY

Merrell, Ellen   June 1, 20xx

CHIEF COMPLAINT: Fatigue

HISTORY OF PRESENT ILLNESS: The patient is a 49-year-old female who complains of feeling very tired for more than a month. She states that she falls asleep within 30 seconds of her head hitting the pillow at night.

PAST MEDICAL HISTORY: The patient has had the usual childhood diseases. No serious injuries or accidents. Allergies: No known drug allergies. Current Medications: Estrace, 0.2 mg q.d. **FAMILY HISTORY:** Both parents, in their 80's, are living and well.
SOCIAL HISTORY: Occasional alcohol consumption. She is a nonsmoker.
OCCUPATIONAL HISTORY: The patient is a retail clothing manager.
REVIEW OF SYSTEMS: HEENT: Occasional sinus headache. CARDIOPULMONARY: Occasional palpitations. No chest pain, cough or shortness of breath. GASTROINTESTINAL: Some increase in weight recently. GENITOURINARY: Recent pap smear and mammogram normal. MUSCULOSKELETAL: Negative. NEUROMUSCULAR: Negative.

PHYSICAL EXAMINATION

GENERAL APPEARANCE: A well-developed, obese female in no acute distress.
VITAL SIGNS: Blood pressure 110/70, pulse 80, respirations 16, temperature 97 degrees F, height 62 inches, weight 206 pounds. **HEENT:** Pupils equal, round and reactive to light and accommodation. Tympanic membranes are normal. No sinus tenderness on percussion. Oropharynx: Clear. **NECK:** Supple; no masses or tenderness. No thyromegaly.
LUNGS: Clear to percussion and auscultation. **HEART:** Rate: 80 and regular; normal sinus rhythm; no murmurs or gallops. **RECTOPELVIC:** Deferred to gynecologist.
EXTREMITIES: No clubbing, cyanosis, or edema. **NEUROLOGICAL:** Physiologic.

LABORATORY DATA: Chest x-ray, ECG, and pulmonary screen are unremarkable.

IMPRESSION: 1. FATIGUE
                            2. HYPOTHYROIDISM
                            3. OBESITY

PLAN/RECOMMENDATION/DISPOSITION: Draw blood today for CBC and thyroid panel. The patient will return to the office in one week for test results.

Reyna James, M.D.

RJ:bst
D: 6/1/20xx
T: 6/2/20xx

Write in the missing abbreviations for the highlighted terms:

1. _____
2. _____
3. _____
4. _____
5. _____
6. _____
7. _____
8. _____
9. _____
10. _____
11. _____
12. _____
13. _____
14. _____
15. _____
16. _____
17. _____
18. _____

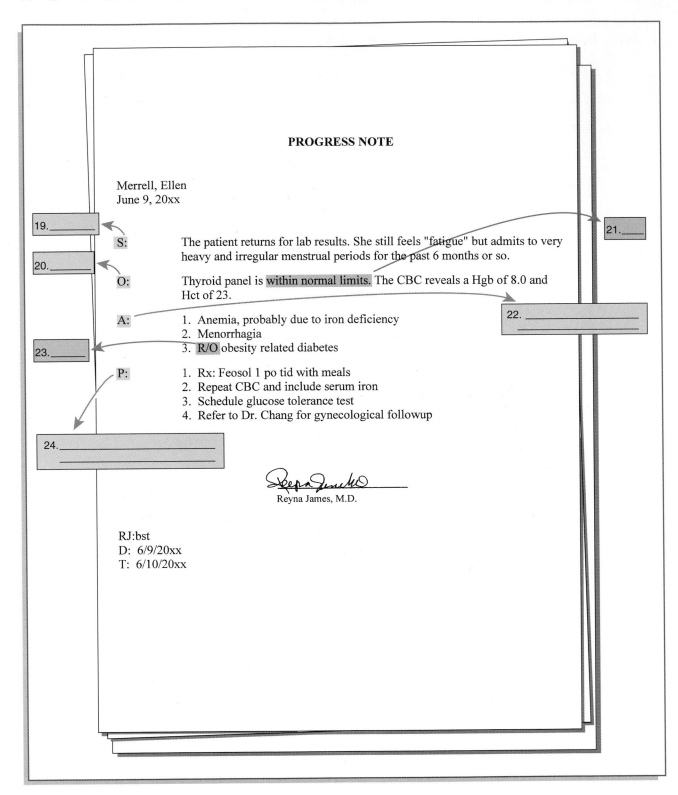

PROGRESS NOTE

Merrell, Ellen
June 9, 20xx

19. _____

S: The patient returns for lab results. She still feels "fatigue" but admits to very
heavy and irregular menstrual periods for the past 6 months or so.

20. _____

O: Thyroid panel is within normal limits. The CBC reveals a Hgb of 8.0 and
Hct of 23.

21. ____

A:
1. Anemia, probably due to iron deficiency
2. Menorrhagia
3. R/O obesity related diabetes

22. _____

23. ____

P:
1. Rx: Feosol 1 po tid with meals
2. Repeat CBC and include serum iron
3. Schedule glucose tolerance test
4. Refer to Dr. Chang for gynecological followup

24. _____

Reyna James, M.D.
Reyna James, M.D.

RJ:bst
D: 6/9/20xx
T: 6/10/20xx

Write in the missing terms for the highlighted abbreviations:

19 _____

20. _____

21. _____

22. _____

23. _____

24. _____

Write the full medical term for the following abbreviations and symbols:

25. CC _____

26. OH _____

27. PR _____

28. BRP _____

29. PAR ___Post anesthetic recovery_____

30. PH _____

31. D/C _____

32. Sig: _____

33. ER _____

34. ICU _____

35. R/O _____

36. NPO _____

37. L&W _____

38. BP _____

39. AU _____

40. Sx _____

41. VS _____

42. ROS _____

43. pt _____

44. OD _____

45. SQ _____

46. H & P ___history & Physical_____

47. Tx _____

48. Dx _____

49. HPI _____

Match the following terms with their meanings:

50. febrile _____

51. syndrome _____

52. chronic _____

53. remission _____

54. etiology _____

55. malignant _____

56. prognosis _____

57. diagnosis _____

58. exacerbation _____

59. localized _____

a. period in which symptoms stop

b. probable outcome of a disease

c. name of a disease based on history, exam and testing

d. elevated temperature

e. set of symptoms characteristic of a particular disease or condition

f. increase in severity with aggravation of symptoms

g. developing slowly over time

h. limited to a definite area or part

i. cancerous

j. the study of the cause of a disease

Match the following definitions with their abbreviations:

60. the route of oral medications _____

61. place for surgery _____

62. as desired _____

63. progress note _____

64. after surgery _____

65. pound _____

66. as needed _____

67. by injection _____

68. before surgery _____

69. immediately _____

a. pre-op

b. prn

c. parenteral

d. po

e. STAT

f. ad lib

g. post op

h. OR

i. SOAP

j. #

Write the meaning for the following pharmaceutical phrases:

70. VS q h x 4 h, then q2h _____

71. † po qid pc hs _____

72. aspirin (ASA) gr ⅱ s̄s̄ qd _____

73. 650 mg po q 4 h prn temp >101° _____

74. ⊤̈ po qod am _____

75. gt ⊤̈ OU tid x 7 d _____

76. cap ⊤̈⊤̈ STAT, then ⊤̈ q 6 h _____

Write the standard pharmaceutical abbreviations for the following:

77. one tablet by mouth three times a day for 7 days

_____

78. one suppository in the vagina at bedtime

_____

79. ½ grain by mouth twice a day

_____

80. one or two by mouth every 3 to 4 hours as needed

_____

81. two drops in left ear every 3 hours

_____

82. one capsule by mouth two times a day, morning and evening

_____

83. two by mouth immediately, then by mouth once every 6 hours

_____

84. thirty milligrams by mouth at bedtime as needed

_____

Give the military times for the following:

85. 1:00 AM _____

86. 2:30 PM _____

87. midnight _____

88. 1:00 PM _____

89. 7:00 PM _____

Match the following chart entries with health record abbreviations:

90. works as a security officer _____   a. UCHD

91. advised to lower salt intake _____   b. HPI

92. father, age 88, L&W; mother, age 78, died, stoke _____   c. PE

93. quit smoking 2 years ago, drinks alcohol socially _____   d. CC

94. Diagnosis: tonsillitis _____   e. OH

95. c/o lower back pain _____   f. SH

96. pain in lower back for two weeks, worse at night _____   g. FH

97. no reaction to any previously administered drug _____   h. P

98. had all commonly contracted childhood diseases _____   i. A

99. Lungs: clear. Heart: regular rate and rhythm _____   j. NKA

From the following list of diagnostic imaging modalities, circle those that <u>use</u> ionizing radiation:

100. computed tomography

101. magnetic resonance imaging

102. radiology

103. radionuclide organ imaging

104. sonography

Match the following:

105. computed tomography _____   a. standard x-rays

106. magnetic resonance imaging _____   b. gamma rays

107. radiology _____   c. ultrasound waves

108. radionuclide organ imaging _____   d. radio waves

109. sonography _____   e. 3-D x-rays

Medical Record Analyses

MEDICAL RECORD 2-1

Progress Note

CC: 37 y.o. ♂ c̄ diabetes c/o swelling of the Ⓡ foot and calf × 3 d

S: There is no Hx of trauma, pain, SOB, or cardiac Sx, smoker × 12 yr, s̄s̄ pkg q d, denies ETOH consumption
Meds: parenteral insulin qd, NKDA

O: Pt is afebrile, BP 140/84, P 72, R 16, lungs are clear; abdomen is benign s̄ organomegaly; muscle tone and strength are WNL; there is swelling of the Ⓡ calf but s̄ erythema or tenderness

A: Edema of Ⓡ calf of unknown etiology

P: Schedule STAT vascular sonogram of lower extremities; pt is to keep the leg elevated × ṫṫ d, then RTC for follow-up and test results on Thursday (or sooner if ↑ edema, SOB, or CP)

1. What is the sex of the patient?
   a. male
   b. female

2. Where was patient seen?
   a. emergency room
   b. outpatient office or clinic
   c. inpatient hospital
   d. not stated

3. What was the condition of the patient's abdomen?
   a. shows signs of cancer
   b. internal organs are enlarged
   c. internal organs are not enlarged
   d. muscle tone and stength are weak

4. How much does the patient smoke per day?
   a. one package
   b. two packages
   c. half a package
   d. none; patient quit smoking 12 years ago

5. How is the patient's insulin administered?
   a. orally
   b. transdermally
   c. infusion through implant
   d. by injection

6. What is the cause of the patient's complaint?
   a. unknown
   b. fever
   c. shortness of breath
   d. trauma

7. When should the sonogram be performed?
   a. immediately
   b. within two days
   c. at the time of follow-up
   d. only if symptoms persist

8. How long should patient's leg be kept elevated?
   a. one week
   b. two weeks
   c. one day
   d. two days

MEDICAL RECORD 2-2

Post-op Meds for Laparotomy

1. Vicodin, ṫ tab p.o. q 3 h prn mild pain, or ṫṫ tab p.o. q 3 h prn moderate pain

2. Demerol, 100 mg IM q 3 h prn severe pain

3. Tylenol (acetaminophen) 650 mg p.o. q 4 h prn oral temp ↑ 100.4°F

4. Dalmane (flurazepam) 30 mg p.o. h.s. prn sleep

5. Mylicon (simethicone) 80 mg, ṫ tab chewed and swallowed q.i.d.

6. Ducolax (bisacodyl) suppos, ṫ PR in a.m.

1. How is the Demerol to be administered?
   a. by mouth
   b. within the vein
   c. under the skin
   d. within the muscle

2. What is the Sig: on the Mylicon?
   a. one every other day
   b. one twice a day
   c. one three times a day
   d. one four times a day

3. What is the Sig: on the Ducolax?
   a. one suppository in the rectum in the morning
   b. one suppository taken orally before noon
   c. two suppositories before breakfast
   d. one suppository as needed in the morning

4. When should the Dalmane be administered?
   a. each night
   b. at bedtime
   c. as needed
   d. every hour

5. What are the instructions for administering Vicodin in the case of moderate pain?
   a. one tablet every three hours
   b. three tablets every hour
   c. two tablets every three hours
   d. three tablets every three hours

6. How should Tylenol be administered?
   a. one dose every four hours as needed
   b. one dose every four hours only if patient has a temperature of 100.4°F or higher
   c. one dose every four hours as long as the patient's temperature does not go over 100.4°
   d. one dose every hour up to four per day

7. Laparotomy refers to
   a. a puncture of the abdomen
   b. excision of the stomach
   c. a puncture of the stomach
   d. an incision in the abdomen

MEDICAL RECORD 2-3 FOR ADDITIONAL STUDY

PROGRESS NOTES

Patient Name: MARSI, Michael

DATE	FINDINGS
2-3-xx	CC: 51 y.o. ♂ c/o dizziness × 3 wk and headaches 5-6 × ī wk. Today he woke c̄ numbness in ® leg and hand.
	S Hx of ↑BP × 4yrs. Smoker × 20yrs - 1 pkg/d MEDS: Dyazide ī q d. ī CP ō SOB occipital headaches ī in am mod fat diet 3 beers q noc. NKDA
	O BP 150/100 ® arm ℓ Ht 68″ WT 198# T 98.7° P 76 R 15 Heart - RRR s̄ ⓜ Lungs clear HEENT - WNL.
	A Hypertension (HTN) R/O Congestive heart failure (CHF)
	P Chest x-ray and electrocardiogram today ↓ ETOH to ī beer q noc DC smoking Rx: Procardia #30 ī P.O. q d. ↑ exercise to 3×/wk for 20-30 min stop if CP, SOB or dizzy ↓ fat and cholesterol in diet re√ BP ī wk R.T.O. sooner if CP, SOB or dizzy
	JR Spaulding MD

MEDICAL RECORD 2-3 FOR ADDITIONAL STUDY

Michael Marsi has had chronic health problems in the last 2 years and has been seeing Dr. Spaulding, his personal physician, regularly in recent months. Dr. Spaulding uses problem-oriented medical records and writes a new SOAP progress note at each patient visit. Mr. Marsi has come to see Dr. Spaulding today because he feels worse than usual.

Read Medical Record 2.3 for Michael Marsi and answer the following questions. This record is the progress note for today's visit, part of Dr. Spaulding's POMR for Mr. Marsi. Dr. Spaulding handwrote it herself during the patient's visit.

1. How old is Mr. Marsi? _____

2. Where was the treatment rendered? _____

3. List the three elements of the patient's complaint

    a. _____

    b. _____

    c. _____

4. In your own words, not using medical terminology, briefly summarize Mr. Marsi's history:

    _____

    _____

    _____

5. Which of the following is not mentioned at all in this history?
    a. The prescription medication Mr. Marsi takes
    b. Mr. Marsi's smoking habit
    c. Mr. Marsi's activity level at work
    d. Mr. Marsi's consumption of alcohol

6. Dr. Spaulding and Mr. Marsi talked at length about Mr. Marsi's symptoms and how they've changed recently, and then Dr. Spaulding examined him. List three objective findings she noted in this examination.

    a._____

    b._____

    c._____

7. Dr. Spaulding's assessment is that he has _____

    But she also wants to make sure Mr. Marsi does not have _____

    _____

8. Dr. Spaulding's treatment plan involves four areas. List the specific plan(s) for each of these.

    Diagnostic tests ordered _____

    _____

Instruct the patient to change (and how) his personal habits: _____

_____

_____

_____

_____

Drug prescribed (and how much and when): _____

_____

Future diagnostic check and/or action to take: _____

_____

9. When is Dr. Spaulding expecting to see Mr. Marsi again? _____

_____

Answers to Practice Exercises

1. H & P
2. Hx
3. CC
4. HPI
5. PMH
6. FH
7. SH
8. OH
9. ROS
10. PE
11. A, IMP, Dx
12. P
13. c/o
14. UCHD
15. NKDA
16. L & W
17. NAD
18. PERRLA
19. Subjective
20. Objective
21. WNL
22. Assessment (Impression, Diagnosis)
23. Rule out
24. Plan (Disposition, Recommendation)
25. chief complaint
26. occupational history
27. per rectum
28. bathroom privileges
29. post anesthetic recovery
30. past history
31. discontinue or discharge
32. instructions to patient
33. emergency room
34. intensive care unit
35. rule out
36. nothing by mouth
37. living and well
38. blood pressure
39. both ears
40. symptom
41. vital signs
42. review of systems
43. patient
44. right eye
45. subcutaneous
46. history and physical
47. treatment or traction
48. diagnosis
49. history of present illness
50. d
51. e
52. g
53. a
54. j
55. i
56. b
57. c
58. f
59. h
60. d
61. h
62. f
63. i
64. g
65. j
66. b
67. c
68. a
69. e
70. vital signs every hour for 4 hours, then every 2 hours
71. one by mouth four times a day, after meals and at bedtime
72. two and one-half grains of aspirin every day
73. 650 mg by mouth every 4 hours as needed for temperature more than 101°
74. one by mouth every other day in the morning
75. one drop in both eyes three times a day for 7 days
76. two capsules immediately, then one every 6 hours
77. tab ⊤ po tid x 7 d or ⊤ tab po tid x 7 d
78. suppos ⊤ PV hs or ⊤ suppos PV hs
79. gr $\overline{ss}$ po bid, or $\overline{ss}$ gr po bid
80. ⊤ or ⊤⊤ po q 3-4 h prn
81. gtt ⊤⊤ AS q 3 h or ⊤⊤ gtt AS q 3 h
82. cap ⊤ po bid am and pm or ⊤ cap po bid am and pm
83. ⊤⊤ po STAT, then ⊤ q 6 h
84. 30 mg po hs prn
85. 0100 hours
86. 1430 hours
87. 2400 hours
88. 1300 hours
89. 1900 hours
90. e
91. h
92. g

93. f
94. i
95. d
96. b
97. j
98. a
99. c
100. yes
101. no
102. yes
103. yes
104. no
105. e
106. d
107. a
108. b
109. c

Answers to Medical Records Analyses

(SEE ACCOMPANYING CD-ROM FOR ANSWERS TO MEDICAL RECORD 2-3 FOR ADDITIONAL STUDY)

PROGRESS NOTES

1. a
2. b
3. c
4. c
5. d
6. a
7. a
8. d

POST-OP MEDS

1. d
2. d
3. a
4. b
5. c
6. b
7. d

CHAPTER 3

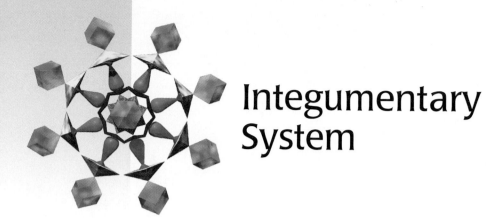

Integumentary System

Integumentary System Overview

Tissues of the integumentary system (Fig. 3-1):

* Skin (also called the *integument*)
* Hair
* Nails
* Sweat glands
* Sebaceous glands

Functions of the integumentary system:

* Protects the body from injury
* Protects the body from intrusion of microorganisms
* Helps regulate body temperature
* Houses receptors for sense of touch, including pain and sensation

The skin has three layers:

* The **epidermis** consists of several layers of stratified squamous (scalelike) epithelium.
   1. Cells are produced in the innermost (basal) layer, moving the older cells up toward the surface.
   2. Cells that are pushed up flatten, fill with a hard protein substance called **keratin,** and die.
   3. Layers of packed dead cells accumulate in the outermost (squamous) layer, where they are sloughed off.
* The **dermis,** the connective tissue layer, contains blood vessels, nerves, and other structures (Fig. 3-1). Collagen fibers make the skin tough and elastic.
* The **subcutaneous layer** below the dermis is composed of loose connective tissue and adipose (fatty) tissue.

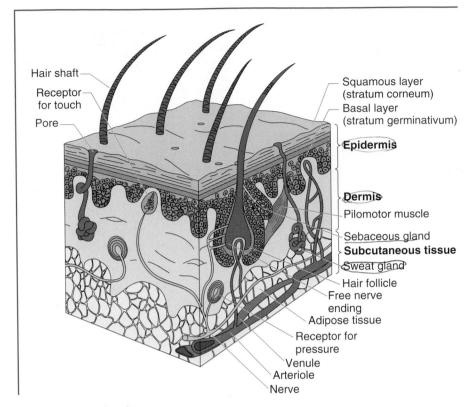

■ **FIGURE 3-1.** The skin.

SELF-INSTRUCTION: COMBINING FORMS

Study the following:

Combining Form	Meaning
adip/o lip/o steat/o	fat
derm/o dermat/o cutane/o	skin
erythr/o	red
hidr/o	sweat
hist/o histi/o	tissue
kerat/o	hard
leuk/o	white
melan/o	black
myc/o	fungus

onych/o	nail
plas/o	formation
purpur/o	purple
seb/o	sebum (oil)
squam/o	scale
trich/o	hair
xer/o	dry
xanth/o	yellow

PROGRAMMED REVIEW: COMBINING FORMS

Answer Column	**Review**

3.1 *Derm/o* and *dermat/o* are Greek combining forms meaning

skin
_____. The medical field specializing in study of the skin is

dermatology
_____. The physician who specializes in the study

dermatologist
and treatment of the skin is called a _____.

skin
Cutane/o is a Latin combining form meaning _____. Subcutaneous

under
therefore pertains to _____ the skin.

cell
3.2 *Cyt/o* means _____. Cells with specialized functions combine

to form varying types of tissue. *Hist/o* is a combining form meaning

tissue, histology
_____. The study of tissues is _____. Histio-

production, tissue
genic pertains to the origin or _____ of _____.

plas/o
3.3 The combining form meaning "formation" is <u>plas</u>. *Dys-* is a

faulty
prefix meaning painful, difficult, or _____, and *-ia* refers to a

condition of
<u>pertaining</u> <del>to</del>. Therefore, the term used to describe a con-

dysplasia
dition of (faulty) <u>abnormal formation of tissue</u> is <u>dysplasia</u>.

upon
3.4 The prefix *epi-*, meaning <u>upon</u>, was used in naming the outer

epi (epidermis)
tissue layer of the skin called the <u>epi</u>dermis. The combining form

scale
squam/o means <u>scale</u>. The suffix *-ous* means

pertaining to	_____pertaining to_____ _____. The flat, scalelike cells of the
squamous	epidermis are aptly called _____ cells.

3.5 The pigment called melanin is found in the basal layer of the epidermis. The combining form *melan/o* means _____, and people

black

darker

with more melanin have _____ skin. Melanocytes are the

cells

_____ in the basal layer that produce melanin.

Kerat/o

3.6 _____ is the combining form that means hard. Keratin

skin

is the hard protein substance found in the basal layer of the _____.
Keratosis is a condition characterized by the overgrowth of cells com-

keratin

posed of much _____.

3.7 Hair follicles are found in the dermis layer of the skin. The com-

trich/o

bining form for hair is _____trich/o_____. Combined with the suffix

hair

meaning rupture, trichorrhexis is the term describing _____hair_____ that is
broken or split.

3.8 Sebaceous glands, which open to the hair follicles in the skin, pro-

sebum, seb/o

duce _____ (oil). The combining form is _____. Seborrhea

sebum

refers to an overproduction of _____ by these glands.

water

3.9 *Hydr/o*, a combining form meaning _____, stems from the
Greek word hydros. A similar component, *hidr/o*, stemming from the

sweat

Greek word hidros, means _____. The formation of sweat is

hidro (hidropoiesis)

termed _____poiesis.

fungus

3.10 Mycosis refers to any condition caused by a _____fungus_____. The

myc/o

term was coined using the combining form _____myc_____.

nail

3.11 The combining form *onych/o* refers to the finger or toe _____nail_____.

softening

The suffix -*malacia* means _____softenig_____. An abnormal soften-

onycho (onychomalacia)	ing of the nails is therefore called ___onycho___ malacia. Onychomyco-sis refers to a ___fungus___ infection (condition) of the nails.
fungus	

3.12 Several combining forms refer to body fat. The term lipid is from

lip/o	the combining form _____. Liposuction, therefore, refers to the
fat	procedure for suctioning _____ from the body tissues. The adjective
adip/o	adipose, meaning fatty, is from the combining form _____.
sub (subcutaneous)	Adipose tissue is found (below the dermis) in the ___sub___ cutaneous
fat	layer of the skin. A third combining form, *steat/o*, also refers to ___fat___.
inflammation, fat	Steatitis refers to an ___inflammation___ of ___fat___.

white	**3.13** The combining form *leuk/o* means _____. It was used to coin the term for a partial or total absence of pigment in the skin,
leuko	known as ___leuko___ derma.

erythr/o	**3.14** The combining form _____ means red. Erythema
red	therefore refers to skin that is _____.
red, skin	Erythroderma is another term referring to ___red___ ___skin___.

	3.15 The meaning of the combining form *purpur/o* is easy to remember because it sounds like the color ___purple___. Purpuric lesions are
purple	
purple	_____ because they result from hemorrhages, or the bursting
blood	forth of ___blood___ into the skin.

blood ~~dis~~
rrhea: discharge

skin	**3.16** Xeroderma is a term meaning dry _____. The combining
xer/o	form for dry is _____. Xerosis is a condition of pathologically
dry	___dry___ skin.

xanth/o	**3.17** The combining form _____ refers to the color yellow.
yellow	A xanthoma is a ___yellow___ skin tumor.

SELF-INSTRUCTION: ANATOMICAL TERMS

Study the following:

Anatomic Terms	Meaning
epithelium *ep-i-thē′lē-ŭm*	cells covering external and internal surfaces of the body
epidermis *ep-i-derm′is*	thin outer layer of the skin
√**squamous cell layer** *skwā′mŭs*	flat, scalelike epithelial cells comprising the outermost epidermis
√**basal layer** *bā′săl*	deepest layer of epidermis
melanocyte *mel′ă-nō-sīt*	cell in the basal layer that gives color to the skin
melanin *mel′ă-nin*	dark brown to black pigment contained in melanocytes
dermis	dense, fibrous connective tissue layer of the skin (also known as corium)
sebaceous glands *sē-bā′shŭs*	oil glands in the skin
sebum *sē′bŭm*	oily substance secreted by the sebaceous glands
sudoriferous glands *sŭ-dō-rif′er-ŭs*	sweat glands (sudor = sweat; ferre = to bear)
subcutaneous layer *sŭb-kyū-tā′nē-ŭs*	connective and adipose tissue layer just under the dermis
collagen *kol′lă-jen*	protein substance in skin and connective tissue (koila = glue; gen = producing)
hair	outgrowth of the skin composed of keratin
nail	outgrowth of the skin at the end of each finger and toe, composed of keratin
keratin *ker′ă-tin*	hard protein material found in the epidermis, hair, and nails

PROGRAMMED REVIEW: ANATOMICAL TERMS

Answer Column	Review

Answer Column

epithelium, upon

-ium

Review

3.18   Cells covering external and internal surfaces of the body are called _____. The prefix *epi-* means _____, and the suffix __*ium*__ means structure or tissue.

epidermis

epi-

skin

dermis

3.19   The outer layer of the skin is called the _____, formed from the prefix __*epi*__ and the combining form *derm/o*, meaning __skin__. The middle layer of skin is called the __dermis__ and is where nerves and blood vessels are located.

squamous

scale

3.20   The __squamous__ cell layer is the outermost layer of the epidermis. The combining form *squam/o* means __scale__, and this layer is so named because the dead skin cells in the outermost layer scale off.

basal

pertaining to

epidermis

3.21   Below the squamous cell layer is the __basal__ cell layer. The suffix *-al* means _____ _____. This layer is therefore the deepest (or (base)) layer of the __epidermis__.

cyt/o

melanin

black

3.22   The combining form for cell is __cyt__. A melanocyte, therefore, is a cell containing __melanin__, the dark pigment of the skin. *Melan/o* means _____.

sebum

adjective

dermis

3.23   The sebaceous glands produce __sebum__, an oily substance. The suffix *-ous* is added to a combining form to create an _____. These glands are located in the skin layer called the __dermis__.

sudoriferous

dermis

3.24   The sweat glands are called the __sudoriferous__ glands, from *sudor* (sweat) and *ferre* (to bear). They are located in the __dermis__ skin layer.

subcutaneous sub- skin	**3.25** Beneath the dermis is the _____ layer. The prefix _____ means below or under, and the combining form _cutane/o_ means _____.
collagen	**3.26** Formed from the roots _koila_ (glue) and _gen_ (producing), _____ is a protein substance found in skin and connective tissue.
keratin nails hard	**3.27** Hair is an outgrowth of the skin composed of _____. The _____ on the fingers and toes are also composed of keratin. The combining form _kerat/o_ means _____.

SELF-INSTRUCTION: SYMPTOMATIC TERMS

Study the following:

Symptomatic Terms	Meaning
lesion _lē′zhŭn_	an area of pathologically altered tissue (two types: primary and secondary) (Fig. 3-2)
primary lesions	lesions arising from previously normal skin

FLAT, NONPALPABLE CHANGES IN SKIN COLOR

macule (macula) (Fig. 3-3, A) _mak′yūl_	a flat, discolored spot on the skin up to 1 cm across (e.g., a freckle)
patch (Fig. 3-3, B)	a flat, discolored area on the skin larger than 1 cm (e.g., vitiligo)

ELEVATED, PALPABLE, SOLID MASSES

papule (Fig. 3-3, C) _pap′yūl_	a solid mass on the skin up to 0.5 cm in diameter (e.g., a nevus or mole)
plaque (Fig. 3-3, D) _plāk_	a solid mass greater than 1 cm in diameter, limited to the surface of the skin
nodule (Fig. 3-3, E) _nod′yūl_	a solid mass greater than 1 cm, extending deeper into the epidermis
tumor (Fig. 3-3, F) _tu′mŏr_	solid mass larger than 1–2 cm
wheal (Fig. 3-3, G) _hwēl_	an area of localized skin edema (swelling) (e.g., a hive)

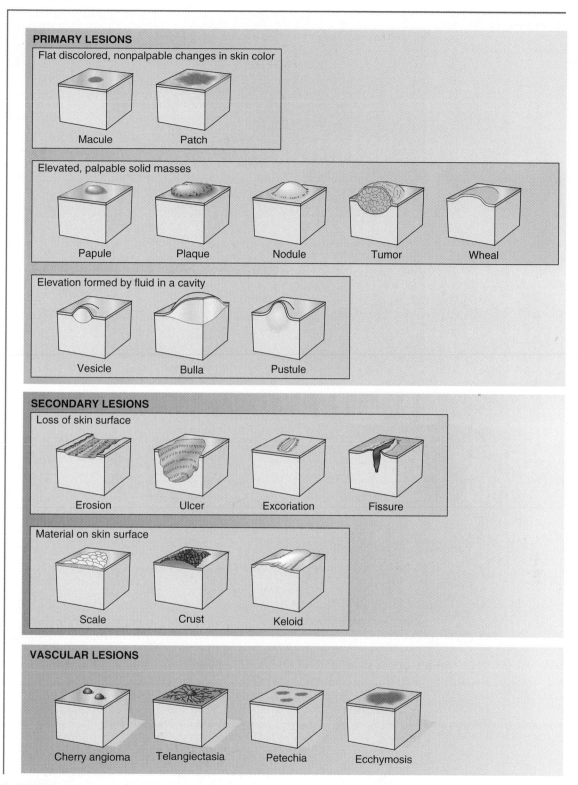

■ FIGURE 3-2. Types of primary, secondary, and vascular lesions.

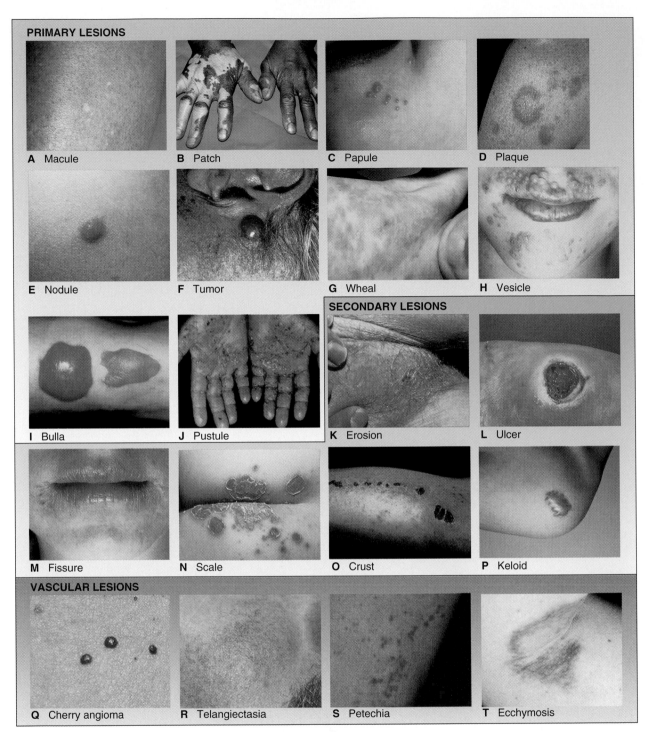

FIGURE 3-3. Skin lesions.

ELEVATION FORMED BY FLUID WITHIN A CAVITY

vesicle (Fig. 3-3, H) *ves' ĭ-kl*	little bladder; an elevated, fluid-filled sac (blister) within or under the epidermis up to 0.5 cm in diameter (e.g., a fever blister)
bulla (Fig. 3-3, I) *bul'ă*	a blister larger than 0.5 cm (e.g., a second-degree burn; bulla = bubble)

pustule (Fig. 3-3, J) *pŭs'chūl*	a pus-filled sac (e.g., a pimple)
secondary lesions	lesions that result in changes in primary lesions

Loss of Skin Surface

erosion (Fig. 3-3, K) *ē-rō'zhŭn*	gnawed away; loss of superficial epidermis leaving an area of moisture but no bleeding (e.g., area of moisture after rupture of a vesicle)
ulcer (Fig. 3-3, L)	an open sore on the skin or mucous membrane that can bleed and scar; sometimes accompanied by infection (e.g., decubitus ulcer)
excoriation *eks-kō'rē-ā'shŭn*	a scratch mark
fissure (Fig. 3-3, M) *fish'ŭr*	a linear crack in the skin

Material on Skin Surface

scale (Fig. 3-3, N)	a thin flake of exfoliated epidermis (e.g., dandruff)
crust (Fig. 3-3, O)	dried residue of serum (body liquid), pus, or blood on the skin (e.g., in impetigo)

Other Secondary Lesions

cicatrix of the skin *sik'ă-triks*	mark left by the healing of a sore or wound, showing the replacement of destroyed tissue by fibrous tissue (cicatrix = scar)
keloid (Fig. 3.3, P) *ke'loyd*	an abnormal overgrowth of scar tissue that is thick and irregular (kele = tumor)
vascular lesions	lesions of a blood vessel
cherry angioma (Fig. 3-3, Q) *chār'e an-jē-ō'mă*	a small, round, bright red blood vessel tumor on the skin, often on the trunk of the elderly
telangiectasia (Fig. 3-3, R) *tel-an'jē-ek-tā'zē-ă*	a tiny, red blood vessel lesion formed by the dilation of a group of blood vessels radiating from a central arteriole, most commonly on the face, neck, or chest (telos = end)
spider angioma *spi'der an-jē-ō'mă* **purpuric lesions** *pŭr'pū-rik*	purpura; lesions resulting from hemorrhages into the skin
petechia (Fig. 3-3, S) *pe-tē'kē-ă*	spot; reddish-brown, minute hemorrhagic spot(s) on the skin that indicate a bleeding tendency; a small purpura

✓**ecchymosis** (Fig. 3-3, T) *ek-i-mō′sis*	bruise; a black and blue mark; a large purpura (chymo = juice)
epidermal tumors	skin tumors arising from the epidermis
nevus (see also Fig. 3-7) *nē′vŭs*	birthmark; a congenital malformation on the skin that can be epidermal or vascular, also called a mole
dysplastic nevus *dis-plas′tik nē′vŭs*	a mole with precancerous changes
verruca *vĕ-rū′kă*	an epidermal tumor caused by a papilloma virus; also called a wart

PROGRAMMED REVIEW: SYMPTOMATIC TERMS

Answer Column	Review
lesion secondary primary secondary	**3.28** A _____ is an area of pathologically altered tissue. There are primary and _____ types. Lesions that arise from previously normal skin are called _____ lesions, whereas those that result in changes in primary lesions are called _____ lesions.
macule (macula) patch, maculae	**3.29** A freckle is an example of a _____, which is a flat discolored spot up to 1 cm across. A larger, flat, discolored spot is called a _____. The plural of macula is _____.
solid plaque nodule small	**3.30** A papule is a _____ mass on the skin up to 0.5 cm in diameter, such as a mole. A _____ is like a papule but is greater than 1 cm in diameter and is limited to the surface of the skin. A _____, like a papule, is greater than 1 cm in diameter but extends deeper into the epidermis. The suffix *-ule* is a diminutive that means _____.
tumor edema	**3.31** Another type of solid mass is a _____, which is larger than 1 to 2 cm. A wheal is an area of localized skin _____ (swelling).

3.32   There are three types of elevated skin lesions with fluid within a cavity. A small elevated blister up to 0.5 cm, such as a fever blister, is a _____. A larger blister, more than 0.5 cm, is a _____, such as may occur with a second-degree burn. The plural form ends in _____. A pus-filled sac, like a pimple, is called a _____.

vesicle, bulla

-ae, pustule

3.33   Some secondary lesions result in a loss of skin surface. If skin is lost, leaving an area of moisture but no bleeding, it is called an _____. An ulcer is an open _____ on the skin or mucous membrane that can bleed. A scratch mark is called an _____. Recall that the prefix *ex-* means _____, and the suffix _____ refers to a process. A crack in the skin is a _____.

erosion, sore

excoriation

out or away, -ation

fissure

3.34   A thin flake of dead epidermis is a _____. A dried residue of serum, pus, or blood is called a _____.

scale

crust

3.35   A healed sore or wound leaves a scar, called a _____ of the skin. An abnormal overgrowth of scar tissue, from the root kele (tumor), is a _____. Recall that the suffix *-oid* means resembling, which in this case implies that a keloid is not actually a _____.

cicatrix

keloid

tumor

3.36   Lesions of a blood vessel are called ___vascular___ lesions. A ___cherry___ angioma is a small, bright red blood vessel tumor on the skin. A ___spider___ angioma is a tiny red blood vessel lesion in a group of vessels radiating from a central arteriole. The suffix *-oma* means _____. Another term for a spider angioma is ___telangiectasia___.

vascular

cherry

spider

tumor

telangiectasia

3.37   ___purpuric___ lesions look purple because of hemorrhages into the skin. The combining form *purpur/o* means _____. A small purpura appearing as a tiny reddish-brown spot on the skin is

Purpuric

purple

petechia, iae

called a _petechia_. The plural form is petech _ae_. A bruise

ecchymosis, es

is called an _ecchymosis_; the plural form is ecchymos _es_.

3.38 Epidermal tumors are skin tumors arising from the

epidermis, nevus

_____. A mole is called a _____. A dysplastic

mole

nevus is a _____ with precancerous changes. The prefix _dys-_ means

painful, difficult, or faulty

_____. A verruca is an epidermal

tumor, wart

_____ caused by a papilloma virus, also called a _____. The

verrucae

plural of verruca is _____.

SELF-INSTRUCTION: GENERAL SYMPTOMATIC TERMS

Study the following:

GENERAL SYMPTOMATIC TERMS

alopecia _al-ō-pē′shē-ă_	fox mange; baldness; natural or unnatural deficiency of hair
comedo (pl. comedos, comedones) _kom′ē-dō_	a blackhead caused by a plug of sebum (oil) within the opening of a hair follicle
eruption _ē-rŭp′shŭn_	appearance of a skin lesion
erythema _er-i-thē′mă_	redness of skin
pruritus _prū-rī′tŭs_	severe itching
rash	a general term for skin eruption, most often associated with communicable disease
skin pigmentation	skin color due to the presence of melanin
depigmentation	loss of melanin pigment in the skin
hypopigmentation	areas of skin lacking color due to deficient amounts of melanin
hyperpigmentation	darkened areas of skin caused by excessive amounts of melanin
suppuration _sŭp′yŭ-rā′shŭn_	production of purulent matter (pus)

urticaria (Fig. 3-3, G) *er'ti-kar'l-a*	hives; an eruption of wheals on the skin accompanied by itch (urtica = stinging nettle)
xeroderma *zēr'ō-der'mă*	dry skin

PROGRAMMED REVIEW: GENERAL SYMPTOMATIC TERMS

Answer Column	Review

alopecia

3.39 Baldness, or an unnatural deficiency of hair, is called

_____.

lesion

rash

urticaria

condition of

3.40 An eruption is the appearance of a skin _____. A _____ is a general term for skin eruption, often associated with a communicable disease. An eruption of wheals on the skin (hives) accompanied by itching is called _____. Remember that the suffix *-ia* means a _____ _____.

pruritus

itch

3.41 Any severe itching is called _____. A pruritic eruption is one that is marked by severe _____.

erythr/o

erythema

pertaining to

3.42 The combining form for red is _____. Redness of the skin is called _____. The adjective erythematous means _____ _____ redness of the skin.

black

color

not

deficient

excessive

de

hypo

hyper

3.43 *Melan/o* is the combining form meaning _____. Melanin is the pigment that gives _____ to the skin. Pigmentation describes the process of skin coloration. Recall the meaning of the following prefixes. *De-* means from, down, or _____; *hypo-* means below or _____; and *hyper-* means above or _____. Each is used to describe a different pigmentation of the skin. Using the prefix meaning from, down, or not, the total loss or absence of melanin is called _____pigmentation. Too little or deficient melanin causes _____pigmentation, and too much or excessive deposits of melanin cause _____pigmentation.

xer/o	**3.44** The combining form meaning dry is _____. The Greek
skin	word derma means _____. Therefore, the term for dry skin is
xeroderma	_____.

SELF-INSTRUCTION: DIAGNOSTIC TERMS

Study the following:

Diagnostic Terms	Meaning
acne *ak'nē*	inflammation of the sebaceous glands and hair follicles of the skin evidenced by comedones (blackheads), pustules, or nodules on the skin (acne = point)
albinism *al'bi-nizm*	a hereditary condition characterized by a partial or total lack of melanin pigment (particularly in the eyes, skin, and hair)
burn	injury to body tissue caused by heat, chemicals, electricity, radiation, or gases
first-degree burn	a burn involving only the epidermis, characterized by erythema (redness) and hyperesthesia (excessive sensation)
second-degree burn	a burn involving the epidermis and the dermis, characterized by erythema, hyperesthesia, and vesications (blisters)
third-degree burn	a burn involving all layers of the skin, characterized by the destruction of the epidermis and dermis with damage or destruction of subcutaneous tissue
dermatitis *der-mă-ti'tis*	inflammation of the skin characterized by erythema, pruritus (itching), and various lesions
dermatosis *der-mă-tō'sis*	any disorder of the skin
exanthematous viral disease *eg-zan-them'ă-tŭs*	eruption of the skin caused by a viral disease (exanthema = eruption)
rubella *rū-bel'ă*	reddish; German measles
rubeola *rū-bē'ō-lă*	reddish; 14-day measles
varicella *var-ĭ-sel'ă*	a tiny spot; chicken pox
eczema *ek'zĕ-mă*	to boil out; term often used interchangeably with dermatitis to denote a skin condition characterized by the appearance of inflamed, swollen papules and vesicles that crust and scale, often with sensations of itching and burning

furuncle *fyū′rŭng-kl*	boil; a painful nodule formed in the skin by inflammation originating in a hair follicle, caused by staphylococcosis
carbuncle *kar′bŭng-kl*	skin infection consisting of clusters of furuncles (carbo = small glowing embers)
abscess *ab′ses*	localized collection of pus in a cavity formed by the inflammation of surrounding tissues, which heals when drained or excised (abscessus = a going away)
gangrene *gang′grēn*	an eating sore; death of tissue associated with a loss of blood supply
herpes simplex virus type 1 (HSV-1) *her′pēz*	transient viral vesicles (e.g., cold sores or fever blisters) that infect the facial area, especially the mouth and nose (herpes = creeping skin disease)
herpes simplex virus type 2 (see Fig. 15-8) (HSV-2)	sexually transmitted, ulcerlike lesions of the genital and anorectal skin and mucosa; after initial infection the virus lies dormant in the nerve cell root and may recur at times of stress
herpes zoster *her′pēz zos′ter*	a viral disease affecting the peripheral nerves, characterized by painful blisters that spread over the skin following affected nerves, usually unilateral; also known as shingles (zoster = girdle)
impetigo *im-pe-tī′go*	highly contagious, bacterial skin inflammation marked by pustules that rupture and become crusted, most often around the mouth and nostrils
keratoses *ker-ă-tō′sez*	thickened areas of epidermis
actinic keratoses *ak-tin′ik* **solar keratoses**	localized thickening of the skin caused by excessive exposure to sunlight, a known precursor to cancer (actinic = ray; solar = sun)
seborrheic keratoses (Fig. 3-4) *seb-ō-rē′ik*	benign, wartlike tumors (more common on elderly skin)
lupus *lū′pŭs*	a chronic autoimmune disease characterized by inflammation of various parts of the body (lupus = wolf)
cutaneous lupus *kyū-tā′nē-ŭs*	limited to the skin; evidenced by a characteristic rash, especially on the face, neck, and scalp
systemic lupus erythematosus (SLE) *sis-tem′ik lū′pŭs er-i-them′ă-tō-sis*	a more severe form of lupus involving the skin, joints, and often vital organs (e.g., lungs or kidneys)
malignant cutaneous neoplasm *mă-lig′nănt kyū-tā′nē-ŭs nē′ō-plazm*	skin cancer

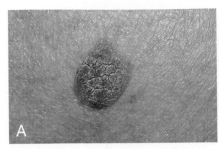

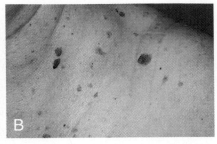

FIGURE 3-4. Seborrheic keratosis. **A.** Lesion with warty, stuck-on appearance. **B.** Multiple lesions showing various colors and sizes.

squamous cell carcinoma (Fig. 3-5) *skwā′mŭs sel kar-si-nō′mă*	malignant tumor of squamous epithelium
basal cell carcinoma (Fig. 3-6) *bā′săl sel kar-si-nō′mă*	malignant tumor of the basal layer of the epidermis (most common type of skin cancer)
malignant melanoma (Fig. 3-7) *mă-lig′nănt mel′ă-n′ōmă*	a malignant tumor composed of melanocytes
Kaposis sarcoma *Kăp′ō-sez sar-kō′mă*	a malignant tumor of the walls of blood vessels appearing as painless, dark bluish-purple plaques on the skin; often spreads to lymph nodes and internal organs
onychia *ō-nik′ē-ă*	inflammation of the fingernail or toenail
paronychia (Fig. 3-8) *par-ō-nik′ē-ă*	inflammation of nail fold
pediculosis *pĕ-dik′yū-lō′sis* **pediculosis capitis** *pĕ-dik′yū-lō′sis kap′i-tis*	infestation with lice that causes itching and dermatitis (pediculo = louse) head lice (capitis = head)

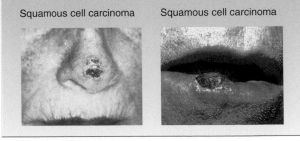

FIGURE 3-5. Squamous cell carcinoma.

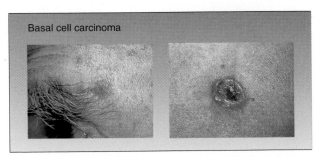

FIGURE 3-6. Basal cell carcinoma.

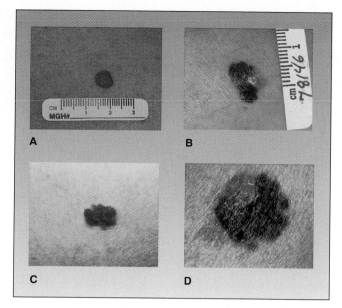

FIGURE 3-7. **A.** Normal mole. **B–D.** Signs of melanoma. Asymmetry: One half does not match the other half **(B).** Border irregularity: The edges are ragged, notched, or blurred **(C).** Color: The pigmentation is not uniform. Shades of tan, brown, and black are present. Red, white, and blue may add to the mottled appearance **(D).** Diameter greater than 6 mm: Any sudden or continuing increase in size should be of special concern (not shown).

pediculosis pubis *pĕ-dik'yū-lō'sis* *pyū'bis*	lice that generally infect the pubic region; sometimes also hair of the axilla, eyebrows, lashes, beard, or other hairy body surfaces; also called crabs (pubis = groin)
psoriasis *sō-rī'ă-sis*	itching; a chronic, recurrent skin disease marked by silver-gray scales covering red patches on the skin; results from overproduction and thickening of skin cells, commonly at elbows, knees, genitals, arms, legs, scalp, and nails
scabies *skā'bēz*	contagious disease caused by a parasite (mite) that invades the skin, causing an intense itch, most often at articulations between the fingers, toes, or elbow (scabo = to scratch)
seborrhea *seb-ō-rē'ă*	skin condition marked by the hypersecretion of sebum from the sebaceous glands

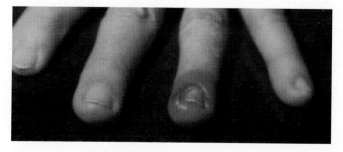

FIGURE 3-8. Chronic paronchia.

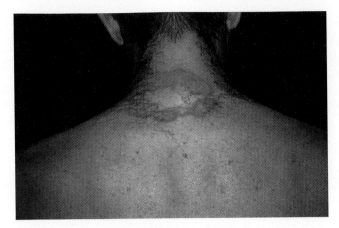

FIGURE 3-9. Tinea corporis.

tinea (Fig. 3-9) *tin′e-ă*	group of fungal skin diseases identified by the body part affected, including tinea corporis (body), commonly called ringworm; and tinea pedis (foot), also called athlete's foot
vitiligo (see Fig. 3-3, B) *vit-i-lī′gō*	the condition caused by the destruction of melanin that results in the appearance of white patches on the skin

PROGRAMMED REVIEW: DIAGNOSTIC TERMS

Answer Column	Review
condition skin dermatosis -itis dermatitis inflammation, skin eczema	**3.45** The suffix *-osis* refers to an increase or _____. *Dermat/o* means _____ Therefore, the general term meaning skin condition is _____. The suffix meaning inflammation is _____. An inflammation of the skin is therefore called _____. There are many forms of dermatitis or _____ of the _____. The term interchangeable with dermatitis characterized by inflamed skin with various lesions accompanied by itching and burning is _____. Eczematous is the adjective form of the term.
comedos or comedones acne	**3.46** An inflammation of the sebaceous glands and hair follicles, often evidenced by blackheads or _____, pustules or nodules on the skin is called _____.

condition of	**3.47** The suffix *-ism* refers to a _____ _____. Albinism is a hereditary condition characterized by a partial or total lack of
melanin	_____ pigment in the body. The condition caused by the destruction of melanin that results in the appearance of white patches on
vitiligo	the skin is called _____.
first-degree	**3.48** A _____-_____ burn involves only the epidermis.
epidermis	A second-degree burn involves both the _____ and the
	dermis. A third-degree burn involves damage to the
subcutaneous	_____ layer.
viral	**3.49** Exanthematous _____ disease is an eruption of the skin caused by a viral infection. One such viral disease, also called German
rubella	measles, is _____. A similar-sounding but different form of
rubeola	measles is _____. Varicella, another viral disease, is com-
chicken pox	monly called _____ _____.
furuncle	**3.50** A painful nodule from inflammation in a hair follicle caused by staphylococcosis is called a _____. A skin infection con-
carbuncle	sisting of clusters of furuncles is a _____, from carbo ("small glowing embers").
abscess	**3.51** Pus that collects in a cavity is called an _____. It usually heals when drained or excised.
	3.52 Gangrene is an eating sore in which tissue dies because of a loss
blood	of _____ supply.
	3.53 There are several forms of herpes disease caused by a
virus	_____. Herpes simplex virus type 1 causes transient
vesicles (blisters)	_____ such as cold sores or fever blisters. Type 2 is sexu-
genital (or anorectal)	ally transmitted and causes lesions in _____ skin.

Herpes vesicles (blisters)	_____ zoster affects the peripheral nerves and is characterized by painful _____ that spread over the skin.
Impetigo scabies fungus pediculosis capitis pubis	**3.54** _____ is a highly contagious bacterial skin inflammation usually occurring around the mouth and nose. Another contagious skin disease, called _____, is caused by a mite that invades the skin and causes intense itching. Tinea is a different group of contagious skin diseases caused by a _____. Lice also can cause an infestation on the skin called _____. Head lice are called pediculosis _____, and lice infesting the pubic region are called pediculosis _____.
hard condition of keratosis keratoses actinic sun, seborrheic	**3.55** Putting together the combining form *kerat/o*, meaning _____, with the suffix *-osis*, meaning a _____ _____, makes the word _____, a condition of thickened epidermis. The plural form of this term is _____. Solar keratoses, or _____ keratoses, are caused by excessive exposure to the _____. Benign, wartlike tumors are called _____ keratoses.
lupus skin systemic erythematosus	**3.56** An autoimmune disease involving inflammation of various parts of the body was named after the Latin word for wolf, _____. Cutaneous lupus is limited to the _____ and causes a characteristic rash. A more serious form, called _____ lupus _____ (SLE), affects many body organs.
condition of fingernail (or toenail) alongside of paronychia	**3.57** In the term onychia, the suffix *-ia* was expanded to indicate a _____ _____ inflammation of a _____. The suffix *para-*, meaning _____ _____, combined with *onych/o* and *-ia*, form the term denoting a condition of inflammation of the nail fold or _____. (Follow the rule that applies by dropping the

final vowel from the prefix before combining it with the combining form that begins with a vowel.)

discharge

3.58 Recall that the suffix *-rrhea* means _____. A skin condition marked by the hypersecretion and discharge of sebum is

seborrhea

called _____.

3.59 A condition in which the skin has silver-gray scales covering red

psoriasis

patches is _____.

new

3.60 Neoplasia is a term describing a condition of _____ formation

malignant

of tissue that is either cancerous (_____), or noncancer-

benign

ous (_____). Several different forms of malignant neoplasia can

squamous cell

involve the skin. A _____ _____ carcinoma is a tumor of the squamous epithelium. A malignant tumor of the basal layer of the

basal cell carcinoma

epidermis is a _____ _____ _____. A tumor

melanoma

composed of melanocytes is malignant _____. Remember

tumors, sarcoma

that the suffix *-oma* means _____. Kaposis _____ is a tumor of the walls of blood vessels.

SELF-INSTRUCTION: DIAGNOSTIC TERMS AND PROCEDURES

Study the following:

Diagnostic Tests and Procedures Terms	Meaning
biopsy (Bx) (Fig. 3-10) *bi′op-sē*	removal of a small piece of tissue for microscopic pathologic examination
excisional Bx	removal of an entire lesion
incisional Bx	removal of a selected portion of a lesion
shave Bx	technique using a surgical blade to "shave" tissue from epidermis and upper dermis

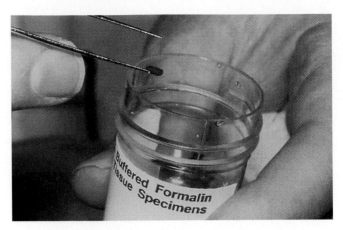

FIGURE 3-10. Collection of a biopsy specimen.

culture and sensitivity (C&S)	technique of isolating and growing colonies of microorganisms to identify a pathogen and to determine which drugs might be effective for combating it
frozen section (FS)	surgical technique involving cutting a thin piece of tissue from a frozen specimen for immediate pathologic examination
skin tests	methods for determining the reaction of the body to a given substance by applying it to, or injecting it into, the skin; commonly used in treating allergies
scratch test	test in which a substance is applied to the skin through a scratch
patch test	test in which a substance is applied topically to the skin on a small piece of blotting paper or wet cloth

PROGRAMMED REVIEW: DIAGNOSTIC TESTS AND PROCEDURES

Answer Column	Review
	3.61 In many different body systems, small samples of tissue are removed for a diagnostic test involving microscopic examination. This is
biopsy	called a _____ (Bx). An excisional biopsy involves removal of
lesion	the entire _____. Remember that the prefix *ex-* means
out or away, incisional	_____. An _____ biopsy, in con-
portion	trast, removes only a _____ of the lesion. Another type,
shave	called a _____ biopsy, uses a surgical blade to "shave" tissue
	from the epidermis and upper dermis.

3.62 A technique for isolating and growing a colony of microorganisms to identify a pathogen is called a _____ and

_____ (C&S). This helps determine what drugs may be effective in fighting the infection.

culture

sensitivity

3.63 A tissue specimen may be frozen and cut thin for examination. This is called a _____ _____ and is abbreviated _____.

frozen section

FS

3.64 Skin tests are commonly used to identify substances to which a person may be allergic. In the _____ test, a small amount of the substance is applied to the skin through a scratch. Applying the substance topically to the skin with a small piece of paper or cloth is called a _____ test.

scratch

patch

SELF-INSTRUCTION: OPERATIVE TERMS

Study the following:

Operative Terms (Fig. 3-11)	Meaning
chemosurgery _kem'ō-ser-jer-ē_ **chemical peel**	technique for restoring wrinkled, scarred, or blemished skin by applying an acid solution to "peel" away the top layers of the skin
cryosurgery _krī-ō-ser'jer-ē_	destruction of tissue by freezing with application of an extremely cold chemical (e.g., liquid nitrogen)
dermabrasion _der-mă-brā'zhŭn_	surgical removal of epidermis frozen by aerosol spray using wire brushes and emery papers to remove scars, tattoos, or wrinkles
debridement _dā-brēd-mon'_	removal of dead tissue from a wound or burn site to promote healing and to prevent infection
curettage _kyū-rĕ-tahzh'_	cleaning; scraping a wound using a spoonlike cutting instrument called a curette; used for debridement
electrosurgical procedures	use of electric currents to destroy tissue; strength of the current and method of application vary
electrocautery _ē-lek'trō-caw'ter-ē_	use of an instrument heated by electric current (cautery) to coagulate bleeding areas by burning the tissue (e.g., to sear a blood vessel)

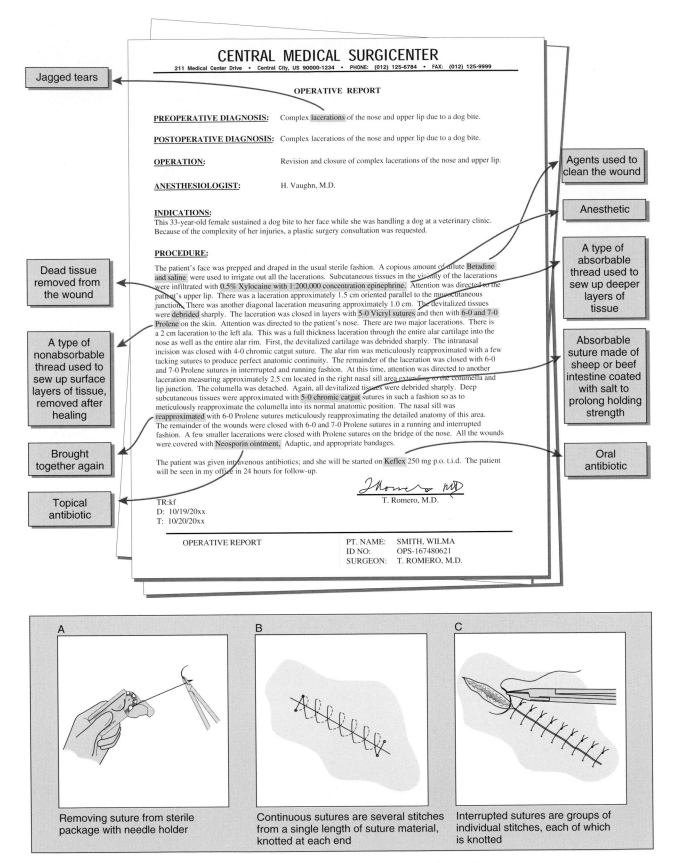

Jagged tears

Dead tissue removed from the wound

A type of nonabsorbable thread used to sew up surface layers of tissue, removed after healing

Brought together again

Topical antibiotic

Agents used to clean the wound

Anesthetic

A type of absorbable thread used to sew up deeper layers of tissue

Absorbable suture made of sheep or beef intestine coated with salt to prolong holding strength

Oral antibiotic

CENTRAL MEDICAL SURGICENTER

211 Medical Center Drive • Central City, US 90000-1234 • PHONE: (012) 125-6784 • FAX: (012) 125-9999

OPERATIVE REPORT

PREOPERATIVE DIAGNOSIS: Complex lacerations of the nose and upper lip due to a dog bite.

POSTOPERATIVE DIAGNOSIS: Complex lacerations of the nose and upper lip due to a dog bite.

OPERATION: Revision and closure of complex lacerations of the nose and upper lip.

ANESTHESIOLOGIST: H. Vaughn, M.D.

INDICATIONS:
This 33-year-old female sustained a dog bite to her face while she was handling a dog at a veterinary clinic. Because of the complexity of her injuries, a plastic surgery consultation was requested.

PROCEDURE:
The patient's face was prepped and draped in the usual sterile fashion. A copious amount of dilute Betadine and saline were used to irrigate out all the lacerations. Subcutaneous tissues in the vicinity of the lacerations were infiltrated with 0.5% Xylocaine with 1:200,000 concentration epinephrine. Attention was directed to the patient's upper lip. There was a laceration approximately 1.5 cm oriented parallel to the mucocutaneous junction. There was another diagonal laceration measuring approximately 1.0 cm. The devitalized tissues were debrided sharply. The laceration was closed in layers with 5-0 Vicryl sutures and then with 6-0 and 7-0 Prolene on the skin. Attention was directed to the patient's nose. There are two major lacerations. There is a 2 cm laceration to the left ala. This was a full thickness laceration through the entire alar cartilage into the nose as well as the entire alar rim. First, the devitalized cartilage was debrided sharply. The intranasal incision was closed with 4-0 chromic catgut suture. The alar rim was meticulously reapproximated with a few tacking sutures to produce perfect anatomic continuity. The remainder of the laceration was closed with 6-0 and 7-0 Prolene sutures in interrupted and running fashion. At this time, attention was directed to another laceration measuring approximately 2.5 cm located in the right nasal sill area extending to the columella and lip junction. The columella was detached. Again, all devitalized tissues were debrided sharply. Deep subcutaneous tissues were approximated with 5-0 chromic catgut sutures in such a fashion so as to meticulously reapproximate the columella into its normal anatomic position. The nasal sill was reapproximated with 6-0 Prolene sutures meticulously reapproximating the detailed anatomy of this area. The remainder of the wounds were closed with 6-0 and 7-0 Prolene sutures in a running and interrupted fashion. A few smaller lacerations were closed with Prolene sutures on the bridge of the nose. All the wounds were covered with Neosporin ointment, Adaptic, and appropriate bandages.

The patient was given intravenous antibiotics; and she will be started on Keflex 250 mg p.o. t.i.d. The patient will be seen in my office in 24 hours for follow-up.

T. Romero, M.D.
T. Romero, M.D.

TR:kf
D: 10/19/20xx
T: 10/20/20xx

OPERATIVE REPORT	PT. NAME: SMITH, WILMA
	ID NO: OPS-167480621
	SURGEON: T. ROMERO, M.D.

A
Removing suture from sterile package with needle holder

B
Continuous sutures are several stitches from a single length of suture material, knotted at each end

C
Interrupted sutures are groups of individual stitches, each of which is knotted

FIGURE 3-11. Typical documentation of a surgical procedure. Suturing is also depicted.

electrodesiccation *ē-lek′trō-des-i-kā′shŭn*	use of high-frequency electric currents to destroy tissue by drying it; the active electrode makes direct contact with the skin lesion (dessicate = to dry up)
fulguration *ful-gŭ-rā′shŭn*	to lighten; use of long, high-frequency, electric sparks to destroy tissue; the active electrode does *not* touch the skin
incision and drainage (I&D)	incision and drainage of an infected skin lesion (e.g., an abscess)
laser surgery *lā′zer*	surgery using a laser in various dermatological procedures to remove lesions, scars, tattoos, etc.
laser	acronym for light amplification by stimulated emission of radiation; the instrument produces a small, extremely intense beam that is precise in depth and diameter; it is applied to body tissues to destroy lesions or to dissect (cutting parts for study)
Mohs surgery *mōz*	technique used to excise tumors of the skin by removing fresh tissue layer by layer until a tumor-free plane is reached
skin grafting	transfer of skin from one body site to another to replace skin lost through a burn or injury
autograft *aw′tō-graft*	graft transfer to a new position in the body of the same person (auto = self)
heterograft *het′er-ō-graft*	graft transfer from one animal species to one of another species (hetero = different)
homograft *hō′mō-graft* **allograft** *al′ō-graft*	donor transfer between persons of the same species, such as human to human (homo = same)

PROGRAMMED REVIEW: OPERATIVE TERMS

Answer Column	Review
chemical peel	**3.65** A special form of chemosurgery, called a _____ _____, uses an acid to peel away the top layers of skin.
freezing	**3.66** Cryosurgery destroys tissue by _____ it, usually with an extremely cold chemical such as liquid nitrogen.

dermabrasion

3.67 Another way to remove skin tissue, particularly scars, tattoos, or wrinkles, is to surgically scrape the skin off with a wire brush or emery paper. This is called _____.

from (or down or not)

debridement

curettage

3.68 Recall that the prefix *de-* means _____. When dead tissue is removed from a wound or burn site, this is called _____. This is often done with a cutting instrument called a curette, and the technique is thus called _____.

electrosurgery

electrocautery

drying

fulguration

process

3.69 Electricity is used in many dermatologic procedures to destroy unwanted tissue. The general term for such operative procedures is _____. The use of an electrically heated instrument to coagulate a bleeding area by burning the tissue is called _____. Electrodesiccation, in contrast, applies an electrical current directly to a skin lesion to destroy the tissue by _____ it. Another process using electrical sparks to destroy tissue is called _____. In both these terms, the suffix *-ation* means a _____.

incision, drainage

3.70 An infected lesion such as an abscess may undergo the surgical procedure called _____ and _____ (I&D).

laser

laser

3.71 An amplified, intense light beam called a _____ is used to remove various kinds of lesions in an operative procedure called _____ surgery.

layer

3.72 Mohs surgery is a technique for removing a tumor one tissue _____ at a time until a tumor-free layer is reached.

graft

autograft

3.73 A skin _____ is used to replace skin at a burn or injury site by transferring it from another site. If the graft is transferred from elsewhere on the same person, this is called an _____

self	("auto" means _____). A homograft is a graft transferred to one
human	human from another _____ ("homo" = same). This is also called
allograft	an _____. A heterograft, in contrast, is transferred from
species, different	a different _____ ("hetero" means _____).

SELF-INSTRUCTION: THERAPEUTIC TERMS

Study the following:

Therapeutic Term	Meaning
chemotherapy *kēm'ō-ther-ă-pē*	treatment of malignancies, infections, and other diseases with chemical agents that destroy selected cells or impair their ability to reproduce
radiation therapy *rā'dē-ā'shŭn*	treatment of neoplastic disease using ionizing radiation to deter proliferation of malignant cells
sclerotherapy *sklēr-ō-ther'ă-pē*	use of sclerosing agents in treating diseases (e.g., injection of a saline solution into a dilated blood vessel tumor in the skin, resulting in hardening of the tissue within and eventual sloughing away of the lesion)
ultraviolet therapy *ŭl-tră-vī'ō-let*	use of ultraviolet light to promote healing of a skin lesion (e.g., an ulcer)

COMMON THERAPEUTIC DRUG CLASSIFICATIONS

anesthetic *an-es-thet'ik*	a drug that temporarily blocks transmission of nerve conduction to produce a loss of sensations (e.g., pain)
antibiotic *an'tē-bī-ot'ik*	a drug that kills or inhibits the growth of microorganisms
antifungal *an-tē-fŭng'ăl*	a drug that kills or prevents the growth of fungi
antihistamine *an-tē-his'tă-mēn*	a drug that blocks the effects of histamine in the body
histamine *his'tă-men*	a regulating body substance released in excess during allergic reactions causing swelling and inflammation of tissues [e.g., in urticaria (hives) or hay fever]
anti-inflammatory *an'tē-in-flam'ă-tor-ē*	a drug that reduces inflammation
antipruritic *an'tē-prū-rit'ik*	a drug that relieves itching
antiseptic *an-tă-sep'tik*	an agent that inhibits the growth of infectious microorganisms

PROGRAMMED REVIEW: THERAPEUTIC TERMS

Answer Column	Review
	3.74 Several different types of therapy are used to treat tumors and other skin lesions. The use of chemical agents as a treatment is called
chemotherapy, radiation therapy	_____. Ionizing _____ is also used on tumors and is called radiation _____. In another form of therapy, sclerosing agents are injected into a lesion to harden
sclerotherapy	the tissue within; this is called _____. Finally,
light	ultraviolet therapy is the use of ultraviolet _____ to promote healing of a skin lesion such as an ulcer.
anesthetic	**3.75** An _____ agent (using the suffix *-tic,* meaning "pertaining to") produces a loss of sensation so that the person undergoing a procedure does not feel pain.
fungus	**3.76** Tinea is a group of skin diseases caused by a _____. A drug that kills or prevents the growth of such infections is called an
antifungal	_____, using the prefix *anti-,* which means
against (or opposed to)	_____.
antibiotic	**3.77** A different sort of drug kills or inhibits the growth of bacteria. This class of drugs is known as an _____.
antihistamine	**3.78** Histamine is a body substance released in excess in an allergic reaction. A drug that blocks the effects of this substance is called an _____. This drug is used to combat allergic reactions such as hives or hay fever.
antipruritic	**3.79** Many other drug classifications are also named according to what they work against, using the prefix *anti-,* meaning against or opposed to. The term for itching is pruritus, and a drug that relieves itching is called an _____. Sepsis is an infection by microorganisms; a drug that inhibits the growth of such microorgan-

antiseptic

anti-inflammatory

isms is an _____. Similarly, a drug that reduces in-flammation is called an _____ drug.

Practice Exercises

For the following terms, on the lines below the term, write out the indicated word parts: prefixes, combining forms, roots, and suffixes. Then define the word.

For example:
hypodermic

hypo/derm/ic
P   R   S

DEFINITION: below or deficient/skin/pertaining to

1. onychomalacia

   _____ / _____
        CF   S

   DEFINITION: _____

2. mycotic

   _____ / _____
    CF   S

   DEFINITION: _____

3. dermatologist

   _____ / _____
        CF   S

   DEFINITION: _____

4. histotrophic

   _____ / _____ / _____
       CF   R   S

   DEFINITION: _____

5. paronychia

   _____ / _____ / _____
      P   R   S

   DEFINITION: _____

6. hyperkeratosis

   _____ / _____ / _____
      P   R   S

   DEFINITION: _____

7. leukotrichia

_____ / _____ / _____
     CF   R   S

DEFINITION: _____

8. mycology

_____ / _____
    CF   S

DEFINITION: _____

9. epidermal

_____ / _____ / _____
    P   R   S

DEFINITION: _____

10. lipoma

_____ / _____
    R   S

DEFINITION: _____

11. subcutaneous

_____ / _____ / _____
    P   R   S

DEFINITION: _____

12. anhidrosis

_____ / _____ / _____
    P   R   S

DEFINITION: _____

13. histopathology

_____ / _____ / _____
    CF   CF   S

DEFINITION: _____

14. dysplasia

_____ / _____ / _____
    P   R   S

DEFINITION: _____

15. adiposis

_____ / _____
    R   S

DEFINITION: _____

16. squamous

_____ / _____
     R   S

DEFINITION: _____

17. erythrodermatitis

_____ / _____ / _____
    CF   R   S

DEFINITION: _____

18. desquamation

_____ / _____ / _____
    P   R   S

DEFINITION: _____

19. histotoxic

_____ / _____ / _____
    CF   R   S

DEFINITION: _____

20. melanocyte

_____ / _____ / _____
    CF   R   S

DEFINITION: _____

21. xerosis

_____ / _____
     R   S

DEFINITION: _____

22. purpuric

_____ / _____
     R   S

DEFINITION: _____

23. seborrhea

_____ / _____
    CF   S

DEFINITION: _____

24. xanthoma

_____ / _____
     R   S

DEFINITION: _____

25. asteatosis

_____ / _____ / _____
    P   R   S

DEFINITION: _____

Write the correct medical term for each of the following:

26. death of tissue associated with loss of blood supply _____

27. transfer of skin to a new position in the body of the same person _____

28. black and blue mark _____

29. itching _____

30. a cluster of furuncles _____

31. fungal skin disease _____

32. hives _____

33. a graft transfer from one animal species to one of another species _____

34. pubic lice _____

35. a boil _____

36. freckle _____

37. flake of exfoliated epidermis _____

38. head lice _____

39. baldness _____

40. virus that causes cold sores _____

41. study of tissue _____

42. redness of skin _____

43. a blackhead _____

44. mark left by healed wound _____

45. a linear crack in the skin _____

46. surgery that freezes tissue _____

47. excision of tissue for microscopic study _____

48. appearance of a skin lesion _____

49. abnormal scar formation _____

Complete the medical term by writing the missing part:

50. _____ oma = black tumor

51. sebo _____ = discharge of oil

52. _____ coriation = scratch mark on skin

53. _____ derma = white skin

54. _____ section = type of microscopic study of fresh tissue

55. _____ derma = red skin

56. _____ derma = hard skin

57. _____ keratoses = thickened skin tumors seen in old age

58. _____ oma = fat tumor

59. _____ derma = yellow skin

60. _____ osis = presence of fungus

61. _____ dermic = pertaining to below the skin

62. _____ angioma = bright red, round blood vessel tumor

63. _____ derma = dry skin

Give the medical terms for the following viral diseases:

64. German measles _____

65. chickenpox _____

66. 14-day measles _____

Match the following terms with the primary lesions described:

67. vesicle _____   a. tiny, flat discolored spot on the skin, up to 1 cm diameter

68. pustule _____   b. a large, flat discolored area on the skin, larger than 1 cm diameter

69. papule _____   c. raised spot on skin less than 0.5 cm in diameter

70. bulla _____   d. a solid mass greater than 1 cm that extends into the epidermis

71. nodule _____   e. a solid mass greater than 1 cm limited to the skin's surface

72. wheal _____   f. a small blister

73. macule _____   g. area of localized skin edema, such as a hive

74. tumor _____   h. a large blister

75. patch _____   i. a pus-filled sac

76. plaque _____   j. a solid mass larger than 1–2 cm in diameter

Write the full medical term from the following abbreviations:

77. HSV-2 _____

78. Bx _____

79. FS _____

80. I&D _____

Write the plural forms of the following terms:

81. keratosis _____

82. ecchymosis _____

83. bulla _____

84. macula _____

85. nevus _____

Match the following terms with their meanings:

86. scabies _____   a. chemical peel

87. cryosurgery _____   b. crabs

88. telangiectasia _____   c. mites

89. nevus _____   d. freezing treatment

90. cicatrix _____   e. intense light

91. actinic keratoses _____ f. desiccation

92. radiation therapy _____ g. spider angioma

93. petechia _____   h. mole

94. liposis _____   i. scar

95. verruca _____   j. cancer treatment

96. chemosurgery _____   k. wart

97. electrosurgery _____   l. solar keratoses

98. pediculosis _____   m. purpuric lesion

99. laser _____   n. adiposis

For each of the following, circle the correct spelling of the term:

100. cicatrix	scicatrix	cicatrex
101. puritis	purritis	pruritus
102. petechia	patechia	petecchia
103. veruca	verucca	verruca
104. eckamosis	ecchymosis	eckemyosis

105. excission	excisison	excision
106. soriasis	psoreyeasis	psoriasis
107. impetigo	infantiego	impatiego
108. eggszema	eczema	ecczema
109. debridemant	debridement	debreedment

Give the noun that was used to form the following adjectives.

110. _____ keratotic

111. _____ bullous

112. _____ nodular

113. _____ seborrheic

114. _____ petechial

115. _____ ecchymotic

116. _____ urticarial

117. _____ eczematous

118. _____ macular

119. _____ suppurative

Write in the missing words on lines in the following illustration of the skin's anatomy:

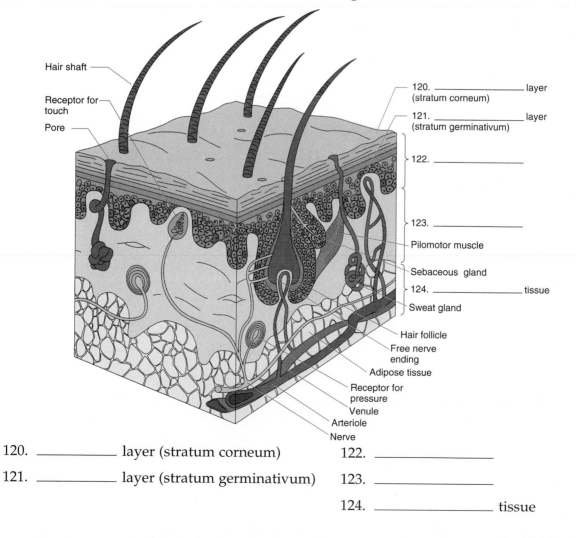

Hair shaft

Receptor for touch

Pore

120. _____ layer (stratum corneum)

121. _____ layer (stratum germinativum)

122. _____

123. _____

Pilomotor muscle

Sebaceous gland

124. _____ tissue

Sweat gland

Hair follicle

Free nerve ending

Adipose tissue

Receptor for pressure

Venule

Arteriole

Nerve

120. _____ layer (stratum corneum)

121. _____ layer (stratum germinativum)

122. _____

123. _____

124. _____ tissue

For each of the following, circle the combining form that corresponds to the meaning given:

125. **fat**	leuk/o	steat/o	seb/o
126. **black**	necr/o	trich/o	melan/o
127. **fungus**	seb/o	myc/o	onych/o
128. **nail**	onych/o	trich/o	squam/o
129. **red**	xanth/o	purpur/o	erythr/o
130. **hair**	trich/o	histi/o	fibr/o
131. **dry**	kerat/o	xer/o	xanth/o
132. **oil**	py/o	hidr/o	seb/o

Medical Record Analyses

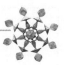

MEDICAL RECORD 3-1

Progress Note

S: This is a 30 y.o. ♀ presents with an erythematous and scaly eruption on the face and ears × 6 mo. Stress and emotional tensions aggravate the rash. Over-the-counter remedies provide no relief.

O: Patchy erythema with greasy, yellowish scaling appears over the nose and along the eyebrows. The external ears are similarly affected. Erythematous papules are scattered across the face, and there is ↑ oiliness around the nose.

A: Seborrheic dermatitis

P: Rx: hydrocortisone cream, s̄s̄ oz tube
     Sig: apply to affected areas t.i.d.

1. What is the sex of the patient?
   a. male
   b. female
   c. not stated

2. What is the patient's CC?
   a. stress and emotional tension
   b. appearance of raised, yellow, pus-filled lesions on the skin
   c. appearance of red areas on the skin with flaking of the outer layers of the skin
   d. appearance of red areas on the skin with open sores
   e. appearance of a communicable rash on the face and ear

3. What is the diagnosis?
   a. inflammation of the sebaceous glands and hair follicles of the skin evidenced by comedones
   b. fungus of the skin
   c. inflammation of the skin with excessive secretion of sebum from the sebaceous glands
   d. highly contagious bacterial skin inflammation marked by pustules that rupture and become crusted
   e. transient, viral cold sores that infect the facial area

4. How much hydrocortisone cream was prescribed?
   a. one ounce
   b. two ounces
   c. one-half dram
   d. one dram
   e. one-half ounce

5. What is the Sig: on the prescription?
   a. apply to affected areas twice a day
   b. apply to affected areas three times a day
   c. apply to affected areas four times a day
   d. apply to affected areas every two hours
   e. apply to affected areas every three hours

MEDICAL RECORD 3-2 FOR ADDITIONAL STUDY

CENTRAL MEDICAL GROUP, INC.
Department of Dermatology

201 Medical Center Drive • Central City, US 90000-1234 • PHONE: (012) 125-8888 • FAX: (012) 125-3434

CHART NOTE

PATIENT: FULLER, ROBERT K.

DATE: October 19, 20xx

SUBJECTIVE: The patient presents with a growth on the right hand, multiple lesions, and other growths.

OBJECTIVE: Ulcerated growth on the right hand, marked A; one verruciform tumor on the left hand; erythematous keratotic patches on the arms.

ASSESSMENT: Basal cell carcinoma, verruca vulgaris, and actinic keratoses.

PLAN: Following full counseling on healing with scarring, keloids, and possible recurrence, the growth from the right hand was excised. The site was anesthetized with Xylocaine 2% without epinephrine, 2 cc. Following excision, the bases of the growths were treated with fulguration and electrodesiccation. Desiccation was also performed on 0.3 cm of normal surrounding skin. The wart was treated with liquid nitrogen, two cycles. Freezing time: 8-10 seconds. Ten erythematous keratotic patches were also treated with liquid nitrogen, two cycles. Freezing time: 10-14 seconds.

D. Luong, M.D.

DL:ti

D: 10/19/20xx
T: 10/20/20xx

MEDICAL RECORD 3-2 FOR ADDITIONAL STUDY

After ignoring various skin problems for months, Robert Fuller consulted his doctor in October when he became alarmed by what he saw happening on his right hand. His doctor referred him to Dr. Luong, a dermatologist, who then diagnosed and treated Mr. Fuller.

Read Medical Record 3.1 for Robert Fuller (page 128) and answer the following questions. This record is a SOAP progress note dictated by Dr. Luong immediately after the treatment of Mr. Fuller and transcribed the next day by his assistant.

1. Below are medical terms used in this record that you have not yet encountered in this text. Underline each where it appears in the record and define below.

   vulgaris _____

   verruciform _____

2. In your own words, not using medical terminology, briefly describe Mr. Fuller's complaint.

   _____

   _____

   _____

3. In your own words, not using medical terminology, briefly describe Dr. Luong's three objective findings:

   _____

   _____

   _____

4. Define the three diagnoses for those three objective findings:

   a. _____

   b. _____

   c. _____

5. Briefly describe the treatments for those three diagnoses:

   a. _____

   b. _____

   c. _____

6. What did Dr. Luong tell Mr. Fuller might occur in the future? Check all that apply:

   _____ scarring where the lesions were

   _____ nausea and possible vomiting from the nitrogen

   _____ red freckle-like spots appearing on right hand

   _____ possible regrowth of lesions

   _____ self-desiccating tissue destruction

Answers to Practice Exercises

1. onycho/malacia
   CF   S
   nail/softening
2. myco/tic
   CF   S
   fungus/pertaining to
3. dermato/logist
   CF   S
   skin/one who specializes in the study or treatment of
4. histo/troph/ic
   CF   R   S
   tissue/nourishment or development/pertaining to
5. par/onych/ia
   P   R   S
   alongside of/nail/condition of
6. hyper/kerat/osis
   P   R   S
   above or excessive/hard/condition or increase
7. leuko/trich/ia
   CF   R   S
   white/hair/condition of
8. myco/logy
   CF   S
   fungus/study of
9. epi/derm/al
   P   R   S
   upon/skin/pertaining to
10. lip/oma
    R   S
    fat/tumor
11. sub/cutane/ous
    P   R   S
    below or under/skin/pertaining to
12. an/hidr/osis
    P   R   S
    without/sweat/condition or increase
13. histo/patho/logy
    CF   CF   S
    tissue/disease/study of
14. dys/plas/ia
    P   R   S
    painful, difficult or faulty/formation/condition of
15. adip/osis
    R   S
    fat/condition or increase
16. squam/ous
    R   S
    scale/pertaining to

17. erythro/dermat/itis
    CF   R   S
    red/skin/inflammation
18. de/squam/ation
    P   R   S
    from, down, or not/scale/process
19. histo/tox/ic
    CF   R   S
    tissue/poison/pertaining to
20. melano/cyt/e
    CF   R   S
    black/cell/noun marker
21. xer/osis
    R   S
    dry/condition or increase
22. purpur/ic
    R   S
    purple/pertaining to
23. sebo/rrhea
    CF   S
    sebum (oil)/discharge
24. xanth/oma
    R   S
    yellow/tumor
25. a/steat/osis
    P   R   S
    without/fat/condition or increase
26. gangrene
27. autograft
28. ecchymosis
29. pruritus
30. carbuncle
31. tinea
32. urticaria
33. heterograft
34. pediculosis pubis
35. furuncle
36. macule or macula
37. scale
38. pediculosis capitis
39. alopecia
40. herpes simplex virus type 1
41. histology
42. erythema
43. comedo
44. cicatrix
45. fissure
46. cryosurgery
47. biopsy
48. eruption
49. keloid
50. melanoma
51. seborrhea
52. excoriation
53. leukoderma
54. frozen section

55. erythroderma
56. keratoderma
57. seborrheic keratoses
58. lipoma or steatoma
59. xanthoderma
60. mycosis
61. hypodermic
62. cherry angioma
63. xeroderma
64. rubella
65. varicella
66. rubeola
67. f
68. i
69. c
70. h
71. d
72. g
73. a
74. j
75. b
76. e
77. herpes simplex virus type 2
78. biopsy
79. frozen section
80. incision and drainage
81. keratoses
82. ecchymoses
83. bullae
84. maculae
85. nevi
86. c
87. d
88. g
89. h
90. i
91. l
92. j
93. m
94. n
95. k
96. a
97. f
98. b
99. e
100. cicatrix
101. pruritus
102. petechia
103. verruca
104. ecchymosis
105. excision
106. psoriasis
107. impetigo
108. eczema
109. debridement
110. keratosis
111. bulla

112. nodule
113. seborrhea
114. petechia
115. ecchymosis
116. urticaria
117. eczema
118. macule or macula
119. suppuration
120. squamous layer (stratum corneum)
121. basal layer (stratum germinativum)

122. epidermis
123. dermis
124. subcutaneous tissue
125. **fat** ——————— steat/o
126. **black** ——————— melan/o
127. **fungus** ——————— myc/o
128. **nail** ——————— onych/o
129. **red** ——————— erythr/o
130. **hair** ——————— trich/o
131. **dry** ——————— xer/o
132. **oil** ——————— seb/o

Answers to Medical Record Analyses

1. b
2. c
3. c
4. e
5. b

CHAPTER 4

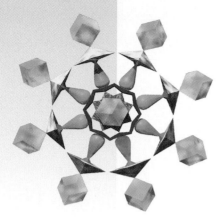

Musculoskeletal System

Musculoskeletal System Overview

Functions of the skeleton (Fig. 4-1):

❉ Provides support and shape to the body

❉ Stores calcium and other minerals

❉ Produces certain blood cells within bone marrow

Functions of the muscles (Fig. 4-2):

❉ Create forces for body movements

❉ Provide a protective covering for internal organs

❉ Produce body heat

Orthopedics is the specialty field most involved with the study and treatment of the musculoskeletal system. "Orthopaedic" is the British spelling of the term, which was accepted for the name of the American Board of Orthopaedic Surgery.

SELF-INSTRUCTION: COMBINING FORMS

Study the following:

Combining Form	Meaning
ankyl/o	crooked or stiff
arthr/o articul/o	joint
brachi/o	arm
cervic/o	neck

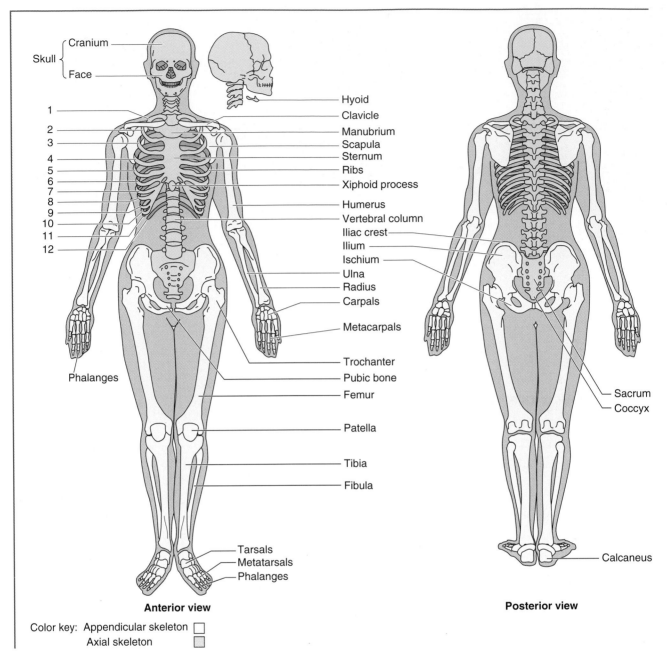

■ FIGURE 4-1. The skeleton.

chondr/o	cartilage (gristle)
cost/o	rib
crani/o	skull
dactyl/o	digit (finger or toe)
fasci/o	fascia (a band)
femor/o	femur
fibr/o	fiber

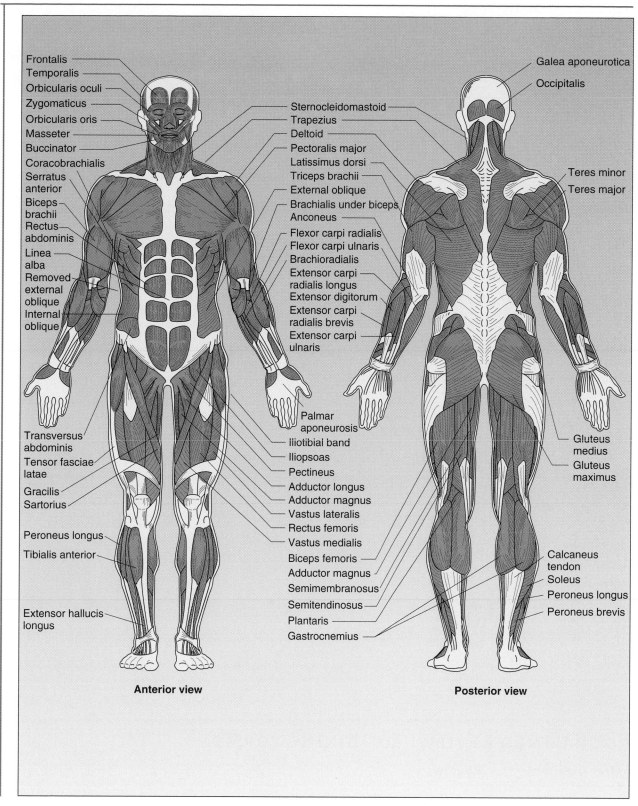

Frontalis
Temporalis
Orbicularis oculi
Zygomaticus
Orbicularis oris
Masseter
Buccinator
Coracobrachialis
Serratus anterior
Biceps brachii
Rectus abdominis
Linea alba
Removed external oblique
Internal oblique

Transversus abdominis
Tensor fasciae latae
Gracilis
Sartorius

Peroneus longus
Tibialis anterior

Extensor hallucis longus

Sternocleidomastoid
Trapezius
Deltoid
Pectoralis major
Latissimus dorsi
Triceps brachii
External oblique
Brachialis under biceps
Anconeus
Flexor carpi radialis
Flexor carpi ulnaris
Brachioradialis
Extensor carpi radialis longus
Extensor digitorum
Extensor carpi radialis brevis
Extensor carpi ulnaris

Palmar aponeurosis
Iliotibial band
Iliopsoas
Pectineus
Adductor longus
Adductor magnus
Vastus lateralis
Rectus femoris
Vastus medialis
Biceps femoris
Adductor magnus
Semimembranosus
Semitendinosus
Plantaris
Gastrocnemius

Galea aponeurotica
Occipitalis

Teres minor
Teres major

Gluteus medius
Gluteus maximus

Calcaneus tendon
Soleus
Peroneus longus
Peroneus brevis

Anterior view

Posterior view

■ **FIGURE 4-2.** Skeletal muscles.

kyph/o	humped-back
lei/o	smooth
lord/o	bent
lumb/o	loin (lower back)
myel/o	bone marrow or spinal cord
my/o **myos/o** **muscul/o**	muscle
oste/o	bone
patell/o	knee cap
pelv/i **pel/o**	hip bone or pelvic cavity
radi/o	radius
rhabd/o	rod shaped or striated (skeletal)
sarc/o	flesh
scoli/o	twisted
spondyl/o **vertebr/o**	vertebra
stern/o	sternum (breastbone)
ten/o **tend/o** **tendin/o**	tendon (to stretch)
thorac/o	chest
ton/o	tone or tension
uln/o	ulna

PROGRAMMED REVIEW: COMBINING FORMS

Answer Column	Review
straight, normal, or correct	**4.1** *Orth/o*, meaning _____, and ped/o, meaning
foot	_____, were combined to form the term orthopedic, pertaining to
	the medical specialty related to the musculoskeletal system. The British
orthopaedic	spelling of this specialty is _____.

oste/o	**4.2** The combining form meaning bone is _____. Since the suffix _____ means inflammation, osteitis therefore refers to inflammation of bone. Inside most bones is bone marrow; the combining form meaning bone marrow is _____, as in the adjective term myeloid.
-itis	
myel/o	

4.3 The three combining forms for muscle are *muscul/o, my/o,* and _____. The musculoskeletal system involves both muscles and bones. Recalling that the suffix *-algia* means pain, myalgia must mean _____ pain. Myositis is an _____ of muscle.

myos/o

muscle, inflammation

4.4 The cranial bones comprise the _____. The combining form that means skull is _____. Neck bones are referred to as the _____ vertebrae, from the combining form *cervic/o,* meaning _____.

skull

crani/o

cervical

neck

4.5 The two combining forms for vertebrae, the bones of the spine, are *vertebr/o* and _____. Spondylitis is inflammation of the _____. *Scoli/o* means _____, and, when combined with the suffix *-osis,* which means _____, forms the word scoliosis, which refers to a condition of having a twisted spine. The combining form meaning bent is _____, and a spine that is bent forward is called lordosis. The condition of a humped back is called kyphosis, from the combining form _____, meaning humped-back. The lower back is the lumbar spine, from the combining form _____. Lumbodynia refers to _____ in the _____ back.

spondyl/o

vertebrae, twisted

condition or increase

lord/o

kyph/o

lumb/o, pain

lower

4.6 The breastbone is the _____, from the combining form *stern/o.* Most of the ribs connect to the breastbone in the front of the body. The combining form *cost/o* means rib. The sternocostal area, therefore, is where the _____ is connected to the _____.

sternum

sternum (or breastbone), ribs

chest thorac/o -ic	**4.7** Thoracic is the adjective referring to the _____, formed from the combining form _____, which means chest, and the adjective-forming suffix _____.
pelvis pelvis, measurement	**4.8** Below the ribs and spine are the bones of the _____, from the combining form *pelv/i*. A pelviscope is used to examine the interior of the _____. Pelvimetry is the _____ of the diameters of the pelvis.
femor/o patell/o	**4.9** Below the pelvis is the longest bone in the body, the femur. The combining form for this term is _____. The femur joins the tibia at the knee joint, where a small bone called the kneecap covers the joint. The medical term for the kneecap is patella, from the combining form _____.
ulna radi/o radius	**4.10** The two bones of the forearm are the radius and the _____, from the combining forms _____ and *uln/o*. Radioulnar is an adjective referring to both the _____ and the ulna.
digit pain	**4.11** The combining form *dactyl/o* refers to _____ (either a finger or toe). Dactylalgia therefore means _____ of the fingers or toes.
brachi/o arm	**4.12** The combining form for arm is _____. The brachial artery, for example, runs through the _____.
articul/o arthr/o inflammation	**4.13** A joint is where two or more bones join together. This is also called an articulation, from the combining form _____. Another combining term for joint is _____, used to form the term arthritis, which means _____ of a joint.
stiff	**4.14** *Ankly/o* is a combining form meaning crooked or _____. Ankylosis therefore is a stiffened joint.

4.15 Cartilage is a gristlelike substance that covers bones where they articulate at joints. Chondroma is a tumor that arises from cartilage, the combining form for which is _____.

chondr/o

4.16 Muscle fibers have the ability to contract, allowing them to move bones and thus body parts. The combining form for fiber is _____, and a common adjective form is fibrous. Muscles are composed of either smooth (*lei/o*) or striated (*rhabd/o*) muscle tissues. A leiomyoma is a tumor of _____ muscle. A rhabdomyoma is a _____ of _____ (skeletal) muscle.

fibr/o

smooth

tumor, striated

4.17 The combining form for tone is _____. Therefore, myotonia refers to a condition of _____ _____.

ton/o

muscle tone

4.18 A tendon connects a muscle to a bone. Three combining forms for tendon are *ten/o*, _____, and *tendin/o*. Tendinitis is _____ of a tendon.

tend/o

inflammation

4.19 Fascia is a band or sheet of fibrous tissue that encloses muscles or groups of muscles. It comes from the combining form _____.

fasci/o

4.20 *Sarc/o* means _____ or a muscular substance. A sarcoma, for example, is a fleshy _____.

flesh

tumor

SELF-INSTRUCTION: ANATOMICAL TERMS RELATED TO BONES

Study the following:

Term	Meaning
appendicular skeleton *ap'en-dik'yū-lăr*	bones of shoulder, pelvis, and upper and lower extremities
axial skeleton *ak'sē-ăl*	bones of skull, vertebral column (Fig. 4-3), chest, and hyoid bone (U-shaped bone at the base of the tongue)
bone	specialized connective tissue composed of osteocytes (bone cells) forming the skeleton

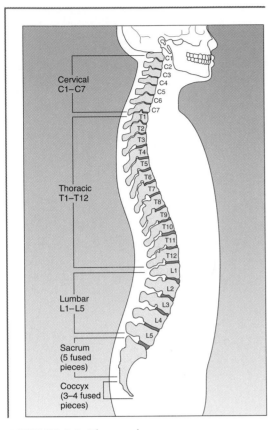

◼ **FIGURE 4-3.** The vertebrae.

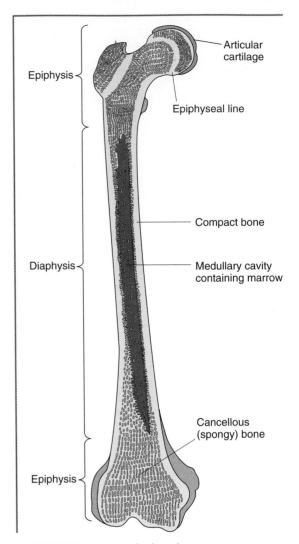

◼ **FIGURE 4-4.** Parts of a long bone.

TYPES OF BONE TISSUE

compact bone	tightly solid, strong bone tissue resistant to bending
spongy (cancellous) bone *spŭn'jē kan'sĕ-lŭs*	mesh-like bone tissue containing marrow and fine branching canals through which blood vessels run

CLASSIFICATION OF BONES

long bones	bones of arms and legs
short bones	bones of wrist and ankles
flat bones	bones of ribs, shoulder blades, pelvis, and skull
irregular bones	bones of vertebrae and face
sesamoid bones *ses'ă-moyd*	round bones found near joints (e.g., patella)

PARTS OF A LONG BONE (FIG. 4-4)

epiphysis _e-pif′i-sis_	wide ends of a long bone (physis = growth)
diaphysis _dī-af′i-sis_	shaft of a long bone
metaphysis _m_e-taf′i-sis_	growth zone between epiphysis and diaphysis during development of a long bone
endosteum _en-dos′tē-ŭm_	membrane lining the medullary cavity of a bone
medullary cavity _med′ŭ-lār-ē_	cavity within the shaft of the long bones filled with bone marrow
bone marrow _mar′ō_	soft connective tissue within the medullary cavity of bones
red bone marrow	functions to form red blood cells, some white blood cells, and platelets; found in cavities of most bones in infants and in the flat bones in adults
yellow bone marrow	gradually replaces red bone marrow in adult bones; functions as storage for fat tissue; and is inactive in formation of blood cells
periosteum _per-ē-os′tē-ŭm_	a fibrous, vascular membrane that covers the bone
articular cartilage _ar-tik′yu-l-ar kar′ti-lij_	a gristlelike substance on bones where they articulate

PROGRAMMED REVIEW: ANATOMICAL TERMS RELATED TO BONES

Answer Column	Review
axial, appendicular skull	**4.21** The skeleton as a whole is divided into the appendicular skeleton and the _____ skeleton. The _____ skeleton includes the shoulders and arms and the pelvis and legs. The axial skeleton includes the spine, chest, and _____.
osteo compact Cancellous	**4.22** Bone cells, or _____cytes, form the skeleton. Tightly solid bone that resists bending is called _____ bone. _____ bone is spongy and contains marrow and canals through which blood vessels run.
arms, legs Short	**4.23** Long bones are found in the _____ and _____. _____ bones are found in the wrists and ankles. The ribs, shoul-

flat round	der blades, and pelvis are _____ bones. Bones of the vertebrae and face are called irregular bones. Sesamoid bones are _____ bones (e.g., the patella) near joints.
end, dia- -physis	**4.24** Long bones have several parts. Several of these parts are named with terms from the root *physis* (growth), referring to how the bones grow. The epiphysis is the wide _____ of a long bone. The _____physis is the shaft. The meta_____ is the growth zone between epiphysis and diaphysis.
within bone marrow, Red marrow, fat periosteum around	**4.25** The prefix *endo-* means _____. The endosteum is a membrane lining the medullary cavity within a _____. Inside the medullary cavity is bone _____. _____ bone marrow makes red blood cells, whereas yellow bone _____ stores _____ tissue. The membrane that covers a bone is called the _____, composed of the combining term for bone (*oste/o*) and the prefix *peri-*, meaning _____.
articular	**4.26** The kind of cartilage on bones where they articulate is called _____ cartilage.

SELF-INSTRUCTION: ANATOMICAL TERMS RELATED TO JOINTS AND MUSCLES

Study the following:

Term	Meaning
articulation (Fig. 4-5) *ar'tik-yū-lā'shŭn*	a joint; the point where two bones come together
bursa *ber'să*	a fibrous sac between certain tendons and bones, lined with a synovial membrane that secretes synovial fluid
disk (disc) (Fig. 4-6)	a flat, platelike structure composed of fibrocartilaginous tissue found between the vertebrae to reduce friction
nucleus pulposus *nu'klē-ŭs pōl-pō'sŭs*	soft, fibrocartilaginous, central portion of intervertebral disc

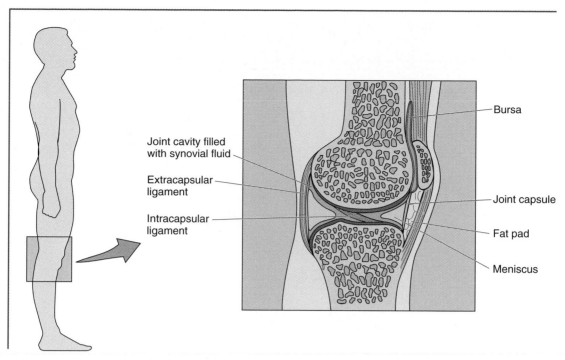

■ **FIGURE 4-5.** Lateral view of knee joint.

ligament *lig′ă-ment*	a flexible band of fibrous tissue that connects bone to bone
synovial membrane *si-nō′vē-ăl mem′brān*	Membrane lining the capsule of a joint
synovial fluid *si-nō′vē-ăl flū′id*	joint-lubricating fluid secreted by the synovial membrane
muscle *mŭs′ĕl*	tissue composed of fibers that can contract, causing movement of an organ or part of the body

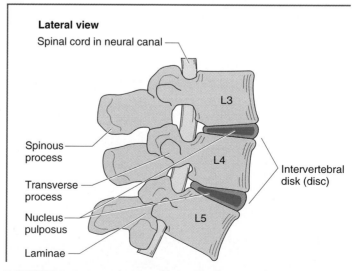

■ **FIGURE 4-6.** Lateral view of lower lumbar vertebrae.

striated (skeletal) muscle *stri′ā-ted (skel′e-tăl)*	voluntary muscle attached to the skeleton
smooth muscle	Involuntary muscle found in internal organs
cardiac muscle	muscle of the heart
origin of a muscle	muscle end attached to the bone that does not move when the muscle contracts
insertion of a muscle	muscle end attached to the bone that moves when the muscle contracts
tendon *ten′dŏn*	a band of fibrous tissue that connects muscle to bone
fascia *fash′ē-ă*	a band or sheet of fibrous connective tissue that covers, supports, and separates muscle

PROGRAMMED REVIEW: ANATOMICAL TERMS RELATED TO JOINTS AND MUSCLES

Answer Column	Review
Muscle Smooth muscle heart striated	**4.27** _____ tissue can contract, causing movement of an organ or body part. There are three types of muscle tissue. _____ muscle is found in internal organs and is also called involuntary muscle because you cannot will it to contract. Cardiac _____ is an involuntary muscle found only in the _____. Skeletal muscle, or _____ muscle, is under voluntary control.
origin insertion tendons fascia	**4.28** Skeletal muscle is attached to bone at both ends of the muscle. The end attached to the bone that does not move when the muscle contracts is called the _____ of the muscle. The other end, attached to the bone that moves with contraction, is called the _____ of the muscle. Muscles are connected to bones by _____. The band or sheet of fibrous tissue that covers muscles is _____.
articulations	**4.29** Muscles come together in joints, also called _____. A fibrous band that connects bone to

ligament	bone is a _____. The joint capsule is lined with a _____ membrane, which secretes a lubricating fluid called synovial _____.
synovial	
fluid	
bursa	**4.30** The fibrous sac between certain tendons and bones is a _____; an inflammation of this tissue is called bursitis. The suffix *-itis* means _____.
inflammation	
disks, discs	**4.31** The flat, platelike structures between the vertebrae are called _____, sometimes also spelled _____.
pulposus	**4.32** The nucleus _____ is a soft fibrocartilaginous tissue in the center of intervertebral discs.

SELF-INSTRUCTION: ANATOMICAL POSITION AND TERMS OF REFERENCE

Study the following:

Term	Meaning
anatomical position	the position of the body to which health professionals refer when noting body planes, positions, or directions: the person is assumed to be standing upright (erect), facing forward, feet pointed forward and slightly apart, with arms at the sides and palms facing forward; the patient is visualized in this pose before applying any other term of reference
body planes (Fig. 4-7)	reference planes for indicating the location or direction of body parts

BODY PLANES

coronal or frontal plane *kōr'ŏ-năl frŭn'tăl*	vertical division of the body into front (anterior) and back (posterior) portions
sagittal plane *saj'i-tăl*	vertical division of the body into right and left portions
transverse plane *trans-vers'*	horizontal division of the body into upper and lower portions

DIRECTIONAL TERMS

anterior (A) (ventral) *an-tēr'ē-ōr ven'trăl*	front of the body

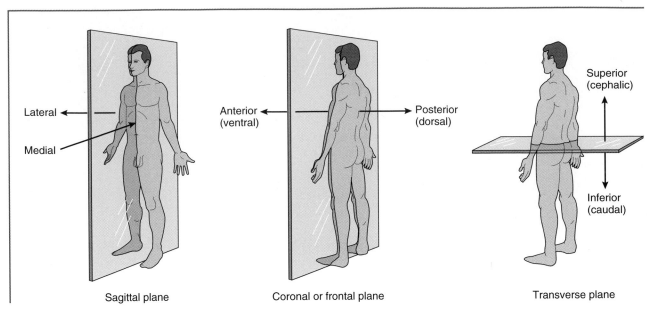

■ **FIGURE 4-7.** Anatomical position with body planes.

posterior (P) (dorsal) *pos-tēr′ē-ōr dor′săl*	back of the body
anterior-posterior (AP)	from front to back; such as in the direction of an x-ray beam
posterior-anterior (PA)	from back to front; such as in the direction of an x-ray beam
superior (cephalic) *su-pēr′ē-ōr se-fal′ik*	situated above another structure, toward the head
inferior (caudal) *in-fē′rē-ōr kaw′dăl*	situated below another structure, away from the head
proximal *prok′si-măl*	toward the beginning or origin of a structure; e.g., the proximal aspect of the femur (thigh bone) is the area closest to where it attaches to the hip.
distal *dis′tăl*	away from the beginning or origin of a structure; e.g., the distal aspect of the femur (thigh bone) is the area at the end of the bone near the knee.
medial *mē′dē-ăl*	toward the middle (midline)
lateral *lat′er-ăl*	toward the side
axis *ak′sis*	line that runs through the center of the body or body part

BODY POSITIONS

erect *ĕ-rĕkt′*	normal standing position
decubitus *dē-kyū′bi-tŭs*	lying down, especially in a bed; i.e., lateral decubitus is lying on the side (decumbo = to lie down).

prone *prōn*	lying face down and flat
recumbent *rē-kŭm′bent*	lying down
supine *sū-pīn′*	horizontal recumbent; lying flat on the back ("on the spine")

BODY MOVEMENTS (FIG. 4-8)

flexion *flek′shŭn*	bending at the joint so that the angle between the bones is decreased
extension *eks-ten′shŭn*	straightening at the joint so that the angle between the bones is increased

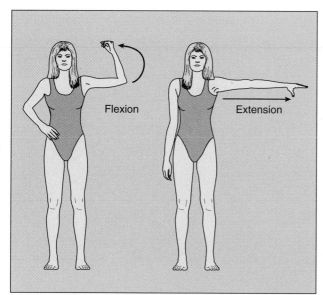
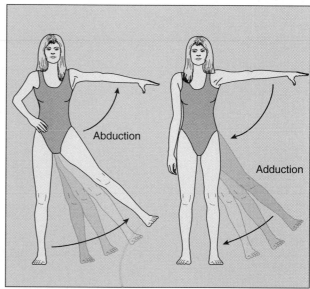
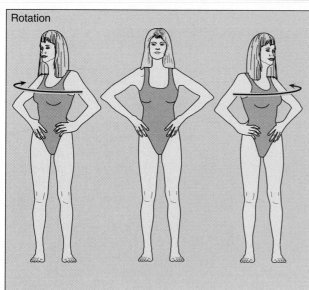
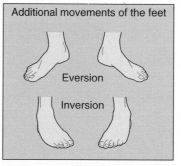
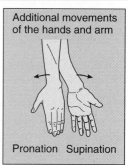
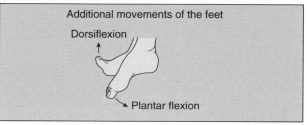

■ **FIGURE 4-8.** Body movements.

abduction *ab-dŭk′shŭn*	movement away from the body
adduction *ă-duk′shŭn*	movement toward the body
rotation *rō-tā′shŭn*	circular movement around an axis
eversion *ē-ver′zhŭn*	turning outward, i.e., a foot
inversion *in-ver′zhŭn*	turning inward, i.e., a foot
supination *sū′pi-nā′shŭn*	turning upward or forward of the palmar surface (palm of the hand) or plantar surface (sole of the foot)
pronation *prō-nā′shŭn*	turning downward or backward of the palmar surface (palm of the hand) or plantar surface (sole of the foot)
dorsiflexion *dōr-si-flek′shŭn*	bending of the foot or the toes upward
plantar flexion *plan′tăr*	bending of the sole of the foot by curling the toes toward the ground
range of motion **(ROM)**	total motion possible in a joint, described by the terms related to body movements, i.e., ability to flex, extend, abduct, or adduct; measured in degrees
goniometer (Fig. 4-9) *gō-nē-om′ĕ-ter*	instrument used to measure joint angles (gonio = angle)

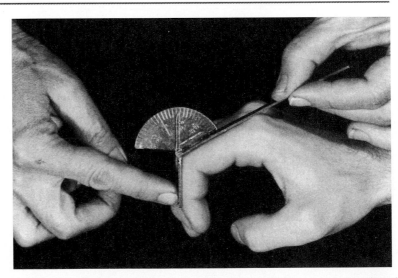

■ **FIGURE 4-9.** Dorsal placement of goniometer used when measuring digital motion.

PROGRAMMED REVIEW: ANATOMICAL POSITION AND TERMS OF REFERENCE

Answer Column	Review

4.33 Health professions describe body part locations relative to the

anatomical

anat position, in which one is standing upright, or

erect, forward

erct , facing _forward_ , feet pointed forward and slightly

sides, forward

apart, with the arms at the _side_ and palms facing _forward_ .

---

planes

4.34 Body _planes_ help one understand directional and position terms. The body is vertically divided into front (anterior) and back

coronal

(posterior) portions by the _coronal_ , or frontal, plane. The

sagittal

Sagittal plane divides the body vertically into right and left

portions. The transverse plane divides the body

horizontally

horizontally into upper and lower portions.

---

before

4.35 Remember that the prefix *ante-* means _____, and the pre-

after

fix *post-* means _____. Using these word parts, the front of the

anterior

body is _anterior_ (also called ventral), and the back of the

posterior

body is _posterior_ (also called dorsal).

4.36 The direction of an x-ray beam from front to back is designated

anterior-posterior

_____-_____, whereas the direction from

posterior-anterior

back to front is _____-_____.

---

superior

4.37 The head is _Superior_ to (above) the shoulders, whereas

inferior

the feet are _inferior_ to (below) the knees.

---

closest

4.38 The proximal aspect of a structure is the area _____

distal

to its origin or attachment. The _____ aspect of a structure is the

proximal

area away from its origin or attachment. The _____ aspect
of the femur (thighbone) is the area closest to where it attaches to the

end

hip. The distal aspect of the femur (thighbone) is the area at the _____
of the bone near the knee.

medial

side

4.39 Toward the middle or midline is called _____, whereas lateral means toward the _____.

axis

4.40 An imaginary line that runs through the center of the body or a body part is called an _____. For example, you can rotate your wrist on its axis.

erect

recumbent

decubitus

lateral

face, supine

4.41 The normal standing position is _____ (as in the anatomical position). Several terms describe different ways the body lies down. The general term for lying down is _reumbent_____. Lying down, especially in bed, is called ____decubitus_____. A patient lying on one side in bed is in a __lateral___ decubitus position. Prone means lying _face_-down flat, and _supine____ means lying face-up flat on the back.

decreases

extension, away

away from

adduction, toward

4.42 Many different terms are used to describe body movements at joints. Flexing a joint (flexion) _____ the angle between the bones; the opposite movement (increasing the angle) is _____. Movement _away_ from the body is called abduction (the prefix *ab*- means _away_ _from_); the opposite movement is __adduction____ (the prefix *ad*- means _toward__).

rotation

eversion

4.43 A circular movement around an axis is called _____. For example, you can rotate your feet inward and outward. The term for inward rotation is inversion; the term for outward rotation begins with the prefix e- (out or away): _____.

supination, pronation

4.44 Turning the palm of the hand upward or forward is called _____; the opposite movement is _____. Note the relationship of these terms to the terms for the body lying supine or prone.

dorsiflexion

plantar flexion

4.45 The foot and toes bend upward in _____ and downward in _____ _____.

range	**4.46** The total amount of motion in a joint is called its _____ of motion. In certain musculoskeletal conditions the range of motion may decrease. The instrument used to measure a joint angle is a
goniometer	_____ .

SELF-INSTRUCTION: SYMPTOMATIC TERMS

Study the following:

Term	Meaning
arthralgia *ar-thral′jē-ă*	joint pain
atrophy *at′rō-fē*	shrinking of muscle size
crepitation *krep-i-tā′shŭn* **crepitus** *krep-i-tŭs*	grating sound sometimes made by movement of a joint or broken bones
exostosis *eks-os-tō′sis*	a projection arising from a bone that develops from cartilage
flaccid *flas′id*	flabby, relaxed, or having defective or absent muscle tone
hypertrophy *hī-per′trō-fē*	increase in the size of a muscle
hypotonia *hī′pō-tō′ne-ă*	reduced muscle tension
myalgia *mī-al′jē-ă* **myodynia** *mī′ō-din′ē-ă*	muscle pain
ostealgia *os-tē-al′jē-ă* **osteodynia** *os-tē-o-din′ē-ă*	bone pain
rigor or rigidity *rig′er ri-jid′i-tē*	stiffness; stiff muscle
spasm *spazm*	drawing in; involuntary contraction of muscle
spastic *spas′tik*	uncontrolled contractions of skeletal muscles causing stiff and awkward movements (resembles spasm)

tetany *tet'ă-nē*	tension; prolonged, continuous muscle contraction
tremor *trem'er*	shaking; rhythmic muscular movement

PROGRAMMED REVIEW: SYMPTOMATIC TERMS

Answer Column	Review
crepitation	**4.47** Broken bones rubbing together may produce a grating sound called crepitus or _____. This sound may also occur in a joint.
outside exostosis	**4.48** The prefix exo- means _____. A term for a cartilage projection growing outside a bone is _____.
-algia osteodynia, ostealgia myodynia myalgia arthralgia	**4.49** Two suffixes for pain are –dynia and _____. Using the combining form for bone, two terms for bone pain are _____ and _____. Two similarly formed terms for muscle pain are _____ and _____. Using the combining form arthr/o, the term for joint pain is _____.
above or excessive increased atrophy	**4.50** The prefix hyper- means _____. Hypertrophy refers to _____ muscle size. Shrinking muscle size is called _____.
deficient hypotonia flaccid	**4.51** The prefix hypo- means below or _____. A condition of reduced muscle tension or tone is called _____. In such a case, the muscle can be said to be flabby or _____.
rhythmic	**4.52** Tremor, from the Latin word for shaking, is a _____ muscular movement. This may result from certain neurologic conditions.

rigor	**4.53** A stiff muscle is called _____ or rigidity.
spasm tetany condition	**4.54** An involuntary contraction of a muscle is a _____. A prolonged, continuous muscle contraction is a condition called _____. Recall that the suffix –y means a _____ or process.

SELF-INSTRUCTION: DIAGNOSTIC TERMS

Study the following:

Term	Meaning
ankylosis *ang'ki-lō'sis*	stiff joint condition
arthritis *ar-thrī'tis*	inflammation of the joints characterized by pain, swelling, redness, warmth, and limitation of motion; there are more than 100 different types of arthritis
osteoarthritis (Fig. 4-10) *os'tē-ō-ar-thrī'tis*	most common form of arthritis, especially affecting weight-bearing joints (e.g., knee or hip) characterized by the erosion of articular cartilage

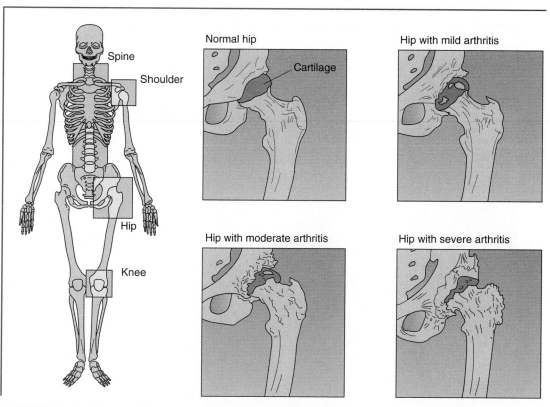

■ **FIGURE 4-10.** Osteoarthritis. **A.** Common sites of osteoarthritis. **B.** How osteoarthritis affects the hip.

degenerative arthritis
dē-jen'er-ă-tiv ar-thrī'tis

degenerative joint disease (DJD)
dē-jen'er-ă-tiv joynt di- zēz'

rheumatoid arthritis (Fig. 4-11)
rū'mă-toyd ar-thrī'tis

most crippling form of arthritis, characterized by chronic, systemic inflammation most often affecting joints and synovial membranes (especially in the hands and feet), causing ankylosis and deformity

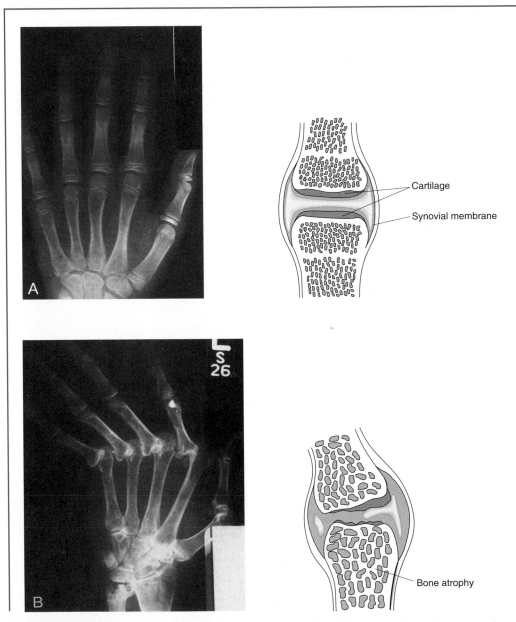

Cartilage

Synovial membrane

Bone atrophy

■ **FIGURE 4-11.** Joints of the hand affected by rheumatoid arthritis. **A.** Radiograph of normal hand. **B.** Radiograph of hand with rheumatoid arthritis.

gouty arthritis *gow'tē ar-thrī'tis*	acute attacks of arthritis usually in a single joint (especially the great toe) caused by hyperuricemia (an excessive level of uric acid in the blood)
bony necrosis *nĕ-krō'sis* **sequestrum** *sē-kwes'trŭm*	bone tissue that has died from loss of blood supply (e.g., after a fracture)
bunion *bŭn'yŭn*	swelling of the joint at the base of the great toe caused by inflammation of the bursa
bursitis *ber-sī'tis*	inflammation of a bursa
chondromalacia *kon'drō-mă-lā'shē-ă*	softening of cartilage
epiphysitis *e-pif-i-sī'tis*	inflammation of epiphyseal regions of the long bone
fracture (Fx) (Fig. 4-12) *frak'chūr*	broken or cracked bone
closed fracture	broken bone with no open wound
open fracture	compound fracture; broken bone with an open wound
simple fracture	a nondisplaced fracture with one fracture line that does not require extensive treatment to repair (e.g., hairline Fx, stress Fx, or a crack)
complex fracture	a displaced fracture that requires manipulation or surgery to repair
fracture line	the line of the break in a broken bone (e.g., oblique, spiral, or transverse)
comminuted fracture *kom'i-nū-ted*	broken in many little pieces
greenstick fracture	bending and incomplete break of a bone—most often seen in children
herniated disk or disc *her'nē-ā-ted*	protrusion of a degenerated or fragmented intervertebral disk so that the nucleus pulposus protrudes, causing compression on the nerve root
myeloma *mī-ă-lō'mă*	bone marrow tumor
myositis *mī-ō-sī'tis*	inflammation of muscle
myoma *mī-ŏ'mă*	muscle tumor
leiomyoma *lī'ō-mī-ŏ'mă*	smooth muscle tumor
leiomyosarcoma *lī'ō-mī-o-sar-kō'mă*	malignant smooth muscle tumor

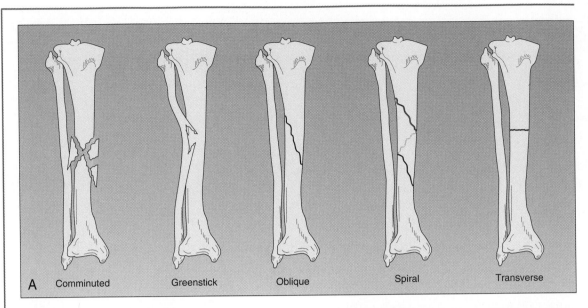

A Comminuted   Greenstick   Oblique   Spiral   Transverse

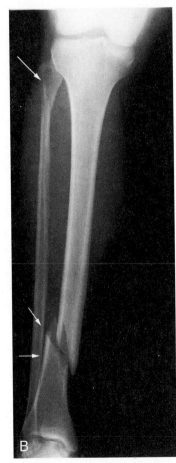

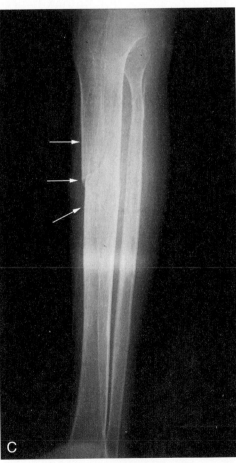

◼ **FIGURE 4-12. A.** Types of common fractures. **B.** Anterior-posterior radiography of lower leg demonstrating open fractures of tibia and fibula *(arrows)*. **C.** Lateral view radiograph demonstrating a closed spiral fracture of tibia *(arrows)*.

rhabdomyoma *rab'dō-mī-o'mă*	skeletal muscle tumor
rhabdomyosarcoma *rab'dō-mī-sar-kō'mă*	malignant skeletal muscle tumor
muscular dystrophy *mŭs'kyū-lăr dis'trō-fē*	a category of genetically transmitted diseases characterized by progressive atrophy of skeletal muscles (Duchenne's type is most common)
osteoma *os-tē-ō'mă*	bone tumor
osteosarcoma *os-tē-ō-sar-kō'mă*	type of malignant bone tumor
osteomalacia *os'tē-ō-mă-lā'shē-ă*	disease marked by softening of the bone caused by calcium and vitamin D deficiency
rickets *rik'ets*	osteomalacia in children (causes bone deformity)
osteomyelitis *os'tē-ō-mī-ĕ-lī'tis*	infection of bone and bone marrow causing inflammation
osteoporosis *os'tē-ō-pō-rō'sis*	condition of decreased bone density and increased porosity, causing bones to become brittle and to more easily fracture (porosis = passage)
spinal curvatures (Fig. 4-13) *spī'năl*	
kyphosis *kī-fō'sis*	abnormal posterior curvature of the thoracic spine (humped-back condition)
lordosis *lōr-dō'sis*	abnormal anterior curvature of the lumbar spine (sway-back condition)
scoliosis *skō-lē-ō'sis*	abnormal lateral curvature (S-shaped curve)
spondylolisthesis *spon'di-lō-lis-thē'sis*	forward slipping of a lumbar vertebra (listhesis = slipping)
spondylosis *spon-di-lō'sis*	stiff, immobile condition of vertebrae
sprain *sprān*	injury to a ligament caused by joint trauma but without joint dislocation or fracture
subluxation *sŭb-lŭk-sā'shŭn*	a partial dislocation (luxation = dislocation)
tendinitis *ten-di-nī'tis* **tendonitis** *ten-dō-nī'tis*	inflammation of a tendon

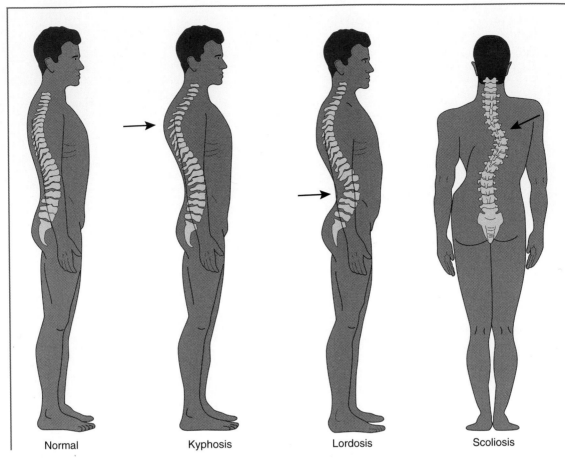

Normal   Kyphosis   Lordosis   Scoliosis

■ **FIGURE 4-13.** Spinal curvatures.

PROGRAMMED REVIEW: DIAGNOSTIC TERMS

Answer Column	Review
condition or increase ankylosis	**4.55**　Formed from the combining form for stiff and the suffix -osis meaning _____, a stiff joint condition is called _____.
inflammation arthritis osteoarthritis joint rheumatoid, Gouty	**4.56**　Formed from the combining form for joint and the suffix -itis meaning _____, the term for inflammation of joints characterized by pain and swelling is _____. The most common form of arthritis, formed using the combining form for bone, is _____. This is also called degenerative arthritis or degenerative _____ disease. The most crippling type of arthritis characterized by chronic systemic inflammation is _____ arthritis. _____ arthritis attacks a single

joint (e.g., the great toe) because of too much uric acid in the blood, or

hyper

_____ uricemia.

-itis

bursa

epiphysitis

muscle

tendonitis (or tendinitis)

bone marrow

4.57   Recall that the suffix _____ refers to inflammation. Bursitis is inflammation of a _____. Inflammation of epiphyseal regions of a long bone is _____. Myositis is inflammation of a _____. Inflammation of a tendon is _____. Osteomyelitis is an infection and inflammation of bone and _____ _____.

swelling

4.58   A bunion is a _____ at the joint at the base of the great toe caused by inflammation of the bursa.

death

condition, increase

necrosis

sequestrum

4.59   The combining form necr/o means _____, and the suffix -osis means _____ or _____. The term for the condition or increase of dead bone tissue caused by a loss of blood supply is bony _____, also called _____.

chrondr/o

cartilage

4.60   Recall that the combining form for cartilage is _____. The term chondromalacia refers to a softening of _____.

fracture

closed

open

simple

complex

Fx

4.61   A broken bone, or _____, can happen in various ways. The skin is not broken in a _____ fracture, whereas there is an open wound with an _____ fracture. If the fracture has only one fracture line and the bones are not displaced, this is a _____ fracture, whereas a displaced fracture that requires manipulation to put the bone pieces in correct position is a _____ fracture. The abbreviation for fracture is _____.

comminuted

4.62   A fracture involving bone broken in many little pieces is a _____ fracture. An incomplete fracture seen usually

greenstick	in children, named for how a living tree branch may break when you bend it, is a _____ fracture.
herniated	**4.63** A degenerated or fragmented intervertebral disk that protrudes and compresses a nerve is called a _____ disk (disc).
tumor myoma osteoma bone marrow malignant	**4.64** Recall that the suffix -oma means _____. Using the combining forms for muscle and bone, a muscle tumor is a _____ and a bone tumor is an _____. A myeloma is a tumor of the _____ _____. An osteosarcoma is a type of _____ bone tumor.
leiomyoma rhabdomyoma rhabdomyosarcoma	**4.65** There are several types of muscle tumors. While the suffix -oma refers to any tumor, a sarcoma is a malignant tumor. (Recall the meanings of the combining forms lei/o and rhabd/o.) A smooth muscle tumor is a _____, whereas a skeletal muscle tumor is a _____. A malignant smooth muscle tumor is a leiomyosarcoma, and a malignant skeletal muscle tumor is a _____.
dystrophy shrinking painful or faulty	**4.66** Muscular _____ is a group of diseases characterized by progressive atrophy of skeletal muscles. Recall that atrophy means _____ of muscle size, and the prefix dys- means _____.
osteomalacia rickets	**4.67** Recall that chondromalacia means softening of cartilage. The term for softening of bone is _____. This is caused by calcium and vitamin D deficiency. In children this is called _____.
condition or increase osteoporosis	**4.68** The suffix -osis means _____. The condition in which bones become less dense and more porous is called _____.

4.69 Joints can be injured by trauma in various ways. If the bones are partially dislocated from their usual position in a joint, this is called

subluxation

_____. An injury to a ligament without dislocation

sprain

or fracture is called a _____.

4.70 Several abnormal spinal curvatures are common. Kyphosis is an

posterior

abnormal _____ curvature of the thoracic region. From the combining form meaning bent, an abnormal anterior curvature of

lordosis

the lumbar region is called _____. From the combining form meaning twisted, an abnormal lateral curvature is called

scoliosis

_____.

4.71 Recall that spondyl/o is the combining form for

vertebra

_____. The term for a stiff, immobile condition of vertebrae

spondylosis

is _____. The term for forward slipping of lumbar

spondylolisthesis

vertebra is _____.

SELF-INSTRUCTION: DIAGNOSTIC TESTS AND PROCEDURES

Study the following:

Test or Procedure	Explanation
electromyogram (EMG) _ē-lek-trō-mī'o-gram_	a neurodiagnostic graphic record of the electrical activity of muscle at rest and during contraction; used to diagnose neuromusculoskeletal disorders (e.g., muscular dystrophy); usually performed by a neurologist
magnetic resonance imaging (MRI) (Fig. 2-13 in Chapter 2) _măg-năt'ik rez'ō-nans im'ă-jing_	a nonionizing (no x-ray) imaging technique using magnetic fields and radio frequency waves to visualize anatomic structures; used in detecting joint, tendon, and vertebral disc disorders
nuclear medicine imaging _nū'klē-er_ **radionuclide organ imaging** _rā'dē-ō-nū'klīd_	a diagnostic imaging technique using injected or ingested radioactive isotopes and a gamma-camera for determining the size, shape, location, and function of various body parts
bone scan (Fig. 2-12 in Chapter 2)	a nuclear scan of bone tissue to detect a tumor, malignancy, etc.

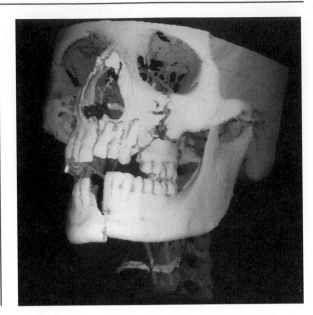

■ **FIGURE 4-14.** Three-dimensional computed tomography reconstruction of a skull showing traumatic injury to facial bones suffered as the result of a motor vehicle accident.

radiography (x-ray) (Fig. 2-10 in Chapter 2) *rā′dē-og′ră-fē*	an imaging modality using x-rays (ionizing radiation) to diagnose condition or impairment somewhere in the body (e.g., extremities, ribs, back, shoulders, joint)
arthrogram *ar′thrō-gram*	a radiograph of a joint taken after injection of a contrast medium
computed tomography (CT) (Fig. 4-14) *tō-mog′ră-fē* **computed axial tomography** (CAT)	a radiologic procedure using a machine called a scanner to take a series of cross-sectional x-ray images in a full circle rotation; a computer then calculates the rates of absorption and density of the radiographs to create the image
sonography *sŏ-nog′ră-fē*	use of high frequency sound waves (ultrasound) to make an image of tissues or structures (e.g., muscles, ligaments, displacements or dislocations, and arthroscopic visualizations)

PROGRAMMED REVIEW: DIAGNOSTIC TESTS AND PROCEDURES

Answer Column	Review

4.72 The combining form *electr/o* refers to electricity, and the suffix -*gram* means a _____. Combine these with the combining form for muscle to create the word for the diagnostic record of the electrical activity of a muscle: _____

record

electromyogram

4.73 The imaging technique using magnetic fields and radio frequency waves to visualize bone and joint structures is called _____ _____ _____ (MRI).

magnetic resonance imaging

4.74 The suffix -*graphy* refers to the _____ of _____. *Radi/o* is the combining form for radiation, from the Latin word for ray. The general imaging modality that records images produced by x-rays is called _____. Recall that the suffix -*gram* means a _____. Using the combining form for joint, an x-ray of a joint (usually taken using a contrast medium) is an _____.

process

recording

radiography

record

arthrogram

4.75 A special imaging modality using an x-ray scanner and a computer to produce cross-sectional images is called _____ _____ (CT). This is also called computed _____ tomography (CAT) because the scanner rotates around the axis of the body to make the image.

computed

tomography

axial

4.76 The Latin word nucleus refers to a little nut, or the inside of a thing. In modern physics, nucleus refers to the inside of an atom and radiation using subatomic particles. Nuclear medicine imaging, also called _____ organ imaging, is a diagnostic technique using radioactive isotopes and a gamma camera instead of x-rays. A _____ _____ is a nuclear scan of bone tissue to detect abnormalities.

radionuclide

bone scan

4.77 The combining form meaning sound is *son/o*. The imaging modality using high-frequency sound (ultrasound) is called

sonography

_____.

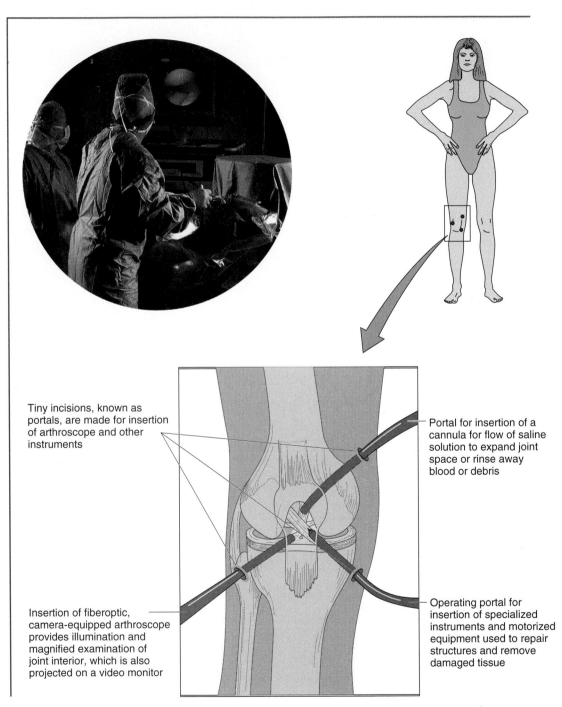

Tiny incisions, known as portals, are made for insertion of arthroscope and other instruments

Portal for insertion of a cannula for flow of saline solution to expand joint space or rinse away blood or debris

Insertion of fiberoptic, camera-equipped arthroscope provides illumination and magnified examination of joint interior, which is also projected on a video monitor

Operating portal for insertion of specialized instruments and motorized equipment used to repair structures and remove damaged tissue

■ **FIGURE 4-15.** Arthroscopic knee surgery, showing projection of surgeon's view on video monitor.

SELF-INSTRUCTION: OPERATIVE TERMS

Study the following:

Term	Meaning
amputation *am-pyū-tā'shŭn*	partial or complete removal of a limb; AKA, above-knee amputation; BKA, below-knee amputation
arthrocentesis *ar'thrō-sen-tē'sis*	puncture for aspiration of a joint
arthrodesis *ăr-thrō-dē'sĭs*	binding or fusing of joint surfaces
arthroplasty *ar'thrō-plas-tē*	repair or reconstruction of a joint
arthroscopy (Fig- 4.15) *ar-thros'kă-pē*	procedure using an arthroscope to examine, diagnose, and repair a joint from within
bone grafting	transplantation of a piece of bone from one site to another to repair a skeletal defect
bursectomy *ber-sek'tō-mē*	excision of a bursa
myoplasty *mī'ō-plas-tē*	repair of muscle
open reduction, internal fixation (ORIF) (Fig. 4-16)	internal surgical repair of a fracture by bringing bones back into alignment and fixing them into place with devices such as plates, screws, and pins

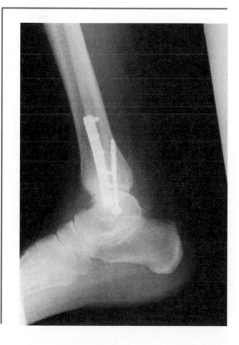

FIGURE 4-16. Radiograph taken after open reduction, internal fixation (ORIF) of right ankle (see Medical Record 4.1).

osteotomy *os-tē-ot'ō-mē*	an incision into bone
osteoplasty *os'tē-ō-plas-tē*	repair of bone
spondylosyndesis *spon'di-lō-sin-dē'sis*	spinal fusion
tenotomy *te-not'ō-mē*	division by incision of a tendon to repair a deformity caused by shortening of a muscle

PROGRAMMED REVIEW: OPERATIVE TERMS

Answer Column	Review
	4.78 Several different operative procedures are performed on joints. Often the term for these procedures is formed using the combining
joint	form *arthr/o*, meaning _____. Remember that the suffix *-desis* means binding; the term for binding or fusing of joint surfaces is there-
arthrodesis	fore _____. The suffix for puncture for aspiration is
-centesis	_____; the term for puncture of a joint for aspiration is
arthrocentesis	therefore _____. The procedure using an
	instrument to examine a joint from within is called
arthroscopy	_____. The suffix *-plasty* means surgical
repair	_____ or reconstruction, and the repair or reconstruction of a
arthroplasty	joint is called _____.
	4.79 A partial or complete removal of a limb is an
amputation	_____.
	4.80 Recall that the suffix *-ectomy* means a surgical
excision or removal	_____. The excision of a bursa is therefore called a
bursectomy	_____.
	4.81 Transplantation of a piece of bone from one site to another is
grafting	called bone _____. This is done, for example, to repair a
	skeletal defect.

-plasty myoplasty osteoplasty	**4.82** The suffix for surgical repair or reconstruction is _____. The repair of a muscle is therefore _____. The repair of a bone is _____.
incision osteotomy tenotomy	**4.83** The suffix *-tomy* refers to a surgical _____. An incision into bone is therefore _____, whereas an incision into a tendon is _____.
binding spondylosyndesis	**4.84** The suffix *-desis* means _____ (or fusing). From the combining form for vertebrae, the term for surgical spinal fusion is _____.
open reduction, internal fixation	**4.85** Some fractures, particularly comminuted fractures, must be surgically repaired by internal (open) surgery using devices such as screws and pins to hold the bone fragments in place. This procedure is called _____ _____ , _____ _____ (ORIF).

SELF-INSTRUCTION: THERAPEUTIC TERMS

Study the following:

Term	Meaning
closed reduction, external fixation of a fracture	external manipulation of a fracture to regain alignment along with application of an external device to protect and hold the bone in place while healing
casting	use of a stiff, solid dressing around a limb or other body part to immobilize it during healing
splinting	use of a rigid device to immobilize or restrain a broken bone or injured body part
traction (Tx) *trak'shŭn*	application of a pulling force to a fractured bone or dislocated joint to maintain proper position for healing
closed reduction percutaneous fixation of a fracture (Fig. 4-17)	external manipulation of a fracture to regain alignment, followed by insertion of one or more pins through the skin to maintain position—often includes use of an external device called a fixator to keep the fracture immobilized during healing
orthosis (Fig. 4-18) *ōr-thsis*	use of an orthopedic appliance to maintain a bone's position or to provide limb support (e.g., back, knee, or wrist brace)

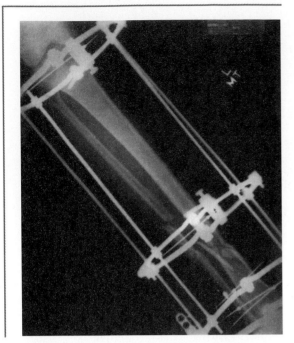

■ **FIGURE 4-17.** This radiograph, taken after closed reduction, percutaneous fixation of an open comminuted distal tibia/fibula fracture, shows placement of an external fixator to maintain pin placement during the healing process. The injury was the result of a gun shot to the lower extremity.

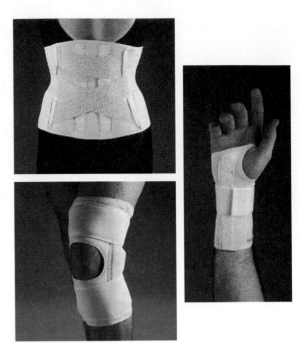

FIGURE 4-18. Examples of orthoses: back, knee, and wrist.

physical therapy (PT) *fiz'i-kăl ther'ă-pē*	treatment to rehabilitate patients disabled by illness or injury, involving many different modalities (methods) such as exercise, hydrotherapy, diathermy, and ultrasound
prosthesis (Fig. 4-19) *pros'thē-sis*	an artificial replacement for a missing body part, or a device used to improve a body function, such as an artificial limb, hip, or joint

COMMON THERAPEUTIC DRUG CLASSIFICATIONS

analgesic *an-ăl-jē'zik*	a drug that relieves pain
narcotic *nar-kot'ik*	a potent analgesic with addictive properties
anti-inflammatory *an'tē-in-flam'ă-tō-rē*	a drug that reduces inflammation
antipyretic *an'tē-pī-ret'ik*	a drug that relieves fever
nonsteroidal anti-inflammatory drug (NSAID) *non-stēr'oy-dăl*	a group of drugs with analgesic, anti-inflammatory, and antipyretic properties (e.g., ibuprofen, aspirin) commonly used to treat arthritis

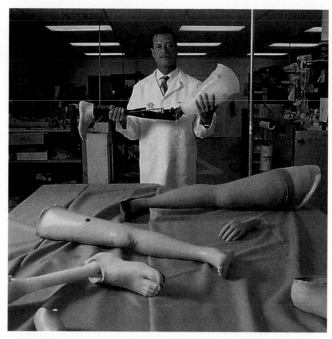

FIGURE 4-19. Prosthetist holding an above-the-knee prosthesis, with an array of prostheses on table in foreground.

PROGRAMMED REVIEW: THERAPEUTIC TERMS

Answer Column	Review
	4.86 Recall that some fractures require open reduction, internal fixation. Other fractures can be reduced (the bone pieces brought into alignment) without surgery and held in place externally. This procedure is
closed reduction, external	called _____ _____, _____
fixation	_____. If the fracture is reduced and one or more pins are inserted through the skin (*cutane/o*) to maintain the bone position, this is
percutaneous	called closed reduction, _____
fixation	_____.
	4.87 With closed reduction, external fixation, the fractured bone must be held immobile in place. The use of a stiff, solid dressing around a
casting	limb to immobilize it is called _____. The use of a rigid device to immobilize a limb with a fracture of injury is called
splinting	_____. Sometimes it is necessary to maintain a pulling force on a fractured bone or dislocated joint for proper positioning during healing; this is called
traction	ing healing; this is called _____.

orthosis

4.88   The combining form *orth/o* means straight. An orthopedic device used to maintain limb support or the position of bones is called an

_____.

physical

4.89   Patients with musculoskeletal injuries or illnesses often receive rehabilitative therapy called _____ therapy, combining exercise and other modalities.

prosthesis

4.90   An artificial limb is an example of a _____.

without

analgesic

narcotic

4.91   The prefix *an-* means _____. The Greek word algesis means sensation of pain. A drug that relieves pain is called an _____. The combining form *narc/o* means benumb or deaden; a type of potent, addictive analgesic drug is a _____.

against

antipyretic

anti-inflammatory

4.92   Many drugs are named according to their action against a condition or symptom. The prefix *anti-* means _____. The Greek word pyr means heat or fire, and a drug that relieves fever is an _____. A drug that reduces inflammation is an _____.

nonsteroidal, anti-

inflammatory

4.93   There are several types of analgesic and anti-inflammatory drugs. The group that includes aspirin and ibuprofen is called _____ _____ drugs (NSAIDs).

Practice Exercises

For the following terms, on the lines below the term, write out the indicated word parts: prefixes, combining forms, roots, and suffixes. Then define the word.

For example:

hypertrophy

<u>hyper/troph/y</u>
P   R   S

DEFINITION: above or excessive/nourishment or development/condition or process of

1. hemipelvectomy

        /   /
   P   R   S

DEFINITION: _____

2. thoracic

        /
   R   S

DEFINITION: _____

3. myofascial

        /   /
   CF   R   S

DEFINITION: _____

4. arthropathy

        /   /
   CF   R   S

DEFINITION: _____

5. spondylolysis

        /
   CF   S

DEFINITION: _____

6. osteogenic

        /   /
   CF   R   S

DEFINITION: _____

7. chondrectomy

        /
   R   S

DEFINITION: _____

8. myonecrosis

_____ / _____ / _____
  CF   R   S

DEFINITION: _____

9. ostealgia

_____ / _____
   R   S

DEFINITION: _____

10. periosteitis

_____ / _____ / _____
  P   R   S

DEFINITION: _____

11. leiomyosarcoma

_____ / _____ / _____ / _____
  CF   CF   R   S

DEFINITION: _____

12. myelocyte

_____ / _____ / _____
  CF   R   S

DEFINITION: _____

13. costovertebral

_____ / _____ / _____
  CF   R   S

DEFINITION: _____

14. spondylomalacia

_____ / _____
  CF   S

DEFINITION: _____

15. osteoarthritis

_____ / _____ / _____
  CF   R   S

DEFINITION: _____

16. intercostal

_____ / _____ / _____
  P   R   S

DEFINITION: _____

17. orthosis

_____ / _____
   R   S

DEFINITION: _____

18. myotonia

_____ / _____ / _____
  CF   R   S

DEFINITION: _____

19. kyphosis

_____ / _____
   R   S

DEFINITION: _____

20. craniectomy

_____ / _____
   R   S

DEFINITION: _____

21. arthrodesis

_____ / _____
  CF   S

DEFINITION: _____

22. fibromyalgia

_____ / _____ / _____
  CF   R   S

DEFINITION: _____

23. rhabdomyoma

_____ / _____ / _____
  CF   R   S

DEFINITION: _____

24. sternocostal

_____ / _____ / _____
  CF   R   S

DEFINITION: _____

25. intraarticular

_____ / _____ / _____
   P   R   S

DEFINITION: _____

26. syndactylism

_____ / _____ / _____
  P   R   S

DEFINITION: _____

27. lumbodynia

_____ / _____
  CF   S

DEFINITION: _____

28. cervicobrachial

_____ / _____ / _____
  CF   R   S

DEFINITION: _____

29. arthroscopy

_____ / _____
  CF   S

DEFINITION: _____

30. lordosis

_____ / _____
  R   S

DEFINITION: _____

Write the correct medical term for each of the following:

31. lateral curvature of the spine _____

32. joint pain _____

33. bone tumor _____

34. muscle tumor _____

35. grating sound made by movement of broken bones _____

36. bone pain _____

37. x-ray of a joint _____

38. line that divides the body into right and left halves

_____

39. surgical reconstruction of bone _____

40. plane that divides the body into front and back portions

_____

41. opposite of hypertrophy _____

42. striated (skeletal) muscle tumor _____

43. test to record muscle response to electrical stimulation _____

44. smooth muscle tumor _____

45. application of a pulling force to a fractured or dislocated joint to maintain proper position during healing

_____

46. flabby (relaxed muscle) _____

47. lying flat on the back _____

48. bone marrow tumor _____

49. arthritis caused by hyperuricemia _____

50. horizontal plane that divides the body into superior and inferior portion

_____

51. turning downward or backward of the palm of the hand or sole of the foot

_____

52. stiff joint _____

53. a partial dislocation _____

54. toward the beginning of a structure _____

55. lying face down and flat _____

56. an artificial replacement for a missing body part _____

57. diagnostic test that uses nuclear imaging techniques to visualize bone tissue

_____

58. above another structure or toward the head _____

59. bending of the foot or toes upward _____

60. internal surgical repair of a fracture by bringing bones into alignment

_____

61. osteomalacia in children _____

62. diagnostic imaging technique using high-frequency sound waves to visualize body tissues and structures

_____

63. physician specializing in x-ray technology _____

64. stiff muscle _____

Complete the medical term by writing the missing part:

65. inter_____ al = pertaining to between the *ribs*

66. _____ myosarcoma = malignant *striated or skeletal* muscle tumor

67. hyper_____ = excessive *nourishment or development* (increase in the size of a muscle)

68. myo_____ = *suture* of a muscle

69. spondylosyn_____ = *binding* together of vertebrae

70. _____myoma = *smooth* muscle tumor

71. osteo_____ = *softening* of bone

72. _____listhesis = slipping of *vertebra*

73. arthro_____ = *radiograph* of a joint

74. _____tomy = incision into *bone*

75. epiphys_____ = *inflammation* of the ends of the long bones

76. _____al = pertaining to the *neck*

77. bone _____osis = *dead* bone tissue

78. _____oma = tumor of *cartilage*

79. arthro_____ = *puncture for aspiration* of a joint

Match the following terms with the appropriate body movements:

80. flexion _____   a. movement toward the body

81. inversion _____   b. straightening

82. adduction _____   c. bending

83. extension _____   d. to turn inward

84. abduction _____   e. to turn outward

85. eversion _____   f. movement away from the body

Define the following abbreviations:

86. CT _____

87. PT _____

88. Tx _____

89. ROM _____

90. Fx _____

For each of the following, circle the correct spelling of the term:

91. spondelosis   spandalosis   spondylosis

92. scholiosis   scoliosis   scoleosis

93. arthrodynia   arthradynia   arthrodenia

94. osteoalgia   ostealgia   osstealgia

95. sagital   saggittal   sagittal

96. flaccid   flacid   flascid

97. sekquestrum   sequestrom   sequestrum

98. anklylosis   ankylosis   anklosis

99. chondral   chrondral   chondrel

100. dorsaflexion   dorsiflexion   dorsflexion

101. osteoparosis   osteoporosis   osteophorosis

102. rabdomyoma   rrhabdomyoma   rhabdomyoma

Write in the missing words on the lines in the following illustrations of the body planes.

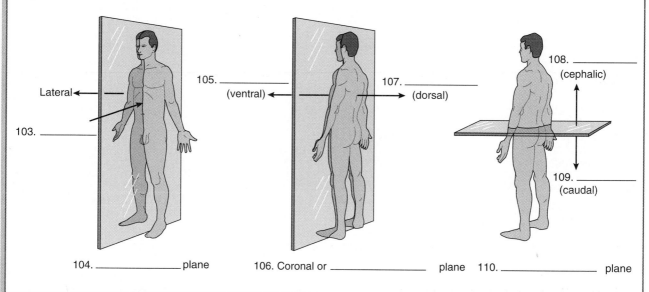

Lateral ←

103. _____

104. _____ plane

105. _____ (ventral) ←

107. _____ (dorsal)

106. Coronal or _____ plane

108. _____ (cephalic)

109. _____ (caudal)

110. _____ plane

Write in the missing words on the lines in the following illustrations of body movements.

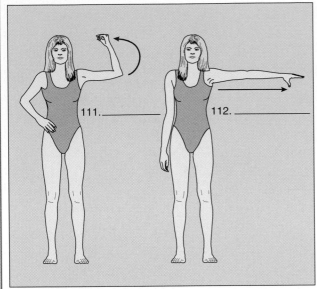

111. _____

112. _____

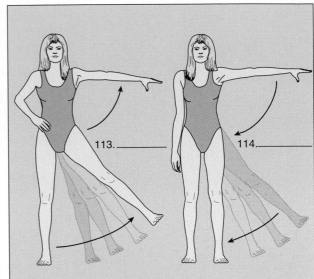

113. _____

114. _____

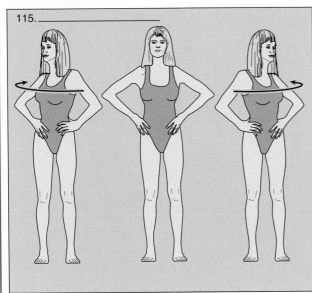

115. _____

Additional movements of the feet

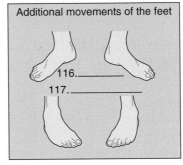

116. _____

117. _____

Additional movements of the hands and arm

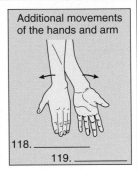

118. _____

119. _____

Additional movements of the feet

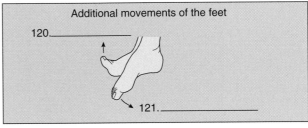

120. _____

121. _____

Write in the missing anatomical terms on the lines in the following illustration.

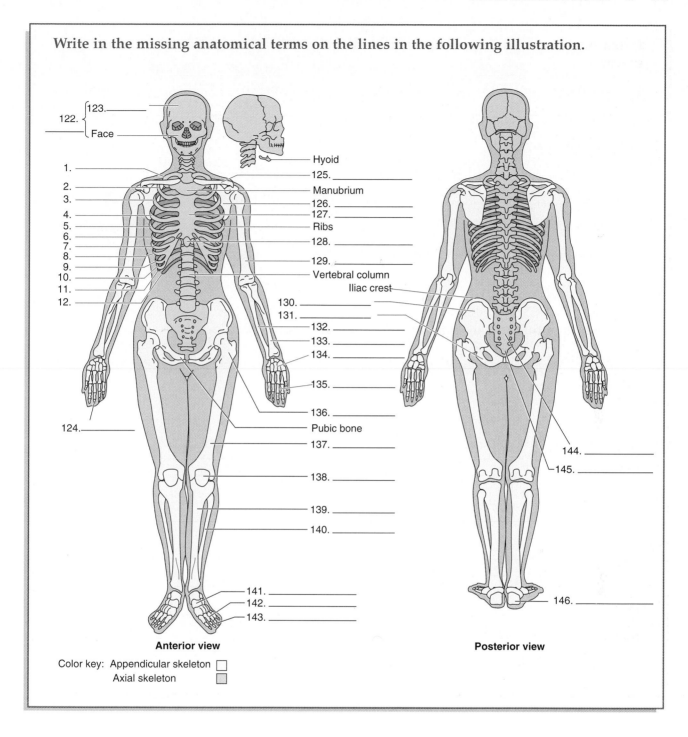

122.
123. _____
Face

1. _____
2. _____
3. _____
4. _____
5. _____
6. _____
7. _____
8. _____
9. _____
10. _____
11. _____
12. _____

124. _____

Hyoid
125. _____
Manubrium
126. _____
127. _____
Ribs
128. _____
129. _____
Vertebral column
Iliac crest
130. _____
131. _____
132. _____
133. _____
134. _____
135. _____
136. _____
Pubic bone
137. _____
138. _____
139. _____
140. _____
141. _____
142. _____
143. _____

Anterior view

144. _____
145. _____
146. _____

Posterior view

Color key: Appendicular skeleton ☐
            Axial skeleton ▨

For each of the following, circle the combining form that corresponds to the meaning given:

147. **cartilage**	crani/o	cost/o	chondr/o
148. **vertebra**	myel/o	spondyl/o	lumb/o
149. **bone marrow**	my/o	myel/o	muscul/o
150. **neck**	thorac/o	crani/o	cervic/o
151. **joint**	oste/o	arthr/o	ankyl/o
152. **chest**	thorac/o	cervic/o	spondyl/o
153. **muscle**	my/o	myel/o	lei/o
154. **rib**	stern/o	chondr/o	cost/o

Give the noun that was used to form the following adjectives.

155. orthotic _____

156. hypertrophic _____

157. radial _____

158. kyphotic _____

159. bursal _____

160. dystrophic _____

161. necrotic _____

162. osteoporotic _____

163. lordotic _____

164. ulnar _____

165. scoliotic _____

166. prosthetic _____

Medical Record Analyses

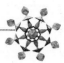

MEDICAL RECORD 4-1

History and Physical Examination

CC: "attacks" of right knee discomfort and instability

HPI: This 19 y/o ♂ presents with "attacks" of right knee pain and instability. Three years ago, while playing basketball, he turned sharply and felt his kneecap pop in and out. It was acutely swollen and painful and required manipulation to reduce it. He had a course of PT and did reasonably well for a few months until resuming athletic activities. Since then he has had recurrent episodes of the knee slipping in and out, all related to twisting and turning while surfing or playing basketball. His primary complaint is the episodic discomfort and the inability to trust the knee. He is asymptomatic at this time.

PMH: NKDA. Hx of right ankle Fx in 20xx. Meds: none. Operations: none.

SH: alcohol rarely used. FH: Father, age 49, Mother, age 43, both L&W.

ROS: noncontributory.

PE: The patient is a cooperative male in NAD.

VS: T 97.2° F., P 64, R 14, BP 118/66
HEENT- WNL. Neck: supple, no tenderness, full ROM, no adenopathy.
Lungs, heart, abdomen: WNL. Back: no tenderness or deformity.
Extremities: unremarkable except for involved knee. Knee ROM is 0-45° equally. There is no parapatellar tenderness.
Neurologic: Negative.
Radiographs show subluxation of the right knee.

IMP: RECURRENT RIGHT KNEE PATELLAR INSTABILITY

RECOMMENDATION: Patelloplasty is being discussed, and the risks and benefits of the procedure have been explained. The patient will return with his parents for further consultation before deciding whether to proceed with treatment.

1. Which describes the patient's symptoms at the time of the initial injury?
   a. severe pain over a short course
   b. pain that comes and goes
   c. pain that progressively gets worse
   d. pain that develops slowly over time
   e. no pain

2. What treatment was provided 3 years ago?
   a. puncture for aspiration of a joint
   b. transplantation of a piece of bone from one site to another
   c. examination of a joint from within
   d. physical rehabilitation including exercise
   e. binding or fusing joint surfaces

3. Which best describes the patient's symptoms at the time of this visit?
   a. severe pain
   b. moderate pain
   c. progressive pain
   d. mild pain
   e. no pain

4. Describe the orthopedic condition noted in the past history:
   a. forward slipping of a vertebra
   b. broken bone
   c. arthritis
   d. bone pain
   e. dislocation

5. What does full ROM indicate?
   a. swelling
   b. spasm
   c. inflammation
   d. bruising
   e. mobility

6. What did the radiographs indicate?
   a. no radiographs were mentioned
   b. patellar instability
   c. partial dislocation
   d. inflammation
   e. joint stiffness

7. What treatment did the physician recommend?
   a. surgical reconstruction of the knee cap
   b. physical therapy
   c. surgical repair of bone
   d. excision of the patella
   e. examination and repair of a joint from within using an endoscope

MEDICAL RECORD 4-2 FOR ADDITIONAL STUDY

CENTRAL MEDICAL CENTER

211 Medical Center Drive • Central City, US 90000-1234 • PHONE: (012) 125-6784 • FAX: (012) 125-9999

OPERATIVE REPORT

PREOPERATIVE DIAGNOSIS: Trimalleolar fracture, right ankle/fracture dislocation.

POSTOPERATIVE DIAGNOSIS: Trimalleolar fracture, right ankle/fracture dislocation.

OPERATION PERFORMED: Open reduction and internal fixation of medial malleolus and lateral malleolus, right ankle.

ANESTHESIOLOGIST: K. Teglam, M.D.

ANESTHESIA: General.

DESCRIPTION OF OPERATION: After successful general anesthesia, the right lower extremity was prepped and draped in a sterile fashion. A pneumatic tourniquet was used in the case at 300 mm Hg (mercury) for 51 minutes. The medial side was opened first; the skin was incised, and this was carried down through the subcutaneous tissue down to the periosteum which was incised enough at the fracture site for visualization of a large transverse medial malleolar fracture. A hematoma was evacuated by curettage and irrigation. Unfortunately, there was some debris within the joint which was articular cartilage destruction and damage on the talus.

Attention was then directed laterally where an incision was made and carried through the skin and subcutaneous tissue. The fracture was brought into full view very easily. The fracture was long and oblique. This was curetted of hematoma and irrigated, and using a bone clamp, it was clamped in a reduced position. A 6-hole semitubular fibular-type plate was then bent to position and placed onto the fibula; and after predrilling, premeasuring, and pretapping, six cortical 3.5 mm diameter screws were used to hold the plate to the fractured fibula.

Attention was then directed medially. The fracture was reduced and held in place with a towel clip, and a 60 mm long malleolar screw was then inserted into the fragment into the distal tibia. X-rays revealed that three of the screws laterally were too long, and these were changed. The medial malleolus screw was also tightened down further. Repeat film revealed very satisfactory position of all the screws. The posterior malleolar fragment was felt to be adequately positioned. All the wounds were then irrigated with goodly amounts of antibiotic solution. Vicryl sutures, 0 and 2-0, were used to close the subcutaneous tissue on both sides; and staples were used for the skin. A bulky Jones dressing was applied with splints anteriorly and posteriorly.

The patient tolerated the procedure well and was transferred to the recovery room with stable vital signs.

R. Rodriguez, M.D.

RR:mb

D: 10/19/20xx
T: 10/20/20xx

OPERATIVE REPORT

PT. NAME: TOOHEY, ALICE M.
ID NO: IP-236701
ROOM NO: 729
ATT. PHYS: R. RODRIGUEZ, M.D.

MEDICAL RECORD 4-2 FOR ADDITIONAL STUDY

As Alice Toohey was playing with her young granddaughter, she stepped on a toy dump truck and fell down her porch steps, wrenching her ankle violently. Because of the sharp pain and immediate swelling, Ms. Toohey was taken immediately to the hospital. After being seen by the emergency room physician, she was admitted and scheduled for surgery.

Read Medical Record 4.1 (page 182) for Alice Toohey and answer the following questions. This record is the operative report dictated by the surgeon, Dr. Ricardo Rodriguez, immediately after the operation and processed by a medical transcriptionist.

1. Below are medical terms used in this record that you have not yet encountered in this text. Underline each where it appears in the record, and define below.

   malleolus _____

   oblique _____

   sterile _____

2. In your own words, not using medical terminology, briefly describe the preoperative diagnosis for Ms. Toohey.

   _____

   _____

   _____

3. Put the following operative steps in correct order by numbering them 1 to 10.

   _____ radiograph of the screws that were too long

   _____ incision on the outer side of the ankle

   _____ plate placed onto fibula

   _____ sewing the incisions

   _____ radiograph of satisfactory screw position

   _____ towel clip positioned

   _____ removal of medial hematoma

   _____ removal of lateral hematoma

   _____ placement of screw into lower tibia

   _____ incision on the inner side of the right ankle

4. In this operation the surgeon redid one step after using a diagnostic procedure to check whether that step was as effective as possible. In your own words, explain what Dr. Rodriguez changed and why.

   _____

   _____

   _____

   _____

5. Describe the fracture line:

_____

6. When Dr. Rodriguez examined the ankle after making the first incision, he found a problem he could not and did not repair. In your own words, what had been destroyed in Ms. Toohey's injury? _____

_____

7. Which of the following actions did *not* occur in this operation?
   a. washing the wound with antibiotic
   b. taping the fracture line
   c. drilling holes in the bone
   d. stapling the skin closed

8. Describe Ms. Toohey's condition when transferred to PAR after the operation:

_____

_____

Answers to Practice Exercises

1. hemi/pelv/ectomy
   P   R   S
   half/hip bone or pelvic
      cavity/excision (removal)
2. thorac/ic
   R   S
   chest/pertaining to
3. myo/fasci/al
   CF   R   S
   muscle/fascia (a band)/
      pertaining to
4. arthro/path/y
   CF   R   S
   joint/disease/condition or
      process of
5. spondylo/lysis
   CF   S
   vertebra/breaking down or
      dissolution
6. osteo/gen/ic
   CF   R   S
   bone/origin or production/
      pertaining to
7. chondr/ectomy
   R   S
   cartilage/excision (removal)
8. myo/necr/osis
   CF   R   S
   muscle/death/condition or
      increase

9. oste/algia
   R   S
   bone/pain
10. peri/oste/itis
    P   R   S
    around/bone/inflammation
11. leio/myo/sarc/oma
    CF   CF   R   S
    smooth/muscle/flesh/tumor
12. myelo/cyt/e
    CF   R   S
    bone marrow or spinal
       cord/cell/noun marker
13. costo/vertebr/al
    CF   R   S
    rib/vertebra/pertaining to
14. spondylo/malacia
    CF   S
    vertebra/softening
15. osteo/arthr/itis
    CF   R   S
    bone/joint/inflammation
16. inter/cost/al
    P   R   S
    between/rib/pertaining to
17. ortho/osis
    R   S
    straight, normal, or
       correct/condition or
       increase
18. myo/ton/ia
    CF   R S
    muscle/tone/condition of

19. kyph/osis
    R   S
    humped/condition or
       increase
20. crani/ectomy
    R   S
    skull/excision (removal)
21. arthro/desis
    CF   S
    joint/binding
22. fibro/my/algia
    CF   R   S
    fiber/muscle/pain
23. rhabdo/my/oma
    CF   R   S
    rod shaped or striated
       (skeletal)/muscle/tumor
24. sterno/cost/al
    CF   R   S
    sternum (breastbone)/rib/
       pertaining to
25. intra/articul/ar
    P   R   S
    within/joint/pertaining to
26. syn/dactyl/ism
    P   R   S
    together or with/digit (finger or toe)/condition of
27. lumbo/dynia
    CF   S
    loin (lower back)/pain
28. cervico/brachi/al
    CF   R   S
    neck/arm/pertaining to

29. <u>arthro/scopy</u>
       CF   S

   joint/process of examination
30. <u>lord/osis</u>
       R   S

   bent/condition or increase
31. scoliosis
32. arthralgia or arthrodynia
33. osteoma
34. myoma
35. crepitation or crepitus
36. ostealgia or osteodynia
37. arthrogram
38. sagittal
39. osteoplasty
40. coronal or frontal
41. atrophy
42. rhabdomyoma
43. electromyogram
44. leiomyoma
45. traction
46. flaccid
47. horizontal recumbent or
   supine
48. myeloma
49. gouty arthritis
50. transverse
51. pronation
52. ankylosis
53. subluxation
54. proximal
55. prone
56. prosthesis
57. bone scan
58. superior (cephalic)
59. dorsiflexion
60. open reduction internal fixation of a fracture (ORIF)
61. rickets
62. sonography
63. radiologist
64. rigor, rigidity
65. intercostal
66. rhabdomyosarcoma
67. hypertrophy
68. myorrhaphy
69. spondylosyndesis
70. leiomyoma
71. osteomalacia
72. spondylolisthesis
73. arthrogram
74. osteotomy

75. epiphysitis
76. cervical
77. bone necrosis
78. chondroma
79. arthrocentesis
80. c
81. d
82. a
83. b
84. f
85. e
86. computed tomography
87. physical therapy
88. traction or treatment
89. range of motion
90. fracture (broken bone)
91. spondylosis
92. scoliosis
93. arthrodynia
94. ostealgia
95. sagittal
96. flaccid
97. sequestrum
98. ankylosis
99. chondral
100. dorsiflexion
101. osteoporosis
102. rhabdomyoma
103. medial
104. sagittal
105. anterior
106. frontal
107. posterior
108. superior
109. inferior
110. transverse
111. flexion
112. extension
113. abduction
114. adduction
115. rotation
116. eversion
117. inversion
118. pronation
119. supination
120. dorsi flexion
121. plantar flexion
122. skull
123. cranium
124. phalanges
125. clavicle
126. scapula

127. sternum
128. xiphoid process
129. Humerus
130. Ilium
131. Ischium
132. Ulna
133. Radius
134. Carpals
135. Metacarpals
136. Trochanter
137. Femur
138. Patella
139. Tibia
140. Fibula
141. Tarsals
142. Metatarsals
143. Phalanges
144. Sacrum
145. Coccyx
146. Calcaneus
147. **cartilage** = chondr/o
148. **vertebra** = spondyl/o
149. **bone marrow** = myel/o
150. **neck** = cervic/o
151. **joint** = arthr/o
152. **chest** = thorac/o
153. **muscle** = my/o
154. **rib** = cost/o
155. orthosis
156. hypertrophy
157. radius
158. kyphosis
159. bursa
160. dystrophy
161. necrosis
162. osteoporosis
163. lordosis
164. ulna
165. scoliosis
166. prosthesis

Answers to Medical Record Analyses

1. a
2. d
3. e
4. b
5. e
6. c
7. a

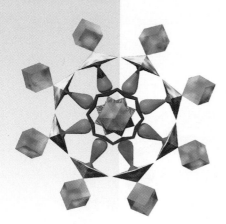

CHAPTER 5

Cardiovascular System

Cardiovascular System Overview

THE HEART (FIG. 5-1)

* The heart is a muscular organ that pumps blood throughout the body.
* The heart consists of four chambers: the *right atrium* and *left atrium* (upper chambers), and the *right ventricle* and *left ventricle* (lower chambers).
* The heart is divided into right and left portions by the *interatrial septum* and the *interventricular septum.*
* Heart valves open and close to maintain the one-way flow of blood through the heart.
* There are three heart layers: the *endocardium* lines the interior cavities of the heart; the *myocardium* is the thick, muscular layer; and the *epicardium* is the outer membrane.
* Enclosing the heart is a loose, protective sac called the *pericardium.*

Blood flow through heart:

1. *Deoxygenated* blood from the body enters the heart through the *superior vena cava* and *inferior vena cava* into the right atrium.
2. With atrial contraction, the tricuspid valve opens, and blood flows into the right ventricle.
3. Contraction of the ventricle pushes blood through the pulmonary semilunar valve into the pulmonary artery.
4. The *pulmonary artery* carries the blood to the lungs and through the *pulmonary circulation* (arteries, capillaries, air sacs, and veins in the lung), where it is oxygenated.
5. Oxygenated blood returns to the heart via the *pulmonary veins* into the left atrium.
6. With atrial contraction, the mitral (bicuspid) valve opens, and blood flows into the left ventricle.
7. Contraction of the left ventricle pushes blood through the aortic valve into the aorta and on to all parts of the body through *systemic circulation* (arteries, arterioles, capillaries, and veins).
8. The heart is first to receive oxygenated blood via the right and left coronary arteries, which distribute blood throughout the entire heart (Fig. 5-2).

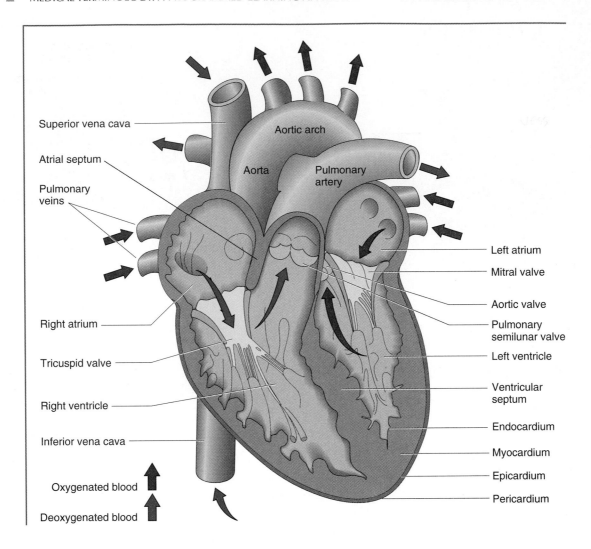

■ **FIGURE 5-1.** Structures of the heart.

SELF-INSTRUCTION: COMBINING FORMS

Study the following:

Combining Form	Meaning
angi/o **vas/o** **vascul/o**	vessel
aort/o	aorta
arteri/o	artery
ather/o	fatty (lipid) paste
atri/o	atrium
cardi/o	heart
coron/o	circle or crown

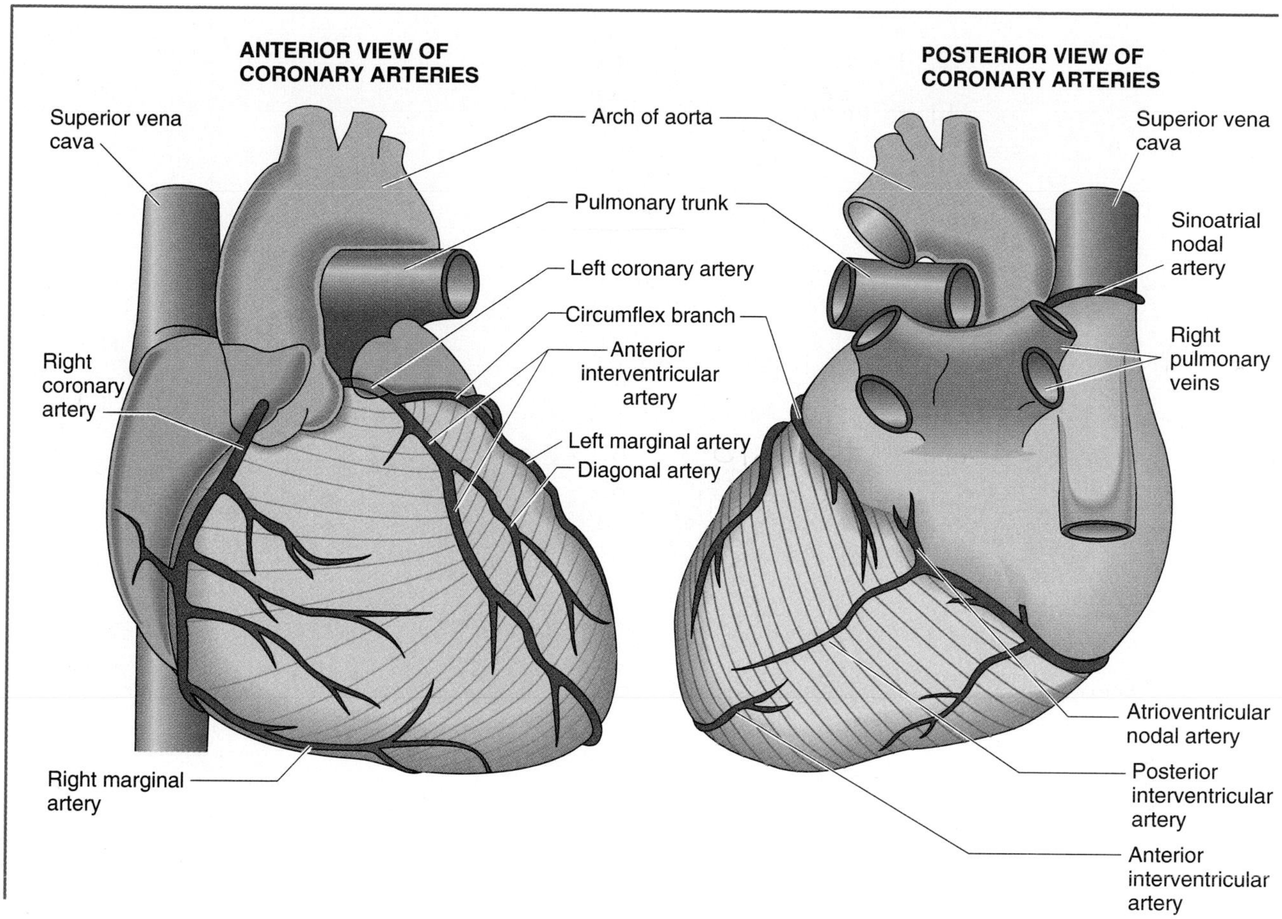

■ **FIGURE 5-2.** Coronary arteries.

my/o	muscle
pector/o steth/o	chest
✓ sphygm/o	pulse
thromb/o	clot
ven/o phleb/o	vein
varic/o	swollen, twisted vein
ventricul/o	ventricle (belly or pouch)

PROGRAMMED REVIEW: COMBINING FORMS

Answer Column	Review
	5.1 A cardiologist is a physician who specializes in the study of the
heart	_____ .

angiogram	**5.2** Formed from *angi/o*, an _____ is an x-ray record of a blood vessel.
vessel	**5.3** Vasospasm is an involuntary contraction of a blood _vessel_.
Cardiology	**5.4** _____ is the medical specialty dealing with the study of the heart.
Thromb/o breaking down or dissolution	**5.5** _thromblo_, the combining form meaning clot, is the subject of thrombolysis, a term referring to the _____ _____ of a clot or clots.
ventricle ventricul/o cardiologist	**5.6** Someone with a congenital ventricular defect is born with an imperfection of a _____ in the heart. (The combining form in this term is _____.) That person would likely be under the care of a _____.
fat (lipids) or fatty paste	**5.7** Atherosclerosis is a condition in which hardened _____ builds up inside blood vessels.
veins phleb/o, vein	**5.8** A phlebotomist is someone trained to draw blood samples from the _____. This title comes from the combining form _____, meaning _____.
varic/o	**5.9** Varicose veins are so named, from the combining form _____, because they are swollen and twisted.
ven/o Arteries	**5.10** Veins, from the combining form _____, return blood to the heart from all around the body. _____, from the root *arteri/o*, carry blood in the other direction—from the heart to the body or lungs.
pector/o	**5.11** The heart is located in the chest, behind the pectoral muscle area. The pectoral muscles get their name from the combining form _____, which means chest. Another combining form that

steth/o

means chest is _____, which is the subject of the term stethoscope, an instrument for listening to the heart or breathing within the chest.

atria

atri/o

ventricul/o

5.12   The heart's four chambers consist of two ventricles and two _____, which is the plural form of atrium. Atrium comes from the combining form _____, and ventricle comes from the combining form _____.

aorta

5.13   The _____, from the combining form *aort/o*, is the large blood vessel through which blood leaves the heart for delivery to all parts of the body. The coronary arteries branch from the aorta and supply the heart muscle tissue, or _____, with blood.

myocardium

circle (or crown)

coronary

The original meaning of *coron/o* refers to a _____. The _____ arteries got their name because they seem to encircle the heart like a crown.

sphygm/o

5.14   Each beat of the heart produces a pulse. The combining form that means pulse is ___Sphygm/o___. This is the key combining form in the term sphygmomanometer, an instrument that measures blood pressure based on its pressurized pulse through an artery. Arteries and

veins

_____ are the two types of larger blood vessels. Along with the capillaries, they are sometimes referred to collectively as the vasculature, from the combining form _____, meaning vessel.

vascul/o

SELF-INSTRUCTION: ANATOMICAL TERMS

Study the following:

Term	Meaning
SEPTA AND LAYERS OF HEART	
atrium ă′ trĕ-ŭm	upper right or left chamber of heart
endocardium en-dō-karēdē-ŭm	membrane lining the cavities of the heart

epicardium *ep-i-kar′dē-ŭm*	membrane forming the outer layer of the heart
interatrial septum *in-ter-ă-trē-ăl sep′tŭm*	partition between right and left atrium
interventricular septum *in-ter-ven-trik′yu-lăr sep′tŭm*	partition between right and left ventricle
myocardium *mī-o-kar′dē-ŭm*	heart muscle
pericardium *per-i-kar′dē-ŭm*	protective sac enclosing the heart composed of two layers with fluid between
ventricle *ven′tri-kăl*	lower right or left chamber of the heart

VALVES OF HEART AND VEINS

heart valves	structures within the heart that open and close with the heartbeat to regulate the one-way flow of blood
aortic valve *ă-or′tik*	heart valve between the left ventricle and the aorta
mitral or bicuspid valve *mī′trăl bī-kŭs′pid*	heart valve between the left atrium and left ventricle (cuspis = point)
pulmonary semilunar valve *pŭl′mō-năr-ē sem-ē-lū′năr*	heart valve opening from the right ventricle to the pulmonary artery (luna = moon)
tricuspid valve *trī-kŭs′pid*	valve between the right atrium and the right ventricle
valves of the veins	valves located at intervals within the lining of veins, especially in the legs, which constrict with muscle action to move the blood returning to the heart

BLOOD VESSELS (FIG. 5-3)

arteries (Fig. 5-4) *ăr′tĕr-ez*	vessels that carry blood from the heart to arterioles
aorta *ă-ōr′tă*	large artery that is the main trunk of the arterial system branching from the left ventricle
arterioles *ăr-tēr′ă-ōlz*	small vessels that receive blood from the arteries

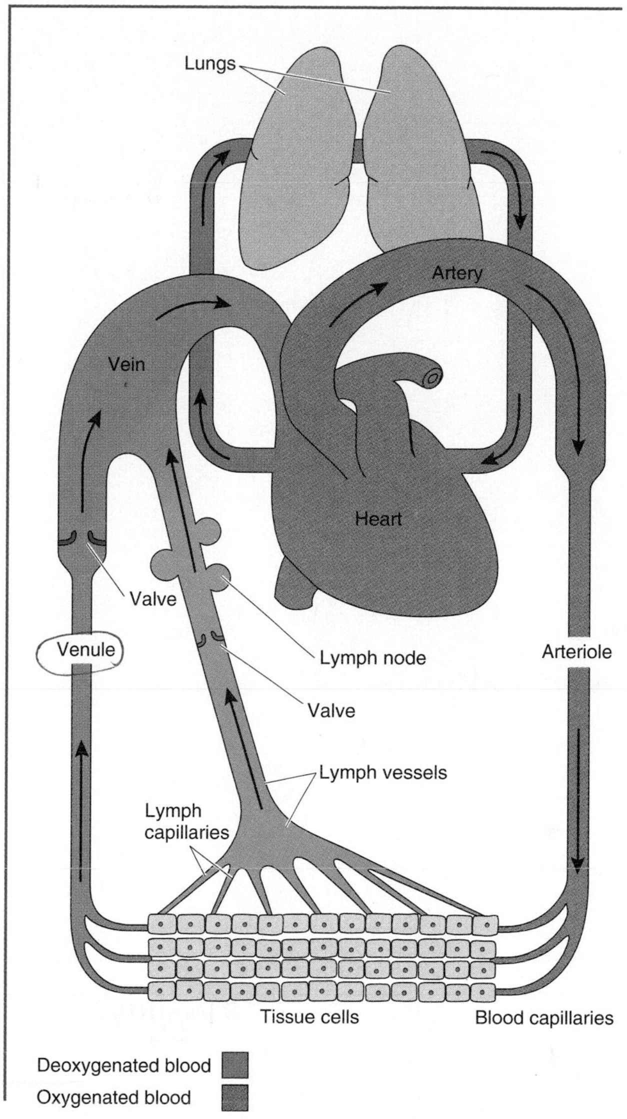

■ FIGURE 5-3. Blood and lymph circulation.

capillaries *kap'I-lār-ēz*	tiny vessels that join arterioles and venules
venules *ven'yūlz*	small vessels that gather blood from the capillaries into the veins
veins (Fig. 5-5) *vānz*	vessels that carry blood to the heart from the venules

CIRCULATION

systemic circulation *sis-tĕm'ik*	circulation of blood throughout the body through arteries, arterioles, capillaries, venules, and veins to deliver oxygen and nutrients to body tissues

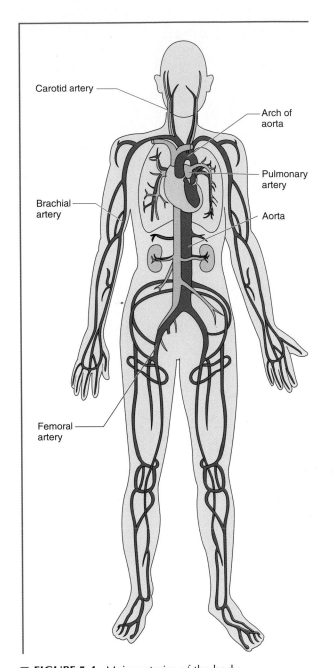

▪ **FIGURE 5-4.** Major arteries of the body.

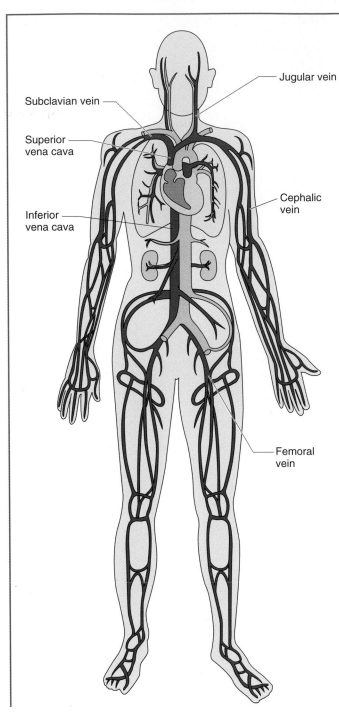

▪ **FIGURE 5-5.** Major veins of the body.

coronary circulation *kor′ō-nār-ē*	circulation of blood through the coronary blood vessels to deliver oxygen and nutrients to the heart muscle tissue
pulmonary circulation *pŭl′mō-nār-ē*	circulation of blood from the pulmonary artery through the vessels in the lungs and back to the heart via the pulmonary vein, providing for the exchange of gases

PROGRAMMED REVIEW: ANATOMICAL TERMS

Answer Column	Review
atri/o atria upper	**5.15** The term atrium is from the combining form _____. The plural form of this word is _____. The right and left atria are the _Upper_ chambers of the heart.
within heart tissue -ium	**5.16** Recall that the prefix *endo-* means _within_. Combined with *cardi/o*, it refers to something within the _heart_. The endocardium is the structure or _____ lining the cavities of the heart. The suffix denoting structure or tissue is _____.
epi- suffix structure, tissue	**5.17** A common prefix, which means upon, is _____. Combined with *cardi/o* and the _____ *-ium*, it forms the term epicardium, which is the _structure_ or _tissue_ forming the outer layer of the heart.
muscle myocardium	**5.18** *My/o* is a combining form meaning _____. The term for heart muscle tissue is _____.
around heart	**5.19** *Peri-* is a prefix that means _____. The pericardium is a protective sac that encloses the _____. It has two layers with fluid between.
ventricul/o lower	**5.20** The ventricles of the heart are so named from the combining form _____, meaning belly or pouch. They are the two _____ chambers of the heart.
between, atria interventricular chambers	**5.21** The term septum refers to an anatomic partition. The interatrial septum is the partition _____ the left and right _____. Between the left and right ventricles is the _____ septum. The two atria and two ventricles are the four _____ of the heart.
valves	**5.22** The one-way blood flow from one heart chamber to another, or from a heart chamber to an artery, is regulated by heart _____,

aortic	which open and close as the heart beats. The valve between the left ventricle and the aorta is the _____ valve.
bicuspid	**5.23** The mitral, or __bicuspid__, valve is between the left atrium and the left ventricle. The tricuspid valve is between the
right, right	__right__ atrium and the _____ ventricle.
pulmonary	**5.24** The pulmonary semilunar valve is between the right ventricle and the _____ artery.
veins	**5.25** Other valves that open and close with muscle action to move blood back to the heart are known as the valves of the _____.
arteries ven/o	**5.26** The names of blood vessels are easy to remember because they are similar to the combining forms. The _____, which carry blood from the heart, are named from arteri/o. The veins, which carry blood to the heart, are named from _____.
arterioles capillaries venules small	**5.27** The _____, also from *arteri/o*, are the small vessels that receive blood from the arteries. The blood then flows to the _____, the tiniest vessels. The blood is then gathered from the capillaries into the _____, small vessels that connect to the veins. The suffixes *-ole* and *-ule* are used to indicate something _____.
aorta	**5.28** The blood leaving the heart for the body first passes through the _____, a large artery that leads to arteries that carry blood throughout the body.
systemic lungs coronary	**5.29** Circulation refers to the flow of the blood through the vessels. The blood flow through the body (except the lungs) is called the _____ circulation. The pulmonary circulation is the blood flow through the _____. The blood flow to the heart muscle, based on the combining form *coron/o*, is the _____ circulation.

SELF-INSTRUCTION: BLOOD PRESSURE TERMS

Study the following:

Term	Meaning
diastole *dī-as′tō-lē*	to expand; period in the cardiac cycle when blood enters the relaxed ventricles from the atria
systole *sis′tō-lē*	to contract; period in the cardiac cycle when the heart is in contraction and blood is ejected through the aorta and pulmonary artery
normotension *nōr-mō-ten′shŭn*	normal blood pressure
hypotension *hī′pō-ten′shŭn*	low blood pressure
hypertension *hī′per-ten′shŭn*	high blood pressure

PROGRAMMED REVIEW: BLOOD PRESSURE TERMS

Answer Column	Review
BP systole diastole	**5.30** Blood pressure, abbreviated _____, is a measurement of the pressure on the walls of the arteries during contraction (_____) and relaxation (_____) of the heart (Fig. 5-6).
blood pressure systole diastole suffix pertaining to systolic diastolic	**5.31** When BP, or _____ _____, is recorded, the contraction phase or _____ is written first, followed by a slash, followed by the relaxation phase or _____. The _____ -ic is used to modify the terms to mean _____ _____. Pertaining to the contraction phase is _____, and pertaining to the relaxation phase is _____.
normo 120, 80 hyper, hypo	**5.32** A blood pressure of 120/80 is considered a normal blood pressure and is termed _normo_tension. The numbers reflect a systolic reading of _____ and a diastolic reading of ____. High blood pressure is _____tension, and low blood pressure is _____tension.

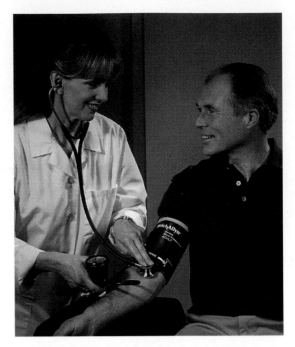

FIGURE 5-6. Blood pressure determination.

SELF-INSTRUCTION: SYMPTOMATIC TERMS

Study the following (Fig. 5-7):

Term	Meaning
arteriosclerosis *ar-tēr´ē´ō´skler-ō´sis*	thickening, loss of elasticity, and calcification (hardening) of arterial walls
atherosclerosis *ath´er-ō-skler-ō´sis*	buildup of fatty substances that harden within the walls of arteries
atheromatous plaque *ath-er-ō´mă-tŭs plak*	a swollen area within the lining of an artery caused by the buildup of fat (lipids)
thrombus *throm´bŭs*	a stationary blood clot

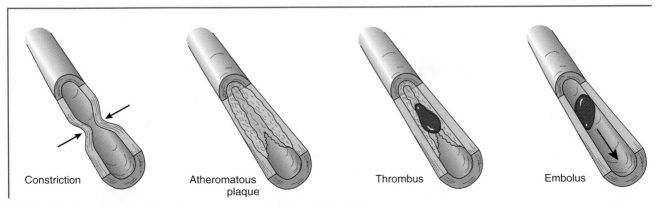

Constriction   Atheromatous plaque   Thrombus   Embolus

■ **FIGURE 5-7.** Examples of conditions causing reduction of blood flow.

embolus *em'bō-lŭs*	a clot (air, fat, foreign object, etc.) carried in the bloodstream that obstructs when it lodges (embolus = a stopper)
<u>**stenosis**</u> *ste-nō'-sis*	condition of <u>narrowing</u> of a part
constriction *kon-strik'shŭn*	compression of a part
occlusion *ŏ-klū'zhŭn*	plugging; obstruction or a closing off
ischemia *to hold back blood* *is-kē'mē-ă*	to hold back blood; decreased blood flow to tissue caused by constriction or occlusion of a blood vessel $\downarrow O_2$
perfusion deficit *per-fyū'zhŭn def'i-sit*	a lack of flow through a blood vessel caused by narrowing, occlusion, etc.
infarct *to stuff* *in'farkt* *chest*	to stuff; a localized area of necrosis (condition of tissue death) caused by ischemia resulting from occlusion of a blood vessel
angina pectoris *an'ji-nă pek'tō-ris*	"chest pain" caused by a temporary loss of oxygenated blood to heart muscle often caused by narrowing of coronary arteries (angina = to choke)
aneurysm (Fig. 5-8) *an'yū-rizm*	a widening; bulging of the wall of the heart, aorta, or artery caused by congenital defect or acquired weakness
saccular aneurysm *săk-ū-lăr*	a saclike bulge on one side
fusiform aneurysm *fū'zŭ-form*	a spindle-shaped bulge
dissecting **aneurysm**	a split or tear of the vessel wall

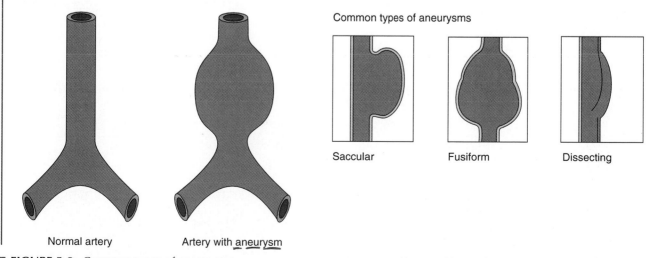

■ **FIGURE 5-8.** Common types of aneurysms.

claudication *klaw-di-kā'shŭn*	to limp; pain in a limb (especially the calf) while walking that subsides after rest; caused by inadequate blood supply
heart murmur *hart mer'mer*	an abnormal sound from the heart produced by defects in the chambers or valves
palpitation *pal-pi-tă'shŭn*	subjective experience of pounding, skipping, or racing heartbeats
vegetation *vej-ĕ-tă'shŭn*	to grow; an abnormal growth of tissue around a valve, generally a result of infection

PROGRAMMED REVIEW: SYMPTOMATIC TERMS

Answer Column	Review
fatty (lipid) paste hard or hardened arteriosclerosis	**5.33** *Ather/o*, you'll recall, means _____. Atherosclerosis is a condition of _____ fatty substances built up within the walls of arteries. The thickening, loss of elasticity, and hardening of arterial walls is called _____.
embolus stationary	**5.34** An ~~embolus~~ → plugge is a clot of any sort carried in the bloodstream that obstructs when it lodges. A (thrombus), on the other hand, is a ___stationary___ blood clot.
stenosis constriction plugging (obstruction)	**5.35** Blood flow through a vessel can be affected by various kinds of restrictions. A _____ is a narrowing, and a _____ is the compression of a vessel. An occlusion also might occur, which is the _____ of a vessel.
ischemia deficit	**5.36** If blood flow is reduced to tissue, ___ischemia___ occurs. When diagnostic tests detect the lack of blood flow from a vessel to tissue cells, it is called a perfusion ___deficit___. Perfusion refers to tissues with an adequate circulation of blood.
angina	**5.37** A heart condition of chest pain may occur when a temporary or transient restriction of blood flow to heart muscle occurs, called ___angina___ pectoris. You'll recall that the combining form

pector/o	_____ refers to the chest. Therefore, this chest pain is called angina pectoris.
death infarct	**5.38** When prolonged or total ischemia occurs in an area, tissue necrosis or __death__ results. The area of scarring from necrosis is called an __infarct__.
bulge (or widen) saccular dissecting	**5.39** An aneurysm can occur in the heart or a blood vessel because of a weakness in the wall. This causes the wall to __buldge__. The type of aneurysm with a saclike bulge is called a __saccular__ aneurysm. If the bulge causes a split or tear of the vessel wall, it is called a __dissecting__ aneurysm.
pain	**5.40** Various symptoms help cardiologists determine what condition a patient is experiencing. Claudication is a __pain__ in a limb, sometimes causing a limp, which results during movement because of an inadequate blood supply to the limb.
palpitation	**5.41** The symptom describing a subjective experience of the heart pounding, skipping, or racing is called __palpitation__. Be careful not to confuse this term with palpation, the word meaning to touch or feel.
murmur	**5.42** The physician, when listening to the heart through a stethoscope, might hear an abnormal sound, called a heart __murmur__, which is produced by a defect in the heart chambers or valves.

Cardiac Conduction

Cardiac conduction provides the electrical stimulus necessary to cause the heart muscle to pump blood by the continual contraction (systole), then relaxation (diastole) of myocardial cells (Fig. 5-9).
   Repeated electrical impulses are conducted:
   1. from the sinoatrial (SA) node (the pacemaker of the heart)
   2. to the atrioventricular (AV) node
   3. to the bundle of His
   4. to the left and right bundle branches
   5. to the Purkinje fibers

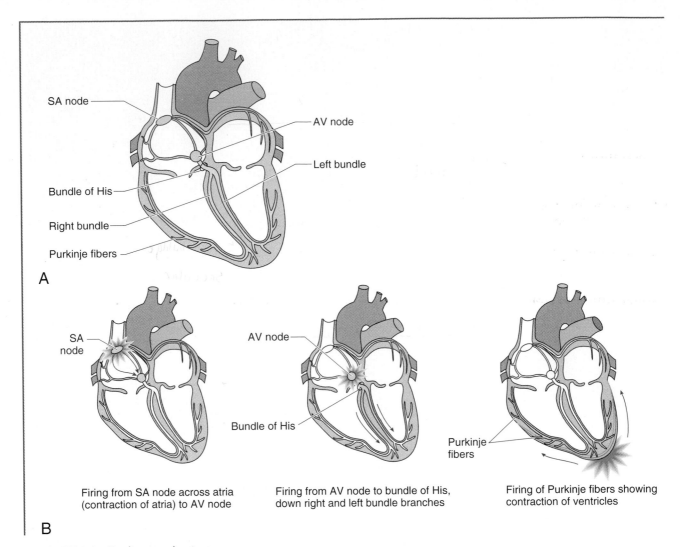

Firing from SA node across atria (contraction of atria) to AV node

Firing from AV node to bundle of His, down right and left bundle branches

Firing of Purkinje fibers showing contraction of ventricles

■ **FIGURE 5-9.** Cardiac conduction.

The impulses cause each myocardial cell to:

1. change from a resting state (polarized)
2. to a state of contraction (depolarized)
3. back to a resting state by recharging (repolarizing)

SELF-INSTRUCTION: CARDIAC CONDUCTION TERMS

Study the following:

Term	Meaning
sinoatrial node (SA node) *sī'nō-ă'trē-ăl nōd*	the pacemaker; highly specialized neurologic tissue impeded in the wall of the right atrium responsible for initiating electrical conduction of the heartbeat, causing the atria to contract and firing conduction of impulses to the AV node
atrioventricular node (AV node) *ă'trē-ō-ven-trik'yū-lăr*	neurologic tissue in the center of the heart that receives and amplifies the conduction of impulses from the SA node to the bundle of His

bundle of His *bŭn'dl*	neurologic fibers extending from the AV node to the right and left bundle branches that fire the impulse from the AV node to the Purkinje fibers
Purkinje fibers (network) *pŭr-kin'jē fi'berz*	fibers in the ventricles that transmit impulses to the right and left ventricles, causing them to contract
polarization *pō'lăr-i-zā'shŭn*	resting; resting state of a myocardial cell
depolarization *dē-pă-lăr-i-zā'shŭn*	change of a myocardial cell from a polarized (resting) state to a state of contraction (de = not; polarization = resting)
repolarization *rē-pō-lăr-i-zā'shŭn*	recharging of the myocardial cell from a contracted state back to a resting state (re = again; polarization = resting)
normal sinus rhythm (NSR)	regular rhythm of the heart cycle stimulated by the SA node (average rate of 60–100 beats per minute) (*see* Fig. 5-14A)

PROGRAMMED REVIEW: CARDIAC CONDUCTION TERMS

Answer Column	Review
sinoatrial AV atri/o, ventricul/o	**5.43** Review Fig. 5-9. SA node refers to the _____ node. Here the heart's electrical impulse originates. This impulse is conducted to the atrioventricular node, or _____ node, a term made from the combining forms _____ and _____.
Purkinje contract	**5.44** The impulse then moves from the Bundle of His down the right and left bundle branches to the _____ fibers, which transmit impulses to the ventricles and cause them to _____. This rhythmic contraction is the heartbeat.
muscle, heart heart muscle	**5.45** *My/o* means _____, and *cardi/o* means _____. Myocardial cells compose the _____ _____.
depolarization repolarization	**5.46** The resting state of myocardial cells is called polarization. When each cell contracts, it changes to a state of _____. The stage of _____ is the change back to a resting state.

	5.47 The normal regular heart rhythm produced by this continued simulation of heart muscle by electrical impulses originating in the
sinoatrial, normal	_____ (SA) node is called _____
sinus	_____ rhythm (NSR).

SELF-INSTRUCTION: DIAGNOSTIC TERMS

Study the following:

Term	Meaning
arrhythmia *ă-rith'mē-ă*	any of several kinds of irregularity or loss of rhythm of the heartbeat (*see* Fig. 5-14)
bradycardia *brad-ē-kar'dē-ă*	slow heart rate (<60 beats/minute) (*see* Fig. 5-14B)
fibrillation *fib-ri-lē'shŭn*	chaotic, irregular contractions of the heart (as in atrial or ventricular fibrillation)
flutter *flŭ'ter*	extremely rapid but regular contractions of the heart (as in atrial or ventricular flutter)
premature ventricular contraction (PVC) *prē-mă-tūr' ven-trik'yū-lăr kon-trak'shŭn*	a ventricular contraction preceding the normal impulse initiated by the SA node (pacemaker)
tachycardia *tak'i'kar'dē-ă*	fast heart rate (>100 beats/minute) (*see* Fig. 5-14C)
arteriosclerotic heart disease (ASHD) *ar-tēr'ē-ō-skler-ot'ik*	a degenerative condition of the arteries characterized by thickening of the inner lining, loss of elasticity, and susceptibility to rupture; seen most often in the aged or smokers
bacterial endocarditis *bak-tēr'ē-ăl en'dō-kar-dī'tis*	a bacterial inflammation that affects the endocardium or the heart valves
cardiac tamponade *kar'dē-ak tam-pŏ-năd'*	compression of the heart produced by the accumulation of fluid in the pericardial sac as can result from pericarditis or trauma, causing rupture of a blood vessel within the heart (tampon = a plug)
cardiomyopathy *kar'dē-ō-mī-op'ă-thē*	a general term for "disease of the heart muscle" [e.g., alcoholic cardiomyopathy (damage to the heart muscle caused by excessive consumption of alcohol)]

congenital anomaly of the heart
kon-jen'i-tăl ă-nom'ă-lē

malformations of the heart present at birth (congenital = born with; anomaly = irregularity)

atrial septal defect (ASD)
ā'trē-ăl sep'tăl dē'fekt

an opening in the septum separating the atria

coarctation of the aorta
kō-ark-tā'shŭn

narrowing of the descending portion of the aorta resulting in a limited flow of blood to the lower part of the body

patent ductus arteriosus
pā'tĕnt dŭk'tŭs ăr-tĕr-ē-ō'sŭs

an abnormal opening between the pulmonary artery and the aorta caused by the failure of the fetal ductus arteriosus to close after birth (patent = open)

ventricular septal defect (VSD)
ven-trik'yū-lăr sep'tăl dē'fekt

an opening in the septum separating the ventricles

congestive heart failure (CHF)
kon-jes'tiv
left ventricular failure

failure of the left ventricle to pump an adequate amount of blood to meet the demands of the body, resulting in a "bottleneck" of congestion in the lungs that may extend to the veins, causing edema in lower portions of the body

cor pulmonale
kō pul-mō-nā'lē
right ventricular failure

enlargement of the right ventricle resulting from chronic disease within the lungs that causes congestion within the pulmonary circulation and resistance of blood flow to the lungs (cor = heart)

coronary artery disease (CAD)
(Fig. 5-10)

a condition affecting arteries of the heart that reduces the flow of blood and delivery of oxygen and nutrients to the myocardium; most often caused by atherosclerosis

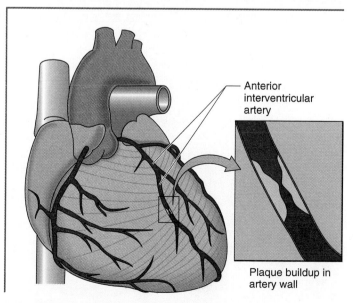

Anterior interventricular artery

Plaque buildup in artery wall

■ **FIGURE 5-10.** Coronary artery disease.

hypertension (HTN) *hī′per-ten′shŭn*	persistently high blood pressure
essential (primary) hypertension *ĕ-sen′shăl hī′per-ten′shŭn*	high blood pressure attributed to no single cause, but risks include smoking, obesity, increased salt intake, hypercholesterolemia, and hereditary factors
secondary hypertension	high blood pressure caused by the effects of another disease (e.g., kidney disease)
mitral valve prolapse (MVP) *mī′trăl*	protrusion of one or both cusps of the mitral valve back into the left atrium during ventricular contraction, resulting in incomplete closure and backflow of blood
myocardial infarction (MI) (Fig. 5-11) *mī-ō-kar′dē-ăl in-fark′shŭn*	heart attack; death of myocardial tissue (infarction) owing to loss of blood flow (ischemia) as a result of an occlusion (plugging) of a coronary artery; usually caused by atherosclerosis
myocarditis *mī′o-kar-dī′tis*	inflammation of myocardium most often caused by viral or bacterial infection
pericarditis *per′i-kar-dī′tis*	inflammation of the pericardium
phlebitis *vein* *flĕ-bī′tis*	inflammation of a vein
rheumatic heart disease *rū-mat′ik*	damage to heart muscle and heart valves by rheumatic fever (a streptococcal infection)

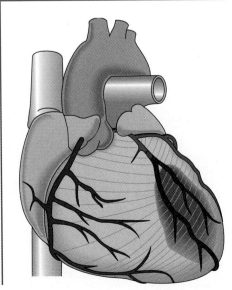

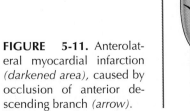

FIGURE 5-11. Anterolateral myocardial infarction *(darkened area)*, caused by occlusion of anterior descending branch *(arrow)*.

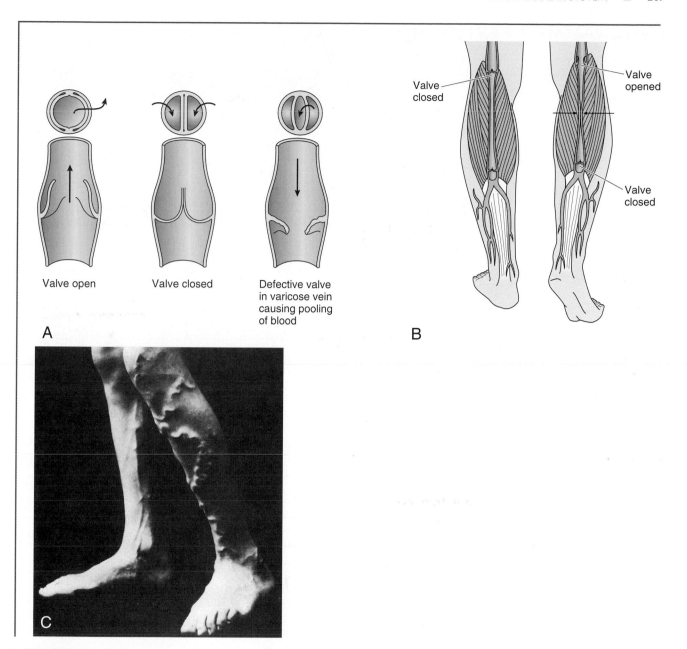

■ **FIGURE 5-12.** Varicose veins. **A.** Function of valves in venous system. **B.** Contraction of skeletal muscle causes valves to open and close, preventing backflow of blood returning to heart. **C.** Varicose veins.

thrombophlebitis *throm'bo-flĕ-bi'tis*	inflammation of a vein associated with a clot formation
varicose veins (Fig. 5-12) *văr'ĭ-kōs*	abnormally swollen twisted veins with defective valves; most often seen in the legs
deep vein thrombosis (DVT) *throm-bō'sis*	formation of a clot in a deep vein of the body, occurring most often in the femoral and iliac veins

PROGRAMMED REVIEW: DIAGNOSTIC TERMS

Answer Column	Review

inflammation

5.48 The suffix *-itis* refers to an _____. Myocarditis therefore means an inflammation of the

myocardium (or heart muscle)

_____. Inflammation of the pericardium is called

pericarditis

_____. Bacterial endocarditis is a bacterial in-

endocardium

flammation affecting the _____ and heart valves.

5.49 The condition of reduced blood flow through the arteries that

coronary artery

supply heart muscle is called _____ _____

disease

_____ (CAD). It most commonly results from a hardened

buildup of fatty substances within the lining of the arteries, a condition

atherosclerosis

known as _____.

5.50 Atherosclerotic buildup within the wall of one or more coronary

arteries can lead to its partial or total obstruction known as an

occlusion

_____. The resulting loss of blood flow, or

ischemia

___*ischemia*___, deprives the affected heart muscle of the oxygen it

death

needs to survive. Necrosis, or condition of ~~myocardial~~ *death* of the myocar-

myocardial

dial tissue, results. This is known as a ___*myocard*___

infarction, heart attack

___*infarctin*___, commonly called a ___*heart*___ ___*attack*___.

muscle

5.51 My*muscle*opathy refers to a condition of diseased _____. The

general term for a condition of diseased heart muscle is

cardiomyopathy

_____.

5.52 The word root tampon means a plug (obstruction), and the term

tamponade refers to an obstruction. A compression of the heart pro-

duced by accumulated fluid in the pericardial sac is called a cardiac

tamponade

_____.

5.53 Another word root that means heart is *cor*. The condition called

pulmonale

cor _____ is caused by congestion in the pulmonary

circulation that results in right ventricular failure. The right ventricle becomes _____ because of the increased effort to pump blood to the diseased lungs.

enlarged

5.54 Congestive _____ failure (CHF) is a failure of the left ventricle to pump out enough blood to the body. This is also called left ventricular _____.

heart

failure

5.55 Anomaly means irregularity (not normal). Congenital pertains to something a person is born _with_. There are several congenital anomalies of the heart. An atrial septal defect is an irregularity in the septum, or _____, that separates the _____. A _____ septal defect is an opening in the septum separating the ventricles.

with

partition, atria

ventricular

5.56 A narrowing of the descending portion of the aorta that restricts blood flow to the lower body is called a _coarctation_ of the aorta.

coarctation

5.57 Patent ductus arteriosus (PDA) is an abnormal opening between the pulmonary artery and the aorta. Patent means open. PDA results if the fetal ductus arteriosus fails to _close_ after birth.

close

5.58 The prefix _a-_ means without. An arrhythmia is a heartbeat _without_ a normal rhythm. The prefix meaning slow is _____. Bradycardia is a condition of _____ heart rate. _Tachy-_ is the prefix meaning _____. _____ is a condition of fast heart rate.

without

brady-, slow

fast, Tachycardia

5.59 Fast, chaotic, irregular contractions of the heart occur in a condition called _fibrillation_. Contractions that are extremely rapid but still regular are called _flutter_.

fibrillation

flutter

contraction

node

5.60 Another common arrhythmia is a premature ventricular _____contraction_____. In this case, the contraction precedes the normal impulse initiated by the SA _node_ .

hypertension, HTN

essential

Secondary

5.61 The condition of persistently high blood pressure is called _____HTN_____ and is abbreviated _____. Primary, or _____essential_____, hypertension cannot be attributed to a single cause. _____Secondary_____ hypertension, however, is caused by another condition, such as kidney disease.

rheumatic

5.62 Rheumatic fever can cause damage to heart muscle and valves. This is called _____rheumatic_____ heart disease.

vein

phlebitis

thrombophlebitis

5.63 *Phleb/o* is a combining term for _vein_ . This, combined with the suffix for inflammation, forms the term _phleb itis_ , which means inflammation of a vein. If that inflammation is associated with a clot formation, the condition is called _thrombo phlebitis_ .

deep vein thrombosis

thrombus

embolus

5.64 The condition of a formed clot in a deep vein of the body is called _deep_ _vein_ _thrombosis_ . The danger of any clot (_thrombus_) formation in a vein is that it can break loose to become a traveling _embolus_ .

SELF-INSTRUCTION: DIAGNOSTIC TESTS AND PROCEDURES

Study the following:

Test or Procedure	Explanation
auscultation *aws-kŭl-tā′shŭn*	a physical examination method of listening to sounds within the body with a stethoscope (e.g., auscultation of the chest for heart and lung sounds)
gallop	an abnormal heart sound that mimics the gait of a horse; related to abnormal ventricular contraction

electrocardiogram (ECG or EKG) (Figs. 5-13 and 5-14) *e-lek-trō-kar'dē-ō-gram*	an electrical picture of the heart represented by positive and negative deflections on a graph labeled with the letters P, Q, R, S, and T, corresponding to events of the cardiac cycle
stress electrocardiogram	an ECG of the heart recorded during the induction of controlled physical exercise using a treadmill or ergometer (bicycle); useful in detecting conditions (e.g., ischemia, infarction)
Holter ambulatory monitor *hōlt er am'byū-lă-tōr-ē mon'i-ter*	a portable electrocardiograph worn by the patient that monitors electrical activity of the heart over 24 hours; useful in detecting periodic abnormalities
magnetic resonance angiography (MRA) *rez'ō-nans an-jē- og'ră-fē*	magnetic resonance imaging of the heart and blood vessels for evaluation of pathology

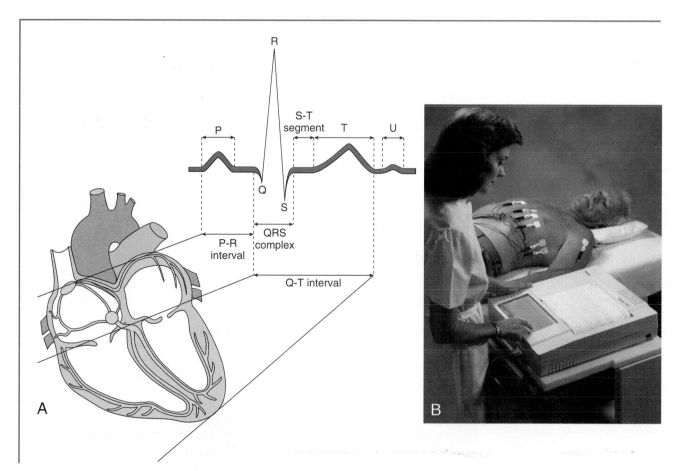

■ **FIGURE 5-13. A.** Electrocardiographic conduction. **B.** Resting electrocardiogram.

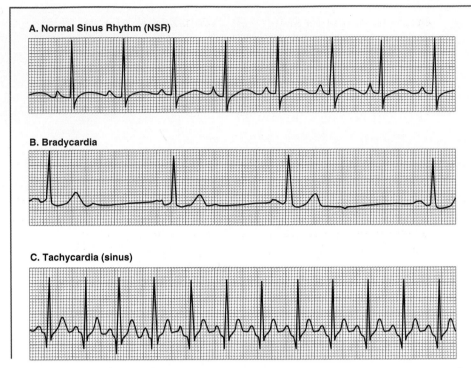

■ FIGURE 5-14. Electrocardiogram tracings showing two types of arrhythmia compared to normal. **A.** Normal sinus rhythm. **B.** Bradycardia. **C.** Tachycardia.

nuclear medicine imaging *nū′klē-ar med′i-sin im′ă-jing*	radionuclide organ imaging
myocardial radionuclide *rā′dē-ō-nū′klīd* **perfusion scan**	a scan of the heart made after an intravenous injection of an isotope (e.g., as thallium) that is absorbed by myocardial cells in proportion to blood flow throughout the heart
myocardial radionuclide perfusion stress scan	nuclear scan of the heart taken before and after the induction of controlled physical exercise (treadmill or bicycle) or a pharmaceutical agent that produces the effect of exercise stress in patients unable to ambulate
radiology	x-ray imaging
angiography *an-jē-og′ră-fē*	the process of x-ray imaging of a blood vessel after injection of contrast medium
angiogram *an′-jē-ō-gram*	record obtained by angiography
coronary angiogram *kōr′o-nār-ē* *an′-jē-ō-gram*	radiograph of the blood vessels of the heart (*see* Fig. 5-20)

Term	Definition
arteriogram *ar-tēr′e-ō-gram*	x-ray of a particular artery (e.g., coronary arteriogram, renal arteriogram)
aortogram *ā-ōr′tō-gram*	x-ray of the aorta
venogram *vē′nō-gram*	x-ray of a vein
cardiac catheterization *kar′dē-ak* *kath′ĕ-ter—zā′shŭn*	introduction of a flexible, narrow tube, or catheter, through a vein or artery into the heart to withdraw samples of blood; to measure pressures within the heart chambers or vessels; and to inject contrast media for fluoroscopic radiography and cine film (motion picture) imaging of the chambers of the heart and coronary arteries. Often includes interventional procedures, such as angioplasty and atherectomy (see endovascular procedures listed under "Operative Terms").
left heart catheterization	x-ray of the left ventricular cavity and coronary arteries
right heart catheterization	measurement of oxygen saturation and pressure readings of the right side of the heart
ventriculogram *ven-trik′ū-lō-gram*	an x-ray visualizing the ventricles
stroke volume (SV)	measurement of amount of blood ejected from a ventricle in one contraction
cardiac output (CO)	measurement of amount of blood ejected from either ventricle of the heart per minute
ejection fraction *ē-jek′shŭn frak′shŭn*	measurement of volume percentage of left ventricular contents ejected with each contraction
sonography	sonographic imaging
echocardiography (ECHO) (Fig. 5-15) *ek′o-kar-de-og″ră-fē*	recording of sound waves through the heart to evaluate structure and motion
stress echocardiogram (stress ECHO)	an echocardiogram of the heart recorded during the induction of controlled physical exercise (treadmill or bicycle) or a pharmaceutical agent that produces the effect of exercise stress in patients unable to ambulate; useful in detecting conditions such as ischemia or infarction
transesophageal echocardiogram (TEE) *trans-ē-sof′ă-jē′ăl*	an echocardiographic image of the heart after placement of an ultrasonic transducer at the end of an endoscope inside the esophagus
Doppler sonography (Fig. 5-16) *Dŏp′lĕr sŏ-nog′ră-fē*	ultrasound technique used to evaluate blood flow to determine the presence of a deep vein thrombosis (DVT) or carotid insufficiency, or to determine flow through the heart, chambers, valves, and so on

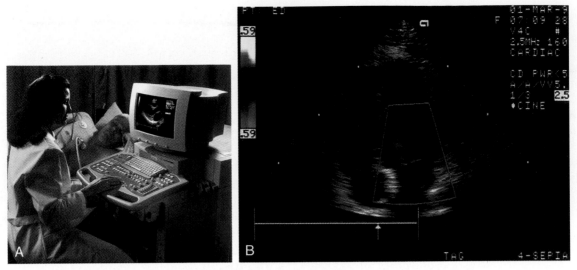

FIGURE 5-15. A. Echocardiography. **B.** Echocardiogram: normal, two-dimensional, apical four-chamber view (standard view of American Society).

PROGRAMMED REVIEW: DIAGNOSTIC TESTS AND PROCEDURE

Answer Column	Review

chest

stethoscope

auscultation

5.65 You'll recall that *steth/o* means _Chest_, and that a

_____ is an instrument for listening to sounds

within the chest or elsewhere in the body. This procedure, from the

Greek word meaning "to listen," is called _auscultation_.

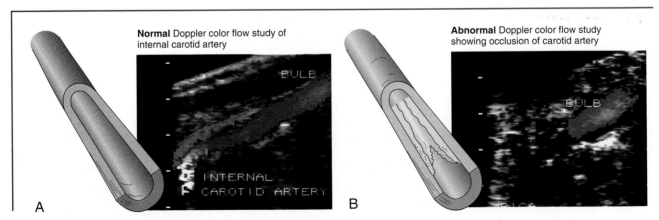

■ **FIGURE 5-16.** Doppler color flow studies. **A.** Normal Doppler color flow study of internal carotid artery. **B.** Abnormal color flow study showing occlusion of carotid artery.

5.66 Auscultation can be used to detect a heart murmur or other abnormal heart sound, such as that which mimics the gait of a horse, called a ___gallop___.

gallop

5.67 The suffix *-gram* refers to a ___record___. *Cardi/o* refers to the ___heart___. A record of the electrical conductivity of the heart is called an _____ (ECG or EKG). A special kind of ECG obtained during the (physical stress of exercise) is called a ___stress___ ___electrocardiogram___.

record

heart

electrocardiogram

stress electrocardiogram

5.68 *Angi/o* refers to a ___vessel___. The suffix *-graphy* refers to the diagnostic process of making a record, such as by x-ray imaging. The process of x-raying a blood vessel is called ___angiography___. The record itself is called an ___angiogram___. A coronary angiogram is an x-ray of the blood vessels encircling the ___heart___.

vessel

angiography

angiogram

heart

5.69 An x-ray of a particular artery is called an arteriogram. An x-ray of the aorta is called an ___aortogram___. An x-ray of a vein is called a ___venogram___.

aortogram

venogram

5.70 A catheter can be introduced into the heart for diagnostic purposes. This is called ___cardiac___ ___catheterization___. Left heart catheterization is usually done to obtain a radiograph of the left ventricular cavity and coronary arteries, and ___right___ heart catheterization is usually done to measure ___oxygen___ saturation and pressure.

cardiac catheterization

right

oxygen

5.71 An x-ray of the <u>ventricles</u> is a _____, from the combining form *ventricul/o* and the suffix _____.

ventriculogram

-gram

5.72 Cardiac catheterization also allows for measurement of stroke volume (SV), or how much blood is ejected from a ventricle in one ___contraction___; cardiac ___output___ (CO) measures the amount of blood ejected from either ventricle per minute; ejection fraction measures the volume percentage of the ___left___ ventricle's contents ___ejected___ with each contraction.

contraction, output

left

ejected

angiography	**5.73** MRA stands for magnetic resonance ___Angiography___, which is a specialized imaging of the heart and blood vessels.
radionuclide organ imaging	**5.74** Nuclear medicine imaging, also known as _____ _____ _____, uses radioactive isotopes to visualize body structures and to analyze
functions, radionuclide	_____. A myocardial _____
heart, intravenous	perfusion scan is made of the ___heart___ after _____
myo	(IV) injection of an isotope is absorbed by ___myo___cardial cells in pro-
blood	portion to ___blood___ flow.
ultrasound	**5.75** Sonography, or diagnostic ___ultrasound___, is the imag-
sound	ing modality using high-frequency ___sound___ waves to visualize body tissues. The recording of sound waves through the heart to evalu-
echo	ate structure and motion is called ___echo___ cardiography.
echocardiogram	**5.76** A record of the heart made with echocardiography is called an _____. Made during controlled exercise, it
stress	is called a _____ echocardiogram. Made after passing the trans- ducer through the esophagus, it is called a
transesophageal	___Trans esophageal___ echocardiogram (TEE).
Doppler	**5.77** The type of sonography using ultrasound to evaluate blood flow is called ___Doppler___ sonography.

SELF-INSTRUCTION: OPERATIVE TERMS

Study the following:

Term	Meaning
Procedures performed in traditional operating room setting	
coronary artery bypass graft (CABG, which is pronounced "cabbage") (Fig. 5-17)	grafting of a portion of a blood vessel retrieved from another part of the body (such as a length of saphenous vein from the leg or mammary artery from the chest wall) to bypass an occluded coronary artery restoring circulation to myocardial tissue

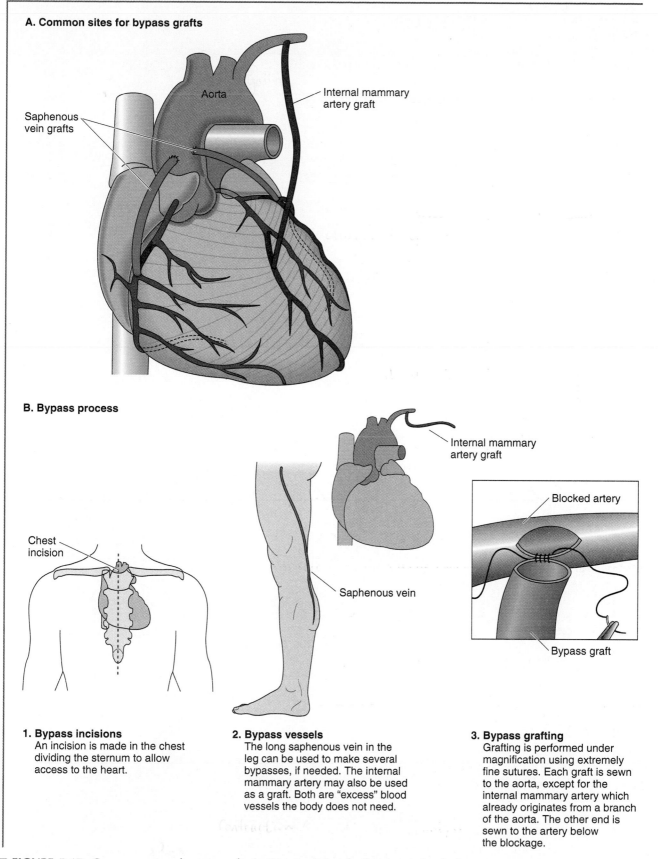

A. Common sites for bypass grafts

Aorta

Internal mammary artery graft

Saphenous vein grafts

B. Bypass process

Internal mammary artery graft

Chest incision

Saphenous vein

Blocked artery

Bypass graft

1. Bypass incisions
An incision is made in the chest dividing the sternum to allow access to the heart.

2. Bypass vessels
The long saphenous vein in the leg can be used to make several bypasses, if needed. The internal mammary artery may also be used as a graft. Both are "excess" blood vessels the body does not need.

3. Bypass grafting
Grafting is performed under magnification using extremely fine sutures. Each graft is sewn to the aorta, except for the internal mammary artery which already originates from a branch of the aorta. The other end is sewn to the artery below the blockage.

■ **FIGURE 5-17.** Coronary artery bypass graft. **A.** Common sites for bypass grafts. **B.** Bypass grafting.

anastomosis *ă-nas'tō-mō'sis*	opening; joining of two blood vessels to allow flow from one to the other
valve replacement	replacement of a diseased heart valve with an artificial one
valvuloplasty *val'vyū-lō-plas-tē*	surgical repair of a heart valve
transmyocardial revascularization (TMR)	a laser technique used to open tiny channels in the heart muscle to restore blood flow, thereby relieving angina in patients who have advanced coronary artery disease
endovascular surgery (Fig. 5-18)	interventional procedures performed at the time of cardiac catheterization in a specialized laboratory setting or "cath lab" instead of the traditional operating room
angioscopy (vascular endoscopy) *an-jē-os'kō-pē*	use of a flexible fiberoptic angioscope (accompanied by an irrigation system, camera, video recorder, and monitor) that is guided through a specific blood vessel to visually assess a lesion and to select the mode of therapy
arteriotomy *ăr-tēr-ē-ot'ō-mē*	an incision into an artery

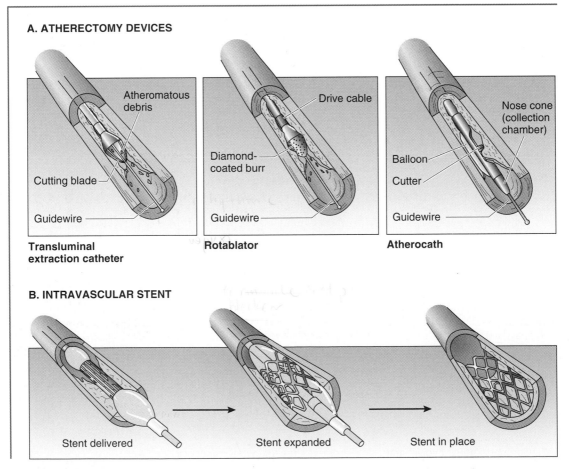

■ **FIGURE 5-18.** Examples of devices used in endovascular interventional procedures. **A.** Atherectomy devices. **B.** Intravascular stent.

atherectomy *ăth-er-ek′tō-mē* (Fig. 5-19, A)	excision of atheromatous plaque from within an artery utilizing a device housed in a flexible catheter that selectively cuts away or pulverizes tissue buildup
embolectomy *em-bō-lek′tō-mē*	incision into an artery for the removal of an embolus
thrombectomy *throm-bek′tō-mē*	incision into an artery for the removal of a thrombus
endarterectomy *end-ar-ter-ek′tō-mē*	surgical removal of the lining of an artery to clear a blockage caused by a clot or atherosclerotic plaque buildup
percutaneous transluminal coronary angioplasty (PTCA) (Fig. 5-19) *per-kyū-tā′nē-ŭs* *trăns-lū′mĭ-năl* *kōr′o- nār-ē* *an′jē-ō-plas-tē*	a method of treating the narrowing of a coronary artery by inserting a specialized catheter with a balloon attachment, then inflating it to dilate and open the narrowed portion of the vessel and restore blood flow to the myocardium
intravascular stent *in′tra-vas′kyū-lăr* (Fig 5-19B)	implantation of a device used to reinforce the wall of a vessel and assure its patency (openness)—most often used to treat a stenosis or a dissection (a split or tear in the wall of a vessel) or to reinforce patency of a vessel after angioplasty

PERCUTANEOUS TRANSLUMINAL CORONARY ANGIOPLASTY (PCTA)

Pre-dilation angiogram revealing 99% stenosis of the right coronary artery (RCA).

PTCA procedure showing catheter placement and straddling of the balloon at the occluded site.

Post-PTCA angiogram showing successful dilation

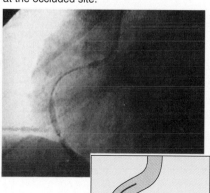
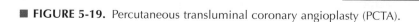
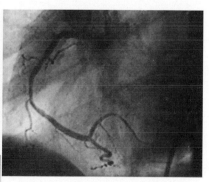

Catheter and wire placement with balloon inflation

■ **FIGURE 5-19.** Percutaneous transluminal coronary angioplasty (PCTA).

PROGRAMMED REVIEW: OPERATIVE TERMS

Answer Column	Review

vessel angioscope	**5.78** The suffix *-scopy* refers to the process of examination. Angioscopy is the examination of a blood _____ using a fiberoptic _____.
incision arteriotomy	**5.79** The suffix *-tomy* refers to an _____. An incision into an artery is called an _____.
-ectomy embolus thrombectomy atherectomy endartectomy	**5.80** The suffix _____ refers to removal or excision. An embolectomy is the surgical removal of an _____ from within an artery. A _____ is the removal of a thrombus. Removal of an atheromatous plaque is called an _____. Surgical removal of the lining of an artery (using the prefix *endo-*) is an _____.
bypass graft	**5.81** CABG is the abbreviation for a coronary artery _____ _____, in which a portion of a blood vessel is grafted in place to bypass an occluded coronary artery.
vessels	**5.82** An anastomosis is the joining of two blood _____ to allow flow from one to the other.
valvuloplasty	**5.83** The suffix *-plasty* refers to a surgical repair. A _____ is the repair of a heart valve.
vessel coronary angioplasty	**5.84** An angioplasty is the surgical repair of a blood _____. A specialized procedure called a percutaneous transluminal _____ _____ (PTCA) is a treatment for a narrowed coronary artery.
stent	**5.85** An intravascular _____ is implanted to keep a blood vessel open and to reinforce the vessel's wall.

Transmyocardial	**5.86** _____
revascularization	_____ (TMR) is a laser technique
	used to open tiny channels in the heart muscle to restore blood flow in
coronary artery	patients with advanced _____ _____
disease	_____ (CAD).

SELF-INSTRUCTION: THERAPEUTIC TERMS

Study the following:

Terms	Meaning
defibrillation _dē-fib-ri-lā'shŭn_	termination of ventricular fibrillation by delivering an electrical stimulus to the heart; most commonly done by applying electrodes of the defibrillator externally to the chest wall but can be performed internally during open heart surgery or via an implanted device
defibrillator _dē-fib-ri-lāter_	device that delivers the electrical stimulus in defibrillation
cardioversion _kar'dē-ō-ver'zhŭn_	termination of tachycardia either by pharmaceutical means or by delivery of electrical energy
implantable cardioverter defibrillator (ICD) _kar'dē-o-ver'ter_ _dē-fib-ri-lā'ter_	an implanted, battery-operated device with rate sensing leads; the device monitors cardiac impulses and initiates an electrical stimulus as needed to stop ventricular fibrillation or tachycardia
pacemaker (Fig. 5-20)	a device used to treat slow heart rates (bradycardia) by electrically stimulating the heart to contract; most often implanted with lead wires and battery circuitry under the skin but can be temporarily placed externally with lead wires inserted into the heart via a vein

PROGRAMMED REVIEW: THERAPEUTIC TERMS

Answer Column	Review
	5.87 The term for a condition of slow heart is
bradycardia	_____. A device that is surgically implanted to
	make a slow heart maintain an adequate pace is called a
pacemaker	_____.

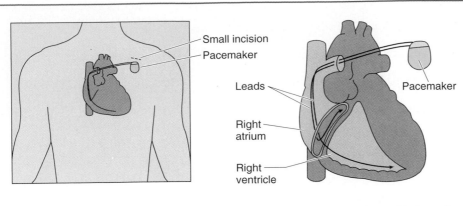

| Small incision |
| Pacemaker |
| Leads |
| Pacemaker |
| Right atrium |
| Right ventricle |

A small incision is made in the upper chest, below the clavicle, to access a large vein nearby.

A

The pacemaker leads are then guided through the vein and into the heart. After proper placement is determined, the leads are secured in position.

A small "pocket" to house the pacemaker is created just under the skin at the incision site. The leads are connected to the pacemaker that is secured in the "pocket." Finally the incision is closed with a few sutures.

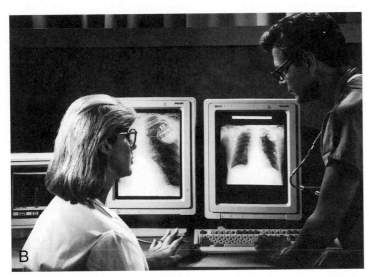

B

■ **FIGURE 5-20.** Pacemaker. **A.** Endocardial pacemaker. **B.** Teleradiology/critical care workstation chest radiographs on screen show pacemaker placement.

---

fast

terminate or stop

5.88 Tachycardia is a condition of _____ heart rate. <u>Cardioversion</u> is a way to _~~terminate or stop~~_ tachycardia, <u>either by use of a drug</u> <u>or by electrical energy.</u>

5.89 Chaotic, irregular contractions of the heart are called

fibrillation

not

defibrillator

_____*fibrillation*_____. *De-* is a prefix that means from, down, or

__*hot*__. A device used on a patient to stop ventricular fibrillation is

called a ___*de fibrillator*___. The process of doing so is

called defibrillation.

5.90 An implantable device that initiates an electrical stimulus to stop ventricular fibrillation or tachycardia is called an

implantable cardioverter

defibrillator

Implantable _cardioverter_ _defibrillator_ (ICD).

SELF-INSTRUCTION: COMMON THERAPEUTIC DRUG CLASSIFICATIONS

Study the following:

Term	Meaning
angiotensin-converting enzyme (ACE) inhibitor _ăn'jē-ō-tĕn'sin kŏn-vĕr'ting ĕn'zĭm_	a drug that suppresses the conversion of angiotensin in the blood by the angiotensin-converting enzyme; used in the treatment of hypertension _ACE_ _Angiotensin → Angioten I_
antianginal _an'tē-an'ji-năl_	a drug that dilates coronary arteries, restoring oxygen to the tissues to relieve the pain of angina pectoris
antiarrhythmic _an'tē-ă-rith'mik_	a drug that counteracts cardiac arrhythmia
anticoagulant _an'tē-kō-ag'yū-lant_	a drug that prevents clotting of the blood.
antihypertensive _an'tē-hī-per-ten'siv_	a drug that lowers blood pressure
beta-adrenergic blocking agents _bā'tă ad-rĕ-ner'jik blok'ing_ **beta blockers** _bā'tă-blok'ers_	agents that inhibit responses to sympathetic adrenergic nerve activity, causing a slowing of electrical conduction and heart rate and a lowering of the pressure within the walls of the vessels; used to treat angina pectoris and hypertension
calcium channel blockers _kal'sē-ŭm chan'l blok'ers_	agents that inhibit the entry of calcium ions in heart muscle cells, causing a slowing of the heart rate, lessening the demand for oxygen and nutrients, and relaxing of the smooth muscle cells of the blood vessels to cause dilation; used to prevent or treat angina pectoris, some arrhythmias, and hypertension
cardiotonic _kar'dē-ō-ton'ik_	a drug that increases the force of myocardial contractions in the heart; commonly used to treat congestive heart failure
diuretic _dī-yū-ret'ik_	a drug that increases the secretion of urine; commonly prescribed in treating hypertension

hypolipidemic *hī-pō-lip′i-dē′mik*	a drug that reduces serum fat and cholesterol
thrombolytic agents	drugs used to dissolve thrombi (blood clots) (e.g., streptokinase or tissue plasminogen activator [TPA or tPA])
vasoconstrictor	a drug that causes a narrowing of the blood vessels, decreasing blood flow
vasodilator	a drug that causes dilation of the blood vessels, increasing blood flow

PROGRAMMED REVIEW: COMMON THERAPEUTIC DRUG CLASSIFICATIONS

Answer Column	Review
against (or opposed to) coagulation (clotting) hypertensive	**5.91** The prefix *anti-* means _____. A class of drugs called anticoagulants work to prevent _____. A drug that lowers high blood pressure is called an anti_____.
chest pain antianginal dilator myocardium	**5.92** Angina pectoris, you'll recall, is _____ _____. Drugs that treat this pain are classified as _____ drugs. Nitroglycerin is a common antianginal medication. It acts as a vaso___*dilator*___, causing the coronary arteries to expand, increasing the <u>flow of blood</u> to the <u>heart muscle tissue</u>, or ___*myocardium*___.
arrhythmic	**5.93** A drug that counteracts a <u>cardiac arrhythmia</u> is called an anti⟩ *arrhythmic* _____.
beta blockers	**5.94** A number of different drug classifications are used to treat hypertension. Beta-adrenergic blocking agents, also called more simply ___*beta*___ ___*blockers*___, work by inhibiting responses to a nerve activity and slowing electrical conduction and heart rate.
calcium channel	**5.95** Another type of antihypertensive drug works by inhibiting the entry of calcium ions in heart muscle cells, <u>therefore slowing the heart and causing other changes.</u> These are called ___*calcium*___ ___*channel*___ blockers.

urine	**5.96** Another antihypertensive drug, called a diuretic, works by increasing the secretion of _____ from the body.
tonic	**5.97** Congestive heart failure is often treated with drugs that increase the force of ventricular contractions. These drugs are called cardio _tonic_ agents.
hypolipid	**5.98** Lipids, you'll recall, are fats. Drugs that lower (term built with the prefix *hypo*-) the amount of fat in the blood are called _____emic agents.
breaking down (dissolution) clots thrombo	**5.99** *-Lysis* is a suffix meaning _____. Drugs that work to dissolve thrombi or _____ in the blood are called _____lytic agents.

Practice Exercises

For the following terms, on the lines below the term, write out the indicated word parts: prefixes, combining forms, roots, and suffixes. Then define the term.

For example:
pericardial

peri/cardi/al
P   R   S

DEFINITION: around/heart/pertaining to

1. angiography

   _____ / _____
      CF   S

   DEFINITION: _____

2. varicosis

   _____ / _____
      R   S

   DEFINITION: _____

3. pectoral

   _____ / _____
      R   S

   DEFINITION: _____

4. vasospasm

_____ / _____
     CF   S

DEFINITION: _____

5. venous

_____ / _____
     R   S

DEFINITION: _____

6. aortocoronary

_____ / _____ / _____
     CF   R   S

DEFINITION: _____

7. thrombophlebitis

_____ / _____ / _____
     CF   R   S

DEFINITION: _____

8. arteriosclerosis

_____ / _____ / _____
     CF   R   S

DEFINITION: _____

9. vasculopathy

_____ / _____ / _____
     CF   R   S

DEFINITION: _____

10. atherogenesis

_____ / _____
     CF   S

DEFINITION: _____

11. stethoscope

_____ / _____
     CF   S

DEFINITION: _____

12. myocardium

_____ / _____ / _____
     CF   R   S

DEFINITION: _____

13. aortoplasty

_____ / _____
     CF   S

DEFINITION: _____

14. venostomy

_____ / _____
     CF   S

DEFINITION: _____

15. arteriostenosis

_____ / _____ / _____
     CF   R   S

DEFINITION: _____

16. phlebotomy

_____ / _____
     CF   S

DEFINITION: _____

17. cardioaortic

_____ / _____ / _____
     CF   R   S

DEFINITION: _____

18. ventriculogram

_____ / _____
     CF   S

DEFINITION: _____

19. phlebitis

_____ / _____
     R   S

DEFINITION: _____

20. angioplasty

_____ / _____
     CF   S

DEFINITION: _____

21. endovascular

_____ / _____ / _____
     P   R   S

DEFINITION: _____

22. cardiotoxic

_____ / _____ / _____
       CF   R   S

DEFINITION: _____

23. arteriogram

_____ / _____
       CF   S

DEFINITION: _____

24. atherectomy

_____ / _____
       R   S

DEFINITION: _____

25. cardiac

_____ / _____
       R   S

DEFINITION: _____

Match the following terms with their meanings:

26. ____ atherosclerosis   a. high blood pressure

27. ____ infarct   b. bulging of a vessel

28. ____ hypotension   c. stationary clot

29. ____ vegetation   d. cramp in leg muscle

30. ____ embolus   e. normal blood pressure

31. ____ occlusion   f. hard, nonelastic condition

32. ____ hypertension   g. traveling clot that obstructs when it lodges

33. ____ thrombus   h. buildup of fat

34. ____ constriction   i. growth of tissue

35. ____ normotension   j. a plugging

36. ____ angina   k. loss of blood flow

37. ____ claudication   l. squeezed

38. ____ ischemia   m. cramp in heart muscle

39. ____ arteriosclerosis   n. low blood pressure

40. ____ aneurysm   o. scar left by necrosis

Write the correct medical term for each of the following:

41. _____ malformations of the heart present at birth

42. _____ thickening, loss of elasticity, and calcification (hardening) of arterial walls

43. _____ irregularity or loss of rhythm of the heartbeat

44. _____ a general term for disease of the heart muscle

45. _____ joining of two blood vessels to allow flow from one to the other

46. _____ an abnormal heart sound that mimics the gait of a horse

47. _____ a recording of sound waves directed through the heart to evaluate structure and motion

48. _____ a condition of enlargement of the right ventricle as a result of chronic disease within the lungs

49. _____ an x-ray of the blood vessels of the heart made with the introduction of a catheter and release of a contrast medium

50. _____ electrocardiogram of the heart recorded during controlled physical exercise

Write in the missing words on the lines in the following illustration of the heart's anatomy:

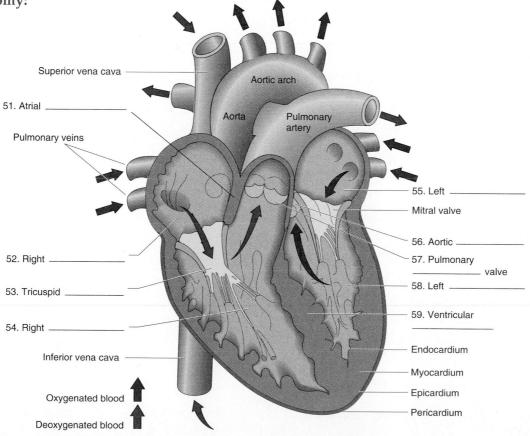

Superior vena cava

Aortic arch

Aorta

Pulmonary artery

51. Atrial _____

Pulmonary veins

55. Left _____

Mitral valve

56. Aortic _____

57. Pulmonary _____ valve

52. Right _____

58. Left _____

53. Tricuspid _____

59. Ventricular _____

54. Right _____

Endocardium

Myocardium

Inferior vena cava

Epicardium

Pericardium

Oxygenated blood

Deoxygenated blood

Write the full medical term for the following abbreviations:

60. PVC _____

61. PDA _____

62. ASHD _____

63. ICD _____

64. CHF _____

65. CAD _____

66. HTN _____

67. MVP _____

68. MRA _____

69. VSD _____

Match the following abbreviations with their meanings:

70. ____ ECG   a. balloon angioplasty

71. ____ tPA   b. magnetic resonance of blood vessels

72. ____ MRA   c. a clot in a vein

73. ____ PTCA   d. heart bypass surgery

74. ____ MI   e. electrical picture of heart

75. ____ DVT   f. echocardiogram directed through the esophagus

76. ____ ASD   g. left ventricular failure

77. ____ CABG   h. thrombolytic drug

78. ____ TEE   i. an abnormal opening in the atrial septum

79. ____ CHF   j. heart attack

For each of the following, circle the correct spelling of the term:

80. ventricel	ventrical	ventricle
81. aorta	aorto	aorrta
82. thrombos	thrombus	thrommbus
83. myocardial	mycardial	myocardiol
84. hypatension	hyptension	hypotension
85. diastolie	diastoly	diastole
86. ischemia	ishchemia	ishemia
87. oclusion	occlusion	ocllusion

88. infart	enfarct	infarct
89. anuerysm	aneurysm	annurysm
90. atherosclerotic	atherosclerrotic	atherasclerotic
91. thromboflebitus	thromboflebitis	thrombophlebitis
92. anngiogram	angiogram	angeogram
93. defibrillation	defibillation	defibrilation
94. antarhythmic	antiarrhythmic	antiarhythmic

Write the term that means the opposite of the terms given:

95. vasoconstriction _____

96. coagulant _____

97. hypotension _____

98. fibrillation _____

99. bradycardia _____

100. normal sinus rhythm _____

101. polarization _____

102. diastole _____

For each of the following, circle the combining form that corresponds to the meaning given:

103. **chest**	phleb/o	sphygm/o	pector/o
104. **vein**	aort/o	phleb/o	varic/o
105. **vessel**	angi/o	arteri/o	coron/o
106. **heart**	ven/o	coron/o	cardi/o
107. **fatty paste**	aort/o	ather/o	atri/o
108. **circle**	cardi/o	coron/o	sphygm/o
109. **pulse**	sphygm/o	steth/o	thromb/o
110. **clot**	atri/o	angi/o	thromb/o
111. **artery**	arteri/o	angi/o	aort/o
112. **belly or pouch**	varic/o	ventricul/o	ven/o

Medical Record Analyses

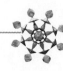

MEDICAL RECORD 5-1

Progress Note

S: This 54 y.o. ♂ was admitted to CCU with onset of acute anterior chest pain radiating to the left shoulder and SOB; pt underwent a CABG x 4 six months ago.

O: BP 190/110, P 100, R 72, T 38°C
On PE, pt was in moderate to severe distress. An ECG showed sinus tachycardia, and a CXR revealed ventricular hypertrophy.

A: R/O MI

P: Order blood enzyme measurement STAT
echocardiogram
CT scan of chest

1. What is the patient's CC?
   a. severe angina
   b. angina developing slowly over time
   c. enlargement of the heart
   d. fast heart rate
   e. slow heart rate

2. Describe the procedure that the patient underwent 6 months ago:
   a. surgery to dilate and open narrowed portions of coronary arteries
   b. replacement of occluded arteries with transplanted portions of vein
   c. replacement of a diseased heart valve
   d. coring of the lining of an artery to remove a clot
   e. heart transplant

3. Where was the patient treated?
   a. outpatient medical office
   b. outpatient emergency room
   c. inpatient intensive care
   d. inpatient coronary care
   e. outpatient cardiology department

4. What type of physician is most appropriate to provide initial care and assessment of this patient?
   a. emergency room physician
   b. internist
   c. gerontologist
   d. cardiovascular surgeon
   e. cardiologist

5. What did the electrical picture of the heart reveal?
   a. extremely rapid but regular contractions of the heart
   b. slow heart rate
   c. chaotic, irregular contractions of the heart
   d. fast heart rate
   e. interference with normal electrical conduction of the heart known as a block

6. What was the assessment?
   a. patient may have had a heart attack
   b. patient may be suffering from right heart failure
   c. patient has congestive heart failure
   d. patient may have high blood pressure
   e. patient may have an enlarged heart

7. What were the objective findings of the chest radiograph?
   a. unknown
   b. enlargement of the heart
   c. vessel disease
   d. dead heart muscle
   e. fast heart rate

8. Identify the x-ray imaging procedure ordered in the plan:
   a. sonogram of heart
   b. chest radiography
   c. blood pressure
   d. computed tomography
   e. biochemistry panel

MEDICAL RECORD 5-2

CENTRAL MEDICAL CENTER
211 Medical Center Drive • Central City, US 90000-1234 • PHONE: (012) 125-6784 • FAX: (012) 125-9999

CARDIAC CATHETERIZATION

DATE OF PROCEDURE: November 3, 20xx

PROCEDURE PERFORMED: Left heart catheterization with left ventriculography, left and right coronary arteriography.

INDICATIONS: Recent onset of angina pectoris.

CATHETERS USED: 6 French pigtail Cordis, 6 French JL4, 6 French JR4.

CONTRAST: Optiray-320.

MEDICATIONS GIVEN: None.

PROCEDURE IN DETAIL:
Informed consent was obtained. The patient was brought to the Cardiac Catheterization Laboratory where the right groin was prepped and draped in the usual sterile fashion. The skin was anesthetized with 1% Xylocaine. The right femoral artery was entered by Seldinger technique and a 7 French Cordis sheath was inserted through which a 7 French angled pigtail catheter was inserted and advanced under fluoroscopic guidance to the descending thoracic aorta. Heparin was administered. Arterial pressures were recorded. The pigtail catheter was then advanced across the aortic valve to the left ventricle. Pressures were recorded, and left ventriculography was performed by power injection of 40 cc of contrast at 12 cc per second with cine in the RAO projection. Post ventriculography pressures were recorded, and pullback across the aortic valve was performed. The pigtail catheter was exchanged for a left coronary catheter as listed above which was advanced to the ostium of the left coronary artery. Left coronary arteriography was performed by hand injections of 8-10 cc of contrast with cine in multiple views. The left coronary catheter was exchanged for the right coronary catheter, as listed above, and it was then advanced to the ostium of the right coronary artery. Right coronary arteriography was performed by hand injections of 8-10 cc of contrast with cine in multiple views. The right coronary catheter and femoral artery sheath were removed, and hemostasis was obtained by C-clamp pressure for 30-45 minutes. Complications: None. Fluoro time: 2.2 minutes. Contrast dose: 76 cc.

(continued)

CARDIAC CATHETERIZATION Page 1	PT. NAME: SMITH, W. ID NO: ROOM NO: ATT. PHYS: R. GALASSO, M.D.

MEDICAL RECORD 5-2 CONTINUED

CENTRAL MEDICAL CENTER

211 Medical Center Drive • Central City, US 90000-1234 • PHONE: (012) 125-6784 • FAX: (012) 125-9999

CARDIAC CATHETERIZATION

FINDINGS:

1. HEMODYNAMICS:
   Left ventricle: 182/0; end-diastolic: 16 mm Hg. Aorta: 190/70; mean: 110 mm Hg.

2. LEFT VENTRICULOGRAPHY:
   The left ventricle is normal in configuration, dimensions, and segmental wall motion with ejection fraction computed at 58% by area-length method. There is no evidence of mitral regurgitation.

3. CORONARY ARTERIOGRAPHY:
   <u>Left Main:</u> Normal.

   <u>Left Anterior Descending:</u> Seventy percent focal stenosis immediately after the first septal perforator branch. The remainder of the left anterior descending is within normal limits.

   <u>Ramus Intermedius:</u> Normal.

   <u>Left Circumflex:</u> Nondominant vessel with one marginal branch, all free of disease.

   <u>Right Coronary Artery:</u> Large dominant vessel free of disease.

CONCLUSIONS:

1. MODERATE STENOSIS OF THE LEFT ANTERIOR DESCENDING CORONARY ARTERY.

2. NORMAL LEFT VENTRICULAR FUNCTION WITH EJECTION FRACTION 56%.

RECOMMENDATIONS:
The patient will be managed medically at this time. Radionuclide perfusion stress testing will be performed. If the patient has progressive anginal symptoms or has marked reversible ischemia in the distribution of the left anterior descending coronary artery, angioplasty of this vessel would be considered.

CARDIAC CATHETERIZATION Page 2	PT. NAME: SMITH, W. ID NO: ROOM NO: ATT. PHYS: R. GALASSO, M.D.

MEDICAL RECORD 5-2 FOR ADDITIONAL STUDY

William Smith woke in the middle of the night with substernal chest heaviness that radiated to both arms. After experiencing no relief from taking aspirin and antacids, he went to the emergency room and was seen by Dr. Roland Galasso. The chest pain subsided only after administration of intravenous nitroglycerin. Dr. Galasso decided to admit Mr. Smith for further cardiac evaluation and treatment. A cardiac catheterization was performed the next day.

Read Medical Record 5.1 and answer the following questions.

1. Below are medical terms used in this record that you have not yet encountered in this text. Underline each where it appears in the record and define the term here:

   ostium _____

   hemodynamic _____

   mitral regurgitation _____

   focal _____

2. In your own words, not using medical terminology, briefly describe the *indications* for performing the cardiac catheterization.

   _____

   _____

   _____

   _____

3. Put the following actions in correct order by numbering them 1 to 14.

   _____ pigtail catheter advanced to the left ventricle

   _____ hemostasis obtained by C-clamp pressure

   _____ right coronary arteriography performed

   _____ pigtail catheter exchanged for left coronary artery catheter

   _____ informed consent signed

   _____ arterial pressures were recorded

   _____ right groin prepped and draped

   _____ left coronary arteriography performed

   _____ right femoral artery entered and Cordis sheath inserted

   _____ right coronary catheter and femoral artery sheath removed

   _____ pigtail catheter inserted through sheath and guided to descending thoracic aorta

   _____ left coronary catheter exchanged for right coronary catheter

   _____ left ventriculography performed

   _____ heparin was administered

4. Briefly describe conclusions of the procedure in nonmedical language:

   a. _____

   b. _____

5. From the recommendations, describe the test that will be performed right away:

   _____

6. Identify the possible future complications:

   _____

   _____

   _____

7. Describe the procedure that is recommended should these complications occur.

   _____

   _____

   _____

Answers to Practice Exercises

1. angio/graphy
   CF   S
   vessel/process of/recording

2. varic/osis
   R   S
   swollen, twisted vein/
   condition or increase

3. pector/al
   R   S
   chest/pertaining to

4. vaso/spasm
   CF   S
   vessel/involuntary contraction

5. ven/ous
   R   S
   vein/pertaining to

6. aorto/coron/ary
   CF   R   S
   aorta/circle or crown/
   pertaining to

7. thrombo/phleb/itis
   CF   R   S
   clot/vein/inflammation

8. arterio/scler/osis
   CF   R   S
   artery/hard/condition or
   increase

9. vasculo/path/y
   CF   R   S
   vessel/disease/condition
   or process of

10. athero/genesis
    CF   S
    fatty paste (lipids)/origin or
    production

11. stetho/scope
    CF   S
    chest/instrument for
    examination

12. myo/card/ium
    CF   R   S
    muscle/heart/structure
    or tissue

13. aorto/plasty
    CF   S
    aorta/surgical repair or
    reconstruction

14. veno/stomy
    CF   S
    vein/creation of an opening

15. arterio/sten/osis
    CF   R   S
    artery/narrow/condition or
    increase

16. phlebo/tomy
    CF   S
    vein/incision

17. cardio/aort/ic
    CF   R   S
    heart/aorta/pertaining to

18. ventriculo/graphy
    CF   S
    ventricle/process of
    recording

19. phleb/itis
    R   S
    vein/inflammation

20. angio/plasty
    CF   S
    vessel/surgical repair or
    reconstruction

21. endo/vascul/ar
    P   R   S
    within/vessel/pertaining to

22. cardio/tox/ic
    CF   R   S
    heart/poison/pertaining to

23. arterio/gram
    CF   S
    artery/record

24. ather/ectomy
    R   S
    fat (lipids)/excision

25. cardi/ac
    R   S
    heart/pertaining to

26. h
27. o
28. n
29. i
30. g
31. j
32. a
33. c
34. l
35. e
36. m
37. d
38. k
39. f
40. b
41. congenital anomalies
42. arteriosclerosis
43. arrhythmia
44. cardiomyopathy
45. anastomosis
46. gallop
47. echocardiogram
48. cor pulmonale or right ventricular failure
49. coronary angiogram
50. stress electrocardiogram
51. atrial septum
52. right atrium
53. tricuspid valve
54. right ventricle
55. left atrium
56. aortic valve
57. pulmonary semilunar valve
58. left ventricle
59. ventricular septum

60. premature ventricular contraction
61. patent ductus arteriosus
62. arteriosclerotic heart disease
63. implantable cardioverter defibrillator
64. congestive heart failure
65. coronary artery disease
66. hypertension
67. mitral valve prolapse
68. magnetic resonance angiography
69. ventricular septal defect
70. e
71. h
72. b
73. a
74. j
75. c
76. i
77. d
78. f
79. g
80. ventricle
81. aorta
82. thrombus
83. myocardial
84. hypotension
85. diastole
86. ischemia
87. occlusion
88. infarct
89. aneurysm
90. atherosclerotic
91. thrombophlebitis

92. angiogram
93. defibrillation
94. antiarrhythmic
95. vasodilation
96. anticoagulant
97. hypertension
98. defibrillation
99. tachycardia
100. arrhythmia
101. depolarization
102. systole
103. pector/o
104. phleb/o
105. angi/o
106. cardi/o
107. ather/o
108. coron/o
109. sphygm/o
110. thromb/o
111. arteri/o
112. ventricul/o

Answers to Medical Record Analyses

1. a
2. b
3. d
4. e
5. d
6. a
7. b
8. d

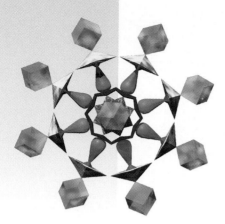

CHAPTER 6

Blood and Lymph Systems

Blood and Lymph Systems Overview

Functions of the blood:

❉ Transports oxygen, nutrients, and hormones to body cells

❉ Carries wastes away from the cells

Functions of the lymphatic system (Fig. 6-1):

❉ Protects the body by filtering microorganisms and foreign particles from the lymph

❉ Supports the activities of the lymphocytes in the immune response

❉ Maintains the body's internal fluid environment as an intermediary between the blood in the capillaries and tissue cells

❉ Carries fats away from the digestive organs

SELF-INSTRUCTION: COMBINING FORMS

Study the following:

Combining Form	Meaning
blast/o **-blast** (also a suffix)	germ or bud
chrom/o **chromat/o**	color
chyl/o	juice
hem/o **hemat/o**	blood
immun/o	safe

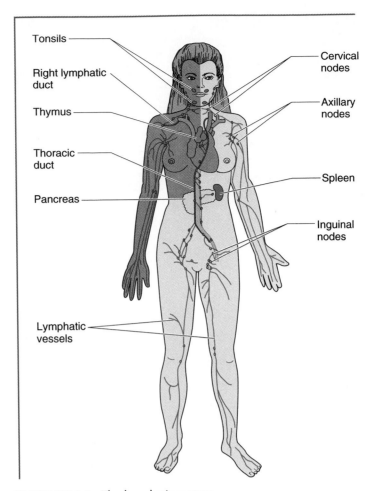

■ **FIGURE 6-1.** The lymphatic system.

lymph/o	clear fluid
morph/o	form
phag/o	eat or swallow
plas/o	formation
reticul/o	a net
splen/o	spleen
thromb/o	clot
thym/o	thymus gland

PROGRAMMED REVIEW: COMBINING FORMS

Answers	Review

Answers

blast/o

-blast

cell, blood

red

chromat/o

color

condition of

juice

blood

chyle

hemat/o

hem/o

formation

blood

immun/o

immunocompromised

Review

6.1   The combining form meaning germ or bud is _____, as in the term blastogenesis, referring to the origin or production of cells by budding. The suffix from this combining form is _____. Hemocytoblasts (a term formed from the combination of *-blast* with *cyt/o* meaning _____ and *hem/o* meaning _____) are the primitive stem cells in the bone marrow that develop into blood cells. An erythroblast develops into an erythrocyte, or _____ blood cell.

6.2   The combining form *chrom/o* or _____ means _____. For example, chromone refers to plant pigments. Recall that the suffix *-ism* means _____ _____; therefore, chromatism is a condition of abnormal pigmentation.

6.3   The combining form *chyl/o* means _____ or fluid. Chyle is a pale yellow fluid from the intestine that is carried by the lymphatic system. The suffix *-emia* refers to a _____ condition, and thus chylemia means the presence of _____ in the blood.

6.4   Hematology, a term made from the combining form _____ for blood, is the medical study of the blood. Another combining form for blood is _____, as in hemostat, an agent or device that stops the flow of blood from a vessel. Recall that the suffix *-poiesis* means _____; therefore, hemopoiesis refers to the process of formation and development of various types of _____ cells.

6.5   The combining form meaning safe is _____. The immune system helps keep the body safe from infectious disease. Both the blood and lymphatic systems are involved in the body's immune system. Someone whose immune system has been compromised by disease is said to be _____.

clear

lymphoma

6.6 The combining form *lymph/o* means _____ fluid. Lymph is a clear fluid collected from body tissues that flows through lymphatic vessels and eventually into the venous blood circulation. Using the suffix that means tumor, a neoplasm of the lymphatic system is a

_____ .

eat

cell, eats

condition

6.7 The combining form *phag/o* means _____ or swallow. The suffix *-cyte* refers to a _____. A phagocyte therefore is a cell that _____ bacteria, foreign particles, and other cells. Using the suffix *-osis*, which generally means increase or _____, phagocytosis is the process or condition of phagocytes ingesting other solid substances.

formation

without

condition of

6.8 *Plas/o* is a combining form meaning _____. Using the prefix *a-*, meaning _____, and the suffix *-ia*, meaning _____ ____, aplasia is a condition in which a formation (tissue or organ) is absent or defective.

form

study of

6.9 *Morph/o* is a combining form meaning _____. Combined with *-logy*, the suffix meaning _____ ____, morphology is the study of form, including the size and shape of a specimen, such as blood cells.

net

erythro

reticulo

red

6.10 *Reticul/o* is a combining form meaning a _____. A network of substances influences the development of red blood cells from the primitive _____blast (red bud or germ) to the immature red blood cell, or _____cyte (from the combining form meaning a net). Reticulocytes are immature _____ blood cells, or erythrocytes.

splen/o

enlargement, spleen

6.11 The spleen is a key organ of the lymphatic system. It filters the blood and performs other functions. The combining form for spleen is _____. Recalling that the suffix *-megaly* means _____, splenomegaly is an enlarged _____.

splenectomy	Using the common suffix for excision or removal, removal of the spleen is called _____.
cells thromb/o clot	**6.12** Thrombocytes are blood _____ that function to clot the blood. The combining form meaning clot is _____. A thrombus is a blood _____ inside a blood vessel.
thym/o, thymoma	**6.13** The thymus is a gland in the lymphatic system, from the combining form _____. A tumor of thymus tissue is a _____.

SELF-INSTRUCTION: ANATOMICAL TERMS IN THE BLOOD SYSTEM

Study the following:

Term	Meaning

TERMS RELATED TO BLOOD FLUID

plasma *plaz'mah*	liquid portion of the blood and lymph containing water, proteins, and cellular components (leukocytes, erythrocytes, and platelets)
serum *sēr'ŭm*	liquid portion of the blood left after clotting

CELLULAR COMPONENTS OF BLOOD (FIG. 6-2)

erythrocyte (Fig. 6-3) *ĕ-rith'rō-sīt*	red blood cell, which transports oxygen and carbon dioxide
hemoglobin *hē-mō-glō'bin*	protein-iron compound contained in erythrocytes that transports oxygen and carbon dioxide
leukocyte (Fig. 6-3) *lu'kō-sĭt*	white blood cell, which protects the body from invading harmful substances
granulocytes *gran'yū-lō-sīts*	a group of leukocytes containing granules in their cytoplasm
neutrophil *nū'trō-fil*	a granular leukocyte, named for the neutral stain of its granules, that fights infection by swallowing bacteria (phagocytosis) (neutr = neither; phil = attraction for)
polymorpho- nuclear leukocyte (PMN) *pol-ē-mōr'fo- nū'klĕ-ăr*	another term for neutrophil, named for the many segments present in its nucleus (poly = many; morpho = form; nucleus = kernel)

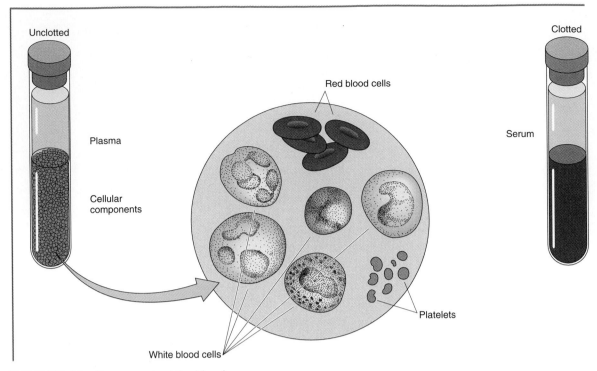

■ FIGURE 6-2. Components of the blood.

CELLULAR COMPONENTS OF THE BLOOD

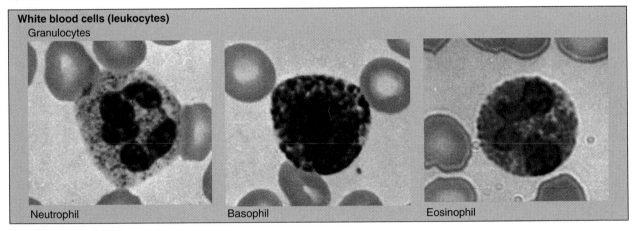

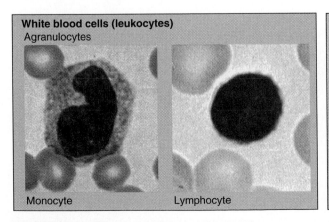
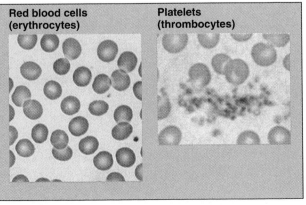

FIGURE 6-3. Cellular components of the blood.

band	an immature neutrophil
eosinophil *ē-ō-sin'ō-fil*	a granular leukocyte, named for the rose-colored stain of its granules, that increases in allergic and some infectious reactions (eos = dawn-colored (rosy); phil = attraction for)
basophil *bā'sō-fil*	a granular leukocyte, named for the dark stain of its granules, that brings anticoagulant substances to inflamed tissues (baso = base; phil = attraction for)
agranulocytes *ă-gran'yū-lō-sīt*	a group of leukocytes without granules in their nuclei
lymphocyte *lim'fō-sīt*	an agranulocytic leukocyte active in the process of immunity; the three categories of lymphocytes are T cells (thymus dependent), B cells (bone marrow–derived), and NK (natural killer) cells
monocyte *mon'ō-sīt*	an agranulocytic leukocyte that performs phagocytosis to fight infection (mono = one)
platelets *plāt'lets*	thrombocytes; cell fragments in the blood essential for blood clotting (coagulation)

PROGRAMMED REVIEW: ANATOMICAL TERMS IN THE BLOOD SYSTEM

Answers	Review
plasma serum	**6.14** The liquid portion of the blood and lymph is called _____. The plasma contains proteins, cells, and other substances. After blood clots, the liquid portion that remains is called _____.
cell red red, cell hemoglobin blood	**6.15** Recall that *cyt/o* is a combining form meaning _____ and *erythr/o* is a combining form meaning _____. Therefore, an erythrocyte is a _____ blood _____. Erythrocytes transport oxygen and carbon dioxide, which bond to the protein-iron compound in them called _____ (from the combining form *hem/o*, meaning _____).
white leukocyte	**6.16** The combining form *leuk/o* means _____; thus, a white blood cell is a _____. There are many types of leukocytes in the blood in two general categories, with or without granules in their cytoplasm. Leukocytes with granules are called

granulocytes	_____. Because the prefix *a-* means
without	_____, the term for leukocytes without granules is
agranulocytes	_____.

6.17   Several types of leukocytes were named by how they appear when stained. For example, a neutrophil is a leukocyte whose granules stain neutrally (phil = attraction for); a neutrophil has an attraction for neither (neutr) color stain. An _____ is a leukocyte

eosinophil

whose granules stain (attract) a rose color (eos = rosy color; phil = attraction for). Finally, another type of leukocyte has granules that stain (attract) a dark base color (baso = base; phil = attraction for); this type

basophil

is a _____.

6.18   Another term for a neutrophil is named for the many segments

polymorphonuclear

present in the nucleus: _____ leukocyte, abbreviated PMN. A band is an _____ neutrophil.

immature

6.19   An agranulocytic leukocyte in the lymphatic system active in the

lymphocyte

process of immunity is the _____. A monocyte, another

infection

agranulocytic leukocyte, performs phagocytosis to fight _____.

platelet

6.20   Another term for a thrombocyte is _____. Because

clot, clotting

thromb/o means _____, platelets function in blood _____

SELF-INSTRUCTION: ANATOMICAL TERMS IN THE LYMPH SYSTEM

Study the following:

Term	Meaning
LYMPH ORGANS	
thymus *thī′mŭs*	primary gland of the lymphatic system, located within the mediastinum, that helps maintain the body's immune response by producing T lymphocytes
spleen *splēn*	organ between the stomach and diaphragm that filters out aging blood cells, removes cellular debris by performing phagocytosis, and provides an environment for lymphocytes to initiate immune responses

LYMPH STRUCTURES (FIG. 6-4)

lymph *limf*	fluid circulated through the lymph vessels
lymph capillaries *limf kap'i-lār-ē*	microscopic vessels that draw lymph from tissues to the lymph vessels
lymph vessels *limf ves'ĕlz*	vessels that receive lymph from the lymph capillaries and circulate it to the lymph nodes
lacteals *lak'tē-ălz*	specialized lymph vessels in the small intestine that absorb fat into the bloodstream (lacteus = milky)
chyle *kīl*	white or pale yellow substance in lymph that contains fatty substances absorbed by the lacteals
lymph nodes *limf nōdz*	several small, oval structures that filter lymph from the lymph vessels; major locations include the cervical, axillary, and inguinal regions

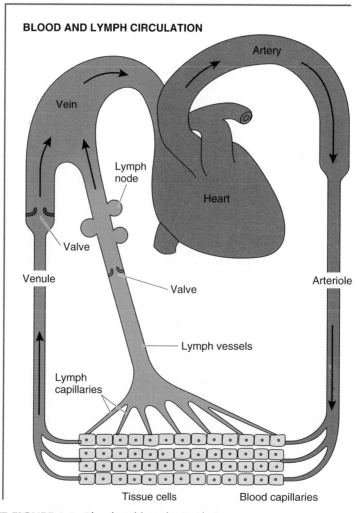

■ FIGURE 6-4. Blood and lymph circulation.

lymph ducts *limf dŭktz*	collecting channels that carry lymph from the lymph nodes to the veins
right lymphatic duct *lim-fat'ik dŭkt*	receives lymph from the right upper part of the body
thoracic duct *thō-ras'ik dŭkt*	receives lymph from the left side of the head, neck, chest, abdomen, left arm, and lower extremities

IMMUNITY

immunity *i-myū'ni-tē*	process of disease protection induced by exposure to an antigen
antigen *an'ti-jen*	a substance that, when introduced into the body, causes formation of antibodies against it
antibody *an'tē-bod-ē*	a substance produced by the body that destroys or inactivates an antigen that has entered the body
active immunity *ak'tiv i-myū'ni-tē*	an immunity that protects the body against a future infection, as the result of antibodies that develop *naturally* in response to an infection or *artificially* after administration of a vaccine
passive immunity *pas'iv i-myū'ni-tē*	an immunity resulting from antibodies that are conveyed *naturally* through the placenta to a fetus or *artificially* by injection of a serum containing antibodies

PROGRAMMED REVIEW: ANATOMIC TERMS IN THE LYMPH SYSTEM

Answers	Review
thymus thym/o	**6.21** Located in the mediastinum, the _____ gland produces T lymphocytes for the body's immune response. This term comes from the combining form _____.
spleen splenectomy	**6.22** Aging blood cells are filtered out in the _____, which also removes cellular debris by performing phagocytosis. The removal of this organ is called a _____.
lymph clear	**6.23** The fluid circulating through the lymph vessels is _____. The meaning of the combining form *lymph/o* reminds us that this fluid is _____.

6.24 The microscopic vessels that draw lymph from body tissues to the lymph vessels are called lymph _____. The same term is used in the circulatory system for the tiny vessels connecting arteries and veins.

capillaries

6.25 In addition to lymph capillaries, which collect lymph from body tissues, special lymph vessels in the intestine, called _____, absorb fat. This liquid in lymph absorbed by the lacteals is called _____.

lacteals

chyle

6.26 Lymph vessels carry lymph to the lymph _____, which filter the lymph. Lymph is then carried from the lymph nodes to the veins via lymph _____. The right _____ duct receives lymph from the right upper part of the body, and the _____ duct receives lymph from the left side of the head, neck, chest, left arm, and lower _____.

nodes

ducts, lymphatic

thoracic

extremities

6.27 The body protects itself from infectious disease in several ways. An antigen is a substance that, when introduced into the body, causes formation of an _____ against it. This process of disease protection is called _____. Exposure to an _____ starts the process, and the _____ destroys or inactivates the antigen.

antibody

immunity

antigen, antibody

6.28 Antibodies that develop naturally after contracting an infection or artificially after administering a vaccine result in _____ immunity. Antibodies that are conveyed naturally through the placenta to a fetus result in passive _____. The difference between active and passive in this case is whether the body itself actively makes the antibodies or passively receives them from outside.

active

immunity

SELF-INSTRUCTION: SYMPTOMATIC TERMS

Study the following:

Term	Meaning
anisocytosis *an-ī'sō-sī-tō'sis*	presence of red blood cells of unequal size (an = not, without; iso = equal) (*see* Fig. 6-6)
pancytopenia *pan'sī-tō-pē'nē-ă*	an abnormally reduced number of all cellular components in the blood
erythropenia *ĕ-rith-rō-pē'nē-ă*	an abnormally reduced number of red blood cells
hemolysis *hē-mol'i-sis*	breakdown of the red blood cell membrane
immunocompromised *im'yū-nō-kom'pro-mīzd*	impaired immunologic defenses caused by an immunodeficiency disorder or therapy with immunosuppressive agents
immunosuppression *im'yū-nō-sŭ-presh'ŭn*	impaired ability to provide an immune response
lymphadenopathy *lim-fad-ĕ-nop'ă-thē*	enlarged (diseased) lymph nodes
lymphocytopenia *lim'fō-sī-tō-pē'nē-ă*	an abnormally reduced number of lymphocytes
macrocytosis *mak'rō-sī-tō'sis*	presence of large red blood cells (*see* Fig 6-6)
microcytosis *mī-krō-sī-tō'sis*	presence of small red blood cells
neutropenia *nū-trō-pē'nē-ă*	decrease in the number of neutrophils
poikilocytosis *poy'ki-lō-sī-tō'sis*	presence of large, irregularly shaped red blood cells (poikilo = irregular) (*see* Fig. 6-6)
reticulocytosis *re-tik'yū-lō-sī-tō'sis*	increased number of immature erythrocytes in the blood
splenomegaly *splē-nō-meg'ă-lē*	enlargement of the spleen

PROGRAMMED REVIEW: SYMPTOMATIC TERMS

Answers	Review
reduction	**6.29** Recall that the suffix *-penia* means abnormal _____. Several symptomatic terms involving blood cells are formed with this suffix. An abnormally reduced number of lymphocytes is called

lymphocytopenia	_____. An abnormally reduced number of erythrocytes is termed erythrocytopenia, but the shorter term
erythropenia	_____ is generally used.

all	**6.30** The prefix *pan-* means _____. An abnormally reduced number
pancytopenia	of all blood cells is therefore _____. Like the shorter term erythropenia, the term for a reduced number of neutrophils uses just one combining form with the suffix *-penia:*
neutropenia	_____.

increase	**6.31** The suffix *-osis* can mean either a condition or _____. In either case, the suffix is used with symptomatic terms to indicate an abnormal or unusual condition. The presence of large red blood cells is
cytosis	macro_____, and the presence of small red blood cells is
microcytosis	called _____.

	6.32 Red blood cells may also be present in unequal sizes. The presence of red blood cells of unequal size (aniso = unequal) is termed
anisocytosis	_____. The presence of large, irregularly shaped
poikilocytosis	(poikilo = irregular) red blood cells is _____.

	6.33 As mentioned earlier, a reticulocyte is a young red blood cell, so named because of the network of substances in the cell. The combining
net	form *reticul/o* means _____. The condition of an increased number of
reticulocytosis	immature erythrocytes in the blood is _____.

	6.34 The suffix meaning breakdown or dissolution is _____.
-lysis	The term for the breakdown of the red blood cell membrane uses the combining form for blood (in effect the blood itself breaks down):
hemolysis	_____.

	6.35 The symptomatic suffix *-megaly* refers to an
enlargement	_____. An enlarged spleen, which may result from
splenomegaly	several different diseases, is _____.

6.36   The combining form *path/o* simply means disease, as in pathology. The combining form *aden/o* means gland (or node). A disease state in which lymph nodes are enlarged is _____.

lymphadenopathy

6.37   Some drugs or disease states suppress the body's ability to provide an immune response; this is called _____. A patient with impaired immunologic defenses caused by a disorder or immunosuppressive agents is said to be _____.

immunosuppression

immunocompromised

SELF-INSTRUCTION: DIAGNOSTIC TERMS

Study the following:

Term	Meaning
acquired immuno-deficiency syndrome (AIDS) *ă-kwĭrd′ i-myŭn′o-dē-fish′en-sē sin′drōm*	a syndrome caused by the human immunodeficiency virus (HIV) that renders immune cells ineffective, permitting opportunistic infections, malignancies, and neurologic diseases to develop; transmitted sexually or through contaminated blood
anemia *ă-nē′mē-ă*	a condition of reduced numbers of red blood cells, hemoglobin, or packed red cells in the blood, resulting in a diminished ability of red blood cells to transport oxygen to the tissues
iron deficiency anemia (Fig. 6-5, B) *i′ern dē-fish′en-sē*	a microcytic-hypochromic type of anemia characterized by a lack of iron, affecting production of hemoglobin and small red blood cells containing low amounts of hemoglobin
pernicious anemia (Fig. 6-6) *per-nish′ŭs*	a macrocytic normochromic type of anemia characterized by an inadequate supply of vitamin B_{12}, causing red blood cells to become large, varied in shape, and reduced in number
aplastic anemia *ā-plas′tik*	a normocytic-normochromic type of anemia characterized by the failure of bone marrow to produce red blood cells
erythroblastosis fetalis *ĕ-rith′rō-blas-tō′sis fē′tă′lis*	a disorder that results from the incompatibility of a fetus with Rh-positive blood and a mother with Rh-negative blood, causing red blood cell destruction in the fetus; a blood transfusion is necessary to save the fetus
Rh factor	the presence or lack of antigens on the surface of red blood cells, which causes a reaction between Rh-positive blood and Rh-negative blood
Rh positive	presence of antigens
Rh negative	absence of antigens

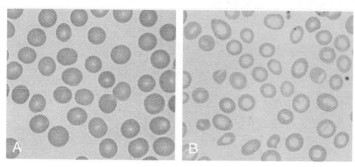

FIGURE 6-5. A blood smear showing normal erythrocytes **(A)** compared with a blood smear revealing microcytic-hypochromic erythrocytes in a patient with iron deficiency anemia **(B).**

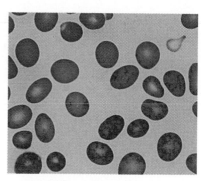

FIGURE 6-6. Photomicrograph of a blood smear from a patient with pernicious anemia reveals macrocytosis, anisocytosis, and poikilocytosis.

hemochromatosis *hē-mō-krō-mă-tō′sis*	hereditary disorder with an excessive buildup of iron deposits in the body
hemophilia *hē-mō-fil′ē-ă*	group of hereditary bleeding disorders with a defect in clotting factors necessary for coagulation of blood
leukemia *lū-kē′mē-ă*	chronic or acute malignant (cancerous) disease of the blood-forming organs, marked by abnormal leukocytes in the blood and bone marrow
myelodysplasia *mā′ĕ-lō-dis-plā′zē-ă*	disorder within the bone marrow characterized by a proliferation of abnormal stem cells (cells that give rise to different types of blood cells); usually develops into a specific type of leukemia
lymphoma *lim-fō′mă*	any neoplastic disorder of lymph tissue, usually malignant, as in Hodgkin's disease
metastasis *mĕ-tas′tĕ-sis*	process by which cancer cells are spread by blood or lymph circulation to a distant organ; "metastases" is the plural form of the term, indicating the spread to two or more distant sites
mononucleosis *mon′ō-nū-klē-ō′sis*	viral condition characterized by an increase in mononuclear cells (monocytes and lymphocytes) in the blood along with enlarged lymph nodes (lymphadenopathy), fatigue, and sore throat (pharyngitis)
polycythemia *pol′ē-sī-thē′mē-ă*	increased number of erythrocytes and hemoglobin in the blood
septicemia *sep-ti-sē′mē-ă*	systemic disease caused by the infection of microorganisms and their toxins in circulating blood
thrombocytopenia *throm′bō-sī-tō-pē′nē-ă*	bleeding disorder characterized by an abnormally decreased number of platelets in the blood, impairing the clotting process

PROGRAMMED REVIEW: DIAGNOSTIC TERMS

Answers	Review

6.38 Recall that *-penia* means abnormal reduction. An abnormal reduction in the number of platelets (thrombocytes) is termed

thrombocytopenia

_____.

blood

6.39 The diagnostic suffix *-emia* refers to a _____ condition. A malignant blood disease marked by abnormal white blood cells (leukocytes) is

leukemia

_____. A disorder in the bone marrow that usually develops into leukemia is built from the combining form for bone marrow (*myel/o*), the prefix *dys-* meaning faulty, and *-plasia*, referring to

formation

a condition of _____. This disorder is called

myelodysplasia

_____.

6.40 Also built with the suffix *-emia,* the term for an increase in the number of erythrocytes and hemoglobin in the blood begins with the

many

prefix *poly-,* which means _____. This disorder is called

polycythemia

_____.

6.41 Sepsis is from the Greek word for putrefaction, indicating infection. A systemic condition caused by infection in the blood is therefore

septicemia

termed _____.

without

6.42 The prefix *an-* means _____ or reduction. The general term for a blood condition in which there is a reduction in the number of red blood cells, the hemoglobin, or the volume of packed red blood

anemia

cells is _____. There are several common types of anemia. Anemia characterized by a lack of iron, affecting production of hemoglobin,

iron deficiency

is called _____ _____ anemia. The anemia char-

pernicious

acterized by an inadequate supply of vitamin B_{12} is _____ anemia. Another type, the term formed in part by word roots meaning

aplastic

without (*a-*) formation (*plas/o*), is _____ anemia.

acquired

immunodeficiency

syndrome

6.43   AIDS is the acronym for _____

_____ _____, a syn-

drome caused by the human immunodeficiency virus (HIV).

6.44   A disorder resulting from incompatibility of a fetus with Rh-positive blood and a mother with Rh-negative blood, named in part because of the large number of erythroblasts found in the fetus's blood,

erythroblastosis fetalis

factor

Rh

negative

is _____ _____. The Rh _____ is said to be positive when Rh antigens are present on the surface of red blood cells. The absence of such antigens is _____ _____.

hemochromatosis

6.45   A hereditary blood disorder results in an excessive buildup of iron deposits in the body. A clue to the term for this condition is that skin pigmentation may change (the term uses the combining form meaning color and the combining form for blood). This condition is _____.

clotting

6.46   Hemophilia is a group of hereditary bleeding disorders with a defect in _____ factors necessary for coagulation.

-oma

lymphoma

6.47   Recall that the suffix meaning tumor is _____. A neoplasm of lymph tissue is a _____.

beyond

metastasis

6.48   The prefix *meta-* means _____, after, or change. The term for the spread of cancer cells beyond the original site of the tumor through blood or lymph is _____.

mononucleosis

increase

6.49   Monocytes and lymphocytes are mononuclear cells. The viral condition characterized by an increase in both types is _____. The suffix *–osis* means condition or _____.

SELF-INSTRUCTION: DIAGNOSTIC TESTS AND PROCEDURES

Study the following:

Test or Procedure	Explanation
BLOOD STUDIES	
phlebotomy *flă-bot'ō-mē* **venipuncture** *ven-i-pŭnk-chūr'*	incision into or puncture of a vein to withdraw blood for testing
blood chemistry *blŭd kem'is-trē*	test of the fluid portion of blood to measure amounts of chemical constituents (e.g., glucose and cholesterol)
blood chemistry panels	specialized batteries of automated blood chemistry tests performed on a single sample of blood; used as a general screen for disease or to target specific organs or conditions, i.e., metabolic panel, lipid panel, arthritis panel
basic metabolic panel	battery of tests used as a general screen for disease: calcium, carbon dioxide (CO_2), chloride, creatinine, glucose, potassium, sodium and blood urea nitrogen (BUN)
comprehensive metabolic panel (Fig. 6-7)	tests in addition to basic panel for expanded screening purpose: albumin, bilirubin, alkaline phosphatase, protein, ALT, and AST
blood culture *blŭd kŭl'chŭr*	test to diagnose an infection in the bloodstream, by culturing a specimen of blood to encourage the growth of microorganisms, which are then identified
erythrocyte sedimentation rate (ESR) *ĕ-rith'trōsīt sed'i-men-tā'shŭn rāt*	timed test that measures the rate at which red blood cells settle through a volume of plasma
partial thromboplastin time (PTT)	test to determine coagulation defects, such as platelet disorders
thromboplastin *throm-bō-plas'tin*	substance present in tissues, platelets, and leukocytes that is necessary for coagulation
prothrombin time (PT)	test to measure activity of prothrombin in the blood
prothrombin *pr–o-throm'bin*	protein substance in the blood that is essential to the clotting process

CENTRAL MEDICAL CENTER
211 Medical Center Drive • Central City, US 90000-1234 • PHONE: (012) 125-6784 • FAX: (012) 125-9999

11/02/20xx
14:27

NAME   : TEST, PATIENT   LOC: TEST   DOB: 02/03/xx   AGE: 38Y
MR#   : TEST-221   SEX: M
ACCT#   : H111111111

M63561 COLL: 11/02/20xx 13:24   REC: 11/02/20xx 13:25

COMPREHENSIVE METABOLIC PANEL

Blood Urea Nitrogen (BUN)	*30	[5 - 25]	mg/dl
Sodium	139	[135 - 153]	mEq/L
Potassium	4.2	[3.5 - 5.3]	mEq/L
Chloride	105	[101 - 111]	mEq/L
Carbon Dioxide (CO_2)	27	[24 - 31]	mmol/L
Glucose, Random	*148	[70 - 110]	mg/dl
Creatinine	*1.5	[< 1.5]	mg/dl
SGOT (AST)	18	[10 - 42]	U/L
SGPT (ALT)	*8	[10 - 60]	U/L
Alkaline Phosphatase	58	[42 - 121]	U/L
Total Protein	6.5	[6.0 - 8.0]	G/dl
Albumin	3.7	[3.5 - 5.0]	G/dl
Amylase	33	[< 129]	U/L
Bilirubin, Total	0.7	[< 1.5]	mg/dl
Calcium, Total	9.7	[8.6 - 10.6]	mg/dl

TEST, PATIENT   TEST-221   END OF REPORT   PAGE 1
11/02/20xx 14:27

INTERIM REPORT COMPLETED

FIGURE 6-7. Comprehensive metabolic panel report (formerly termed biochemistry or SMA panel). Note: Normal ranges are in brackets [ ].

complete blood count (CBC) (Fig. 6-8)	a common laboratory blood test performed as a screen of general health or for diagnosis, including the following four component tests (Note: CBC results are usually reported along with normal values so that the clinician can interpret the results based on the instrumentation used by the laboratory. Normal ranges also may vary depending on the region, climate, etc.)
white blood count (WBC)	a count of the number of white blood cells per cubic millimeter, obtained by manual or automated laboratory methods
red blood count (RBC)	a count of the number of red blood cells per cubic millimeter, obtained manually or via automated laboratory methods
hemoglobin (HGB or Hgb) *hē-mō-glō′bin*	a test to determine the blood level of hemoglobin (expressed in grams)
hematocrit (HCT or Hct) *hē′mă-tō-krit*	a measurement of the percentage of packed red blood cells in a given volume of blood

CENTRAL MEDICAL CENTER
211 Medical Center Drive • Central City, US 90000-1234 • PHONE: (012) 125-6784 • FAX: (012) 125-9999

11/02/20xx
14:27

NAME   : TEST, PATIENT   LOC: TEST   DOB: 2/2/xx   AGE: 27Y
MR#   : TEST-221   SEX: M
ACCT#   : H111111111

M63558 COLL: 11/2/20xx 13:23   REC: 11/2/20xx 13:24

HEMOGRAM
CBC
WBC	*11.5	[4.5 - 10.5]	K/UL
RBC	5.84	[4.6 - 6.2]	M/UL
HGB	17.2	[14.0 - 18.0]	G/DL
HCT	50.8	[42.0 - 52.0]	%
MCV	87	[82 - 92]	FL
MCH	29.5	[27 - 31]	PG
MCHC	33.9	[32 - 36]	G/DL
PLT	202	[150 - 450]	K/UL

Auto Lymph %	15	[20 - 40]	%
Auto Mono %	2	[1 - 11]	%
Auto Neutro %	82	[50 - 75]	%
Auto Eos %	1	[0 - 6]	%
Auto Baso %	0	[0 - 2]	%
Auto Lymph #	1.7	[1.5 - 4.0]	K/UL
Auto Mono #	0.2	[0.2 - 0.9]	K/UL
Auto Neutro #	9.4	[1.0 - 7.0]	K/UL
Auto Eos #	0.1	[0 - 0.7]	K/UL
Auto Baso #	0.0	[0 - 0.2]	K/UL

TEST, PATIENT   TEST-221   END OF REPORT   PAGE 1
11/02/20xx   14:27   INTERIM REPORT

INTERIM REPORT COMPLETE

FIGURE 6-8. Complete blood count (CBC) report. Note: Normal ranges are in brackets [ ].

blood indices *in'di-sēz*	calculations of RBC, HGB, and HCT results to determine the average size, hemoglobin concentration, and content of red blood cells to classify an anemia
mean corpuscular (cell) volume (MCV) *kōr-pŭs'kyū-lăr*	calculation of the volume of individual cells in cubic microns using HCT and RBC results: MCV = HCT/RBC
mean corpuscular (cell) hemoglobin (MCH) *kōr-pŭs'kyū-lăr* *hē-mō-glō'bin*	calculation of the content in weight of hemoglobin in the average red blood cell using HGB and RBC results: MCH = HGB/RBC

mean corpuscular (cell) hemoglobin concentration (MCHC) *hē-mō-glō′bin kon-sen-trē′shŭn*	calculation of the average hemoglobin concentration in each red blood cell using HGB and HCT results: MCHC = HGB/HCT Note: "corpuscular" pertains to a blood cell
differential count	determination of the number of each type of white blood cell (leukocyte) in a stained blood smear; each type is counted and reported as a percentage of the total examined *Type of Leukocyte* *Normal Range* lymphocytes 25–33% monocytes 3–7% neutrophils 54–75% eosinophils 1–3% basophils 0–1%
red cell morphology *mōr-fol′ō-jē*	as part of identifying and counting the WBCs, the condition, size, and shape of red blood cells in the background of the smeared slide are noted (e.g., anisocytosis, poikilocytosis)
platelet count (PLT) *plāt′let*	calculation of the number of thrombocytes in the blood: normal range is between 150,000 to 450,000 per cubic millimeter

BONE AND LYMPH STUDIES

bone marrow aspiration *bōn mar′ō as-pi-rā′shŭn*	needle aspiration of bone marrow tissue for pathologic examination
lymphangiogram *lim-fan′jē-ō-gram*	an x-ray of a lymph node or vessel taken after injection of a contrast medium

PROGRAMMED REVIEW: DIAGNOSTIC TESTS AND PROCEDURES

Answers	Review
	6.50 Blood studies are tests performed with samples of blood. The blood sample, often drawn by a phlebotomist, is obtained through a
venipuncture	needle puncture (or incision) of a vein called a _____
phlebotomy	or a _____. Recall that the suffix *-tomy* refers to an
incision	_____.
	6.51 Blood studies generally examine the chemical constituents of the blood or the physical properties of different kinds of blood cells. A test of the fluid portion of blood for the presence of chemical constituents is

chemistry, panel	called blood _____. A blood chemistry _____ includes a battery of chemistry tests using a single sample of blood. Some panels target specific organs or conditions, such as a lipid or arthritis panel. There are two panels of chemistry tests that are used as a general
metabolic	or expanded screen for disease: basic _____ panel and
comprehensive metabolic panel	_____ _____ _____ (formerly termed biochemistry or SMA panel).
culture	**6.52** To determine the presence and type of an infection in the blood, a blood sample may be put in an environment that encourages the growth of microorganisms. This test is called a blood _____.
erythrocytes	**6.53** Red blood cells are _____. A diagnostic test that measures how fast they settle through plasma is called the
erythrocyte sedimentation	_____ _____ rate.
thromb/o	**6.54** The combining form for clot is _____. That root is part of the term for the substance present in tissues, platelets, and leukocytes that is necessary for coagulation, called
thromboplastin	_____. The test for coagulation defects is
partial thromboplastin	_____ _____ time (PTT). The term for a protein substance in blood essential for clotting comes simply from a prefix meaning before, along with the combining form for clot:
prothrombin	_____. The diagnostic test that measures the ac-
prothrombin time	tivity of this protein is _____ _____ (PT).
blood count	**6.55** A complete _____ _____ (CBC) is a diagnostic test often performed as a general screen. It typically includes four component
red blood	tests. The RBC is a count of the number of _____ _____ cells per
white	cubic millimeter. A WBC is a count of the number of _____ blood
cells	_____. The test of the blood level of hemoglobin is often called sim-
HGB, Hgb	ply a hemoglobin, abbreviated _____ or _____. The measurement of the percentage of packed red blood cells in a given volume of blood is
hematocrit	called the _____ (abbreviated HCT or Hct).

6.56   Different values in the CBC are used to calculate the size, makeup, and content of red blood cells in order to classify an anemia. These calculations are called blood _____. The calculation of the volume of individual cells is called the _____ _____ volume (MCV). "Mean" refers to average. The calculation of the weight of hemoglobin in an average red blood cell is _____ corpuscular (cell) _____ (MCH). The calculation of the mean hemoglobin concentration in each cell is the mean corpuscular (cell) _____ _____ (MCHC).

indices

mean

corpuscular (cell)

mean, hemoglobin

hemoglobin

concentration

6.57   Thrombocytes are also counted in blood samples. Another term for thrombocyte is _____. Thus, this measure is simply called a _____ _____ (PLT).

platelet

platelet count

6.58   Recall that there are several kinds of leukocytes (_____ blood cells), such as lymphocytes, mono_____, neutrophils, eosino_____, and basophils. The determination of the percentage of each type in the total of all types is called a _____ _____.

white

cytes (monocytes)

phils (eosinophils)

differential

count

6.59   When the differential count is done, the size and shape of red blood cells in the sample are also noted. This is called the red cell _____.

morphology

6.60   The removal of bone marrow tissue by a needle for pathologic examination is called bone marrow _____.

aspiration

6.61   The combining form *angi/o* refers to either blood or lymph vessels. The suffix meaning a record is _____. Using these two roots along with the combining form for lymph, the term _____ is an x-ray of a lymph node or vessel.

-gram

lymphangiogram

SELF-INSTRUCTION: OPERATIVE TERMS

Study the following:

Term	Meaning
bone marrow transplant *bōn mar'ō tranz'plant*	transplantation of healthy bone marrow from a compatible donor to a diseased recipient to stimulate blood cell production
lymphadenectomy *lim-fad-ĕ-nek'tō-mē*	removal of a lymph node
lymphadenotomy *lim-fad-ĕ-not'ă-mē*	incision into a lymph node
lymph node dissection *limf nōd di-sek'shŭn*	removal of possible cancer-carrying lymph nodes for pathologic examination
splenectomy *splē-nek'tō-mē*	removal of the spleen
thymectomy *thī-mek'tō-mē*	removal of the thymus gland

PROGRAMMED REVIEW: OPERATIVE TERMS

Answers	Review
removal splenectomy thymectomy lymphadenectomy	**6.62** The suffix *-ectomy* means _____ or excision. The removal of the spleen is a _____. The removal of the thymus gland is a _____. The removal of a lymph node is a _____.
incision lymphadenotomy	**6.63** The suffix *-tomy*, on the other hand, means _____. An incision into a lymph node is a _____.
dissection	**6.64** Removal of possible cancer-carrying lymph nodes for pathologic examination is called a lymph node _____.
bone marrow	**6.65** To stimulate blood cell production inside bones, a _____ transplant is made from a compatible donor to a diseased recipient.

SELF-INSTRUCTION: THERAPEUTIC TERMS

Study the following:

Term	Meaning
blood transfusion	introduction of blood products into the circulation of a recipient whose blood volume is reduced or deficient in some manner
autologous blood *aw-tol'ŏ-gŭs blud*	blood donated by and stored for a patient for future personal use (e.g., upcoming surgery) (auto = self)
homologous blood *hŏ-mol'ō-gŭs blud*	blood voluntarily donated by any person for transfusion to a compatible recipient (homo = same)
blood component therapy	transfusion of a specific blood component, such as packed red blood cells, platelets, or plasma
crossmatching	a method of matching a donor's blood to the recipient by mixing a sample in a test tube to determine compatibility
chemotherapy *kem'ō-thĕr-ă-pē*	treatment of malignancies, infections, and other diseases with chemical agents to destroy selected cells or impair their ability to reproduce
plasmapheresis *plaz'mă-fĕ-rē'sis*	removal of plasma from the body with separation and extraction of specific elements (such as platelets) followed by reinfusion (apheresis = a withdrawal)

COMMON THERAPEUTIC DRUG CLASSIFICATIONS

anticoagulant *an'tē-kō-ag'yū-lant*	a drug that prevents clotting of the blood
hemostatic *hē-mō-stat'ik*	a drug that stops the flow of blood within the vessels
vasoconstrictor *vā'sō-kon-strik'ter*	a drug that causes a narrowing of blood vessels, thereby decreasing blood flow
vasodilator *vā'sō-dī-lā'ter*	a drug that causes dilation of blood vessels, thereby increasing blood flow

PROGRAMMED REVIEW: THERAPEUTIC TERMS

Answers	Review
transfusion	**6.66** The general term for giving blood or blood products to a recipient whose blood is deficient in some way is blood _____. There are several types of blood transfusions. A patient's own blood removed for his or her own personal use in a later transfusion is called
autologous	_____ blood (auto = self). Blood from a compatible

homologous	(same blood type) donor is called _____ blood (homo = same).
component	**6.67** The transfusion of specific blood components, such as platelets or plasma, is called blood _____ therapy.
crossmatching	**6.68** The process of determining compatibility between donated blood and the recipient's blood is called _____. This must be done to ensure the recipient does not suffer a potentially fatal transfusion reaction.
chemotherapy	**6.69** The treatment of neoplasms and other diseases with chemical agents that destroy the targeted cells is _____. Chemotherapy is used with many forms of cancer in virtually all body systems.
plasmapheresis	**6.70** The root apheresis means withdrawal. The withdrawal of blood plasma from the body to separate out specific components before rein-fusing the plasma is _____.
against anticoagulant	**6.71** Recall that the prefix *anti-* means _____. Drug classes are often named by their actions against something. A drug that prevents blood clotting or coagulation is an _____.
vasoconstrictor vasodilator	**6.72** Drug classes are also named for their specific actions. The combining form for blood vessel is *vas/o*. A drug that narrows or constricts blood vessels is a _____. A drug that widens or dilates blood vessels is a _____.
-stasis hem/o hemostatic	**6.73** Recall that the suffix that means stop or stand is _____. The combining form for blood is *hemat/o* or _____. A type of drug that stops blood from flowing within a vessel is a _____.

Practice Exercises

For the following terms, on the lines below the term, write out the indicated word parts: prefixes, combining forms, roots, and suffixes. Then define the word.

Example:
dyshematopoiesis

<u>dys/hemato/poiesis</u>
P   CF   S

DEFINITION: painful, difficult or faulty/blood/formation

1. erythroblastosis

———————— / ———————— / ————————————
    CF   R   S

DEFINITION: _____

2. chylopoiesis

———————— / ————————————
    CF   S

DEFINITION: _____

3. hemocytometer

———————— / ———————— / ————————————
    CF   CF   S

DEFINITION: _____

4. splenorrhagia

———————— / ————————————
    CF   S

DEFINITION: _____

5. lymphadenitis

———————— / ———————— / ————————————
    R   R   S

DEFINITION: _____

6. immunotoxic

———————— / ———————— / ————————————
    CF   R   S

DEFINITION: _____

7. reticulocytosis

———————— / ———————— / ————————————
    CF   R   S

DEFINITION: _____

8. thymopathy

_____ / _____ / _____
CF   R   S

DEFINITION: _____

9. leukocytic

_____ / _____ / _____
CF   R   S

DEFINITION: _____

10. lymphangiogram

_____ / _____ / _____
R   CF   S

DEFINITION: _____

11. splenomegaly

_____ / _____
CF   S

DEFINITION: _____

12. promyelocyte

_____ / _____ / _____ / _____
P   CF   R   S

DEFINITION: _____

13. leukocytopenia

_____ / _____ / _____
CF   CF   S

DEFINITION: _____

14. splenectomy

_____ / _____
R   S

DEFINITION: _____

15. dialysis

_____ / _____
P   S

DEFINITION: _____

16. lymphoma

_____ / _____
R   S

DEFINITION: _____

17. cytomorphology

_____ / _____ / _____
     CF   CF   S

DEFINITION: _____

18. hemolysis

_____ / _____
     CF   S

DEFINITION: _____

19. anemia

_____ / _____
     P   S

DEFINITION: _____

20. metastasis

_____ / _____
     P   S

DEFINITION: _____

Name the blood studies that are part of the blood indices:

21. _____

22. _____

23. _____

Fill in the blanks with the appropriate medical terms and abbreviations:

24. The procedure of counting the number of leukocytes in the blood is called a

_____ _____ _____ and is abbreviated _____.

25. The blood study that determines the amount of pigment present in RBCs is called a

_____ and is abbreviated _____.

26. The blood study that determines packed red blood cell volume is called a

_____ and is abbreviated _____.

27. The classification of WBCs is performed in a _____ _____.

Write the full medical term for the following abbreviations:

28. PT _____

29. ESR _____

30. PTT _____

31. CBC _____

Match the following terms with their meanings:

32. microcytosis _____

33. poikilocytosis _____

34. neutrophil _____

35. monocyte _____

36. eosinophil _____

37. lymphocyte _____

38. basophil _____

39. platelet _____

40. erythrocyte _____

41. granulocyte _____

42. anisocytosis _____

43. macrocytosis _____

a. large red blood cells

b. thrombocyte

c. WBC with rose-stained granules

d. RBC

e. an agranulocyte active in immunity

f. WBC with dark stained granules

g. WBC termed "one cell"

h. RBCs of unequal size

i. WBC with granules

j. large, irregular RBCs

k. a polymorphonuclear WBC

l. small red blood cells

Write the correct medical term for each of the following:

44. a decrease in the number of neutrophils _____

45. blood donated by a person and stored for his or her future use _____

46. impaired ability to provide an immune response _____

47. test tube method of matching a donor's blood to the recipient _____

48. syndrome caused by HIV _____

49. removal of plasma from the body, extraction of specific elements, then reinfusion

_____

50. blood voluntarily donated by any person for transfusion _____

For each of the following, circle the combining form that corresponds to the meaning given:

51. **eat or swallow**	phas/o	phag/o	plas/o
52. **clot**	thromb/o	thym/o	lymph/o
53. **juice**	lymph/o	hemat/o	chyl/o
54. **formation**	plas/o	troph/o	thromb/o
55. **color**	hem/o	chrom/o	cyan/o
56. **blood**	erythr/o	hem/o	lymph/o
57. **safe**	toxic/o	reticul/o	immun/o
58. **germ or bud**	blast/o	gen/o	crin/o

For each of the following, circle the correct spelling of the term:

59. hematopoesis	hematopoiesis	hematoepoisis
60. platelets	plattelets	plateletts
61. anissocytosis	aniscocytosis	anisocytosis
62. polkulocytosis	poikilocytosis	poiekilocytosis
63. hemalysis	hemoliesis	hemolysis
64. lymphadenpathy	lymphadenopathy	lymphoadenopathy
65. myelodysplasia	mylodysplaszia	myelodysphazia
66. thrombocytopnea	thrombocytopenia	throbocytpenia
67. hematocrit	hemacrit	hematocrete
68. splenecktomy	splenectomy	spleenectomy
69. plasmapheresis	plazmaphoresis	plasmophoresis
70. vasodialator	vasodilater	vasodilator

Give the noun that was used to form the following adjectives.

71. leukemic

72. immunosuppressive

73. plasmapheretic

74. thymic

75. hematopoietic

76. splenic

77. septicemic

78. hemophilic

79. myelodysplastic

80. thrombocytopenic

Write in the missing words on lines in the following illustrations of the components of blood

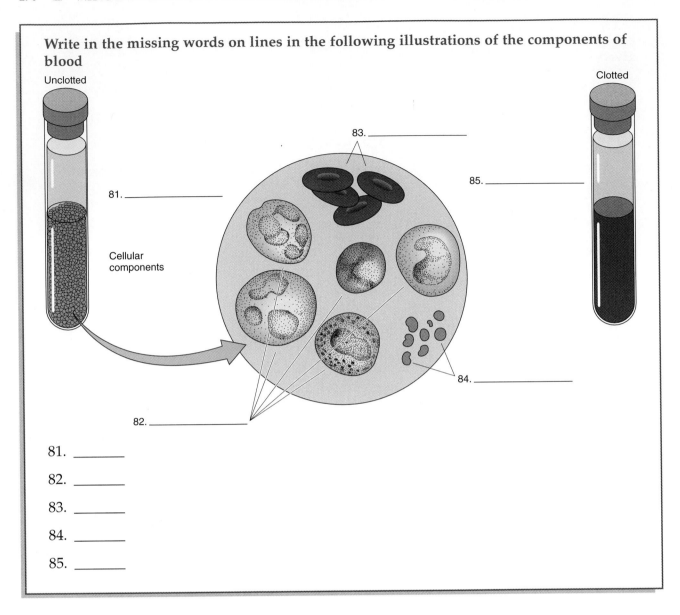

81. _____

82. _____

83. _____

84. _____

85. _____

Medical Record Analyses

MEDICAL RECORD 6-1

Progress Note

CC: fatigue

S: This 43 y/o female c/o feeling run down with lack of energy x 1 mo.
Pt denies fever, chills, nausea, vomiting, diarrhea, constipation and reports no weight loss. She has had very heavy menstrual periods lasting 5 days since DC of birth control pills 1 year ago.
PMH: mononucleosis at age 14, NKDA. FH: father, age 68, died of MI
Mother, age 74, has myelodysplasia; sister, age 45, L&W
SH: married x 8 yr, no children; ETOH—wine with dinner, denies smoking.

O: VS: T 98.8°F, P 81, R 15, BP 136/62. WDWN female in NAD. HEENT-WNL
Neck: supple /s̄ lymphadenopathy. Lungs: clear. Heart: RRR /s̄ murmur
Abdomen: soft and tender /s̄ organomegaly. Extremities: no edema.

A: Etiology of fatigue and decreased energy unclear. Possible iron deficiency anemia in light of heavy menstrual periods.

P: Blood studies to include comprehensive metabolic panel, CBC /c̄ differential.
RTO in 1 wk for lab results.

1. Which of the following is not mentioned in the history?
   a. type of treatment the patient received for mononucleosis
   b. patient's consumption of alcohol
   c. how long the patient had been married
   d. health status of the patient's sister

2. Describe the condition of the patient's mother:
   a. she has leukemia
   b. she has a bleeding disorder characterized by an abnormally decreased number of platelets in the blood
   c. she has a hereditary disorder characterized by an excessive buildup of iron deposits in the body
   d. she has a disorder within the bone marrow characterized by a proliferation of abnormal stem cells, which usually develops into leukemia

3. Which of the following describes the findings of the physical examination?
   a. swollen lymph glands
   b. normal examination
   c. fast heart rate
   d. heart murmur

4. What is the possible cause of the patient's fatigue?
   a. viral condition characterized by an increase in mononuclear cells (monocytes and lymphocytes) in the blood
   b. macrocytic normochromic type of anemia characterized by an inadequate supply of vitamin B_{12}, causing red blood cells to become large, varied in shape, and reduced in number
   c. microcytic-hypochromic type of anemia characterized by small red blood cells containing low amounts of hemoglobin because of lack of iron in the body
   d. normocytic-normochromic type of anemia characterized by the failure of bone marrow to produce red blood cells

5. Identify the subjective information most significantly linked to the assessment:
   a. enlarged lymph glands
   b. heavy menstrual periods
   c. fatigue
   d. the patient quit taking birth control pills

6. Which test of the following tests is part of the plan?
   a. test to determine coagulation defects such as platelet disorders
   b. test to diagnose an infection in the bloodstream, by culturing a specimen of blood
   c. needle aspiration of bone marrow tissue for pathologic examination
   d. expanded battery of automated blood chemistry tests used as a general screen for disease

MEDICAL RECORD 6-2 FOR ADDITIONAL STUDY

Henry Lin went to his personal physician after a period of generally not feeling well, losing his appetite, and starting to lose weight. His doctor then admitted him to Central Medical Center hospital for additional tests after conducting a physical examination and blood tests. He is now being treated as an outpatient by his internist, Dr. Bradley, and an oncologist, Dr. Ellison, to whom he was referred for consultation and concurrent care.

Read Medical Record 6-2 for Mr. Lin (pages 273-274) and answer the following questions.

The progress note is the oncology/hematology progress note dictated by Dr. Ellison, the oncologist treating Mr. Lin, at the time of follow-up visit two weeks after Mr. Lin's hospitalization. The second document is a hematology lab report, submitted before a second follow-up with Dr. Ellison two weeks later.

Write your answers in the spaces provided.

1. Below are medical terms used in the progress note you have not yet encountered in this text. Underline each where it appears in the record and define below.

   edema _____

   scaphoid _____

   anorexia _____

2. In your own words, not using medical terminology, translate Mr. Lin's diagnosis:

   _____

3. Name the diagnostic test that confirmed this diagnosis:

   _____

4. Write the medical term for Mr. Lin's enlarged spleen: _____

5. Dr. Ellison's March 31 record includes the results of two CBC component tests from the earlier March 23 lab report, as well as results from the same tests for March 31. The April 15 lab report also contains the CBC component tests. In the spaces below, write the name of the tests and their results at these three times. Do not use abbreviations. Be sure to include units of measure.

Test	Result		
	March 23	March 31	April 15
_____	_____	_____	_____
_____	_____	_____	_____

6. What are the three elements Dr. Ellison includes in Mr. Lin's treatment plan?

   a. _____

   b. _____

   c. _____

MEDICAL RECORD 6-2

CENTRAL MEDICAL GROUP, INC.
Department of Oncology/Hematology
201 Medical Center Drive • Central City, US 90000-1234 • PHONE: (012) 125-8888 • FAX: (012) 125-3434

PROGRESS NOTE

PATIENT: LIN, HENRY N.

DATE: March 31, 20xx

Mr. Lin is a 69-year-old man seen for myelodysplasia while hospitalized on March 17, 20xx. He was transfused with 4.0 U of packed cells during that hospitalization. A bone marrow revealed histology consistent with chronic myelomonocytic leukemia (myelodysplasia).

A follow-up blood count was obtained through Dr. Bradley's office on March 23, 20xx, and revealed a hemoglobin of 11.0 G/DL and a hematocrit of 31.0%.

There have been no fevers, sweats, or anorexia; but he has noted some weight loss. There has been no bleeding. There has been no nausea, vomiting, or dark and bloody stools.

Exam: Weight: 172 lb. Blood Pressure: 120/50. Temperature: 98.6°F. Pulse: 88. Respirations: 18.

HEENT: Mild gum atrophy and inflammation. NECK: Supple. LYMPH NODES: There is no cervical or supraclavicular adenopathy. LUNGS: Clear. CARDIOVASCULAR: Normal. ABDOMEN: Scaphoid, soft, and nontender. The spleen is enlarged. EXTREMITIES: Without edema or petechiae.

TODAY'S LAB: Complete blood count reveals a total leukocyte count of 6600/cu mm, a hemoglobin of 8.0 G/DL, a hematocrit of 23.0%, and a platelet count of 149,000/cu mm.

CLINICAL DIAGNOSIS:
Chronic myelomonocytic leukemia (myelodysplastic syndrome). The patient is transfusion dependent.

The patient will be typed and crossmatched today and will be transfused with 2.0 U of packed red blood cells through the Oncology Day Facility tomorrow on April 1, 20xx

I have asked the patient to follow up with Dr. Bradley next week and with me in two weeks.

A. Ellison, M.D.

AE:gds
cc: Blair Bradley, M.D.

D: 3/31/20xx
T: 4/3/20xx

CENTRAL MEDICAL CENTER
211 Medical Center Drive • Central City, US 90000-1234 • PHONE: (012) 125-6784 • FAX: (012) 125-9999

04/15/20xx
14:27

NAME : Lin, Henry	LOC: TEST	DOB: 2/2/xx	AGE: 69Y
MR# : TEST-226			SEX: M
ACCT# : 168946701			

M63558 COLL: 04/15/20xx 13:23   REC: 04/15/20xx 13:25

HEMOGRAM

CBC

WBC	4.1	[4.5 - 10.5]	K/UL
RBC	2.93	[4.6 - 6.2]	M/UL
HGB	9.1	[14.0 - 18.0]	G/DL
HCT	25.3	[42.0 - 52.0]	%
MCV	86.2	[82 - 92]	FL
MCH	31.1	[27 - 31]	PG
MCHC	36.0	[32 - 36]	G/DL
PLT	90	[150 - 450]	K/UL

Auto Lymph %	8.3	[20 - 40]	%
Auto Mono %	32.6	[1 - 11]	%
Auto Neutro %	57.8	[50 - 75]	%
Auto Eos %	1.0	[0 - 6]	%
Auto Baso %	0.3	[0 - 2]	%
Auto Lymph #	0.3	[1.5 - 4.0]	K/UL
Auto Mono #	1.3	[0.2 - 0.9]	K/UL
Auto Neutro #	2.4	[1.0 - 7.0]	K/UL
Auto Eos #	0.0	[0 - 0.7]	K/UL
Auto Baso #	0.0	[0 - 0.2]	K/UL

TEST, PATIENT   TEST-221   END OF REPORT   PAGE 1
04/15/20xx 14:27   INTERIM REPORT

INTERIM REPORT COMPLETE

7. Study the April 15 laboratory report carefully and complete the following table of selected test results. Write the name of the measurement that is abbreviated and an N if the result for Mr. Lin is within the normal range or an A (abnormal) if the result is outside the normal range.

a. WBC _____

b. RBC _____

c. HGB _____

d. HCT _____

e. MCV _____

f. MCH _____

g. MCHC _____

h. PLT _____

i. lymph _____

j. mono _____

k. neutro _____

l. eos _____

m. baso _____

Answers to Practice Exercises

1. erythro/blast/osis
   CF   R   S
   red/germ or bud/condition or increase
2. chylo/poiesis
   CF   S
   juice/formation
3. hemo/cyto/meter
   CF   CF   S
   blood/cell/instrument for measuring
4. spleno/rrhagia
   CF   S
   spleen/to burst forth
5. lymph/aden/itis
   R   R   S
   clear fluid/gland/inflammation
6. immuno/tox/ic
   CF   R   S
   safe/poison/pertaining to
7. reticulo/cyt/osis
   CF   R   S
   a net/cell/condition or increase

8. thymo/path/y
   CF   R   S
   thymus gland/disease/condition or process of
9. leuko/cyt/ic
   CF   R   S
   white/cell/pertaining to
10. lymph/angio/gram
    R   CF   S
    clear fluid/vessel/record
11. spleno/megaly
    CF   S
    spleen/enlargement
12. pro/myelo/cyt/e
    P   CF   R   S
    before/bone marrow/cell/noun marker
13. leuko/cyto/penia
    CF   CF   S
    white/cell/abnormal reduction
14. splen/ectomy
    R   S
    spleen/excision (removal)
15. dia/lysis
    P   S
    across or through/breaking down or dissolution

16. lymph/oma
    R   S
    clear fluid/tumor
17. cyto/morpho/logy
    CF   CF   S
    cell/form/study of
18. hemo/lysis
    CF   S
    blood/breaking down or dissolution
19. an/emia
    P   S
    without/blood condition
20. meta/stasis
    P   S
    beyond, after, or change/stop or stand
21. mean corpuscular (cell) volume (MCV)
22. mean corpuscular (cell) hemoglobin (MCH)
23. mean corpuscular (cell) hemoglobin concentration (MCHC)
24. white blood count, WBC
25. hemoglobin, HGB, or Hgb
26. hematocrit, HCT, or Hct
27. differential count

28. prothrombin time
29. erythrocyte sedimentation rate
30. partial thromboplastin time
31. complete blood count
32. l
33. j
34. k
35. g
36. c
37. e
38. f
39. b
40. d
41. i
42. h
43. a
44. neutropenia
45. autologous blood
46. immunosuppression
47. crossmatching
48. acquired immunodeficiency syndrome, AIDS
49. plasmapheresis

50. homologous blood
51. phag/o
52. thromb/o
53. chyl/o
54. plas/o
55. chrom/o
56. hem/o
57. immun/o
58. blast/o
59. hematopoiesis
60. platelets
61. anisocytosis
62. poikilocytosis
63. hemolysis
64. lymphadenopathy
65. myelodysplasia
66. thrombocytopenia
67. hematocrit
68. splenectomy
69. plasmapheresis
70. vasodilator
71. leukemia
72. immunosuppression
73. plasmapheresis

74. thymus
75. hematopoiesis
76. spleen
77. septicemia
78. hemophilia
79. myelodysplasia
80. thrombocytopenia
81. plasma
82. leukocytes
83. erythrocytes
84. thrombocytes
85. serum

Answers to Medical Record 6-1

1. a
2. d
3. b
4. c
5. b
6. d

CHAPTER 7

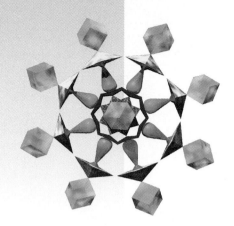

Respiratory System

Respiratory System Overview

Functions of the respiratory system (Fig. 7-1):

* Brings oxygen into the body as the lungs inhale air (inspiration) and passes oxygen into the blood
* Rids the body of carbon dioxide by exhaling it (expiration) as the lungs receive carbon dioxide diffused out of the blood

SELF-INSTRUCTION: COMBINING FORMS

Study the following:

Combining Form	Meaning
alveol/o	alveolus (air sac)
bronch/o bronchi/o	bronchus (airway)
bronchiol/o	bronchiole (little airway)
capn/o carb/o	carbon dioxide
laryng/o	larynx (voice box)
lob/o	lobe (a portion)
nas/o rhin/o	nose
or/o	mouth

THE RESPIRATORY SYSTEM

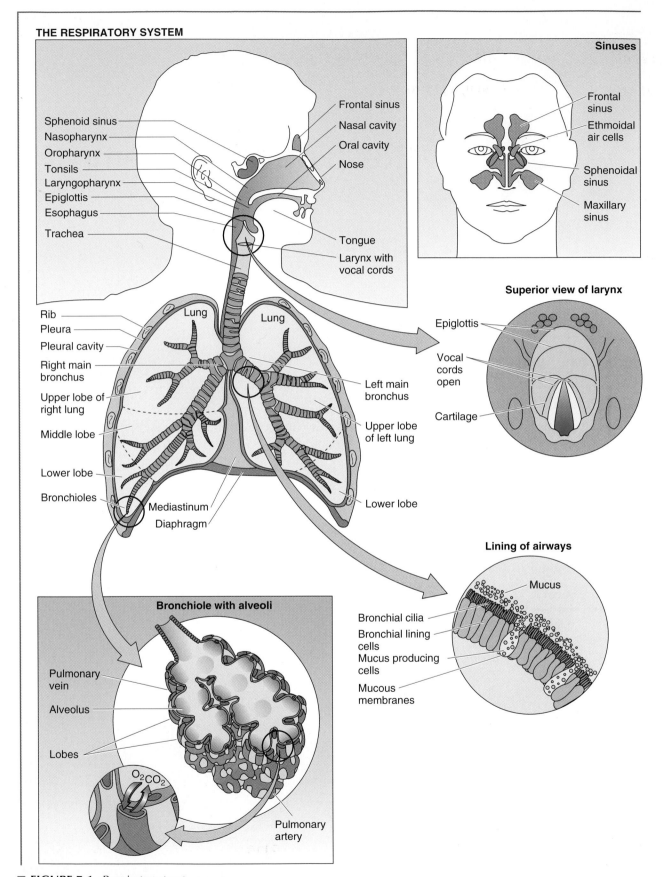

■ **FIGURE 7-1.** Respiratory tract.

ox/o	oxygen
palat/o	palate
pharyng/o	pharynx (throat)
phren/o	diaphragm (also mind)
pleur/o	pleura (lining of lungs)
pneum/o pneumon/o	air or lung
pulmon/o	lung
sinus/o	sinus (cavity)
spir/o	breathing
thorac/o pector/o steth/o	chest
tonsill/o	tonsil
trache/o	trachea (windpipe)
uvul/o	uvula
-pnea (additional suffix)	breathing

PROGRAMMED REVIEW: COMBINING FORMS

Answers	Review

7.1 The lungs are the primary organs of the respiratory system. A pulmonologist is a medical specialist concerned with the lungs. The combining form for lung is _____. The two combining forms that can refer to either air or lung are _____ and

pulmon/o

pneum/o

pneumon/o

inflammation

_____. For example, pneumothorax describes air in the chest (pleural cavity). Pneumonitis is an _____ of the lung.

lob/o

excision

lobectomy

7.2 The combining form for lobe (as in a lung lobe) is _____. Because the suffix *-ectomy* means an _____ or removal, the removal of a lung lobe is a _____.

7.3 Several different combining forms refer to the chest and are therefore the basis of terms related to the respiratory system. A thoracotomy

incision

thorac/o

is an _____ into the chest (the term uses the combining

form _____). A stethoscope is an instrument used to listen to

lung sounds through the chest wall, from the combining form

steth/o, pain

pector/o

_____. Because the suffix *-algia* refers to _____, pectoralgia

means chest pain, from the combining form _____.

ox/o

deficient or below

condition of

hypoxia

blood

hypoxemia

7.4 The combining form meaning oxygen is _____. Using the prefix

hypo-, which means _____, and the suffix *-ia*, which

means _____ _____, the term for a condition of deficient

oxygen levels is _____. Because the suffix *-emia* refers to a

_____ condition, the term for a condition of deficient oxygen in

the blood is _____.

capn/o

carb/o

much

7.5 The lungs move oxygen into the blood and carbon dioxide out of

the blood. The combining forms for carbon dioxide are _____

and _____. Hypercapnia, for example, is a condition of too

_____ carbon dioxide in the blood; hypercarbia is a synonym. The

term for a condition of too little carbon dioxide in the blood is

hypocapnia, hypocarbia

_____ or _____.

breathing

measuring

spirometry

-pnea

difficult (painful, faulty)

7.6 The combining form *spir/o* means _____. Because

-metry refers to the process of _____ something, the

term for the measuring of breathing is _____. A suffix related to breathing is _____, as in the term dyspnea, meaning

_____ breathing.

7.7 Many combining forms are the basis of anatomic terms related to

the respiratory system. The combining form meaning mouth or oral

or/o

nas/o

cavity is _or/o_. The combining form meaning nose or nasal cavity is

nas/o. From the Greek word rhis comes a second combining

rhin/o	term for nose: ___rhin/o___. Rhinitis, for example, is an
inflammation	___inflammation___ of the nose.

sinus/o	**7.8** The combining form for sinus is ___sinus/o___. Because the suffix
-itis	meaning an inflammation is ___-itis___, the term for an inflammation of
sinusitis	a sinus is ___sinus itis___ (remember that a combining vowel is *not* used before a suffix that begins with a vowel).

	7.9 The palate is the roof of the mouth, from the combining form
palat/o	___palat/o___. Recalling that the suffix *-plasty* refers to a surgical repair or reconstruction, the term for reconstruction of the palate is
palatoplasty	___palatoplasty___.

pharyng/o	**7.10** The combining form for the pharynx (throat) is ___pharyng/o___.
pharyngitis	An inflamed pharynx is ___pharyngitis___. Beneath the
	pharynx is the larynx (voice box), from the combining form
laryng/o, laryngitis	___laryng/o___. An inflamed larynx is ___laryngitis___.

	7.11 Many anatomic terms are virtually identical to their combining
	forms. The combining term for tonsil is ___tonsill/o___. The com-
tonsill/o	
uvul/o	bining term for uvula is ___uvul/o___. The combining term for trachea
trache/o	(windpipe) is ___trache/o___. These are all structures of the airway.

bronch/o	**7.12** The combining form for bronchus (airway) is _____ or
bronchi	*bronchi/o*. The plural of bronchus is _____. A related term,
bronchiol/o	bronchiole (little airway), is from the combining form _____.

	7.13 An alveolus is a small air sac in the lungs, from the combining
alveol/o	form _____. The common adjective form is alveolar.

	7.14 Pleura is a membrane enclosing the lungs, and the combining
pleur/o, pleurae	form is _____. The plural of pleura is _____.

	7.15 The Greek word phren can mean either the mind or the diaphragm, a muscular partition below the lungs. The combining form for
phren/o	diaphragm is _____. Using the common suffix for pain, the
phrenalgia or phrenodynia	term for pain in the diaphragm is _____.

SELF-INSTRUCTION: ANATOMICAL TERMS

Study the following:

Term	Meaning
nose *nōz*	structure that warms, moistens, and filters air as it enters the respiratory tract; also houses the olfactory receptors for the sense of smell
sinuses *sī'nŭ-ĕz*	air-filled spaces in the skull that open into the nasal cavity
palate	the roof of the mouth; divided into the hard and soft palate
pharynx *far'ingks*	throat; passageway for food to the esophagus and air to the larynx
nasopharynx *nā-zō-far-ingks*	part of the pharynx directly behind the nasal passages
oropharynx *ŏr'ō-far-ingks*	central portion of the pharynx between the roof of the mouth and the upper edge of the epiglottis
laryngopharynx *lă-ring'gō-far-ingks*	lower part of the pharynx just below the oropharynx opening into the larynx and esophagus
tonsils *ton'silz*	oval lymphatic tissues on each side of the pharynx that filter air to protect the body from bacterial invasion; also called palatine tonsils
adenoid *ad'ĕ-noyd*	lymphatic tissue on the back of the pharynx behind the nose; also called pharyngeal tonsil
uvula	small projection hanging from the back middle edge of the soft palate, named for its grapelike shape
larynx lar'ingks	voice box; passageway for air moving from pharynx to trachea; contains vocal cords
glottis *glot'is*	opening between the vocal cords in the larynx
epiglottis *ep-i-glot'is*	a lidlike structure that covers the larynx during swallowing to prevent food from entering the airway
trachea *trĕ'kē-ă*	windpipe; passageway for air from the larynx to the area of the carina, where it splits into right and left bronchus

bronchial tree *brong′kē-ăl*	branched airways that lead from the trachea to the microscopic air sacs called alveoli
right and left bronchus *brong′kŭs*	two primary airways branching from the area of the carina into the lungs
bronchioles *brong′kē-ōl*	progressively smaller tubular branches of the airways
alveoli *al-vē′ō-lī*	thin-walled microscopic air sacs that exchange gases
lungs *lŭngz*	two spongy organs in the thoracic cavity enclosed by the diaphragm and rib cage, responsible for respiration
lobes *lōbz*	subdivisions of the lung; two on the left and three on the right
pleura *plū″ă*	membranes enclosing the lung (visceral pleura) and lining the thoracic cavity (parietal pleura)
pleural cavity *plūr′ăl kav′i-tē*	potential space between visceral and parietal layers of the pleura
diaphragm *dī′ă-fram*	muscular partition that separates the thoracic cavity from the abdominal cavity and moves up and down to aid respiration
mediastinum *me′dē-as-tī′nŭm*	partition that separates the thorax into two compartments (containing the right and left lungs) and encloses the heart, esophagus, trachea, and thymus gland
mucous membranes *myū′kŭs mem′brān*	thin sheets of tissue that line respiratory passages and secrete mucus, a viscid (sticky) fluid
cilia *sil′ē-ă*	hairlike processes from the surface of epithelial cells, such as those of the bronchi, to move mucus cell secretions upward
parenchyma *pă-reng′ki-mă*	functional tissues of any organ, such as the tissues of the bronchioles, alveoli, ducts, and sacs that perform respiration

PROGRAMMED REVIEW: ANATOMICAL TERMS

Answers	Review
	7.16 Air enters the respiratory system at the mouth and nose, which filters and warms the air. The air-filled cavities in the skull that open
sinuses	into the nasal cavity are called _____. The roof of the mouth
palate	is called the _____, which is divided into two parts: the hard
soft	and _____ palate.

pharynx

7.17 Air then passes through the throat, or _____. The part of this structure behind the nasal passages, a term using the combining

nasopharynx

form for nose, is called the _____nasopharynx_____. The part of the pharynx between the roof of the mouth, a term using the combining

oropharynx

form for mouth, is the _____oropharynx_____.

larynx

7.18 The air moves from the pharynx to the structure called the voice box, the medical term for which is _____larynx_____. Appropriately, the lower part of the pharynx where it meets the larynx is the

laryngopharynx

_____. The oval lymphatic tissues on each side of the pharynx that help "filter bacteria from the air" are the

tonsils

_____tonsil_____. Another area of lymphatic tissue on the back of the

adenoid

pharynx behind the nose is the _____adenoid_____. Hanging from the back middle edge of the soft palate is a small tissue projection called the

uvula

_____uvula_____.

vocal cords

7.19 The glottis is the opening between the _____ _____ in the larynx. A related term for the lidlike structure that covers the larynx during swallowing to prevent food from entering the trachea is the

epiglottis, upon

_____. The prefix *epi-* means _____ (the epiglottis lies upon the trachea to close it like a lid during swallowing).

trachea

7.20 The air then enters the windpipe, or _____, which

bronchi

splits into the right and left _____, the two primary airways to the lungs. Notice in Figure 7-1 how the bronchi soon split into more and more branches. This branching structure is called the

bronchial

_____ tree. The smallest tubular branches are the

bronchioles, -ole

_____. The suffix _____ means small.

7.21 At the ends of the bronchioles are thin-walled microscopic air

alveoli

sacs called _____, where oxygen and carbon dioxide are exchanged. The singular form of this term is _____. The

alveolus

alveoli comprise much of the right and left _____. The left lung is

lungs

lobes	divided into two sections called _____, whereas the right lung
three	has _____ lobes.

7.22 The membranes enclosing the lung and lining the thoracic cavity

pleura	are called _____. Between these two layers of pleura is a po-
pleural	tential space called the _____ cavity.

7.23 The lungs are in the thoracic cavity. Between this area and the ab-

dominal cavity below is the muscular partition that moves up and

diaphragm	down to help breathing, called the _____.

7.24 The term medial means relating to the middle; using the same

combining form, the term for the partition in the middle of the thorax

that separates the thorax into two compartments is the

mediastinum	_____.

7.25 Lining the inside of respiratory passages are membranes that se-

mucous membranes	crete mucus, called _____ _____. Note the dif-
mucous	ference between the noun mucus and the adjective form _____.
	Mucus traps microorganisms and other materials, and tiny, hairlike
cilia	processes called _____ move this mucus up out of the respiratory
	tract to be expelled from the body.

tissue	**7.26** The term parenchyma refers to functional _____ of any
	organ. In the lungs, the parenchyma includes the bronchioles and, most
alveoli	importantly, the _____, where gas exchange takes place.

SELF-INSTRUCTION: SYMPTOMATIC TERMS

Study the following:

Term	Meaning

BREATHING (FIG. 7-2)

eupnea yūp-nē′ă	normal breathing

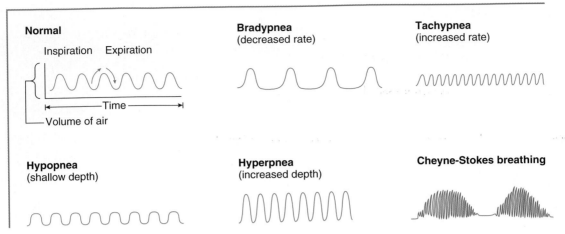

■ **FIGURE 7-2.** Examples of breathing patterns.

bradypnea *brad-ip-nē'ă*	slow breathing
tachypnea *tak-ip-nē'ă*	fast breathing
hypopnea *hī-pop'nē'ă*	shallow breathing
hyperpnea *hi-perp'nē'ă*	deep breathing
dyspnea *disp-nē'ă*	difficulty breathing
apnea *ap'nē-ă*	inability to breathe
orthopnea *ōr-thop-nē'ă*	ability to breathe only in an upright position
Cheyne-Stokes respiration *res-pi-rā'shŭn*	pattern of breathing characterized by a gradual increase of depth and sometimes rate to a maximum level, followed by a decrease, resulting in apnea

Lung Sounds

crackles *krak'ĕelz* **rales** *rahlz*	popping sounds heard on auscultation of the lung when air enters diseased airways and alveoli; occurs in disorders such as bronchiectasis or atelectasis
wheezes *hwēz'ez* **rhonchi** *rong'kī*	high-pitched, musical sounds heard on auscultation of the lung as air flows through a narrowed airway; occurs in disorders such as asthma or emphysema
stridor *strī'dōr*	a high-pitched crowing sound that occurs with an obstruction in the upper airway (trachea or larynx)

GENERAL SYMPTOMATIC TERMS

cyanosis *sī- ă -nō'sis*	a bluish coloration of the skin caused by a deficient amount of oxygen in the blood
dysphonia *dis-fō'nē-ă*	~~hoarseness~~ (phon/o = voice or sound)
epistaxis *ep'i-stak'sis*	~~nosebleed (epi = upon; stazo = to drip)~~
expectoration *ek-spek-tō-rā'shŭn*	coughing up and spitting out of material from the lungs
sputum *spū'tŭm*	material expelled from the lungs by coughing
hemoptysis *hē-mop'ti-sis*	coughing up and spitting out blood originating in the lungs (ptysis = to spit)
hypercapnia *hī-per-kap'nē-ă* **hypercarbia** *hī-per-kar'bē-ă*	excessive level of carbon dioxide in the blood (capno = smoke; (carbo = coal)
hyperventilation *hī'per-ven-ti-lā'shŭn*	excessive movement of air in and out of the lungs, causing hypocapnia
hypoventilation *hī'pō-ven-ti-lā'shŭn*	deficient movement of air in and out of the lungs, causing hypercapnia
hypoxemia *hī-pok-sē'mē-ă*	deficient amount of oxygen in the blood
hypoxia *hī-pok'sē-ă*	deficient amount of oxygen in tissue cells
obstructive lung disorder (Fig. 7-3) *lŭng dis-ōr'der*	condition blocking the flow of air moving out of the lungs
restrictive lung disorder (Fig. 7-3)	condition limiting the intake of air into the lungs
caseous necrosis *kā'sē-ŭs nĕ-krō'sis*	degeneration and death of tissue with a cheeselike appearance
pulmonary edema *pŭl'mō-nār-ē e-dē'mă*	fluid filling of the spaces around the alveoli and eventually flooding into the alveoli
pulmonary infiltrate *pŭl'mō-nār-ē in-fil'trāt*	density on an x-ray representing the consolidation of matter within the air spaces of the lungs, usually resulting from an inflammatory process
rhinorrhea *rī-nō-rē'ă*	thin, watery discharge from the nose (~~runny nose~~)

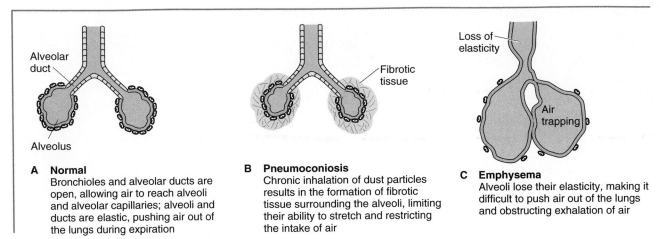

A Normal
Bronchioles and alveolar ducts are open, allowing air to reach alveoli and alveolar capillaries; alveoli and ducts are elastic, pushing air out of the lungs during expiration

B Pneumoconiosis
Chronic inhalation of dust particles results in the formation of fibrotic tissue surrounding the alveoli, limiting their ability to stretch and restricting the intake of air

C Emphysema
Alveoli lose their elasticity, making it difficult to push air out of the lungs and obstructing exhalation of air

FIGURE 7-3. Comparison of normal alveoli (**A**) with alveoli in restrictive (**B**) and obstructive (**C**) lung disorders.

PROGRAMMED REVIEW: SYMPTOMATIC TERMS

Answers	Review
breathing fast brady-, tachypnea bradypnea	**7.27** Again, the suffix *-pnea* refers to _____. Many symptomatic terms use this suffix to identify different breathing problems. Recall that the prefix *tachy-* means _____, and the prefix for slow is _____. Therefore, fast breathing is _____, and slow breathing is _____.
deficient hyper- hypopnea hyperpnea	**7.28** The prefix *hypo-* means below or _____, and the opposite prefix meaning above or excessive is _____. The term for shallow (or deficient) breathing is therefore _____, and the term for deep (or excessive) breathing is _____.
normal difficult eupnea dyspnea	**7.29** The prefix *eu-* means good or _____, and the prefix *dys-* means painful, faulty, or _____. Therefore, the term for normal breathing is _____, and the term for difficulty breathing is _____.
without apnea stopped upright	**7.30** The prefix *a-* means _____. The term for an inability to breathe is _____, and in an apneic patient breathing has _____ entirely. Orthopnea refers to an inability to breathe in any but an _____ position.

Cheyne-Stokes

7.31 A pattern of breathing in which depth and sometimes rate gradually increase and then decrease is called _____-_____ respiration.

7.32 Recall that with a stethoscope one can listen to sounds in the

chest

_____. Lung sounds are often symptomatic of respiratory problems. The popping sounds causes by air entering diseased airways and

crackles

alveoli are called _____ or rales. High-pitched musical sounds resulting from air flowing through a narrowed airway, such as

rhonchi

in asthma or emphysema, are called wheezes or _____. The high-pitched crowing sound occurring with an obstructed upper airway

stridor

is called _____.

7.33 The two combining forms for carbon dioxide are *carb/o* and

capn/o

_____. Using the prefix meaning above or excessive and the suf-

condition of

fix *-ia* meaning _____ ____, the term describing a condition of having too much carbon dioxide in the blood is called

hypercapnia, hypercarbia

_____ or _____.

7.34 *Hypo-* is a prefix meaning below or _____. The

deficient

condition of

suffix *-ia* means _____ ____. Joined with the combin-

ox/o

ing form for oxygen, or _____, the term describing a condition of defi-

hypoxia

cient oxygen (in the tissues) is therefore _____. Hypoxemia is the term that describes the initial effect or condition of the

blood, deficient

_____ when there is a _____ amount of

oxygen

_____. A related term links *cyan/o*, the combining form mean-

blue

ing _____, with *-osis*, the suffix meaning condition or

increase

_____, to form the term describing a bluish coloration of the skin caused by a deficient amount of oxygen in the blood:

cyanosis, cyanotic

_____. The adjective form is _____.

hyperventilation

hypoventilation

7.35 Ventilation is the movement of air in and out of the lungs. Excessive movement of air is called _____,

whereas deficient movement of air is _____.

dys-

dysphonia

7.36 The prefix meaning difficult, painful, or faulty is _dys_. Combined with the combining form *phon/o* meaning voice or sound, and the suffix for condition, the term for a condition of hoarseness (difficult or painful voice) is ___dysphonia___.

epi-

epistaxis

7.37 The term for nosebleed does *not* use the combining form for nose. It literally means "drip upon," combining the prefix for (upon) _epi_, with *stazo*, a root meaning to (drip). The medical term for nosebleed is ___epistaxis___.

expectoration.

sputum

hemoptysis

7.38 The cilia lining the structures of the airway move mucus and other material up out of the airway and lungs, where it can be coughed up and spit out of the body. The process of coughing up and spitting out such material is termed _____. The material expelled from the lungs by coughing is called _____. Using the combining form for blood (*hem/o*), the term for coughing up blood from the lungs is _____.

obstructive

restrictive lung

7.39 A condition blocking the flow of air moving out of the lungs is an _____ lung disorder. A condition limiting the intake of air into the lungs is a _____ _____ disorder.

pulmonary

7.40 Edema is the presence of excessive watery fluid. Edema in the lungs is called _____ edema.

infiltrate

inflammation

7.41 Density on an x-ray representing the consolidation of matter within the air spaces of the lungs is called a pulmonary _____. Pulmonary infiltrates usually indicate a process of _____ in the lung.

necro/o	**7.42** The word caseous means cheeselike in appearance. Recall that the combining form meaning death is _____. The term for dead and degenerating tissue with a cheeselike appearance is
caseous necrosis	_____ _____. The suffix -*osis* means
condition or increase	_____.
discharge	**7.43** Recall that the suffix -*rrhea* means ___*discharge*___. This suffix joins with the Greek combining form for nose to create the term
rhinorrhea	for watery discharge from the nose: ___*rhinorrhea*___.

SELF-INSTRUCTION: DIAGNOSTIC TERMS

Study the following:

Term	Meaning
asthma (Fig. 7-4) *az'mă*	panting; obstructive pulmonary disease caused by a spasm of the bronchial tubes or by swelling of their mucous membrane, characterized by paroxysmal (sudden, periodic) attacks of wheezing, dyspnea, and cough
atelectasis *at-ĕ-lek'tă-sis*	collapse of lung tissue (alveoli) (atele = imperfect; -ectasis = expansion or dilation)
bronchitis *brong-kī'tis*	inflammation of the bronchi
bronchogenic carcinoma *brong-kō-jen'ik kar-si-nō'mă*	lung cancer; cancer originating in the bronchi

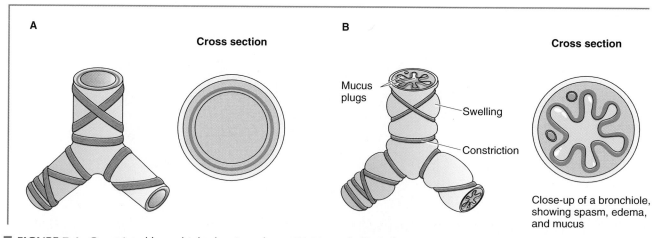

■ FIGURE 7-4. Constricted bronchial tubes in asthma. **(A)** Normal. **(B)** Asthma.

bronchospasm *brong'kō-spazm*	constriction of bronchi caused by spasm (involuntary contraction) of the peribronchial smooth muscle
bronchiectasis (Fig. 7-5) *brong-kē-ek'tă-sis*	abnormal dilation of the bronchi with accumulation of mucus
emphysema (Fig. 7-3C) *em-fi-sē'mă*	obstructive pulmonary disease characterized by overexpansion of the alveoli with air and destructive changes in their walls resulting in loss of lung elasticity and gas exchange (emphysan = to inflate)
chronic obstructive pulmonary disease (COPD) *kron'ik pūl'mō-nār-ē di-zēz'*	permanent, destructive pulmonary disorder that is a combination of chronic bronchitis and emphysema
laryngitis *lar-in-jī'tis*	inflammation of the larynx
laryngotracheo- bronchitis (LTB) *lăr-ing'gō-trā'kē-o- brong-kī'tis* **croup** *krūp*	inflammation of the upper airways with swelling that creates a funnel--shaped elongation of tissue causing a distinct, "seal bark" cough
laryngospasm *lă-ring'gō-spazm*	spasm of laryngeal muscles, causing a constriction

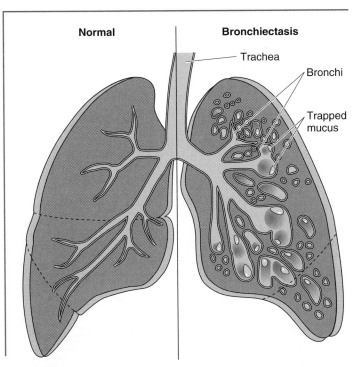

■ **FIGURE 7-5.** Bronchiectasis.

nasal polyposis *nā'zăl pol'i-pō'sis*	presence of numerous polyps in the nose (a polyp is a tumor on a stalk)
pharyngitis *far-in-jī'tis*	inflammation of the pharynx
coryza *kŏ-rī'ză*	head cold; inflammation of the nasal mucous membranes
pleural effusion (Fig. 7-6) *plŭr'ăl e-fū'zhŭn*	accumulation of fluid within the pleural cavity
empyema *em-pī-ē'mă* **pyothorax** *pī-ō-thōr'aks*	accumulation of pus in the pleural cavity
hemothorax *hē-mō-thōr'aks*	blood in pleural cavity
pleuritis *plū-rī'tis* **pleurisy** *plūr'i-sē*	inflammation of pleura
pneumoconiosis (Fig. 7-3 B) *nū'mō-kō-nē-ō'sis*	chronic restrictive pulmonary disease resulting from prolonged inhalation of fine dusts such as coal, asbestos (asbestosis), or silicone (silicosis) (conio = dust)

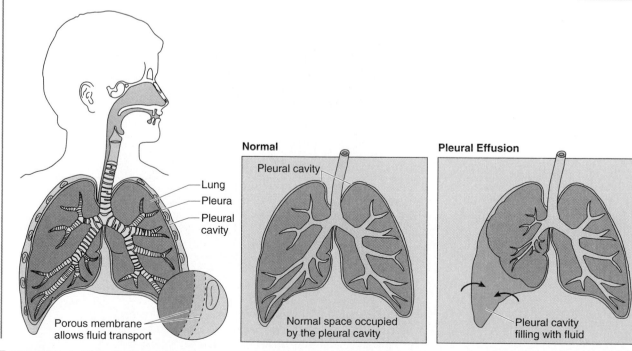

■ FIGURE 7-6. Pleural effusion.

pneumonia (Fig. 7-7) *nū-mō′nē-ă*	an inflammation in the lung caused by infection from bacteria, viruses, fungi, or parasites, or resulting from aspiration of chemicals
Pneumocystis pneumonia *nū-mō-sis′tis nū-mō′nē-ă*	pneumonia caused by the *Pneumocystis carinii* organism, a common opportunistic infection seen in those with positive human immunodeficiency virus
pneumothorax (Fig. 7-8) *nū-mō-thōr′aks*	air in the pleural cavity caused by a puncture of the lung or chest wall
pneumohemothorax *nū′mō-hē-mō-thōr′aks*	air and blood in the pleural cavity
pneumonitis *nū-mō-nī″tis*	inflammation of the lung often caused by hypersensitivity to chemicals or dusts
pulmonary embolism *pŭl′mō-nār-ē em′bō-lizm*	occlusion in the pulmonary circulation, most often caused by a blood clot
pulmonary tuberculosis (TB) *pŭl′mō-nār-ē tū-ber-kyū-lō-sis*	disease caused by the presence of *Mycobacterium tuberculosis* in the lungs, characterized by the formation of tubercles, inflammation, and necrotizing caseous lesions (caseous necrosis)
sinusitis *sī-nŭ-sī′tis*	inflammation of the sinuses

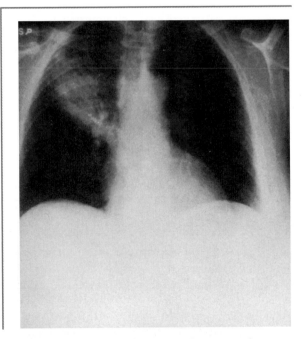

■ **FIGURE 7-7.** Chest radiograph showing pulmonary infiltrates in right upper lobe consistent with lobar pneumonia. Dense material (inflammatory exudate) absorbs radiation, whereas normal alveoli do not.

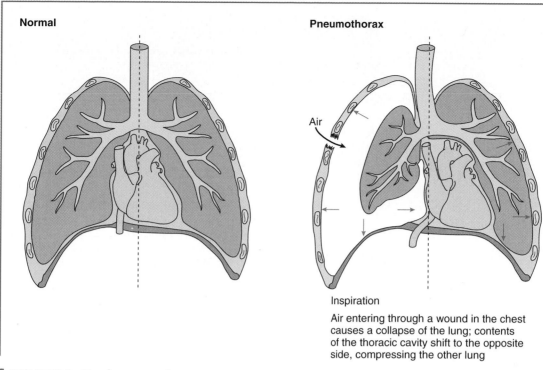

Normal   **Pneumothorax**

Air

Inspiration

Air entering through a wound in the chest
causes a collapse of the lung; contents
of the thoracic cavity shift to the opposite
side, compressing the other lung

■ **FIGURE 7-8.** Simple pneumothorax.

sleep apnea	periods of breathing cessation (10 seconds or more) that occur during sleep, often causing snoring
~~**tonsillitis**~~ *ton'si-lī'tis*	~~acute or chronic inflammation of the tonsils~~
upper respiratory infection (URI) *res'pi-ră-tōr-ē in-fek'shŭn*	infectious disease of the upper respiratory tract involving the nasal passages, pharynx, and bronchi

PROGRAMMED REVIEW: DIAGNOSTIC TERMS

Answers	Review
upper respiratory infection	**7.44** URI is the abbreviation for _Upper_ _Respiratory_ _Infection_, an infection of the upper respiratory tract involving the nasal passages, pharynx, and bronchi.
-itis sinusitis tonsillitis	**7.45** Recall that the suffix for inflammation is _itis_. Many individual structures of the respiratory system can become inflamed, often by an infection. Inflammation of the sinuses is _sinusitis_. Inflammation of the tonsils is _____ Inflammation of

pharyngitis	the pharynx is _____. Inflammation of the larynx
laryngitis	is _____. Inflammation of the bronchi is
bronchitis	_____.

pleuritis	**7.46** Inflammation of the pleura is _____. Another
pleurisy	term for this condition is _____.

7.47   The term for inflammation of the lung is built from the combining form meaning either air or lung. This term is _____.

pneumonitis

Another "itis" inflammation involving the larynx, trachea, and bronchi causes a distinctive, seal-like bark; the longer term for this condition

laryngotracheobronchitis

uses all three combining forms, _____,

croup

and the shorter term for this condition is _____.

7.48   Several other diagnostic terms are built from the combining form meaning air or lung. Using a suffix indicating a condition, the term for an infection of the lung caused by bacteria, viruses, or chemicals is

pneumonia

_____. A particular kind of pneumonia caused by the

Pneumocystis

Pneumocystis carinii organism is _____ pneumonia. A chronic restrictive disease resulting from inhaling dust (conio =

pneumoconiosis

dust) is _____.

7.49   This same combining form for air is used to make terms referring to air in a body cavity. Air in the thorax caused by a puncture of the

pneumothorax

lung or chest wall is _____. The term for both air and blood (hem/o = blood) in the thorax is

pneumohemothorax

_____. The presence of blood alone in

hemothorax

the pleural cavity of the chest is _____.

7.50   In addition to inflammation of the bronchi, called

bronchitis

_____, several other diagnostic conditions can occur in the bronchi. Recall that the suffix for an involuntary contraction is

-spasm

_____. A constriction of the bronchi caused by contraction of the

bronchospasm	smooth muscle around the bronchi is _____. Recall that the diagnostic suffix for expansion or dilation is
-ectasis	_____; thus, the condition of abnormal dilation of the
bronchiectasis	bronchi with an accumulation of mucus is _____.
carcinoma	Recall that _____ means cancer tumor. Lung cancer
bronchogenic	originating in the bronchi is called _____
carcinoma	_____.

-spasm

7.51 Again, the suffix for an involuntary contraction is _____. A contraction of laryngeal muscles, causing a constriction, is termed

laryngospasm

_____.

-ectasis

7.52 Again, the suffix for expansion or dilation is _____. The term for a collapse of lung tissue uses this suffix with the root *atele*

atelectasis

(imperfect): _____.

7.53 There are several types of obstructive pulmonary disease. Caused by a spasm of the bronchial tubes or by swelling of their mucous membrane, _____ is characterized by sudden attacks of wheezing,

asthma

dyspnea, and cough. Another condition, characterized by overexpansion of the alveoli with air and destructive changes in their walls, is

emphysema

_____. The permanent destructive pulmonary disorder that is a combination of emphysema and chronic bronchitis is

chronic obstructive pulmonary

_____ _____ _____

disease

_____ (COPD).

condition

7.54 The diagnostic suffix *-osis* means ___condition___ or increase. The condition of numerous polyps present in the nose is

nasal polyposis

___nasal___ ___polyposis___.

7.55 The medical term for a head cold, or inflammation of the nasal

coryza

mucous membranes, is _____.

hemothorax

pyothorax

pleural

effusion

7.56 Fluid, pus, blood, or air can accumulate in the pleural cavity. The term for blood in this cavity in the thorax is _____. The combining form meaning pus is *py/o*, and thus the accumulation of pus in the pleural cavity is _____, or empyema. An accumulation of fluid in the pleural cavity is called a _____ _____.

apnea

sleep apnea

7.57 Recall that the term for an inability to breathe is _____. The condition in which this happens for short periods during sleep is called _____ _____.

pulmonary tuberculosis

7.58 The bacteria *Mycobacterium tuberculosis* causes this lung disease: _____ _____.

pulmonary embolism

7.59 A blood clot that lodges in the pulmonary circulation causing an occlusion is called a _____ _____.

SELF-INSTRUCTION: DIAGNOSTIC TESTS AND PROCEDURES

Study the following:

Test or Procedure	Explanation
arterial blood gases (ABGs) *ar-tēr–rē-ăl*	analysis of arterial blood to determine adequacy of lung function in the exchange of gases
pH	a measure of blood acidity or alkalinity
PaO$_2$	partial pressure of oxygen measuring the amount of oxygen in the blood
PaCO$_2$	partial pressure of carbon dioxide measuring the amount of carbon dioxide in the blood
endoscopy *en-dos'kŏ-pē*	examination inside a body cavity with a flexible endoscope for diagnostic or treatment purposes
bronchoscopy (Fig. 7-9) *brong-kos'kŏ-pē*	use of a flexible endoscope, called a bronchoscope, to examine the airways

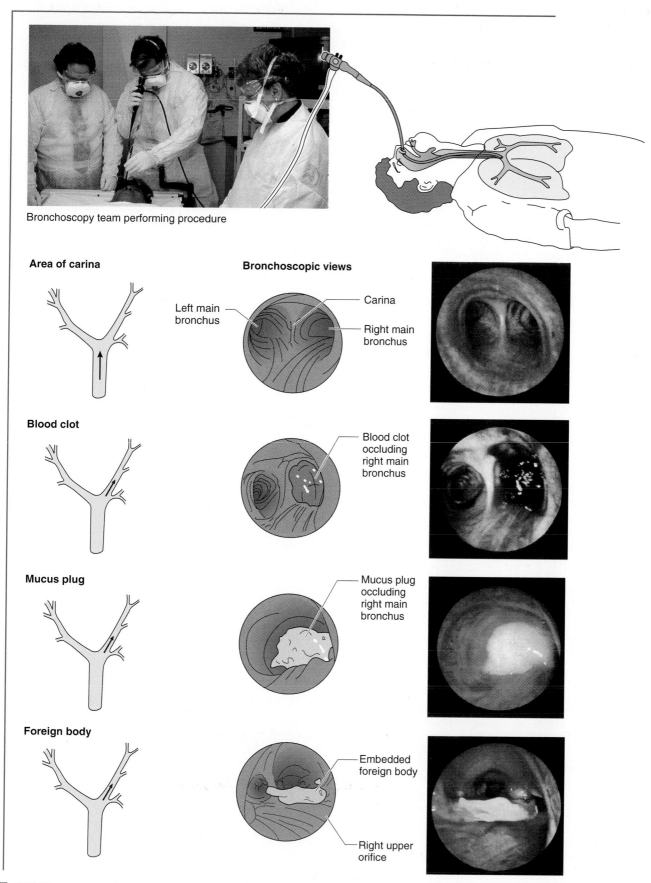

Bronchoscopy team performing procedure

Area of carina

Bronchoscopic views

Left main bronchus

Carina

Right main bronchus

Blood clot

Blood clot occluding right main bronchus

Mucus plug

Mucus plug occluding right main bronchus

Foreign body

Embedded foreign body

Right upper orifice

■ **FIGURE 7-9.** Bronchoscopy procedure.

nasopharyngoscopy *nā′zō-far′ing-gos′kō-pē*	use of a flexible endoscope to examine the nasal passages and the pharynx (throat) to diagnose structural abnormalities such as obstructions, growths, and cancers

examination methods

auscultation *aws-kŭl-tā′shŭn*	to listen; a physical examination method of listening to the sounds within the body with the aid of a stethoscope, such as auscultation of the chest for heart and lung sounds
percussion *per-kŭsh′ŭn*	a physical examination method of tapping over the body to elicit vibrations and sounds to estimate the size, border, or fluid content of a cavity, such as the chest
lung biopsy (Bx) *lŭng bī′op-sē*	removal of a small piece of lung tissue for pathologic examination
lung scan (Fig. 7-10) *lŭng skan*	a two-part nuclear scan of the lungs to detect abnormalities of ventilation (respiration) or perfusion (blood flow) made after radioactive material is: 1) injected in the patient's blood, and 2) as the patient breathes radioactive material into the airways. Comparison of the two scans indicates whether an abnormality exists in the airways or the pulmonary circulation; commonly called a V/Q scan referring to ventilation/perfusion
magnetic resonance image (MRI) *mag-net′ic rez′ō-nans im′ij*	nonionizing image of the lung to visualize lung lesions
polysomnography (PSG)	recording of various aspects of sleep (eye and muscle movements, respiration, brain wave patterns) for diagnosis of sleep disorders (*somn/o* = sleep)

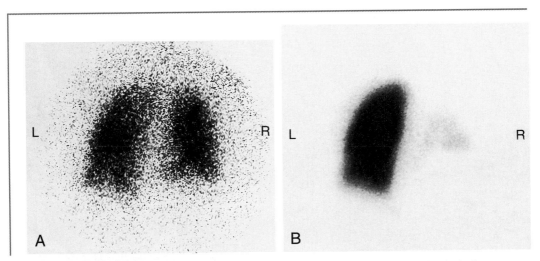

■ **FIGURE 7-10.** Posterior nuclear lung scan in a patient with an embolus in the right lung. Ventilation image **(A)** shows a normal pattern. Absence of blood flow to the right lung is apparent on perfusion scan **(B).** L, left; R, right.

pulmonary function testing (PFT) *pŭl'mō-nār-ē fŭngk'shŭn*	direct and indirect measurements of lung volumes and capacities
spirometry (Fig. 7-11) *spī-rom'ĕ-trē*	a direct measurement of lung volume and capacity
tidal volume (TV or V_T) *tī'dăl vol'yŭm*	amount of air exhaled after a normal inspiration
vital capacity (VC) *vīt-ăl kă-pas'i-tē*	amount of air exhaled after a maximal inspiration
peak flow (PF) **peak expiratory flow rate (PEFR)** *ek-spī'rătō-rē flō rāt*	measure of the fastest flow of exhaled air after a maximal inspiration
radiology *rā-dē-ol'ō-jē*	x-ray imaging
chest x-ray (CXR)	x-ray image of the chest to visualize the lungs; directional terms identify the path of the x-ray beam to produce the radiograph: PA (posterior-anterior): from back to front AP (anterior-posterior): from front to back lateral: toward the side, e.g., left lateral
computed tomography (CT) *tō-mog'ră-fē*	CT of the thorax is used to detect lesions in the lung; CT of the head is used to visualize the structures of the nose and sinuses
pulmonary angiography (Fig. 7-12) *pŭl'mō-nār-ē an-jē-og'ră-fē*	x-ray of the blood vessels of lungs after injection of contrast material

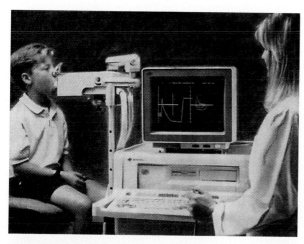

FIGURE 7-11. Spirometry.

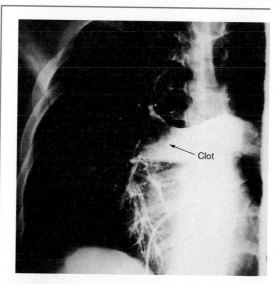

■ **FIGURE 7-12.** Pulmonary angiogram: embolus obstructing pulmonary circulation (*arrow*).

PROGRAMMED REVIEW: DIAGNOSTIC TESTS AND PROCEDURES

Answers	Review
-scopy endoscopy bronchoscopy nasopharyngoscopy	**7.60** Recall that the suffix meaning process of examination (with an instrument) is _____. Because *endo-* is the prefix for within, the general term for examination within a body cavity using a scope is _____. Use of a special endoscope to examine the airways and bronchi is _____. Examination of the throat and nasal passages is _____.
chest auscultation	**7.61** A stethoscope is used to listen to _____ sounds. The physical examination procedure for doing this is called _____.
percussion	**7.62** Another physical examination procedure uses tapping over the body to listen to the resulting sounds and vibrations to make observations about underlying organs and masses. This is called _____.
gases pH PaO$_2$, PaCO$_2$	**7.63** Laboratory tests analyze arterial blood _____ (ABGs) to determine the adequacy of their function in the lung. The _____ is a measure of blood acidity or alkalinity. The amount of oxygen in the blood is measured as the partial pressure of oxygen and is referred to as _____. The partial pressure of carbon dioxide is _____.
biopsy	**7.64** Removal of a small sample of lung tissue for pathologic examination is called lung _____. Many different organs and tissues in the body can be biopsied.
many -graphy polysomnography	**7.65** The combining form *somn/o* means sleep, and the prefix *poly-* means _____. The suffix referring to the process of recording is _____. Using these three word parts, the term for the procedure of recording many aspects of sleep (respiration, muscle movements, and so on) is called _____.

7.66   Measurement of lung volumes and capacities is called

pulmonary function

_____ _____ testing (PFT). Formed from

the combining term for breathing and the suffix for process of measur-

ing, the term for the direct measurement of lung volume and capacity is

spirometry

_____. The amount of air exhaled after a normal in-

tidal

spiration is called _____ volume. The amount of air exhaled after

vital capacity

a maximal inspiration is called _____ _____. The

measure of the fastest flow of exhaled air after a maximal inspiration is

peak expiratory flow

peak flow or _____ _____ _____ rate.

7.67   Several different imaging modalities are used to visualize the

lungs and other respiratory structures. A two-part nuclear scan of the

lungs to detect perfusion or ventilation abnormalities is simply called a

lung scan

_____ _____, also known as a V/Q scan. V stands for

ventilation

_____ (breathing), and Q stands for

perfusion

_____ (blood flow). A nonionizing image of the lungs

magnetic resonance

using magnetic fields and radio frequency waves is produced in a

image

_____ _____ _____ (MRI).

7.68   Using *radi/o*, a combining form referring to x-ray, and the suffix

radiology

meaning study of, the term for x-ray imaging is _____.

record

Radiogram refers to an x-ray _____; however, recall that the

graph

suffix meaning instrument for recording, _____, is used in the

radiograph

preferred term for x-ray image: _____. An x-ray of

chest x-ray

the full thorax to visualize the lungs is a _____ _____

posterior-anterior

(CXR). Abbreviations such as PA, _____-_____,

anterior-posterior

or AP, _____-_____, indicate the path of

the x-ray beam in producing the radiograph. Anterior indicates a path

front

from the _____ of the chest, and posterior indicates a path from

back

the _____ of the chest. A left lateral CXR is taken from the left

side

_____ of the chest. X-ray imaging of the blood vessels of the lungs

taken after injection of a contrast medium is called pulmonary

| angiography | _____. The form of x-ray imaging in which a computer creates cross-sectional images of structures such as the lungs is |
| computed tomography | _____ _____ (CT). |

SELF-INSTRUCTION: OPERATIVE TERMS

Study the following:

Term	Meaning
adenoidectomy *ad'ĕ-noy-dek'tō-mē*	excision of adenoids
lobectomy *lō-bek'tō-mē*	removal of a lobe of a lung
nasal polypectomy *nā'zăl pol-i-pek'tō-mē*	removal of a nasal polyp
pneumonectomy *nū'mō-nek'tō-mē*	removal of an entire lung
thoracentesis (Fig. 7-13) *thōr'ă-sen-tē'sis*	puncture for aspiration of the chest (pleural cavity)
thoracoplasty *thōr'ă-kō-plas-tē*	repair of the chest involving fixation of the ribs
thoracoscopy *thōr-ă-kos'kŏ-pē*	endoscopic examination of the pleural cavity using a thoracoscope

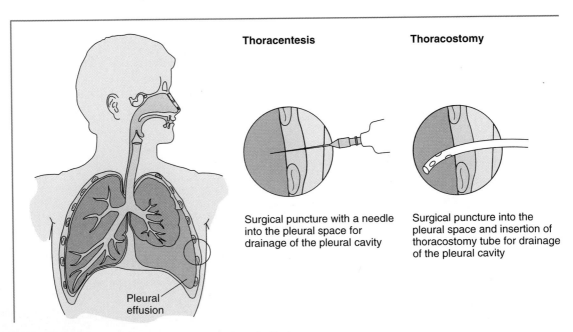

Thoracentesis

Surgical puncture with a needle into the pleural space for drainage of the pleural cavity

Thoracostomy

Surgical puncture into the pleural space and insertion of thoracostomy tube for drainage of the pleural cavity

Pleural effusion

■ **FIGURE 7-13.** Common treatments of pleural effusion.

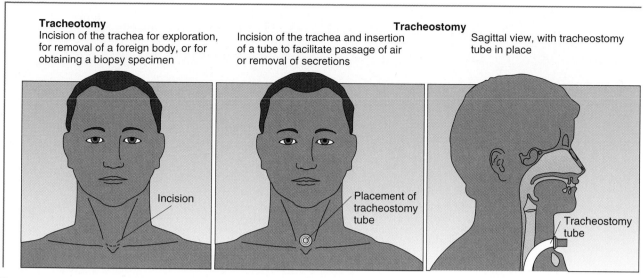

Tracheotomy
Incision of the trachea for exploration, for removal of a foreign body, or for obtaining a biopsy specimen

Tracheostomy
Incision of the trachea and insertion of a tube to facilitate passage of air or removal of secretions

Sagittal view, with tracheostomy tube in place

Incision

Placement of tracheostomy tube

Tracheostomy tube

■ **FIGURE 7-14.** Operative procedures related to the trachea.

thoracostomy (Fig. 7-13) *thōr-ă-kos'tō-mē*	creation of an opening in the chest, usually to insert a tube
thoracotomy *thōr-ă-kot'ō-mē*	incision into chest
tonsillectomy *ton'si-lek'tō-mē*	excision of palatine tonsils
tonsillectomy and adenoidectomy (T & A) *ad'ĕ-noy-dek'tō-mē*	excision of tonsils and adenoids
tracheostomy (Fig. 7-14) *trā'kē-os'tō-mē*	creation of an opening in the trachea, usually to insert a tube
tracheotomy (Fig. 7-14) *trā'kē-ot'ō-mē*	incision into the trachea

PROGRAMMED REVIEW: OPERATIVE TERMS

Answers	Review

excision

7.69 Recall the suffix *-ectomy* means _____ or removal. The term for surgical removal of the adenoids is

adenoidectomy

_____. The term for removal of a nasal polyp

nasal polypectomy

is _____ _____. Formed from the combining form that means either air or lung, the removal of an entire lung is

pneumonectomy	_____. The removal of the tonsils is
tonsillectomy	_____. Sometimes the tonsils and adenoids
tonsillectomy and	are removed at the same time in a procedure called a
adenoidectomy	_____ _____ _____
lobectomy	(T&A). The removal of a lung lobe is a _____

incision	**7.70** The suffix -*tomy* refers to an _____. An incision into
thoracotomy	the chest is called a _____. An incision into the tra-
tracheotomy	chea is a _____.

7.71 The operative suffix -*stomy* means surgical creation of an

opening	_____. The creation of an opening into the trachea, most often
tracheostomy	to insert a tube, is called a _____. The surgical
thoracostomy	creation of an opening into the chest is a _____. Note

that -*tomy* and -*stomy* have related but distinctly different meanings.

7.72 The suffix denoting surgical repair or reconstruction is

-plasty	_____. Thus, the surgical repair of the chest that involves fix-
thoracoplasty	ing the ribs is _____.

puncture	**7.73** The suffix -*centesis* means a_____ for aspiration. A
	puncture surgically made for aspiration of fluid or air from the chest
	(pleural cavity) is called a _____. Note that tho-
thoracentesis	racocentesis is an acceptable term but is used less often than the short-
	ened form thoracentesis.

7.74 Recall that the suffix -*scopy* means process of

examination	_____. The endoscopic examination of the pleural
thoracoscopy	cavity is called _____. Thoracoscopy is a surgical

procedure because an incision must be made for insertion of the endoscope, whereas bronchoscopy and nasopharyngoscopy are diagnostic
procedures because the scope is inserted through natural body openings.

SELF-INSTRUCTION: THERAPEUTIC TERMS

Study the following:

Term	Meaning
cardiopulmonary resuscitation (CPR) *kar′dē-ō-pŭl′mo-nār ē rē-sŭs′i-tā′shŭn*	a method of artificial respiration and chest compressions to move oxygenated blood to vital body organs when breathing and the heart have stopped
continuous positive airway pressure (CPAP)	a device that pumps a constant pressurized flow of air through the nasal passages, commonly used during sleep to prevent airway closure in sleep apnea
endotracheal intubation *en′dō-trā′kē-ăl in-tū-bā′shŭn*	passage of a tube into the trachea via the nose or mouth to open the airway for delivering gas mixtures to the lungs (e.g., oxygen, anesthetics, or air)
incentive spirometry (Fig. 7-15) *in-sen′tiv spī-rom′ĕ-trē*	a common postoperative breathing therapy using a specially designed spirometer to encourage the patient to inhale and hold an inspiratory volume to exercise the lungs and prevent pulmonary complications
mechanical ventilation *mĕ-kan′i-kĕl ven-ti-lā′shŭn*	mechanical breathing using a ventilator

COMMON THERAPEUTIC DRUG CLASSIFICATIONS

antibiotic *an′tē-bī-ot′ik*	a drug that kills or inhibits growth of microorganisms
anticoagulant *an′tē-kō-ag′yū-lant*	a drug that dissolves, or prevents the formation of, thrombi or emboli in the blood vessels (e.g., heparin)

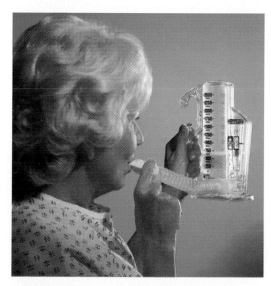

FIGURE 7-15. Incentive spirometer.

antihistamine *an-tē-his′tă-mēn*	a drug that neutralizes or inhibits the effects of histamine
histamine *his′tă-mēn*	a compound in the body that is released by injured cells in allergic reactions, inflammation, and so on, causing constriction of bronchial smooth muscle and dilation of blood vessels
bronchodilator *brong-kōdīlā′ter*	a drug that dilates the muscular walls of the bronchi
expectorant *ek-spek′tō-rănt*	a drug that breaks up mucus and promotes coughing

PROGRAMMED REVIEW: THERAPEUTIC TERMS

Answers	Review
cardiopulmonary resuscitation	**7.75** CPR stands for _____ _____, a method of artificial respiration and chest compressions to move oxygenated blood to vital body organs when breathing and the heart have stopped.
continuous positive airway stopped	**7.76** A patient with sleep apnea may use a device that pumps pressurized air through the nasal passages to prevent airway closure during sleep. This device is called _____ _____ _____ pressure (CPAP). Recall that apnea means _____ breathing.
within endotracheal intubation	**7.77** The prefix *endo-* means _____. The passage of a tube within the trachea via the nose or mouth to deliver oxygen to the lungs is called _____ _____.
measurement incentive spirometry	**7.78** As we saw earlier, spirometry is the direct _____ of lung volume and capacity. A similar spirometer is used in postoperative breathing therapy to motivate the patient to inhale and hold a larger inspiratory volume. This therapy is called _____ _____.

7.79 Mechanical breathing using a ventilator machine is called

mechanical ventilation

_____ _____ .

against

7.80 Recall that the prefix _anti-_ means _____ or opposed to. Drug classes are commonly named for their actions, such as acting against some thing or process. A drug that acts to prevent the process of

anticoagulant

coagulation (forming blood clots) is an _____ . The same prefix joined with the combining form for life (bio) denotes a drug class that acts to kill or inhibit microbial life. This drug is an

antibiotic

_____ .

7.81 A substance in the body that is released in allergic reactions, and

histamine

that causes constriction of bronchial muscles, is _____ . A drug that acts to inhibit the effects of histamine is an

antihistamine

_____ .

7.82 A person who has asthma may experience constriction of the bronchi during an attack. A therapeutic drug that counteracts this constriction by dilating the muscular walls of the bronchi is a

bronchodilator

_____ .

coughing

7.83 Recall that expectoration means _____ up and spitting out material from the lungs. A type of drug that breaks up mucus

expectorant

to promote coughing is an _____ .

Practice Exercises

For the following terms, on the lines below the term, write out the indicated word parts: prefixes, combining forms, roots, and suffixes. Then define the word.

Example:
intranasal

$$\frac{intra/nas/al}{P \quad R \quad S}$$

Definition: within/nose/pertaining to

1. pulmonology

   _____ / _____
        CF   S

   DEFINITION: _____

2. thoracocentesis

   _____ / _____
        CF   S

   DEFINITION: _____

3. nasosinusitis

   _____ / _____ / _____
        CF   R   S

   DEFINITION: _____

4. hypoxemia

   _____ / _____ / _____
        P   R   S

   DEFINITION: _____

5. pleuritis

   _____ / _____
        R   S

   DEFINITION: _____

6. hypercarbia

   _____ / _____ / _____
        P   R   S

   DEFINITION: _____

7. alveolar

   _____ / _____
        R   S

   DEFINITION: _____

8. tracheotomy

_____ / _____
      CF   S

DEFINITION: _____

9. oronasal

_____ / _____ / _____
      CF   R   S

DEFINITION: _____

10. rhinorrhea

_____ / _____
      CF   S

DEFINITION: _____

11. thoracostomy

_____ / _____
      CF   S

DEFINITION: _____

12. tonsillectomy

_____ / _____
      R   S

DEFINITION: _____

13. tracheobronchitis

_____ / _____ / _____
      CF   R   S

DEFINITION: _____

14. bronchospasm

_____ / _____
      CF   S

DEFINITION: _____

15. laryngostenosis

_____ / _____ / _____
      CF   R   S

DEFINITION: _____

16. spirogram

_____ / _____
      CF   S

DEFINITION: _____

17. lobectomy

_____ / _____
     R   S

DEFINITION: _____

18. peripleural

_____ / _____ / _____
     P   R   S

DEFINITION: _____

19. stethoscope

_____ / _____
     CF   S

DEFINITION: _____

20. pneumonic

_____ / _____
     R   S

DEFINITION: _____

21. nasopharyngoscopy

_____ / _____ / _____
     CF   CF   S

DEFINITION: _____

22. bronchiolectasis

_____ / _____
     R   S

DEFINITION: _____

23. phrenoptosis

_____ / _____
     CF   S

DEFINITION: _____

24. pectoral

_____ / _____
     R   S

DEFINITION: _____

25. uvulopalatopharyngoplasty

_____ / _____ / _____ / _____
     CF   CF   CF   S

DEFINITION: _____

Write the correct medical term for each of the following:

26. air in pleural space _____

27. pus in pleural space _____

28. blood in pleural space _____

29. listening to sounds within the body _____

30. endoscope used to examine the airways _____

31. coughing up and spitting out material from lungs _____

32. inflammation of the pleura _____

33. to elicit sounds or vibrations by tapping _____

34. deficient movement of air in and out of the lungs _____

35. puncture for aspiration of the chest _____

36. type of technology used in a lung scan _____

37. hoarseness _____

38. inflammation of the voice box _____

39. deficient amount of oxygen in tissue cells _____

40. disease characterized by overexpansion of the alveoli with air _____
_____

41. nosebleed _____

42. cancer originating in the bronchus _____

43. head cold _____

44. a collapse of lung tissue _____

45. material expelled from the lungs by coughing _____

46. a high-pitched crowing sound that signals obstruction in the upper airway _____
_____

47. blood clot in the lungs _____

48. surgical creation of an opening in the trachea _____

49. disease characterized by paroxysmal wheezing, dyspnea, and cough _____
_____

50. excessive movement of air in and out of lungs _____

51. common lung infection seen in those who are HIV positive _____

52. name referring to a combination of emphysema and chronic bronchitis _____
_____

Complete the medical term by writing the missing part:

53. _____coni_____ = lung condition caused by prolonged dust inhalation

54. bronchi_____ = dilation of bronchus

55. _____plasty = surgical repair of the chest

56. _____itis = inflammation of the lung

57. _____metry = measured breathing

58. _____pnea = normal breathing

59. _____pnea = slow breathing

60. _____pnea = difficulty breathing

61. _____pnea = inability to breathe except in an upright position

62. _____pnea = inability to breathe

63. _____pnea = fast breathing

Write the full medical term for the following abbreviations:

64. PEFR _____

65. VC _____

66. TB _____

67. CPR _____

68. COPD _____

69. PaCO$_2$ _____

70. URI _____

71. V$_T$ _____

72. PFT _____

73. PSG _____

74. CPAP _____

Write the standard abbreviations for the following:

75. chest x-ray _____

76. analysis of blood to determine the adequacy of lung function in exchange of gases ___

77. surgical removal of the tonsils and adenoids _____

Match the following terms with the appropriate right column term:

78. crackles _____   a. naso

79. wheezes _____   b. hyperventilation

80. pleurisy _____   c. hypercarbia

81. pneumoconiosis _____   d. thoraco

82. empyema _____   e. rales

83. hemothorax _____   f. asbestosis

84. stetho _____   g. pleuritis

85. hypercapnia _____   h. rhonchi

86. hyperpnea _____   i. pyothorax

87. rhino _____   j. thoracentesis

For each of the following, circle the correct spelling of the term:

88. auskucation	auscultation	ascultation
89. tackypnea	tachypenia	tachypnea
90. eupnea	eupenia	eupneia
91. plurisy	plurisey	pleurisy
92. hemathorax	hemothorax	hematothorex
93. stethoscope	stethescope	stethascope
94. epitaxes	epistaxes	epistaxis
95. ronchi	rhonchi	rhonkhi
96. hemoptysis	hemaptysis	hemoptsis
97. rhinorhea	rhinorrhea	rinorhea
98. imphasema	emphysema	emphasema
99. atelectasis	atalexisis	attelexis

Give the noun that was used to form the following adjectives.

100. _____ orthopneic   104. _____ pharyngeal

101. _____ asthmatic   105. _____ apneic

102. _____ hypoxic   106. _____ tracheal

103. _____ dyspneic   107. _____ pleuritic

Fill in the blanks for the missing terms.

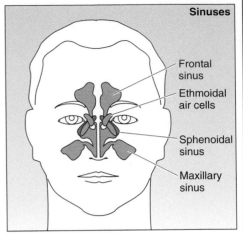

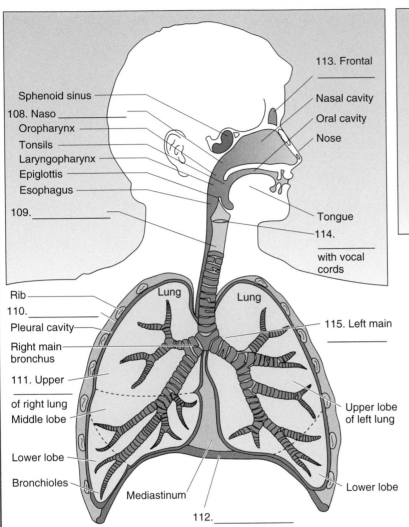

For each of the following, circle the meaning that corresponds to the combining form given:

116. **nose**	ren/o	rhin/o	nos/o
117. **air or lung**	aden/o	pneum/o	thorac/o
118. **throat**	thorac/o	laryng/o	pharyng/o
119. **chest**	thorac/o	pneum/o	lapar/o
120. **voice box**	laryng/o	trache/o	pharyng/o
121. **breathing**	aer/o	spir/o	crin/o
122. **diaphragm**	phren/o	pleur/o	pneumon/o
123. **mouth**	ox/o	or/o	spir/o

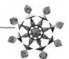

Medical Record Analyses

MEDICAL RECORD 7-1

S: This is a 26 y.o. ♀ c/o a nonproductive cough, dyspnea, and fever × 2 d; pt does not smoke and has otherwise been in good health.

O: T 101°F, BP 100/64, R 25, P 104
Tachypnea is accompanied by mild cyanosis, and inspiratory crackles are noted upon auscultation. WBC 31,000, Hct 37%, platelet count 109,000. CXR shows diffuse infiltrates at the bases of both lungs. An ABG taken while the patient was breathing room air showed a pH of 7.54, $PaCO_2$ of 20, PaO_2 of 74, sputum specimen contains 3+ WBC but no bacteria.

A: Pneumonia of unknown etiology

P: IV erythromycin STAT
admit to ICU
deliver O_2 by face mask and monitor for hypoxemia

1. What is the patients chief complaint?
    a. afebrile with a dry cough and difficulty breathing
    b. febrile with a dry cough and difficulty breathing
    c. cannot breathe, fever, and coughing up material from the lungs
    d. hoarse throat, dry cough, and fever
    e. febrile, coughing up sputum, and breathing fast

2. What are the findings upon PE?
    a. slow breathing, blue skin, and rhonchi heard in the lungs as the patient exhales
    b. fast breathing, blue skin, and musical sounds heard in the lungs as the patient inhales
    c. slow breathing, blue skin, and rales heard in the lungs as the patient holds her breath
    d. fast heart, blue skin, and rales heard in the lungs as the patient inhales
    e. fast breathing, blue skin, and popping sounds heard in the lungs as the patient inhales

3. What did the chest x-ray show?
    a. tuberculosis
    b. asthma
    c. density representing solid material usually indicating inflammation
    d. fluid filling of spaces around the lungs
    e. lung cancer

4. What is the impression?
    a. dilation of the bronchi with an accumulation of mucus
    b. inflammation of the bronchi
    c. inflammation of the pleura
    d. inflammation of the lungs due to sensitivity to dust or chemicals
    e. inflammation of the lungs of unknown cause

5. What is an ABG?
    a. analysis of blood to determine the adequacy of lung function in the exchange of gases
    b. measurement of lung volume and capacity
    c. measure of the flow of air during inspiration
    d. scan to detect breathing abnormalities
    e. image of the lungs used to visualize lung lesions

6. Describe the condition for which the patient was monitored while undergoing oxygen therapy
    a. blockage of airflow out of the lungs
    b. excessive movement of air in and out of the lungs
    c. deficient amount of oxygen in the blood
    d. deficient amount of oxygen in the tissue cells
    e. excessive level of carbon dioxide in the blood

7. What is the Sig: on the erythromycin?
    a. not mentioned
    b. inject into a vein immediately
    c. take four immediately
    d. insert into the vagina immediately
    e. inject into a muscle immediately

MEDICAL RECORD 7-2 FOR ADDITIONAL STUDY

Angelica Torrance, a retired painter who for years has boasted to friends that she has the good health of a 30-year-old, suffered a broken ankle when she slipped off a footstool in her basement. The surgical repair of her fracture at Central Medical Center was routine, but soon after surgery, Ms. Torrance developed other problems, and a pulmonologist was eventually called in for a consultation.

Read Medical Record 7-2 (Pages 320-322) for Ms. Torrance, and answer the following questions. This record is the history and physical examination report from Dr. Carl Brownley, the pulmonologist who consulted with Ms. Torrance's doctors after she developed breathing problems.

Write your answers in the spaces provided.

1. Below are medical terms used in this record that you have not yet encountered in this text. Underline each where it appears in the record and define below.

   morphine _____

   heparin _____

   obese _____

2. In your own words, not using medical terminology, describe what surgery Ms. Torrance had for her broken ankle.

   _____

   _____

   _____

3. Describe in your own words the four symptoms that Ms. Torrance developed postsurgically:

   a. _____

   b. _____

   c. _____

   d. _____

4. Before Ms. Torrance's acute "sense of suffocating," she was being treated with what three pharmacologic treatments?

   a. _____

   b. _____

   c. _____

5. Immediately after her reported "sense of suffocating," she was given what two treatments?

   a. _____

   b. _____

6. Put the following events that occurred in the hospital in correct order by numbering them 1 to 8:

   _____ postoperative pulmonary symptoms

   _____ transport to intensive care

_____ sense of suffocation

_____ episode of tachycardia

_____ nuclear lung scan showing high probability of embolus

_____ evaluation for complications in the lungs

_____ open reduction, internal fixation

_____ intravenous drugs first administered

7. In your own words, not using medical terminology, describe the two diagnostic imaging studies performed the morning of 10/24:

   a. _____

   b. _____

8. Name and describe the test that was performed to monitor Ms. Torrance's heparin therapy:

   _____

   _____

   _____

   _____

9. Translate into lay language Dr. Brownley's first four assessments from the examination:

   a. _____

   b. _____

   c. _____

   d. _____

10. Dr. Brownley's recommendations include requests for certain tests to be run (or run again) and certain other actions to be taken while Ms. Torrance stays in the hospital. Without using abbreviations, list the tests to be performed and the actions to be taken:

    Tests:

    a. _____

    b. _____

    c. _____

    d. _____

    e. _____

    f. _____

    Actions:

    g. _____

    h. _____

MEDICAL RECORD 7-2

CENTRAL MEDICAL CENTER

211 Medical Center Drive • Central City, US 90000-1234 • PHONE: (012) 125-6784 • FAX: (012) 125-9999

HISTORY

DATE OF CONSULTATION:
October 24, 20xx

HISTORY:
The patient is a 75-year-old woman who is admitted to this hospital on October 18, 20xx, after having fractured her right ankle. She underwent an ORIF of this lesion. Upon emerging from surgery, it was noted that she was quite wheezy and was having copious, purulent secretions. She was started on antibiotics; however, fever, cough, and breathlessness persisted. Finally, she was evaluated on October 20, 20xx, for possible pulmonary complications. A V/Q scan at that time showed a high probability for pulmonary emboli, and she was started on IV Heparin along with her antibiotics and bronchodilators. The patient did well with resolution of symptoms and fever and was progressing to the point of discharge.

Late yesterday evening, however, the patient developed the acute onset of "a sense of suffocating." This lasted for about 20-30 minutes and did resolve somewhat with the application of nasal oxygen and morphine sulfate 2 mg. The patient denies any cough, mucus, or actual chest pressure or pain. She denies any wheezing during this episode. Her heart rate went as high as 115-120; however, she was normotensive.

She was transported to ICU for further evaluation and management. An ECG obtained at that time revealed slight ST segment depression and T wave flattening at V4-6 with sinus tachycardia. Arterial blood gases done during the episode on 7 L O_2 showed a PaO_2 of 78, a pH of 7.44, and a $PaCO_2$ of 35. This morning, a chest x-ray revealed continuing resolution of the right upper and right lower lobe infiltrates. A V/Q scan showed evidence of resolving multiple perfusion defects on the right that appeared to actually match the defects noted on the chest x-ray. PTT, which had been continually in control during her Heparin therapy, was as high as 150 on 7 units of Heparin per hour.

PAST MEDICAL HISTORY:
The patient denies a past history of chronic respiratory disease but did have severe pneumonia about 30 years ago. The patient is a nonsmoker who has never smoked, and she has an essentially negative past medical history.

ALLERGIES:
The patient denies any personal allergies, but her family all suffer from chronic post nasal drip.

(continued)

PULMONARY CONSULTATION
Page 1

PT. NAME:	TORRANCE, ANGELICA W.
ID NO:	IP-228904
ROOM NO:	663
ATT. PHYS.	C. BROWNLEY, M.D.

MEDICAL RECORD 7-2 CONTINUED

CENTRAL MEDICAL CENTER

211 Medical Center Drive • Central City, US 90000-1234 • PHONE: (012) 125-6784 • FAX: (012) 125-9999

PHYSICAL EXAMINATION

GENERAL:
Well-nourished, somewhat overweight woman in no acute distress, having recently come back from x-ray with no undue dyspnea.

VITAL SIGNS:
BP: 110/70. Respirations: 16. Heart Rate: 80 and regular. Temperature: 99°.

CHEST:
LUNGS: Fair expansion bilaterally. Percussion node is normal. There are rare, distant end inspiratory rales at both bases

HEART: No clinical cardiomegaly. There are no murmurs or gallops.

ABDOMEN:
Obese, soft, nontender.

EXTREMITIES:
1+ pretibial edema on the left with a cast on the right.

ASSESSMENT:
1. ACUTE ONSET OF SHORTNESS OF BREATH OF UNCLEAR ETIOLOGY.
2. HYPOXIA.
3. HYPOTHROMBINEMIA (PATIENT ON HEPARIN).
4. STATUS POST PULMONARY EMBOLISM WITH RESOLUTION AND NO EVIDENCE OF RECURRENCE.
5. STATUS POST OPEN REDUCTION INTERNAL FIXATION OF TRIMALLEOLAR FRACTURE ON THE RIGHT.
6. RULE OUT ACUTE MYOCARDIAL INFARCTION VERSUS ISCHEMIA.
7. POSSIBLE MUCOUS PLUG.

(continued)

PULMONARY CONSULTATION Page 2	PT. NAME: TORRANCE, ANGELICA W. ID NO: IP-228904 ROOM NO: 663 ATT. PHYS. C. BROWNLEY, M.D.

MEDICAL RECORD 7-2 CONTINUED

CENTRAL MEDICAL CENTER

211 Medical Center Drive • Central City, US 90000-1234 • PHONE: (012) 125-6784 • FAX: (012) 125-9999

PHYSICAL EXAMINATION

RECOMMENDATIONS:
Cardiac enzymes should be obtained, and the ECG should be repeated as well. Recheck ABGs. Recheck PTT and discontinue Heparin until PTT diminishes to the 60s. Check CBC and comprehensive metabolic panel. Continue to observe in the ICU.

It is somewhat unclear as to what is the etiology of the episode of dyspnea. A possibility might be a mucous plug which has mobilized into the central airway and momentarily caused increased respiratory distress.

Thank you for the opportunity to assist in the management of this patient.

C.Brownley, M.D.
Pulmonologist

CB:im

D: 10/24/20xx
T: 10/25/20xx

PULMONARY CONSULTATION Page 3	PT. NAME: TORRANCE, ANGELICA W. ID NO: IP-228904 ROOM NO: 663 ATT. PHYS. C. BROWNLEY, M.D.

Answers to Practice Exercises

1. pulmono/logy
   <u>CF</u>   <u>S</u>
   lung/study of

2. thoraco/centesis
   <u>CF</u>   <u>S</u>
   chest/puncture for aspiration

3. naso/sinus/itis
   <u>CF</u>   <u>R</u>   <u>S</u>
   nose/sinus/inflammation

4. hyp/ox/emia
   <u>P</u>   <u>R</u>   <u>S</u>
   below or deficient/oxygen/
   blood condition

5. pleur/itis
   <u>R</u>   <u>S</u>
   pleura/inflammation

6. hyper/carb/ia
   <u>P</u>   <u>R</u>   <u>S</u>
   above or excessive/carbon
   dioxide/condition of

7. alveol/ar
   <u>R</u>   <u>S</u>
   alveolus (air sac)/pertaining
   to

8. tracheo/tomy
   <u>CF</u>   <u>S</u>
   trachea/incision

9. oro/nas/al
   <u>CF</u>   <u>R</u>   <u>S</u>
   mouth/nose/pertaining to

10. rhino/rrhea
    <u>CF</u>   <u>S</u>
    nose/discharge

11. thoraco/stomy
    <u>CF</u>   <u>S</u>
    chest/creation of an opening

12. tonsill/ectomy
    <u>R</u>   <u>S</u>
    tonsil/excision (removal)

13. tracheo/bronch/itis
    <u>CF</u>   <u>R</u>   <u>S</u>
    trachea (windpipe)/
    bronchus/inflammation

14. broncho/spasm
    <u>CF</u>   <u>S</u>
    bronchus(airway)/
    involuntary contraction

15. laryngo/sten/osis
    <u>CF</u>   <u>R</u>   <u>S</u>
    larynx(voice box)/narrow/
    condition or increase

16. spiro/gram
    <u>CF</u>   <u>S</u>
    breathing/record

17. lob/ectomy
    <u>R</u>   <u>S</u>
    lobe (a portion)/excision
    (removal)

18. peri/pleur/al
    <u>P</u>   <u>R</u>   <u>S</u>
    around/pleura/pertaining to

19. stetho/scope
    <u>CF</u>   <u>S</u>
    chest/instrument for
    examination

20. pneumon/ic
    <u>R</u>   <u>S</u>
    air or lung/pertaining to

21. naso/pharyngo/scopy
    <u>CF</u>   <u>S</u>
    nose/pharynx(throat)/
    process of examination

22. bronchiol/ectasis
    <u>R</u>   <u>S</u>
    bronchiole (little airway)/
    expansion or dilation

23. phreno/ptosis
    <u>CF</u>   <u>S</u>
    diaphragm/falling or
    downward displacement

24. pector/al
    <u>R</u>   <u>S</u>
    chest/pertaining to

25. uvulo/palato/
    <u>CF</u>   <u>CF</u>
    pharyngo/plasty
    <u>CF</u>   <u>S</u>
    uvula (grape)/palate/
    throat/surgical repair or
    reconstruction

26. pneumothorax
27. empyema or pyothorax
28. hemothorax
29. auscultation
30. bronchoscope
31. expectoration
32. pleurisy or pleuritis
33. percussion
34. hypoventilation
35. thoracentesis or
    thoracocentesis
36. nuclear medicine
37. dysphonia
38. laryngitis
39. hypoxia
40. emphysema
41. epistaxis
42. bronchogenic carcinoma
43. coryza
44. atelectasis
45. sputum

46. stridor
47. pulmonary embolism
48. tracheostomy
49. asthma
50. hyperventilation
51. *Pneumocystis* pneumonia
52. chronic obstructive
    pulmonary disease
53. pneumoconiosis
54. bronchiectasis
55. thoracoplasty
56. pneumonitis
57. spirometry
58. eupnea
59. bradypnea
60. dyspnea
61. orthopnea
62. apnea
63. tachypnea
64. peak expiratory flow rate
65. vital capacity
66. tuberculosis
67. cardiopulmonary
    resuscitation
68. chronic obstructive
    pulmonary disease
69. partial pressure of carbon
    dioxide
70. upper respiratory infection
71. tidal volume
72. pulmonary function testing
73. polysomnography
74. continuous positive airway
    pressure
75. CXR
76. ABG
77. T&A
78. e
79. h
80. g
81. f
82. i
83. j
84. d
85. c
86. b
87. a
88. auscultation
89. tachypnea
90. eupnea
91. pleurisy
92. hemothorax
93. stethoscope
94. epistaxis
95. rhonchi
96. hemoptysis

97. rhinorrhea
98. emphysema
99. atelectasis
100. orthopnea
101. asthma
102. hypoxia
103. dyspnea
104. pharynx
105. apnea
106. trachea
107. pleurisy
108. pharynx
109. trachea
110. pleura

111. lobe
112. diaphragm
113. sinus
114. larynx
115. bronchus
116. rhin/o
117. pneum/o
118. pharyng/o
119. thorac/o
120. laryng/o
121. spir/o
122. phren/o
123. or/o

Answers to Medical Records Analyses

1. b
2. e
3. c
4. e
5. a
6. c
7. b

CHAPTER 8

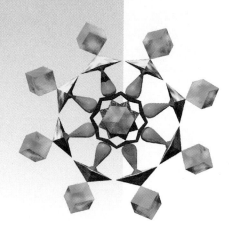

Nervous System

Nervous System Overview

The nervous system is an intricate communication network of neurons and other structures (Fig. 8-1) that activates and controls all functions of the body and receives all input from the environment. The nervous system has three divisions:

* The central nervous system consists of the brain and spinal cord.
* The peripheral nervous system consists of nerves branching from the central nervous system to all parts of the body.
* The autonomic nervous system consists of nerves that carry involuntary impulses to smooth muscle, cardiac muscle, and various glands.

SELF-INSTRUCTION: COMBINING FORMS

Study the following:

Combining Form	Meaning
cerebr/o	cerebrum (largest part of brain)
cerebell/o	cerebellum (little brain)
crani/o	skull
encephal/o	entire brain
esthesi/o	sensation
gangli/o	ganglion (knot)
gli/o	glue
gnos/o	knowing

NEURON

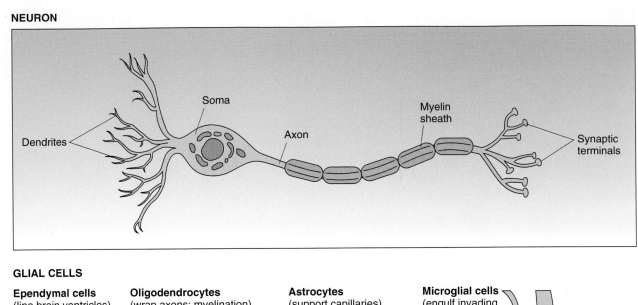

GLIAL CELLS

Ependymal cells
(line brain ventricles)

Oligodendrocytes
(wrap axons: myelination)

Astrocytes
(support capillaries)

Microglial cells
(engulf invading
microorganisms
and dead tissues)

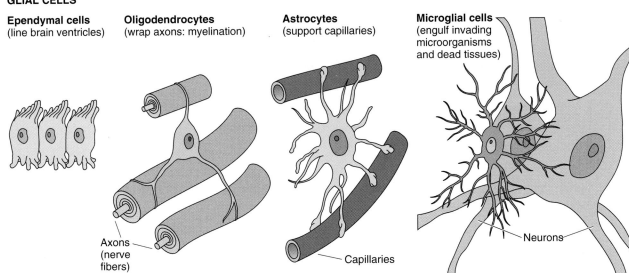

■ **FIGURE 8-1.** Basic components of the nervous system.

kinesi/o	movement
lex/o	word or phrase
mening/o meningi/o	meninges (membrane)
myel/o	spinal cord or bone marrow
narc/o	stupor, sleep
neur/o	nerve
phas/o	speech
phob/o	exaggerated fear or sensitivity
phor/o	carry, bear

phren/o psych/o thym/o	mind
schiz/o	split
somat/o	body
somn/o somn/i hypn/o	sleep
spin/o	spine (thorn)
spondyl/o vertebr/o	vertebra
stere/o	three dimensional or solid
ton/o	tone, tension
tax/o	order or coordination
thalam/o	thalamus (a room)
top/o	place
ventricul/o	ventricle (belly or pouch)

PREFIX

cata-	down

SUFFIXES

-asthenia	weakness
-lepsy	seizure
-mania	abnormal impulse (attraction) toward
-paresis	slight paralysis
-plegia	paralysis

PROGRAMMED REVIEW: COMBINING FORMS

Answers	Review
cerebrum	**8.1** The combining form *cerebr/o* means _____ (largest part of the brain). Thus, the adjective cerebrospinal refers to something
cerebrum, spine	involving both the _____ and the _____. The com-

encephal/o	bining form referring to the entire brain is _____, such as is used in the term encephalography. Recall that the suffix -graphy
recording	means the process of __recording__.

8.2 The brain is housed inside the skull, the combining form for which is __crani/o__. The cranium, for example, is the term for the bones of the skull.

crani/o	

8.3 Another part of the brain is the cerebellum, the combining form for which is __cerebell/o__ (meaning "little brain"). The suffix

cerebell/o	
adjective	-ar is an _____ ending. A common adjective referring
cerebellar	to the cerebellum is __cerebellar__.

8.4 Within the brain are interconnected cavities called ventricles. The

ventricul/o	combining form meaning ventricle is __ventricul/o__. Recall
-stomy	that the surgical suffix for the creation of an opening is __stomy__.
	Thus, a ventriculo<u>stomy</u> is the <u>creation of an opening</u> in a
ventricle	__ventricle__.

8.5 The thalamus is a part of the brain. The combining form meaning

thalam/o, incision	thalamus is _____. A <u>thalam</u>otomy is an _____ into the thalamus.

8.6 The brain and spinal cord are covered with a membrane called meninges. The two combining forms for meninges are *mening/o* and

meningi/o	__meningi/o__. Recall that the suffix -cele means a hernia or
pouching	__pouching__. Therefore, a meningo<u>cele</u> is a pouching of the
meninges, inflammation	_____. Meningitis is _____ of the meninges.

spin/o	**8.7** The combining form meaning the spine is __spin/o__. The com-
spinal	mon adjective form is __spinal__.

8.8 Inside the spine is the spinal cord, a bundle of nerves coming down from the brain and ultimately connecting to all areas of the body. The combining form for the spinal cord (and also for bone marrow) is

myel/o

myel/o, as in the term myelitis, meaning inflammation of the

spinal cord

spinal _cord_.

8.9 The bones of the spine are <u>vertebrae</u>, the plural form of the term

vertebra

vertebra. The two combining forms meaning vertebra are

spondyl/o

vertebr/o and _spondyl/o_. For example, a common adjective

vertebral

form made with the first combining form is _____.

<u>Spondylosyndesis</u>, meaning spinal fusion, is an example of a term using

the second combining form; <u>syndesis</u> is a surgical technique of

binding (joining), vertebra

binding together, and _spondyl/o_ means _vertebra_.

8.10 Nerve cells exist in the brain, in the spinal cord, and throughout the nervous system. The combining form meaning (nerve)is

neur/o

neur/o. The medical specialty studying the <u>nervous system</u> is

neurology

therefore called _neurology_.

8.11 A ganglion is a <u>structure of nerves</u> in the peripheral nervous system. The combining form for ganglion is

gangli/o

gangli/o, as in the

term <u>ganglio</u>neuroma, a neoplasm affecting ganglions. The other plural

ganglia

form of ganglion is _ganglia_.

8.12 Glial cells in the nervous system help hold together (glue together) the neurons, which are the primary nervous system cells. The

gli/o

combining term for glue is _gli/o_. A common adjective form is

glial

glial.

8.13 Almost all functions in the body are regulated through the nervous system. The combining form meaning body is

somat/o

somat/o, as

in the term <u>psycho</u>somatic, which refers to <u>influences of the mind on</u>

body

the _body_.

psych/o, thym/o

mind

mind

faulty

8.14 The three combining forms meaning mind are *phren/o*, ___psych/o___, and ___thym/o___, as in the terms schizophrenia, psychiatry, and dysthymia. Schizophrenia refers to a split ___mind___. Psychiatry is the medical specialty field centered on the diagnosis, treatment, and prevention of disorders of the ___mind___. A dysthymia is a psychiatric disorder; the prefix *dys-* means painful, difficult, or _____.

schiz/o

split

8.15 The combining form meaning split is _____. The thoughts of a patient with schizophrenia are said to be ___split___ from reality.

gnos/o

8.16 The combining form that means knowing, which is the basis of the term gnosia, referring to the ability to perceive and recognize, is ___gnos/o___.

esthesi/o

excessive

8.17 All physical sensations throughout the body are perceived by the brain. The combining form meaning sensation is ___esthesi/o___, as in the term hyperesthesia, an abnormally heightened sensitivity to sensations. The prefix *hyper-* means above or ___excessive___.

kinesi/o

movement

8.18 The nervous system also controls body movement. The combining form meaning movement is ___kinesi/o___, as in the term kinesiology, which is the study of body ___movement___.

phas/o

unable

without, difficulty

faulty, word

phrase

8.19 Speech involves complex mental and motor functions. The combining form meaning speech is ___phas___. Aphasia is a condition of being ___unable___ to speak (recall that the prefix *a-* means ___without___). Dyslexia means a ___difficulty___ understanding written words or phrases (recall that the prefix *dys-* means painful, difficult, or ___faulty___ and lex/o means ___word___ or ___phrase___).

8.20   Someone with a phobia has an exaggerated fear of or sensitivity to something. The combining form for phobia is _____ .

phob/o

8.21   There are three specific combining forms that mean sleep: *somn/o*, _____ , and *hypn/o*. Polysomnography, for example, makes a _record_ of various physiologic changes that occur during _sleep_ . Recall that the prefix *poly-* means _many_ . Hypnosis is the condition of being in a _sleep_ like state by suggestion. Recall that the suffix *-osis* means increase or _Condition_ .

somn/i

record

sleep, many

sleep

condition

8.22   Different from the sleep state, a state of stupor can result in various conditions. The combining form meaning stupor is _narco_ , as in the term narcotic, referring to a class of drugs that induce _stupor_ .

narc/o

stupor

8.23   The combining form *phor/o* means to bear or _carry_ . Recall that the prefix *eu-* means normal or _good_ (well). Thus, the term euphoria, meaning an exaggerated sense of well-being, originated from terms meaning to carry well.

carry

good

8.24   The combining form meaning three-dimensional or solid is _stere/o_ , as in the term stereotaxic, referring to an apparatus allowing precise localization in space.

stere/o

8.25   The combining term meaning tone or tension is _____ , as in the term monotone, which refers to speaking in an unchanging single _____ . Recall that the prefix *mono-* means _____ .

ton/o

tone, one

8.26   The combining form *tax/o* means order or _coordination_ . For example, ataxia is a condition of inability to _coordinate_ muscle movements. The prefix *a-* means _without_ , and the suffix *-ia* means _condition of_ .

coordination

coordinate

without, condition of

top/o place	**8.27** The combining form for place is __top__ . For example, the *→ sensation* term topesthesia refers to the ability to localize the __place__ on which the skin is touched.
down	**8.28** The prefix *cata-* means __down__ . The term catatonia, for exam- ple, which means a state of being unresponsive and unmoving, comes from word roots meaning all muscle activity is down.
-asthenia weakness	**8.29** The suffix meaning weakness is _____ , as in the term myasthenia, which is a condition involving _____ of the muscles. (my/o = muscle).
sleep -lepsy	**8.30** The term narcolepsy is made from the secondary meaning of the combining form *narc/o*, which is __sleep__ , and the suffix __-lepsy__ , which means seizure. In narcolepsy, sleep comes on unex- pectedly and suddenly, as in a seizure.
impulse (or attraction) death fear	**8.31** The noun term *mania* means a state of abnormal elation and in- creased activity. The suffix *-mania*, however, refers to an abnormal *necrosis : cell death* __attraction__ toward. For example, necromania is an abnormal at- traction to __death__ . Compare this with necrophobia, which is an abnormal __fear__ of death.
-paresis half hemi-	**8.32** The suffix meaning a slight paralysis is __-paresis__ , as in the term hemiparesis, meaning a slight paralysis in __half__ of the body (right or left). Recall that the prefix meaning half is _____ .
paralysis	**8.33** The suffix *-plegia* means __paralysis__ , as in the term paraplegia, referring to paralysis of the legs and lower trunk.

SELF-INSTRUCTION: ANATOMICAL TERMS

Study the following:

Term	Meaning
central nervous system (CNS)	brain and spinal cord
brain (Fig. 8-2)	portion of the central nervous system contained within the cranium
cerebrum *sĕr-ē'brum*	largest portion of the brain; divided into right and left halves, known as *cerebral hemispheres,* that are connected by a bridge of nerve fibers called the *corpus callosum;* lobes of the cerebrum are named after the skull bones they underlie
frontal lobe *frŭn'tăl lōb*	anterior section of each cerebral hemisphere responsible for voluntary muscle movement and personality
parietal lobe *pă-rī'ĕ-tăl lōb*	portion posterior to the frontal lobe, responsible for sensations such as pain, temperature, and touch
temporal lobe *tem'pŏ-răl lōb*	portion that lies below the frontal lobe, responsible for hearing, taste, and smell
occipital lobe *ok-sip'i-tăl lōb*	portion posterior to the parietal and temporal lobes, responsible for vision
cerebral cortex *ser'ĕ-brăl kōr'teks*	outer layer of the cerebrum consisting of gray matter, responsible for higher mental functions (cortex = bark)

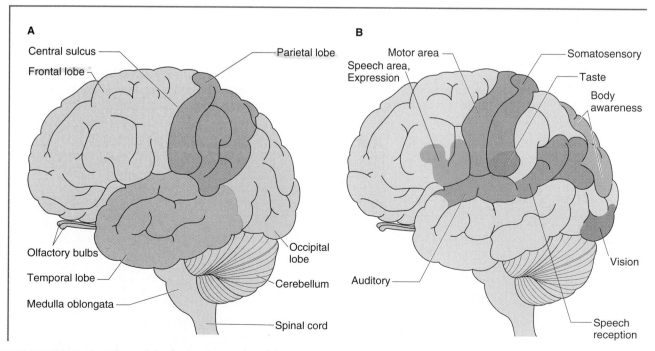

■ **FIGURE 8-2. A.** Lobes of the brain. **B.** Localized functions of the cerebrum.

thalamus (diencephalon) *thal′ă-mŭs* *dī-en-sef′ă-lon*	each of two gray matter nuclei deep within the brain responsible for relaying sensory information to the cortex
gyri *jī′rī*	convolutions (mounds) of the cerebral hemispheres
sulci *sŭl′sī*	shallow grooves that separate gyri
fissures *fish′ŭrz*	deep grooves in the brain
cerebellum (Fig. 8-3) *ser- ĕ-bel′ŭm*	portion of the brain located below the occipital lobes of the cerebrum, responsible for control and coordination of skeletal muscles
brainstem *brān′stem*	region of the brain that serves as a relay between the cerebrum, cerebellum, and spinal cord; responsible for breathing, heart rate, and body temperature; the three levels are the mesencephalon (midbrain), pons, and medulla oblongata
ventricles (Fig. 8-4) *ven′tri-klz*	series of interconnected cavities within the cerebral hemispheres and brainstem filled with cerebrospinal fluid
cerebrospinal fluid (CSF) *ser′ĕ-bro-spī-năl flu′id*	plasmalike clear fluid circulating in and around the brain and spinal cord
spinal cord *spī-năl kord*	column of nervous tissue from the brainstem through the vertebrae, responsible for nerve conduction to and from the brain and the body
meninges *mĕ-nin′jēz*	three membranes that cover the brain and spinal cord, consisting of the dura mater, pia mater, and arachnoid mater
peripheral nervous system(PNS)	nerves that branch from the central nervous system, including nerves of the brain (cranial nerves) and spinal cord (spinal nerves)
cranial nerves *krā̄nē-ăl nervz*	12 pairs of nerves arising from the brain
spinal nerves	31 pairs of nerves arising from the spinal cord
sensory nerves *sen′sŏ-rē nervz*	nerves that conduct impulses from body parts and carry sensory information to the brain; also called afferent nerves (ad = toward; ferre = carry)
motor nerves	nerves that conduct motor impulses from the brain to muscles and glands; also called efferent nerves (e = out; ferre = carry)
autonomic nervous system (ANS)	nerves that carry involuntary impulses to smooth muscle, cardiac muscle, and various glands

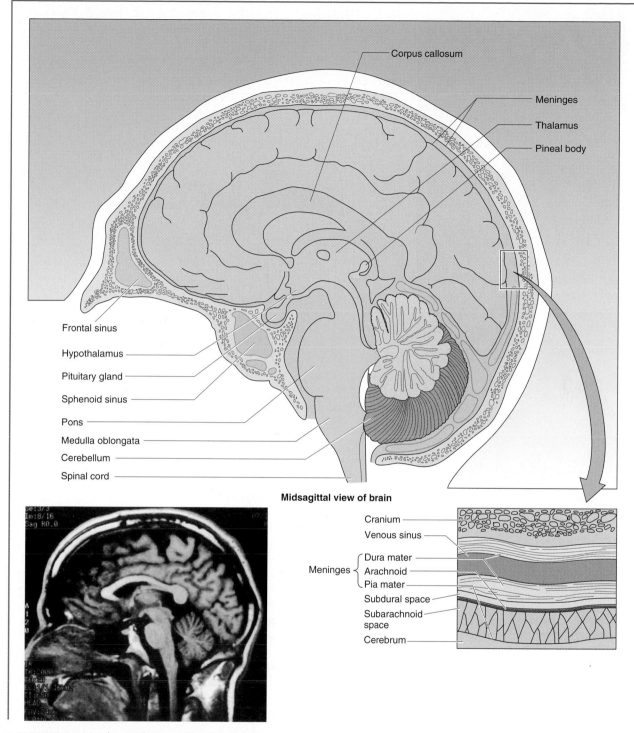

Midsagittal view of brain

■ **FIGURE 8-3.** Midsagittal view of brain.

hypothalamus *hī′pō-thal′ă-mŭs*	control center for the autonomic nervous system located below the thal-amus (diencephalon)
sympathetic nervous **system** *sim-pă-thet′ik*	division of the ANS concerned primarily with preparing the body in stressful or emergency situations

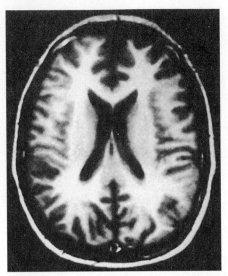

Magnetic resonance image, horizontal view A

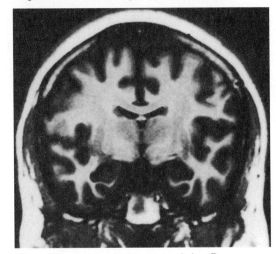

Magnetic resonance image, coronal view B

■ **FIGURE 8-4.** Ventricles of the brain.

parasympathetic nervous system *par-ă-sim-pă-thet'ik*	division of the ANS that is most active in ordinary conditions; it counterbalances the effects of the sympathetic system by restoring the body to a restful state after a stressful experience

PROGRAMMED REVIEW: ANATOMICAL TERMS

Answers	Review
central

brain | **8.34** The brain and spinal cord comprise the _____ nervous system. The _____ is the part of the central nervous system within the cranium. |

cerebrum

8.35 The largest portion of the brain, the _____, is divided into the two cerebral hemispheres. The lobe at the front of each cerebral hemisphere, called the _____ _____, controls

frontal lobe

muscle movement and personality. Behind the frontal lobe is the parietal lobe.

parietal

8.36 The lobe behind the frontal lobe, called the _____ lobe, is responsible for sensations such as pain, temperature, and touch. Below the frontal lobe is the temporal lobe.

temporal

8.37 The lobe below the frontal lobe, called the _____ lobe, is responsible for hearing, taste, and smell. Posterior to the parietal and temporal lobes is the occipital lobe.

8.38 The lobe posterior to the parietal and temporal lobes, the

occipital

_____ lobe, is responsible for vision.

8.39 The Latin word cortex means bark, referring to an outer layer. The outer layer of the cerebrum is the cerebral _____, which is

cortex

the gray matter responsible for higher mental functions. Sensory information is relayed to the cortex by the thalamus (diencephalon).

8.40 The two gray matter nuclei deep within the brain that relay sensory information to the cortex are called the _____ or

thalamus

diencephalon

_____. The plural of thalamus is

thalami

_____.

8.41 Gyri, sulci, and fissures are physical characteristics of the cerebral hemispheres. Convolutions (mounds) of the hemispheres are called

gyri, gyrus

_____. The singular of gyri is _____. The shallow grooves

sulci

that separate gyri are called _____. The singular of sulci is

sulcus

_____. The deep grooves in the brain are called

fissures

_____.

cerebellum

8.42 Below the occipital lobes is the cerebellum. The _____ is responsible for controlling skeletal muscles. The cerebellum and cerebrum both communicate with the spinal cord through the brainstem.

brainstem

8.43 The spinal cord communicates with the cerebrum and cerebellum through the _____, which is also responsible for breathing, heart rate, and body temperature. Interconnected cavities within the brainstem and cerebral hemispheres are called ventricles.

ventricles

cerebrospinal

8.44 Cerebrospinal fluid fills the _____, the cavities in the cerebral hemispheres and brainstem. The plasmalike fluid circulating in and around the brain and spinal cord is _____ fluid.

spinal cord

8.45 The column of nervous tissue that descends from the brainstem through the vertebrae of the spine is the _____ _____. The spinal cord and brain are covered by membranes called meninges.

meninges

8.46 The three membranes covering the brain are called _____.

peripheral

cranial

spinal

8.47 Nerves branch from the central nervous system to the peripheral nervous system to reach all areas of the body. Cranial nerves, spinal nerves, sensory nerves, and motor nerves are all part of the _____ nervous system. The 12 pairs of nerves arising from the brain are the _____ nerves. The 31 pairs of nerves arising from the spinal cord are the _____ nerves.

sensory

motor

8.48 The nerves in the peripheral nervous system that carry sensory information to the brain are the _____ nerves. The nerves that carry motor impulses from the brain to muscles and glands are the _____ nerves.

8.49   The autonomic nervous system controls involuntary functions of smooth muscle, cardiac muscle, and various glands. The hypothalamus

autonomic

is the control center for the _____ nervous system.

8.50   The autonomic nervous system is controlled by the

hypothalamus

_____, which is located below the thalamus.

below

Recall that the prefix *hypo-* means _____ or deficient.

8.51   The sympathetic nervous system and the parasympathetic nervous system are divisions of the autonomic nervous system. In stressful

sympathetic

or emergency situations, the _____ nervous system prepares the body. In most ordinary conditions, the

parasympathetic

_____ nervous system is more active, counterbalancing the effects of the sympathetic nervous system.

SELF-INSTRUCTION: NERVOUS SYSTEM SYMPTOMATIC TERMS

Study the following:

Term	Meaning
aphasia *ă-fā′zē-ă*	inability to speak
dysphasia *dis-fā′zē-ă*	difficulty speaking
coma *kō′mă*	a deep sleep; a general term referring to levels of decreased consciousness with varying responsiveness; a common method of assessment is the Glasgow coma scale
delirium *dē-lir′ē-ŭm*	a state of mental confusion caused by disturbances in cerebral function; the many causes include fever, shock, or drug overdose (deliro = to draw the furrow awry when plowing, i.e., to go off the rails)
dementia *dē-men′shē-ă*	an impairment of intellectual function characterized by memory loss, disorientation, and confusion (dementio = to be mad)
motor deficit *mō′ter def′i-sit*	loss or impairment of muscle function
sensory deficit *sen′sŏ-rē def′i-sit*	loss or impairment of sensation

neuralgia nū-ral′jē-ă	pain along the course of a nerve
paralysis	temporary or permanent loss of motor control
flaccid paralysis flas′sid pă-ral′i-sis	defective (flabby) or absent muscle control caused by a nerve lesion
spastic paralysis spas′tik pă-ral′i-sis	stiff and awkward muscle control caused by a central nervous system disorder
hemiparesis hem-ē-pa-rē′sis	partial paralysis of the right or left half of the body
sciatica sī-at′i-kă	pain that follows the pathway of the sciatic nerve caused by compression or trauma of the nerve or its roots
seizure sē′zher	sudden, transient disturbances in brain function resulting from abnormal firing of nerve impulses (may or may not be associated with convulsion)
convulsion kon-vŭl′shŭn	to pull together; type of seizure that causes a series of sudden, involuntary contractions of muscles
syncope sin′kŏ-pē	fainting
tactile stimulation tak′til	evoking a response by touching
hyperesthesia hī′per-es-thē′zē-ă	increased sensitivity to stimulation such as touch or pain
paresthesia par-es-thē′zē-ă	abnormal sensation of numbness and tingling without objective cause

PROGRAMMED REVIEW: NERVOUS SYSTEM SYMPTOMATIC TERMS

Answers	Review
condition of without phas/o aphasia	**8.52** Recall that the suffix *-ia* means _____, and the prefix *a-* means _____. The combining form for speech is _____. Made from this combining form, the medical term for the condition of being without speech (unable to speak) is _____.
faulty dysphasia	**8.53** The prefix *dys-* means painful, difficult, or _____. The condition of difficulty speaking is termed _____.

coma

8.54 A decreased level of consciousness, measured with the Glasgow coma scale, is called a _____ .

delirium

dementia

8.55 Mental and intellectual function can be disturbed by medical or psychiatric conditions or drugs. A state of mental confusion due to disturbed cerebral function is called __*delirium*__ . The impairment of intellectual function characterized by memory loss and disorientation is __*dementia*__ .

motor

sensory

8.56 A deficit is a loss or impairment related to a nervous system problem. The loss of muscle function is called a __*motor*__ deficit. The loss of sensation is called a _____ deficit.

neur/o

pain

neuralgia

8.57 The combining form meaning nerve is _____ . Recall that the suffix *-algia* means __*pain*__ . Therefore, the term for pain along the course of a nerve is __*neuralgia*__ .

paralysis

flaccid

spastic

8.58 A temporary or permanent loss of motor control is called __*paralysis*__ . A nerve lesion that causes a lack of muscle control, resulting in flabby muscles that do not move, is called __*flaccid*__ paralysis. Stiff, awkward muscle control caused by a central nervous system disorder is called __*spastic*__ paralysis.

-paresis

hemi-

hemiparesis

8.59 The suffix meaning partial paralysis is __*paresis*__ . Recall that the prefix meaning half is _____ . The term for partial paralysis of the right or left half of the body is __*hemiparesis*__ .

sciatica

8.60 The sciatic nerve runs down the leg. Pain along its pathway caused by compression or trauma to this nerve is called __*sciatica*__ .

seizure

convulsion

8.61 A sudden transient disturbance of brain function that results from an abnormal firing of nerval impulses is called a _____ . A type of seizure that involves sudden involuntary muscle contractions is termed __*convulsion*__ .

fainting

syncope

8.62 The Greek word synkope means cutting short or swoon. From this word, the medical term for fainting is ___*syncope*___.

tactile

8.63 The process of evoking a response by touching a person's skin is called ___*tactile*___ stimulation.

condition of

esthesi/o

excessive

hyperesthesia

8.64 Again, the suffix *-ia* means ___*condition*___ *of*. The combining form meaning sensation is ___*esthesi/o*___. The prefix *hyper-* means above or _____. From these three word parts comes this term meaning a condition of increased sensitivity to the sensations of touch and pain: _____.

abnormal

paresthesia

8.65 Recall that the prefix *para-* means alongside of or ___*abnormal*___. The term for a condition of an abnormal sensation of numbness and tingling is ___*paresthesia*___.

SELF-INSTRUCTION: NERVOUS SYSTEM DIAGNOSTIC TERMS

Study the following:

Term	Meaning
agnosia *ag-nō′sē-ă*	any of many types of loss of neurologic function involving interpretation of sensory information
astereognosis *ă-stēr′ē-og-nō′sis*	inability to judge the form of an object by touch (e.g., a coin from a key)
atopognosis *ă-top-og-nō′sis*	inability to locate a sensation properly, such as to locate a point touched on the body
Alzheimer disease	disease of structural changes in the brain resulting in an irreversible deterioration that progresses from forgetfulness and disorientation to loss of all intellectual functions, total disability, and death
cerebral palsy (CP) *ser′ĕ-brăl pawl′ze*	condition of motor dysfunction caused by damage to the cerebrum during development or injury at birth; characterized by partial paralysis and lack of muscle coordination (palsy = paralysis)
cerebrovascular disease	disorder resulting from a change within one or more blood vessels of the brain
cerebral arteriosclerosis *ar-ter′ē-ō-skler-ō′sis*	hardening of the arteries of the brain

cerebral atherosclerosis *ath'er-ō-skler-ō'sis*	condition of lipid (fat) buildup within the blood vessels of the brain (ather/o = fatty [lipid] paste)
cerebral aneurysm *an'yū-rizm*	dilation of a blood vessel in the brain (aneurysm = dilation or widening)
cerebral thrombosis *throm-bō'sis*	presence of a stationary clot in a blood vessel of the brain
cerebral embolism *em'bo-lizm*	obstruction of a blood vessel in the brain by an embolus transported through the circulation
cerebrovascular accident (CVA) (Fig. 8-5) **stroke**	damage to the brain caused by cerebrovascular disease; e.g., occlusion of a blood vessel by an embolus or thrombus or intracranial hemorrhage after rupture of an aneurysm
transient ischemic attack (TIA) (Fig. 8-6) *tran'zē-ĕnt is-kē'mik*	brief episode of loss of blood flow to the brain; usually caused by a partial occlusion that results in temporary neurologic deficit (impairment); often precedes a CVA
encephalitis *en-sēf-ă-lī'tis*	inflammation of the brain
epilepsy *ep'i-lep'sē*	disorder affecting the central nervous system, characterized by recurrent seizures
tonic-clonic *ton'ik-klon'ik*	stiffening-jerking; a major motor seizure involving all muscle groups; previously termed grand mal (big bad) seizure

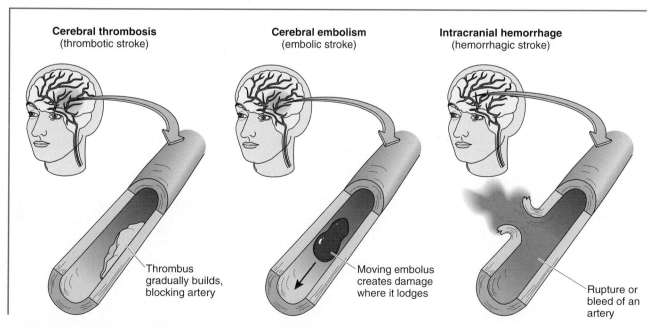

Cerebral thrombosis (thrombotic stroke)

Cerebral embolism (embolic stroke)

Intracranial hemorrhage (hemorrhagic stroke)

Thrombus gradually builds, blocking artery

Moving embolus creates damage where it lodges

Rupture or bleed of an artery

■ **FIGURE 8-5.** Cerebrovascular accident.

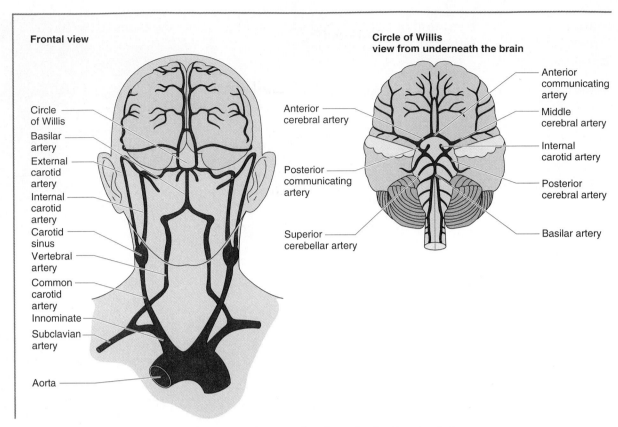

FIGURE 8-6. Sites of transient ischemic attack: carotid and vertebrobasilar circulation.

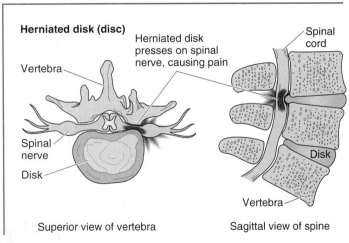

FIGURE 8-7. Herniated disk (disc).

absence *ab'sens*	seizure involving a brief loss of consciousness without motor involvement; previously termed petit mal (little bad) seizure
partial	seizure involving only limited areas of the brain with localized symptoms
glioma *glī-o'mă*	tumor of glial cells graded by degree of malignancy
herniated disk (disc) (Fig 8-7) *her'nē-ā-ted*	protrusion of a degenerated or fragmented intervertebral disk so that the nucleus pulposus protrudes, causing compression on the nerve root

herpes zoster *her'pēz zos'ter*	viral disease affecting the peripheral nerves characterized by painful blisters that spread over the skin following the affected nerves, usually unilateral; also known as shingles
Huntington chorea *kōr-ē'ă* **Huntington disease (HD)**	hereditary disease of the central nervous system characterized by bizarre involuntary body movements and progressive dementia (choros = dance)
hydrocephalus (Fig. 8-8) *hī-drō-sĕf'ă-lŭs*	abnormal accumulation of cerebrospinal fluid in the ventricles of the brain as a result of developmental anomalies, infection, injury, or tumor
meningioma *mĕ-nin'jē-ō'mă*	benign tumor of the coverings of the brain (meninges)
meningitis *men-in-jī'tis*	inflammation of the meninges
migraine headache *mī'gran*	paroxysmal (sudden, periodic) attacks of mostly unilateral headache often accompanied by disordered vision, nausea, or vomiting, lasting hours or days, and caused by dilation of arteries
multiple sclerosis (MS) (Fig. 8-9) *sklĕ-rō'sis*	disease of the central nervous system characterized by the demyelination (deterioration of the myelin sheath) of nerve fibers, with episodes of neurologic dysfunction (exacerbation) followed by recovery (remission)
myasthenia gravis *mī-as-thē'nē-ă grā'văs*	autoimmune disorder that affects the neuromuscular junction causing a progressive decrease in muscle strength; activity resumes and strength returns after a period of rest

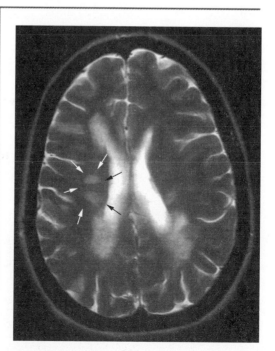

■ **FIGURE 8-9.** Magnetic resonance image of the brain showing plaque formation (*arrows*) in a patient with multiple sclerosis.

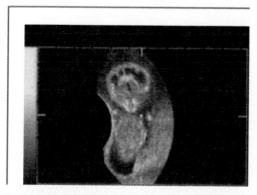

■ **FIGURE 8-8.** Sonogram showing hydrocephalus in early pregnancy.

myelitis *mī-ĕ-lī′tis*	inflammation of the spinal cord
narcolepsy *nar′kō-lep-sē*	sleep disorder characterized by a sudden, uncontrollable need to sleep, attacks of paralysis (cataplexy), and dreams intruding while awake (hypnagogic hallucinations)
Parkinson disease parkinsonism	slowly progressive degeneration of nerves in the brain characterized by tremor, rigidity of muscles, and slow movements (bradykinesia), usually occurring later in life
plegia *plē′jē-ă*	paralysis
hemiplegia *hem-ē-plē′jē-ă*	paralysis on one side of the body
paraplegia *par-ă-plē′jē-ă*	paralysis from the waist down
quadriplegia *kwah′dri-plē′jē-ă*	paralysis of all four limbs
poliomyelitis *po′lē-ō-mi′ĕ-lī′tis*	inflammation of the gray matter of the spinal cord caused by a virus, often resulting in spinal and muscle deformity and paralysis (polio = gray)
polyneuritis *pol′ē-nū-ri-tis*	inflammation involving two or more nerves, often caused by a nutritional deficiency such as lack of thiamine
sleep apnea *ap′nē-ă*	periods of breathing cessation (10 seconds or more) that occur during sleep, often causing snoring
spina bifida (Fig. 8-10) *spī′nă bi′fă-dă*	congenital defect in the spinal column characterized by the absence of vertebral arches, often resulting in pouching of spinal membranes or tissue

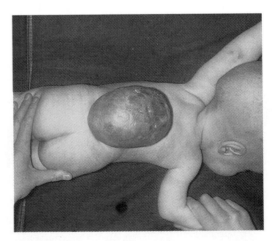

FIGURE 8-10. Spina bifida with myelomeningocele. The infant also has hydrocephaly.

PROGRAMMED REVIEW: NERVOUS SYSTEM DIAGNOSTIC TERMS

Answers	Review

gnos/o

without

agnosia

stere/o

astereognosis

top/o

atopognosis

8.66   Recall that the combining form meaning knowing is _gnos/o_. The prefix *a-* means _____. The general term for many types of loss of neurologic function, generally meaning not knowing, is therefore _agnosia_. The combining form meaning three-dimensional is _____. The type of agnosia in which a person cannot judge the shape of an object by touch is termed _astereo gnosis_. Recall that the combining form meaning place or location is _top_. The type of agnosia in which a person cannot locate a sensation on the body is _atopognosis_.

Alzheimer

8.67   Named for the German neurologist who researched dementia, _____ disease causes structural changes in the brain resulting in mental deterioration.

cerebral palsy

8.68   Palsy means a partial paralysis. The condition of partial paralysis and lack of muscle coordination caused by damage to the cerebrum is _cerebral_ _palsy_ (CP).

cerebrovascular

condition

arteriosclerosis

cerebral atherosclerosis

8.69   The combining form *vascul/o* refers to blood vessels. A disease affecting blood vessels in the cerebrum is called _____ disease. The combining form *scler/o* means hard. Recall that the suffix *-osis* means increase or _____. The term for a condition of hardening of the arteries in the brain is cerebral _arterio sclerosis_. The combining form *ather/o* means fatty paste. The condition of a hardening of a pasty lipid buildup in the blood vessels of the brain is called _____.

aneurysm

8.70   The dilation of a blood vessel in the brain is a cerebral _aneurysm_. The Greek word thrombos means a clot. A stationary blood clot in a blood vessel in the brain is called a

cerebral thrombosis	_____ _~stationary~_ ~thrombosis~ _____. A blood clot carried in the circulation that obstructs a blood vessel in the brain is called a cere-
embolism	bral ___*embolism*___.

8.71 Occlusion of a brain blood vessel by a thrombus or embolus or bleeding after rupture of an aneurysm can cause brain damage known

cerebrovascular accident	as a stroke or _____ _____ (CVA).

8.72 Ischemia is a condition in which blood flow to an area is re-duced. A brief episode of loss of blood flow to the brain caused by a

transient	partial occlusion of a blood vessel is called a _____
ischemic attack	_____ _____.

8.73 Recall that the combining form meaning meninges is

mening/o, -itis	_____. The suffix meaning inflammation is _____. Therefore, the term for inflammation of the meninges is
meningitis	_____.

8.74 Formed from the combination of *en-* meaning in and *cephal/o*

head	meaning ___*head*___, *encephal/o* is a combining form meaning
brain	_____. The term for inflammation of the brain is
encephalitis	_____.

myel/o	**8.75** The combining form for the spinal cord is ___*myel/o*___. Inflam-
myelitis	mation of the spinal cord is termed _____. The combin-ing form *poli/o* means gray. An inflammation of the gray matter of the
poliomyelitis	spinal cord, caused by a virus, is called _____.

neur/o	**8.76** The combining form meaning nerve is ___*neur*___. The prefix
many	*poly-* means _____. The term for inflammation of two or more
polyneuritis	nerves is _____.

8.77 The disorder of the central nervous system characterized by re-

epilepsy	current seizures is _____. Recall that the combining form
tone	*ton/o* refers to muscle ___*tone*___. The type of epileptic seizure in which

tonic-clonic

muscles stiffen and jerk is called ___tonic___-___clonic___. A type of epileptic seizure in which a brief loss of consciousness occurs (the person seems absent for a moment) is called _____. A

absence

partial

_____ seizure affects only limited areas of the brain with localized symptoms.

gli/o

8.78 The combining form meaning glue is _____, the origin of the name of glial cells, thought to "glue" together neurons. The suffix meaning tumor is _____. A malignant (cancerous) tumor of glial cells

-oma

glioma

is called a _____. A benign (noncancerous) tumor of the

meningioma

meninges is called _____. (Note: Word structuring alone does not indicate whether a tumor is cancerous. Rely on a good medical dictionary or oncology reference for clarification.)

8.79 A hernia is a protrusion of a part from its normal location. A degenerated or fragmented intervertebral disk that protrudes and compresses a nerve is called a ___herniated___ disk (disc).

herniated

8.80 A herpes virus causes skin blisters following an affected nerve, often in a beltlike pattern on the skin. The Greek word zoster means girdle or belt. This condition is called _____ _____.

herpes zoster

8.81 The term chorea comes from a Greek word meaning dance. A chorea is a spasmodic involuntary movement of muscles. A hereditary type of chorea characterized by bizarre body movements and progressive dementia is ___Huntington___ ___chorea___ or

Huntington chorea

Huntington disease

___Huntington___ ___Disease___ (HD).

8.82 The combining form *hydr/o* means water or fluid. The combining form *cephal/o* means head. These two combining forms are the origin of the term for an abnormal accumulation of cerebrospinal fluid in the

hydrocephalus

brain: _____.

8.83 The kind of severe headache accompanied by disordered vision,

migraine

nausea, and vomiting is a _____ headache.

hard

8.84 Recall that *scler/o* is the combining form meaning _hard_. A disease of the central nervous system involving deterioration of the myelin sheath of nerve fibers and multiple patches of hard plaques in

multiple sclerosis

the brain and spinal cord is _____ _____.

weakness

8.85 The combining form *my/o* means muscle, and the suffix *-asthenia* means _weakness_. Thus, a term for muscle weakness is

myasthenia

myasthenia. An autoimmune disorder that causes a pro-gressive decrease in muscle strength is myasthenia _gravis_.

gravis

sleep, seizure

8.86 Recall that the combining form *narc/o* means stupor or _____. The suffix *-lepsy* means _____. A sleep disor-der in which the person falls asleep as quickly as if in a seizure is called

narcolepsy

_____.

8.87 Named after a British physician, this disease involves a progres-sive degeneration of nerves in the brain characterized by tremor, rigid-

Parkinson

ity of muscles, and slow movements: _____ disease, also known as parkinsonism.

paralysis

8.88 Recall that the suffix *-plegia* means _paralysis_. The prefix *hemi-* means _half_, and paralysis of one half (one side) of the

half

hemiplegia

body is called _hemiplegia_. Paralysis from the waist down

paraplegia

is called _paraplegia_. Recall that the prefix meaning four

quadri-

is _____. Therefore, the term for paralysis of all four limbs is

quadriplegia

quadriplegia.

8.89 The Greek word *apnoia* means want of breath. The term for a condition in which breathing stops for short periods during sleep is

sleep apnea

apnea.

8.90 The congenital defect in the spinal column characterized by the

bifida

absence of vertebral arches is called spina _____.

SELF-INSTRUCTION: NERVOUS SYSTEM DIAGNOSTIC TESTS AND PROCEDURES

Study the following:

Test or Procedure	Explanation
electrodiagnostic procedures *ē-lek'trō-dī-ag-nō'sis*	
electroencephalogram (EEG) (Fig.8-11) *ē-lek'trō-en-sef'ă-lō-gram*	record of the minute electrical impulses of the brain, used to identify neurologic conditions that affect brain function and level of consciousness
evoked potentials *ē vokt' pō-ten'shăls*	minute electrical waves that are sorted out of ongoing EEG activity to diagnose auditory, visual, and sensory pathway disorders
polysomnography (PSG) (Fig. 8-12) *pol'ē-som-nog'ră-fē*	recording of various aspects of sleep (e.g., eye and muscle movements, respiration, and EEG patterns) to diagnose sleep disorders
lumbar puncture (LP) *lŭm'bar pŭnk'chur*	introduction of a specialized needle into the spine in the lumbar region for diagnostic or therapeutic purpose, such as to obtain cerebrospinal fluid for testing; also called spinal tap

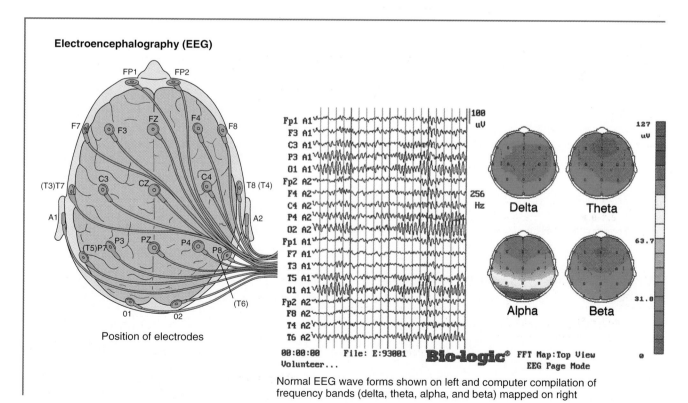

Normal EEG wave forms shown on left and computer compilation of frequency bands (delta, theta, alpha, and beta) mapped on right

■ **FIGURE 8-11.** Electroencephalography.

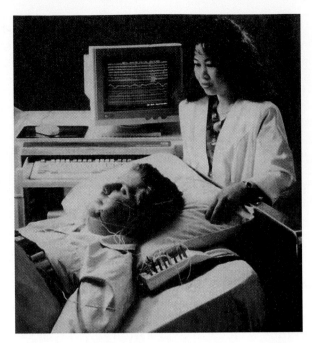

FIGURE 8-12. Polysomnography.

magnetic resonance imaging (See Figs. 8-3, 8-4, and 8-10) *mag-net'ic rez'ō-nans im'ă-jing*	nonionizing imaging technique using magnetic fields (MRI) and radio frequency waves to visualize anatomic structures (especially soft tissue) such as the tissues of the brain and spinal cord
magnetic resonance angiography (MRA) *mag-net'ic rez'ō-nans an-jē-og'ră-fē*	magnetic resonance imaging of the blood vessels, for detecting pathologic conditions such as thrombosis and atherosclerosis
intracranial MRA (*see* reference to anatomy in Fig. 8-6) *in'tră-krā'nē-ăl*	magnetic resonance image of the head to visualize the vessels of the circle of Willis (common site of cerebral aneurysm, stenosis, or occlusion)
extracranial MRA *eks-tră-krā'nē-ăl*	magnetic resonance image of the neck to visualize the carotid artery
nuclear medicine imaging	radionuclide organ imaging
SPECT brain scan (single photon emission computed tomography)	scan combining nuclear medicine and computed tomography to produce images of the brain after administration of radioactive isotopes

positron emission tomography (PET) (Fig. 8-13) *poz'i-tron ē-mish'ŭn tō-mog'ră-fē*	technique combining nuclear medicine and computed tomography to produce images of brain anatomy and corresponding physiology; used to study stroke, Alzheimer disease, epilepsy, metabolic brain disorders, chemistry of nerve transmissions in the brain, and so on; provides greater accuracy than SPECT but is used less often because of cost and limited availability of the radioisotopes
radiography *rā'dē-og'ră-fē*	x-ray imaging
cerebral angiogram *ser'ĕ-brăl an'jē-ō-gram*	x-ray of blood vessels in the brain after intracarotid injection of contrast medium
computed tomography (of the head)	computed tomographic x-ray images of the head used to visualize abnormalities, such as brain tumors and malformations
myelogram	x-ray of the spinal cord made after intraspinal injection of contrast medium
reflex testing	test performed to observe the body's response to a stimulus
deep tendon reflexes (DTR)	involuntary muscle contraction after percussion at a tendon (e.g., patella, Achilles) indicating function; positive findings are either no reflex response or an exaggerated response to stimulus; numbers are often used to record responses: no response 1+ diminished response 2+ normal response 3+ more brisk than average response 4+ hyperactive response

Positron emission tomography (PET) scans

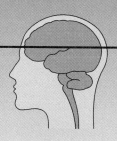

Warm colors (red and yellow) indicate a higher rate of metabolism and brain activity in the normal brain when compared with the brain of the Alzheimer's patient

Area of scan

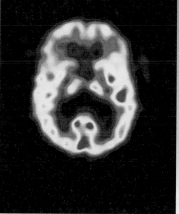

PET scan of healthy brain

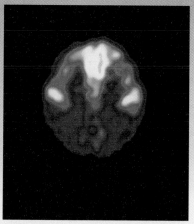

PET scan of Alzheimer's brain

■ **FIGURE 8-13.** Positron emission tomography scans.

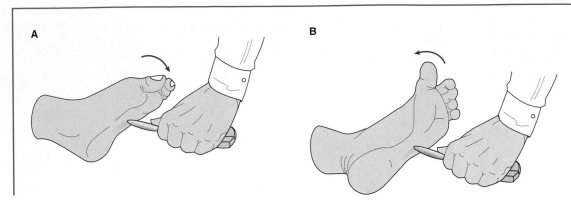

A   **B**

■ **FIGURE 8-14.** Reflex testing. **A.** Normal plantar reflex. **B.** Babinski sign.

Babinski sign or reflex (Fig. 8-14)	pathologic response to stimulation of the plantar surface of the foot; a positive sign is indicated when the toes dorsiflex (curl upward)
transcranial sonogram *trans-krā′nē-ăl*	image made by sending ultrasound beams through the skull to assess blood flow in intracranial vessels; used in diagnosis and management of stroke and head trauma

PROGRAMMED REVIEW: NERVOUS SYSTEM DIAGNOSTIC TESTS AND PROCEDURES

Answers	Review
	8.91 A wide variety of tests and procedures are used to diagnose conditions of the nervous system, including several electrodiagnostic procedures. The combining form referring to electricity is *electr/o*. The combining form referring to the entire brain is _____.
encephal/o	
record	Recall that the suffix *-gram* means __record__. The EEG is a record of electrical impulses in the brain; EEG is an abbreviation for
electroencephalogram	_____. Minute electrical waves sorted out of EEG activity to diagnose specific nerve pathway
evoked	disorders are called _____ potentials (potential is a term referring to electrical charges).
	8.92 In addition to *hypn/o* and *somn/i*, a combining form meaning
somn/o, poly-	sleep is __Somn/o__. The prefix meaning many is _____. The suf-
recording	fix *-graphy* means process of _____. From these three

components comes the term for another electrodiagnostic procedure that measures various physiological aspects of sleep:

polysomnography

_____ (PSG).

8.93 The procedure in which a specialized needle is introduced into the lumbar spine, such as to obtain a sample of cerebrospinal fluid for

lumbar puncture

examination, is called a _lumbar_ _puncture_ (LP).

8.94 A nonionizing imaging technique using magnetic fields to visualize structures such as tissues of the brain and spinal cord is

magnetic resonance

_____ _____ imaging (MRI).

magnetic resonance
  angiography

8.95 An MRI technique for imaging blood vessels is termed

_____ _____ _____

crani/o

(MRA). The combining form for skull is _crani/o_. The prefix _in-_

within

tra- means _within_. The magnetic resonance image of the head to visualize the vessels of the circle of Willis is an

intracranial

_____ MRA. The prefix _extra-_ means

outside

_____. The term for magnetic resonance image of the neck

extracranial

to image the carotid arteries is called an _extra cranial_ MRA.

8.96 Imaging a structure after administration of a radionuclide is

medicine

called nuclear _____ imaging. A specialized brain scan that combines nuclear medicine with computed tomography is called

photon emission

single _photon_ _emission_ computed

tomography

_____ (SPECT).

8.97 Another technique that combines nuclear medicine and computed tomography used to study brain anatomy and physiology is

emission tomography

positron _____ _____ (PET).

process	**8.98** Recall that the suffix *-graphy* means _____ of
recording	_____. The process of recording x-ray images is called
radiography	_____. The adjective form of cerebrum, pertaining
cerebral	to the largest part of the brain, is _____. Again, the com-
angi/o	bining form for blood vessel is _____. An x-ray of the blood ves-
cerebral angiogram	sels of the cerebrum is called a _____ _____.
	8.99 Cross-sectional x-ray images of the brain produced by
computed tomography	_____ _____ (CT) are also used to vi-
	sualize abnormalities such as brain tumors.
myel/o	**8.100** The combining form meaning spinal cord is _____.
record	Again, the suffix *-gram* means _____. An x-ray record of the
	spinal cord using an intraspinal contrast medium is a
myelogram	_____.
	8.101 A reflex is the body's automatic response to a stimulus.
Reflex	_____ testing is performed to observe such responses. Reflexes
	that involve involuntary muscle contraction after percussion at a tendon
deep tendon	are called _deep_ _tendon_ reflexes (DTR).
	8.102 A response to stimulation of the plantar surface of the foot is a
Babinski	pathologic reflex called _Babinski_ sign, named for the physi-
	cian who discovered it. Babinski was a French neurologist.
	8.103 Ultrasound is also called sonography. The prefix *trans-* means
across	_across_ or through. The record of an ultrasound image made by
	sending ultrasound waves through the skull is called a
transcranial sonogram	_transcranial_ _sonogram_.

SELF-INSTRUCTION: NERVOUS SYSTEM OPERATIVE TERMS

Study the following:

Term	Meaning
craniectomy *krā′nē-ek′tō-mē*	excision of part of the skull to approach the brain
craniotomy *krā′nē-ot′ō-mē*	incision into the skull to approach the brain
diskectomy **(discectomy)** (Fig. 8-15) *dis-ek′tō-mē*	removal of a herniated disk; often done percutaneously (per = through; cutaneous = skin)
laminectomy *lam′i-nek′tō-mē*	excision of one or more laminae of the vertebrae to approach the spinal cord
vertebral lamina	flattened posterior portion of the vertebral arch
microsurgery (Fig. 8-16) *mī-krō′-sēr′jer-ē*	use of a microscope to dissect minute structures during surgery
neuroplasty *nur′ō-plas-tē*	surgical repair of a nerve
spondylosyndesis (Fig. 8-17) *spon′di-lō-sin-dē′sis*	spinal fusion

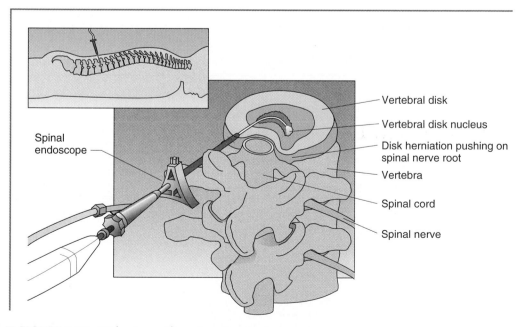

■ **FIGURE 8-15.** Diskectomy (discectomy).

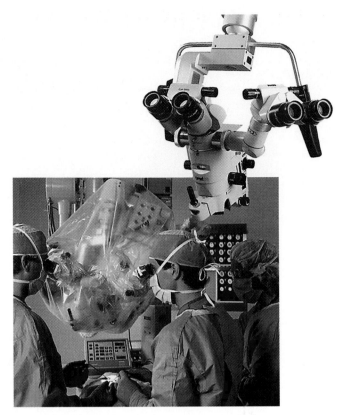

FIGURE 8-16. Microscope for neurological surgery.

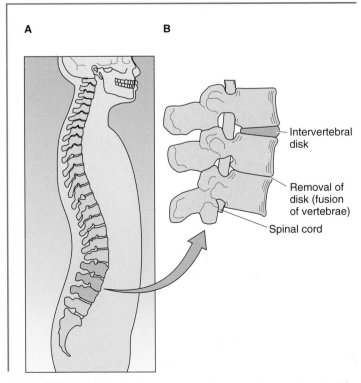

▪ **FIGURE 8-17.** Spondylosyndesis. **A.** Spinal column. **B.** Spinal fusion.

PROGRAMMED REVIEW: NERVOUS SYSTEM OPERATIVE TERMS

Answers	Review
-ectomy	**8.104** The operative suffix meaning excision is _____. The excision of part of the skull, needed to reach the brain surgically, is
craniectomy	termed _____.
diskectomy (discectomy)	**8.105** The excision of a herniated spinal disc is termed a _____.
lamina	**8.106** The flattened posterior portion of the vertebral arch is called a _____. The excision of one or more laminae is termed a
laminectomy	_____.
incision	**8.107** The operative suffix *-tomy* means _____. An inci-
craniotomy	sion into the skull to approach the brain is a _____.
microsurgery	**8.108** Use of a microscope to dissect minute structures during surgery is called _____.
neur/o	**8.109** The combining form meaning nerve is _____. Recall that
-plasty	the suffix for surgical repair or reconstruction is _____. The
neuroplasty	surgical repair of a nerve is termed _____.
spondyl/o	**8.110** The two combining forms meaning vertebra are *vertebr/o* and _____. Syndesis is a surgical technique of joining bones together. The medical term for spinal fusion, or surgically joining verte-
spondylosyndesis	brae together, is _____.

SELF-INSTRUCTION: NERVOUS SYSTEM THERAPEUTIC TERMS

Study the following:

Term	Meaning
chemotherapy *kem'ō-thār-ă-pē*	treatment of malignancies, infections, and other diseases with chemical agents to destroy selected cells or impair their ability to reproduce

radiation therapy (Fig. 8-18) *rā´dē-ā´shŭn thār´ă-pē*	treatment of neoplastic disease using ionizing radiation to impede proliferation of malignant cells
stereotactic (stereotaxic) radiosurgery *ster´ē-ō-tak´tik (ster´ē-ō-tak´sik) rā´dē-ō-sēr´jer-ē*	radiation treatment to inactivate malignant lesions, using multiple, precise external radiation beams focused on a target with the aid of a stereotactic frame and imaging such as CT, MRI, or angiography; used to treat inoperable brain tumors and other lesions
stereotactic (stereotaxic) frame (Fig. 8-19)	mechanical device used to localize a point in space targeting a precise site

COMMON THERAPEUTIC DRUG CLASSIFICATIONS

analgesic *an-ăl-jē´zik*	agent that relieves pain
anticonvulsant *an´tē-kon-vŭl´sant*	agent that prevents or lessens convulsions
antidepressant *an´tē-dē-pres´ănt*	agent that counteracts depression
sedative *sed´ă-tiv*	agent that quiets nervousness
hypnotic *hip-not´ik*	agent that induces sleep

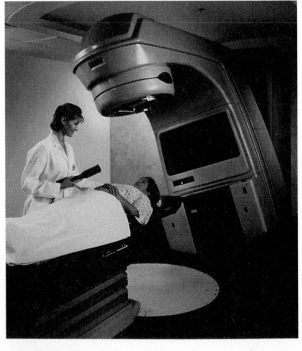

FIGURE 8-18. Radiation therapy linear accelerator.

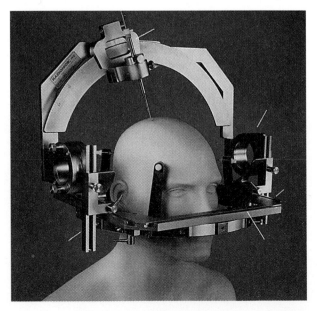

FIGURE 8-19. Stereotactic frame.

PROGRAMMED REVIEW: NERVOUS SYSTEM THERAPEUTIC TERMS

Answers	Review

Answers

chemotherapy

radiation

therapy

stere/o

stereotactic radiosurgery

without

analgesic

against

anticonvulsant

antidepressant

sedative

hypn/o

hypnotic

Review

8.111   The combining form referring to chemical agents is *chem/o*. The treatment of malignancies, infections, and other diseases with chemical agents that destroy targeted cells is called _____.

8.112   Some kinds of cancer are treated with radiation, which deters the proliferation of malignant cells. This is called _____ _____.

8.113   The combining form meaning three-dimensional or solid is _____, as in the term stereotactic (stereotaxic) frame, an apparatus allowing precise localization in space. Radiation therapy given with precise localization of the radiation beam using a stereotactic frame is called _____ _____.

8.114   The prefix *an-* means _____. The Greek word algesis means sensation of pain. A drug that relieves pain is called an _____.

8.115   Many drugs are named according to their action against a condition or symptom. The prefix *anti-* means _____. A drug that works to prevent or lessen convulsion is an _____.

8.116   A drug that counteracts (works against) depression is an _____.

8.117   A patient can be sedated to calm his or her anxious state. A drug that quiets nervousness is called a _____.

8.118   The combining forms meaning sleep are *somn/i, somn/o,* and _____. Formed from the last of these, an agent that induces sleep is termed a _____.

SELF-INSTRUCTION: PSYCHIATRIC SYMPTOMATIC TERMS

Study the following:

Term	Meaning
affect	emotional feeling or mood
flat affect	significantly dulled emotional tone or outward reaction
apathy	a lack of interest or display of emotion
catatonia	a state of unresponsiveness to one's outside environment, usually including muscle rigidity, staring, and inability to communicate
delusion	persistent belief that has no basis in reality
grandiose delusion	a person's false belief that he or she possesses great wealth, intelligence, or power
persecutory delusion	a person's false belief that someone is plotting against him or her with intent to harm
dysphoria	a restless, dissatisfied mood
euphoria	an exaggerated, unfounded feeling of well-being
hallucination	a false perception of the senses for which there is no reality, most commonly hearing or seeing things (alucinor = to wander in mind)
ideation	the formation of thoughts or ideas, for example, suicidal ideation (thoughts of suicide)
mania	state of abnormal elation and increased activity
neurosis	a psychologic condition in which anxiety is prominent
psychosis	a mental condition characterized by distortion of reality resulting in the inability to communicate or function within one's environment
thought disorder	thought that lacks clear processing or logical direction

PROGRAMMED REVIEW: PSYCHIATRIC SYMPTOMATIC TERMS

Answers	Review
affect emotional	**8.119** An emotional feeling or mood is called an ___affect___. A flat affect is a significantly dulled ___emotional___ tone or outward reaction.
apathy	**8.120** A lack of interest or display of emotion is termed ___apathy___.

cata-

ton/o

catatonia

8.121 Recall that the prefix meaning down is ___Cata___, and the combining term for tone is ___ton/o___. The original Greek term katatonos meant stretching down. The medical term for a state of unresponsiveness that includes muscle rigidity is _____.

false

grandiose

persecutory delusion

8.122 A delusion is a persistent _____ belief that has no basis in reality. A delusion that one has great wealth, intelligence, or power is a _____ delusion. A delusion that one is being persecuted by others plotting against him or her is a _____ _____.

carry

dysphoria

normal

euphoria

8.123 The combining form *phor/o* means to bear or ___Carry___. Recall that the prefix *dys-* means painful, difficult, or faulty. Thus, the term dysphoria originated from terms meaning to carry poorly. The medical term for a <u>restless</u>, dissatisfied mood is ___dysphoria___. Incorporating eu-, the prefix meaning good or ___normal___, the term for an exaggerated, unfounded feeling of well-being is ___euphoria___.

hallucination

process

8.124 From the Latin word alucinor, meaning to wander in mind, this medical term means a false perception of the senses: _____. Recall that the suffix *-ation* refers to _____.

ideation

8.125 The process of forming thoughts or ideas is called _____ (for example, thoughts of suicide are called suicidal ideation).

condition of

mania

8.126 Again, the suffix *-ia* means _____ ____. A condition of abnormal elation and increased activity is called ___mania___. The original Greek word mania means frenzy.

increase

nerve

8.127 The suffix *-osis* means condition or ___increase___. The combining form *neur/o* usually means ___nerve___, or in this case, ner-

neurosis	vousness. The term for a psychologic condition in which anxiety is prominent is called _neurosis_, its meaning referring to the condition of nervousness.
psych/o	**8.128** The combining forms meaning mind are *phren/o,* thym/o, and _psych/o_. The last of these is used with a suffix meaning condition to make this term for a mental condition characterized by a distortion of reality resulting in an inability to function within one's environment:
psychosis	_psychosis_.
thought disorder	**8.129** A disorder of thinking in which there is no clear processing or logical direction is a _____ _____.

SELF-INSTRUCTION: PSYCHIATRIC DIAGNOSTIC TERMS

Study the following:

Term	Meaning
MOOD DISORDERS	
major depression **major depressive illness** **clinical depression** **major affective disorder** **unipolar disorder**	a disorder causing periodic disturbances in mood that affect concentration, sleep, activity, appetite, and social behavior; characterized by feelings of worthlessness, fatigue, and loss of interest
dysthymia	a milder affective disorder characterized by a chronic depression
manic depression **bipolar disorder (BD)**	affective disorder characterized by mood swings of mania and depression (extreme up and down states)
seasonal affective disorder (SAD)	an affective disorder marked by episodes of depression that most often occur during the fall and winter and remit in the spring
ANXIETY DISORDERS	
generalized anxiety disorder (GAD)	the most common anxiety disorder, characterized by chronic, excessive, uncontrollable worry about everyday problems; affects the ability to relax or concentrate but does not usually interfere with social interactions or employment; physical symptoms include muscle tension, trembling, twitching, fatigue, headaches, nausea, and insomnia

panic disorder (PD)	a disorder of sudden, recurrent attacks of intense feelings, including physical symptoms that mimic a heart attack (rapid heart rate, chest pain, shortness of breath, chills, sweating, and dizziness), with a general sense of loss of control or feeling that death is imminent; often progresses to agoraphobia
phobia	exaggerated fear of a specific object or circumstance that causes anxiety and panic; named for the object or circumstance, such as agoraphobia (marketplace), claustrophobia (confinement), and acrophobia (high places)
posttraumatic stress disorder (PTSD)	a condition resulting from an extremely traumatic experience, injury, or illness that leaves the sufferer with persistent thoughts and memories of the ordeal; may occur after a war, violent personal assault, physical or sexual abuse, serious accident, or natural disaster; symptoms include feelings of fear, detachment, exaggerated startle response, restlessness, nightmares, and avoidance of anything or any one who triggers the painful recollections
obsessive-compulsive disorder (OCD)	an anxiety disorder featuring unwanted, senseless obsessions accompanied by repeated compulsions; can interfere with all aspects of a person's daily life, for example, the thought that a door is not locked with repetitive checking to make sure it is locked, or thoughts that one's body has been contaminated causing repetitive washing
hypochondriasis	a preoccupation with thoughts of disease and concern that one is suffering from a serious condition that persists despite medical reassurance to the contrary

DISORDERS USUALLY DIAGNOSED IN CHILDHOOD

autism	a developmental disability commonly appearing during the first three years of life, resulting from a neurologic disorder affecting brain function, evidenced by difficulties with verbal and nonverbal communication, and an inability to relate to anything beyond oneself (auto = self) in social interactions; persons with autism often exhibit body movements such as rocking and repetitive hand movements; they commonly become preoccupied with observing parts of small objects or moving parts or performing meaningless rituals
dyslexia	a developmental disability characterized by a difficulty understanding written or spoken words, sentences, or paragraphs, affecting reading, spelling, and self-expression
attention-deficit/ hyperactivity disorder (ADHD)	a dysfunction characterized by consistent hyperactivity, distractibility, and lack of control over impulses, which interferes with ability to function normally at school, home, or work
mental retardation	a condition of subaverage intelligence characterized by an IQ of 70 or below, resulting in the inability to adapt to normal social activities

EATING DISORDERS

anorexia nervosa	a severe disturbance in eating behavior caused by abnormal perceptions about one's body weight, evidenced by an overwhelming fear of becoming fat that results in a refusal to eat and body weight well below normal
bulimia nervosa	an eating disorder characterized by binge eating followed by efforts to limit digestion through induced vomiting, use of laxatives, or excessive exercise

SUBSTANCE ABUSE DISORDERS

Substance abuse disorders	mental disorders resulting from abuse of substances such as drugs, alcohol, or other toxins, causing personal and social dysfunction; identified by the abused substance, such as alcohol abuse, amphetamine abuse, opioid (narcotic) abuse, and polysubstance abuse

PSYCHOTIC DISORDERS

schizophrenia	a disease of brain chemistry causing a distorted cognitive and emotional perception of one's environment; symptoms include distortions of normal function such as disorganized thought, delusions, hallucinations, and catatonic behavior; negative symptoms (normal reactions missing in persons with schizophrenia) include flat affect, apathy, and withdrawal from reality

PROGRAMMED REVIEW: PSYCHIATRIC DIAGNOSTIC TERMS

Answers	Review
	8.130 Psychiatrists use a number of terms referring to major depression, a disorder causing mood disturbances affecting concentration, sleep, and activity and characterized by feelings of worthlessness and
clinical	apathy. Other terms include major depressive illness, _____
affective	depression, major _____ disorder, and unipolar
disorder	_____.
	8.131 The disorder in which a person experiences mood swings between depression and mania is called _____ depression or
manic	
bipolar, one	_____ disorder (BD). Note how "unipolar" refers to _____
bipolar	mood, whereas _____ refers to two moods.

thym/o

faulty, dysthymia

8.132 Recall that the three combining forms meaning mind are *phren/o, psych/o,* and _____. The prefix *dys-* means painful, difficult, or _____. Another mood disorder, _____, is a milder affective disorder characterized by chronic depression, is made with the third combining form.

seasonal

affective disorder

8.133 An affective disorder in which episodes of depression occur in seasonal cycles is called _____ _____ _____ (SAD).

generalized

anxiety

8.134 There are several anxiety disorders. The most common occurs generally, not resulting from a specific anxiety-producing situation. It causes excessive and uncontrollable worrying and may produce physical symptoms. This disorder is called _____ _____ disorder (GAD).

panic disorder

8.135 Another anxiety disorder produces sudden attacks of intense feelings of anxiety and panic with often dramatic physical symptoms. This disorder is called _____ _____ (PD).

phob/o

condition of

phobia

8.136 Recall that the combining form that means an exaggerated fear or sensitivity is _____. The suffix *-ia* means _____ _____. The psychiatric condition in which one experiences an exaggerated fear of something is termed a _____ .

post-, posttraumatic

stress disorder

8.137 After a traumatic experience, a person may develop a stressful condition involving persistent thoughts of the ordeal, fear, and other symptoms. Recall that a common prefix meaning after or behind is _____. This condition is termed _____ _____ _____ (PTSD).

8.138 An obsession is a persistent, uncontrollable thought. A compulsion is a persistent, uncontrollable behavior. An anxiety disorder characterized by obsession and compulsions that often interfere with all aspects of an individual's life is called _____

obsessive-
compulsive disorder

_____ _____ (OCD).

below

8.139   The combining form *chondr/o* refers to cartilage of the ribs. The prefix *hypo-* means deficient or _____. Thus, the term hypochondrium refers to the abdomen (beneath the ribs)—once thought to be the place where sensations of a distressing nature were experienced, such as the concern that one is suffering from a serious condition despite medical reassurance to the contrary. Recall that the suffix *-iasis* means for-

presence

mation of or _____ of. The term for the condition when

hypochondriasis

this concern is present is _____.

8.140   The prefix *auto-* means self. Recall that the suffix *-ism* means

condition of

_____ _____. A developmental condition in which the person is unable to relate to anyone other than himself or herself is

autism

called _____.

lex/o
difficult

8.141   The combining form meaning word or phrase is _____.
The prefix *dys-* means painful, faulty, or _____. The term for the developmental disability of difficulty understanding writ-

dyslexia

ten words or phrases is _____. The suffix *-ia* means

condition of

_____ _____.

attention-deficit
hyperactivity disorder
excessive

8.142   ADHD is typically diagnosed in childhood, when the child has difficulty paying attention to things, is easily distracted, and is generally hyperactive. ADHD is the abbreviation for _____-
_____ / _____ _____.
Recall that the prefix *hyper-* means above or _____.

mental retardation

8.143   The Latin word mens refers to the mind, and the Latin verb retardo means to hinder. The condition of limited intelligence is called

_____ _____.

8.144   The Greek word orexis means appetite. Recall that the prefix

without	*an-* means _____, and the suffix *-ia* means
condition of	_____ _____. Thus, the term for the condition of being
anorexia	without an appetite is _____. When this condition is
	caused by a psychological disturbance ("nervous" condition) and fear of
nervosa	being fat, it is called anorexia _____.

8.145 Another eating disorder, characterized by binge eating followed

bulimia by efforts to limit digestion of food, is called _____ nervosa.

Bulimia comes from two Greek words meaning hungry as an ox.

8.146 Substance abuse disorders are mental disorders resulting from

abuse an _____ of substances such as drugs or alcohol that leads to

dysfunction.

split **8.147** The combining form *schiz/o* means _____, and the com-

mind bining form *phren/o* means _____. Thus, the term for a disease of

brain chemistry that causes disorganized thinking, delusions, hallucina-

schizophrenia tions, and other symptoms is _____. Some

people mistakenly believe that schizophrenia means a mind split in two

personalities (multiple personality disorder), but the term actually origi-

split nally meant a mind _____ from reality.

SELF-INSTRUCTION: PSYCHIATRIC THERAPEUTIC TERMS

Study the following:

Term	Meaning
electroconvulsive therapy (ECT)	electrical shock applied to the brain to induce convulsions; used to treat severely depressed patients
light therapy	use of specialized illuminating light boxes and visors to treat seasonal affective disorder
psychotherapy	treatment of psychiatric disorders using verbal and nonverbal interaction with patients, individually or in a group, employing specific actions and techniques

| **behavioral therapy** | treatment to decrease or stop unwanted behavior |
| **cognitive therapy** | treatment to change unwanted patterns of thinking |

COMMON THERAPEUTIC DRUG CLASSIFICATIONS

psychotropic drugs	medications used to treat mental illnesses (trop/o = a turning)
antianxiety agents anxiolytic agents	drugs used to reduce anxiety
neuroleptic agents	drugs used to treat psychosis, especially schizophrenia

PROGRAMMED REVIEW: PSYCHIATRIC THERAPEUTIC TERMS

Answers	**Review**
electroconvulsive	**8.148** The combining form *electr/o* refers to electricity. Therapy for severely depressed patients that uses a shock to the brain that induces convulsions is called _____ therapy (ECT).
light	**8.149** One theory for the depression of seasonal affective disorder is that the person suffers from reduced amounts of sunlight in the fall and winter. A treatment for this is therefore _____ therapy.
psych/o psychotherapy	**8.150** This treatment modality for psychiatric patients using verbal and nonverbal interactions was originally named to mean therapy of the mind. Three combining forms meaning mind are *phren/o, thym/o,* and _____. Made with the third form, this therapy is termed _____.
behavioral	**8.151** Treatment emphasizing behavioral changes is called _____ therapy.
cognitive	**8.152** Treatment directed to change unwanted patterns of thinking is called _____ therapy. The term cognitive refers to thought processes.

psychotropic

8.153 The suffix *-tropic* pertains to turning. The term for this class of drugs for treating mental illnesses literally means turning of the mind: _____ drugs.

anti-

antianxiety

anxiolytic

8.154 Drug classes are frequently named for their actions that cause something or their actions against something. A common prefix meaning against or opposed to is _____. Drugs that work against anxiety, therefore, are termed _____ drugs. Another term for these drugs uses the suffix *-lytic*, pertaining to breaking down something. Thus, this term for these drugs literally means breaking down anxiety: _____ agents

neur/o

neuroleptic

8.155 The combining form meaning nerve is _____. Drugs used to treat psychosis, especially schizophrenia, are called _____ agents.

Practice Exercises

For the following terms, on the lines below the term, write out the indicated word parts: prefixes, combining forms, roots, and suffixes. Then define the word.

Example:
anencephaly

<u>an/encephal/y</u>
  P   R   S

DEFINITION: without/brain/condition or process of

1. ganglioma

   _____ / _____
       R   S

   DEFINITION: _____

2. atopognosia

   _____ / _____ / _____ / _____
       P   CF   R   S

   DEFINITION: _____

3. catatonic

——————— / ——————————— / ————
　　　P　　　　　　　　　R　　　　　　S

DEFINITION: _____

4. dystaxia

——————— / ——————————— / ————
　　　P　　　　　　　　　R　　　　　　S

DEFINITION: _____

5. bradykinesia

——————— / ——————————— / ————
　　　P　　　　　　　　　R　　　　　　S

DEFINITION: _____

6. meningocele

————— / ——————————
　　CF　　　　　　　S

DEFINITION: _____

7. dysthymia

——————— / ——————————— / ————
　　　P　　　　　　　　　R　　　　　　S

DEFINITION: _____

8. polysomnogram

——————— / ——————————— / ————
　　　P　　　　　　　　　CF　　　　　S

DEFINITION: _____

9. spondylosyndesis

——————— / ——————————— / ————
　　　CF　　　　　　　　P　　　　　　S

DEFINITION: _____

10. hemiplegia

——————— / ————
　　　P　　　　S

DEFINITION: _____

11. craniotomy

——————— / ——————————— / ————
　　　P　　　　　　　　　R　　　　　　S

DEFINITION: _____

12. thalamic

——————— / ———
R　　　　　　S

DEFINITION: _____

13. neuroglial

——————— / ——————— / ———
CF　　　　　　　　R　　　　　　S

DEFINITION: _____

14. dyslexia

——————— / ——————— / ———
P　　　　　　　　R　　　　　　S

DEFINITION: _____

15. somnipathy

——————— / ——————— / ———
CF　　　　　　　　R　　　　　　S

DEFINITION: _____

16. hydrocephalic

——————— / ——————— / ———
CF　　　　　　　　R　　　　　　S

DEFINITION: _____

17. necromania

——————— / ———————
CF　　　　　　　　S

DEFINITION: _____

18. acrophobia

——————— / ——————— / ———
CF　　　　　　　　R　　　　　　S

DEFINITION: _____

19. hypnotic

——————— / ———————
CF　　　　　　　　S

DEFINITION: _____

20. euphoria

——————— / ——————— / ———
P　　　　　　　　R　　　　　　S

DEFINITION: _____

21. parasomnia

—————————— / —————————————— / ———————
      P   R   S

DEFINITION: _____

22. narcolepsy

—————————— / ———————
     CF   S

DEFINITION: _____

23. stereotaxy

—————————— / —————————————— / ———————
     CF   R   S

DEFINITION: _____

24. hemiparesis

—————————— / ———————
     P   S

DEFINITION: _____

25. neurasthenia

—————————— / ———————
     R   S

DEFINITION: _____

26. myelopathy

—————————— / —————————————— / ———————
     CF   R   S

DEFINITION: _____

27. intracranial

—————————— / —————————————— / ———————
     P   R   S

DEFINITION: _____

28. aphasia

—————————— / —————————————— / ———————
     P   R   S

DEFINITION: _____

29. schizophrenia

—————————— / —————————————— / ———————
     CF   R   S

DEFINITION: _____

30. cerebrospinal

_____ / _____ / _____
      CF   R   S

DEFINITION: _____

Write the correct medical term for each of the following:

31. inflammation of the meninges _____

32. excision of a herniated disc _____

33. inability to locate a sensation properly, such as locating a point touched on the body

_____

34. a slowly progressive degeneration of nerves in the brain characterized by tremor, rigidity of muscles, and slow movements

_____

35. a pathologic response to stimulation of the plantar surface of the foot indicated by dorsiflexion of the toes

_____

36. numbness and tingling _____

37. state of unconsciousness _____

38. a type of seizure that causes a series of sudden, involuntary contractions of muscles

_____

39. congenital defect of the spinal column resulting in pouching of spinal membranes

_____

40. a type of agnosia indicating an inability to judge the form of an object by touch, e.g., to tell a coin from a key

Complete the medical term by writing the missing part:

41. electro_____gram = record of electrical brain impulses

42. _____syndesis = spinal fusion

43. crani_____ = excision of part of the skull

44. cerebral _____sclerosis = fat buildup in blood vessel of brain

45. hyper_____ = increased sensations

46. dys_____ = difficulty speaking

47. _____algesia = loss of sense of pain

Match the following terms with the appropriate terms in the right column:

48. herpes zoster _____   a. tonic-clonic

49. spinal tap _____   b. CVA

50. faint _____   c. Alzheimer disease

51. grand mal _____   d. PSG

52. petit mal _____   e. flaccid

53. cerebral thrombus _____   f. absence

54. flabby _____   g. clot

55. stroke _____   h. LP

56. dementia _____   i. shingles

57. sleep study _____   j. syncope

Write the full medical term for the following abbreviations:

58. CT _____

59. MRI _____

60. PET _____

61. MS _____

62. CNS _____

63. CP _____

64. TIA _____

65. EEG _____

66. DTR _____

67. SPECT _____

68. PSG _____

69. ANS _____

70. PNS _____

71. CSF _____

72. MRA _____

73. CVA _____

For each of the following, circle the combining form that corresponds to the meaning given:

74. brain   encephal/o   crani/o   neur/o

75. movement   esthesi/o   kinesi/o   somat/o

76. speech	phas/o	plas/o	phag/o
77. body	somn/o	somat/o	phren/o
78. spinal cord	vertebr/o	spondyl/o	myel/o
79. mind	cerebr/o	thym/o	thalm/o
80. sensation	esthesi/o	neur/o	kinesi/o
81. place	top/o	tax/o	phor/o
82. sleep	somat/o	hypn/o	esthesi/o
83. knowing	phren/o	phas/o	gnos/o

Write in the missing words on lines in the following illustration of brain anatomy:

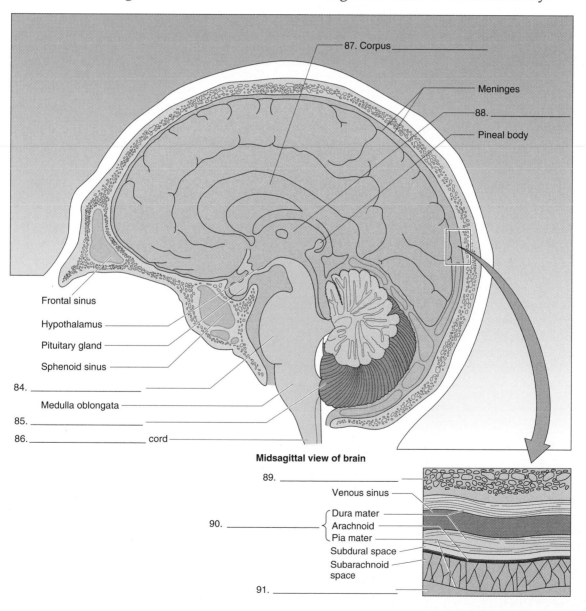

87. Corpus _____

Meninges

88. _____

Pineal body

Frontal sinus

Hypothalamus

Pituitary gland

Sphenoid sinus

84. _____

Medulla oblongata

85. _____

86. _____ cord

Midsagittal view of brain

89. _____

Venous sinus

Dura mater

Arachnoid

Pia mater

Subdural space

Subarachnoid space

90. _____

91. _____

For each of the following, circle the correct spelling of the term:

92. Alsheimer   Alzheimer   Alshiemer

93. skitzoprenia   skizophrenia   schizophrenia

94. polysomnography   polysonography   polysolemography

95. parenoia   paranoia   paranoyea

96. quadraplegia   quadriplega   quadriplegia

97. atopagnosis   atopegnosis   atopognosis

98. demensha   dementia   dimentia

99. epilapsey   epilepsey   epilepsy

100. catonia   catatonia   catetonia

101. delushion   dilusion   delusion

102. hellucination   hallucination   hallucinashun

103. poliomyalitis   poliomyelitis   poleiomyalitis

Give the noun that was used to form the following adjectives.

104. epileptic   _____

105. euphoric   _____

106. cerebellar   _____

107. delusional   _____

108. syncopal   _____

109. autistic   _____

110. psychotic   _____

111. cerebral   _____

112. dysphasic   _____

113. paranoid   _____

MATCHING: Psychiatric Symptoms

Match the following terms with the appropriate terms in the right column:

114. hallucination _____

115. persecutory delusion _____

116. catatonia _____

117. apathy _____

118. euphoria _____

119. mania _____

120. flat affect _____

121. dysphoria _____

122. thought disorder _____

123. grandiose delusion _____

a. an exaggerated, unfounded feeling of well-being

b. dull emotional tone or outward reaction

c. false belief that one is very wealthy, intelligent or powerful

d. false belief that one is being plotted against

e. state of abnormal elation and increased activity

f. a lack of interest or display of emotion

g. thoughts that lack clear process or logical direction

h. state of unresponsiveness that includes muscle rigidity, staring, and inability to communicate

i. restless, dissatisfied mood

j. hearing or seeing things

Write the full medical term for the following abbreviations

124. GAD _____

125. ADHD _____

126. OCD _____

127. ECT _____

128. PD _____

129. BD _____

130. PTSD _____

MATCHING: Psychiatric diagnoses

Match the following terms with the appropriate terms in the right column:

131. unipolar disorder _____

132. anxiety disorder _____

133. bipolar disorder _____

134. psychosis _____

135. disorder identified in childhood _____

136. eating disorder _____

137. mild depression _____

a. hypochondriasis

b. bulimia nervosa

c. clinical depression

d. dysthymia

e. schizophrenia

f. manic depression

g. autism

Write the correct term for each of the following:

138. General term for a psychological condition in which anxiety is a featured characteristic: _____

139. Depression that occurs most in fall and winter: _____

140. Exaggerated fear of a specific object or circumstance: _____

141. Milder affective disorder characterized by mild depression: _____

142. Class of drugs used to treat psychosis, especially schizophrenia: _____

143. General term for a mental condition characterized by a distortion of reality resulting in an inability to communicate or function within one's environment: _____

144. Disorder characterized by chronic excessive worry: _____

145. Affective disorder marked by mood swings from depression to mania: _____

146. Anxiety disorder characterized by intense fearful attacks with physical symptoms that mimic a heart attack: _____

147. Class of drugs used to treat mental illness: _____

MATCHING: Psychiatric therapeutic terms

Match the following terms with the appropriate terms in the right column:

148. anxiety _____   a. behavioral therapy

149. schizophrenia _____   b. light therapy

150. seasonal affective disorder _____   c. anxiolytic agent

151. major affective disorder _____   d. electroconvulsive therapy

152. bulimia _____   e. neuroleptic agent

Medical Record Analyses

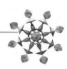

MEDICAL RECORD 8-1

Progress Note

OP H&P

Neurological Services

CC: numbness and tingling in feet and hands

HPI: This 54 y.o. right-handed female c/o numbness in her feet for the past two weeks with "pockets" of numbness in the abdomen. Her legs feel heavy and numb. Her hands started tingling a week ago and she is feeling very nervous. She has had similar episodes over the past 3 years, lasting about a week at a time, often after stressful events, or during hot weather.

PMH: Operations: none. No serious illnesses/accidents
  FH: Father, age 71, L&W; Mother, age 66, is bipolar;
  Her only sibling, a sister, age 28, has cerebral palsy.
  SH: Denies smoking or use of street drugs, but drinks socially
  OH: certified public accountant. Marital Status: single
  ROS: noncontributory.
  VS: T 98.2° F., P 82, R 16, BP 110/68, Ht 5'2", Wt 138#

PE: HEENT: WNL. Neck: negative. Heart/Lungs: normal.
  Cranial nerves intact. Reflexes: DTR's are increased, greater on the left than the right without spasticity. Toes upgoing bilaterally.
  There is numbness to tactile pin stimulation over both extremities. She has no finger-to-nose ataxia. Her gait is steady.

A: R/O MS

P: Schedule MRI of the brain with and without gaolinium (contrast)
  RTO for report and further evaluation × 1 wk

1. Which medical term best describes the patient's symptoms:
   a. hypersthesia
   b. paresthesia
   c. ataxia
   d. hemiparesis
   e. neuralgia

2. What is noted in the history about the patient's mother?
   a. she is alive and well
   b. she suffers from depression
   c. she has mood swings of mania and depression
   d. she suffers from generalized anxiety
   e. she is a hypochondriac

3. Describe the sister's condition
   a. disorder affecting the central nervous system characterized by seizures
   b. hereditary disease of the central nervous system characterized by bizarre involuntary body movements and progressive dementia
   c. abnormal accumulation of cerebrospinal fluid in the ventricles of the brain as a result of developmental abnormality
   d. condition of motor dysfunction caused by damage to the cerebrum during development or injury at birth
   e. slowly progressive degeneration of nerves in the brain characterized by tremor, rigidity and slow movements

4. Which medical term describes the positive finding of the "toes upgoing" bilaterally?
   a. Babinski sign
   b. neuralgia
   c. hemiparesis
   d. spastic paralysis
   e. flaccid paralysis

5. What is the doctor's impression?
   a. the patient has multiple sclerosis
   b. the patient does not have multiple sclerosis
   c. the patient may have multiple sclerosis
   d. the patient may have hardening of the arteries in the brain
   e. the patient does not have hardening of the arteries in the brain

6. Describe the test noted in the Plan:
   a. x-ray
   b. nuclear image
   c. ultrasound scan
   d. tomographic radiograph
   e. scan produced by magnetic fields and radio frequency waves

MEDICAL RECORD 8-2 FOR ADDITIONAL STUDY

CENTRAL MEDICAL GROUP, INC.

Department of Neurology

201 Medical Center Drive • Central City, US 90000-1234 • PHONE: (012) 125-8888 • FAX: (012) 125-3434

June 9, 20xx

Paul Jiang, M.D.
1409 West Ninth Street
Central City, US 90000-1233

Dear Dr. Jiang:

RE: Anne Cross

I had the pleasure of meeting Mrs. Cross today. As you know, she is a 65-year-old right-handed female who began to have difficulties on or about April 17, 20xx. She experienced dizziness that she described as occurring in the midday; there was also some associated slurring of speech. By the next morning, she seemed to have some disorientation with putting on her clothes, and she had some difficulties using the left side of her body. She had no headache or other problems. Prior to that time, she denied having any symptomatology. She was admitted to the hospital, as you are aware, and underwent a series of studies. A CT scan was reviewed and showed evidence of a right ischemic occipital infarct. In addition, she underwent an echocardiogram that was normal and an electroencephalogram that showed some right-sided slowing. A carotid ultrasound study suggested 60-70% stenosis of the bifurcation and/or internal carotids.

The patient was discharged on a combination of Persantine 50 mg t.i.d, enteric-coated aspirin 1 q d, Proventil 1 q 12 h p.r.n. for chronic obstructive pulmonary disease, and Procardia XL 1 q d for hypertension. The patient also has stopped smoking.

The patient reports that in the past, she has been essentially well except for some eye surgery. Additionally, after her discharge, she underwent visual field studies which confirmed the presence of an incomplete left-sided homonymous hemianopsia.

By way of family background, her brother died from complications of a stroke at age 78. Her mother died from liver cancer, and her father died from a myocardial infarction.

The patient has no specific allergy to drugs.

The patient's risk factors have been otherwise unremarkable.

On examination today, the patient is a slender female in no acute distress.

Blood pressure from the left arm in a sitting position is 130/95 and from the right arm in the sitting position is 145/95. Her pulse rate is 76 and regular.

No bruits are present over the carotid distributions. The temporal arteries are not enlarged or tender.

On examination of the eyes, the patient showed some mild arteriolar narrowing without hemorrhage or exudate. Gross visual confrontation suggests a neglect of left hemianopsia. The extraocular movements are full. The pupils are symmetrical. There is no ptosis. Facial movements are normal, and speech is normal.

CENTRAL MEDICAL GROUP, INC.

Department of Neurology

201 Medical Center Drive • Central City, US 90000-1234 • PHONE: (012) 125-8888 • FAX: (012) 125-3434

There is no drift to the outstretched hands. Finger-to-nose test is performed symmetrically.

The patient does not have any asymmetrical topagnosis. She has no evidence of apraxia.

The patient's reflexes are physiologic: they are 2+ at the biceps, triceps, and brachioradialis. The knee and ankle jerks are 2+. No clonus is elicited.

Gait and stance are normal.

OVERALL ASSESSMENT:

Without prior warning, this woman had a new onset of a cerebral infarct. By her description, it is likely that she had a posterior circulatory infarct in the area of the occipital lobe. There may have been an association zone in the parietal area as well. Since that time, she has had some residual hemianopsia as described.

PLAN:

At this time, it is suggested that the most prudent approach would be to do an MRA and an MRI. This should include the great vessels of the neck and the vertebrobasilar system. The MRI would allow us to see the nature of residuals of the stroke, the distribution of the stroke, and would allow us to determine if there are any asymptomatic lesions, including microvascular infarcts which would not be seen on the CAT scan. The MRA would allow us to determine the overall anatomy of the vasculature--including the neck, the bifurcations, and the posterior circulation--in a noninvasive way. Depending on the results of both of these studies, we would have to consider if she needs a full angiogram done with selective views. If, in fact, she has had an infarct of the posterior occipital lobe, then the current treatment with aspirin and Persantine would be adequate. If, by the nature of the MRA, it is determined that there are significant changes or irregularity of the contour of the intima of the vessels at the bifurcations, then there may be an indication for prophylaxis for an endarterectomy despite not having a stroke in that distribution of the vessels. This, of course, would all be determined by the results of this study. The advantage of the MRA-MRI combined would allow us to visualize adequately the vessels combined with the detailed evaluation of her brain.

I think this would be the patient's best and most prudent approach to the patient's health and would help to prevent recurrence of this problem.

Please do not hesitate to call me if there are any questions regarding this patient's evaluation.

Sincerely,

Melvin Classen, M.D.
Department of Neurology
(012) 125-6899

MC:mar
DOT:6/10/20xx

cc: Mrs. Anne Cross

MEDICAL RECORD 8-2 FOR ADDITIONAL STUDY

Anne Cross has been fairly healthy until she had a stroke about 2 months ago. She was treated by Dr. Paul Jiang, her personal physician, at that time, and discharged from the hospital on medication. At the request of Ms. Cross, Dr. Jiang called for a consultation from a neurologist, Dr. Melvin Classen.

Read Medical Record 8-2 (pages 382–383) for Ms. Cross, and answer the following questions. This record is a consultation report written by Dr. Classen as a letter back to Ms. Cross's physician, Dr. Jiang, after his consultation.

Write your answers in the spaces provided.

1. Below are medical terms used in this record you have not yet encountered. Underline each where it appears in the record, and define below.

   homonymous hemianopsia _____

   finger-nose test _____

   apraxia _____

   clonus _____

2. In your own words, not using medical terminology, briefly describe Ms. Cross's symptoms in April before she was admitted to the hospital.

   _____

   _____

   _____

3. Write the missing parts in this table summarizing the diagnostic tests performed in April.

Test	Definition of Test	Findings
CT	_____	_____
_____	sound waves through heart	_____
carotid ultrasound	_____	_____
_____	_____	_____
_____	_____	slowed electrical pulse on right side

4. What family member had a problem perhaps similar to Ms. Cross's?

   _____

5. For each of the following medications given Ms. Cross, translate the dosage instructions:

   Persantine

   _____

   aspirin

   _____

Proventil

_____

Procardia

_____

6. Dr. Classen recommends two diagnostic studies. Describe both in your own words:

   a. _____

   b. _____

   In one sentence, describe Dr. Classen's rationale for recommending the combination of these two tests:

   _____

   _____

7. Name the preventive surgical procedure Dr. Classen suggests that may be appropriate if changes are found in the carotid blood vessels:

   _____

   Describe that procedure in your own words:

   _____

   _____

Answers to Practice Exercises

1. gangli/oma
   <u>R   S</u>
   ganglion (knot)/tumor
2. a/topo/gnos/ia
   <u>P CF   R   S</u>
   without/place/knowing/
   condition of
3. cata/ton/ic
   <u>P   R   S</u>
   down/tone or tension/
   pertaining to
4. dys/tax/ia
   <u>P R S</u>
   painful, difficult or faulty/
   order or coordination/
   condition of
5. brady/kines/ia
   <u>P   R   S</u>
   slow/movement/condition of
6. meningo/cele
   <u>CF   S</u>
   meninges (membrane)/
   pouching or hernia

7. dys/thym/ia
   <u>P   R   S</u>
   painful, difficult or faulty/
   mind/condition of
8. poly/somno/gram
   <u>P   CF   S</u>
   many/sleep/record
9. spondylo/syn/desis
   <u>CF   P   S</u>
   vertebra/together or with/
   binding
10. hemi/plegia
    <u>P   S</u>
    half/paralysis
11. cranio/tomy
    <u>CF   S</u>
    skull/incision
12. thalam/ic
    <u>R   S</u>
    thalamus (a room)/pertaining
    to
13. neuro/gli/al
    <u>CF   R   S</u>
    nerve/glue/pertaining to

14. dys/lex/ia
    <u>P   R   S</u>
    painful, difficult or faulty/
    word or phrase/condition
    of
15. somni/path/y
    <u>CF   R   S</u>
    sleep/disease/condition or
    process of
16. hydro/cephal/ic
    <u>CF   R   S</u>
    water/head/pertaining to
17. necro/mania
    <u>CF   S</u>
    death/condition of abnormal
    impulse toward
18. acro/phob/ia
    <u>CF   R   S</u>
    topmost/exaggerated
    fear/condition of
19. hypno/tic
    <u>CF   S</u>
    sleep/pertaining to
20. eu/phor/ia
    <u>P   R   S</u>
    good or normal/carry or
    bear/condition of

21. para/somn/ia
    P   R   S
    abnormal/sleep/condition of

22. narco/lepsy
    CF   S
    stupor/seizure

23. stereo/tax/y
    CF   R   S
    three-dimensional or solid/
    order or coordination/
    condition or process of

24. hemi/paresis
    P   S
    half/slight paralysis

25. neur/asthenia
    R   S
    nerve/weakness

26. myelo/path/y
    CF   R   S
    spinal cord/disease/
    condition or process of

27. intra/crani/al
    P   R   S
    within/skull/pertaining to

28. a/phas/ia
    P   R   S
    without/speech/condition of

29. schizo/phren/ia
    CF   R   S
    split/mind/condition of

30. cerebro/spin/al
    CF   R   S
    cerebrum/spine/pertaining to

31. meningitis
32. diskectomy
33. atopognosis
34. Parkinson disease or parkinsonism
35. Babinski sign or reflex
36. paresthesia
37. coma
38. convulsion
39. spina bifida
40. astereognosis
41. electroencephalogram
42. spondylosyndesis
43. craniectomy
44. cerebral atherosclerosis

45. hyperesthesia
46. dysphasia
47. analgesia
48. i
49. h
50. j
51. a
52. f
53. g
54. e
55. b
56. c
57. d
58. computed tomography
59. magnetic resonance imaging
60. positron emission tomography
61. multiple sclerosis
62. central nervous system
63. cerebral palsy
64. transient ischemic attack
65. electroencephalogram
66. deep tendon reflexes
67. single photon emission computed tomography
68. polysomnography
69. autonomic nervous system
70. peripheral nervous system
71. cerebrospinal fluid
72. magnetic resonance angiography
73. cerebrovascular accident
74. encephal/o
75. kinesi/o
76. phas/o
77. somat/o
78. myel/o
79. thym/o
80. esthesi/o
81. top/o
82. hypn/o
83. gnos/o
84. pons
85. cerebellum
86. spinal
87. callosum
88. thalamus
89. cranium
90. meninges

91. cerebrum
92. Alzheimer
93. schizophrenia
94. polysomnography
95. paranoia
96. quadriplegia
97. atopognosis
98. dementia
99. epilepsy
100. catatonia
101. delusion
102. hallucination
103. poliomyelitis
104. epilepsy
105. euphoria
106. cerebellum
107. delusion
108. syncope
109. autism
110. psychosis
111. cerebrum
112. dysphasia
113. paranoia
114. j
115. d
116. h
117. f
118. a
119. e
120. b
121. i
122. g
123. c
124. generalized anxiety disorder
125. attention deficit/hyperactivity disorder
126. obsessive-compulsive disorder
127. electroconvulsive therapy
128. panic disorder
129. bipolar disorder
130. posttraumatic stress disorder
131. c
132. a
133. f
134. e
135. g
136. b

137. d
138. neurosis
139. seasonal affective disorder
140. phobia
141. dysthymia
142. neuroleptic agents
143. psychosis
144. generalized anxiety
    disorder (GAD)

145. manic depression or bipolar
    disorder (BD)
146. panic disorder (PD)
147. psychotropic drugs
148. c
149. e
150. b
151. d
152. a

Answers to Medical Records Analyses

1. b
2. c
3. d
4. a
5. c
6. e

CHAPTER 9

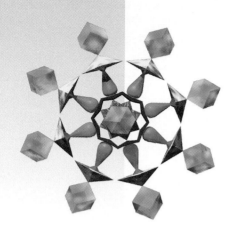

Endocrine System

Endocrine System Overview

The endocrine system secretes hormones and other substances from ductless glands and other structures (Fig. 9-1). Figure 9-2 describes these functions.

SELF-INSTRUCTION: COMBINING FORMS

Study the following:

Combining Form	Meaning
aden/o	gland
adren/o, adrenalo	adrenal gland
andr/o	male
crin/o	to secrete
dips/o	thirst
gluc/o **glyc/o**	sugar
hormon/o	hormone (an urging on)
ket/o **keton/o**	ketone bodies
pancreat/o	pancreas
thym/o	thymus gland
thyr/o, thyroid/o	thyroid gland (shield)

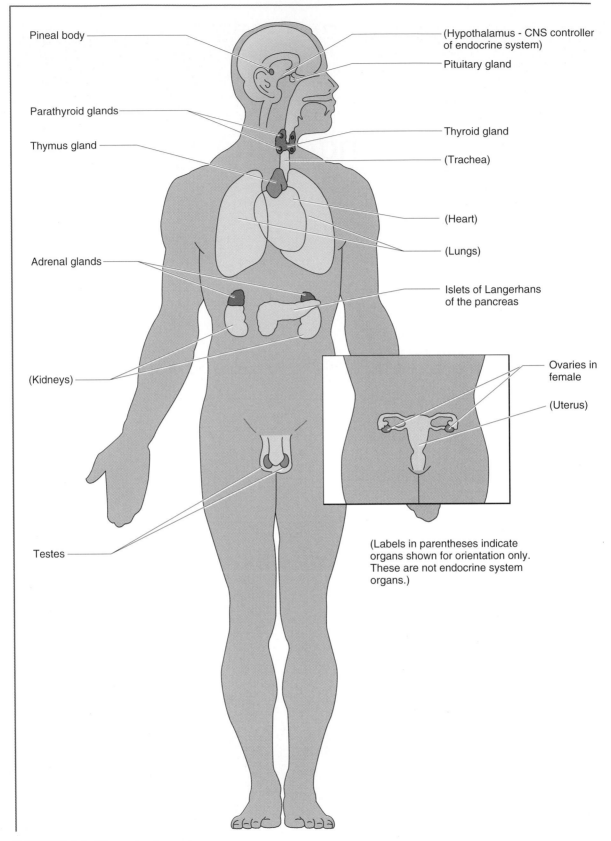

Pineal body

(Hypothalamus - CNS controller of endocrine system)

Pituitary gland

Parathyroid glands

Thyroid gland

Thymus gland

(Trachea)

(Heart)

(Lungs)

Adrenal glands

Islets of Langerhans of the pancreas

(Kidneys)

Ovaries in female

(Uterus)

Testes

(Labels in parentheses indicate organs shown for orientation only. These are not endocrine system organs.)

■ FIGURE 9-1. The endocrine system.

Endocrine gland	Secretions	Function
*Anterior pituitary (adenohypophysis) 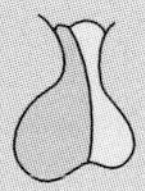	Thyroid-stimulating hormone (TSH)	Stimulates secretion from thyroid gland
	Adrenocorticotrophic hormone (ACTH)	Stimulates secretion from adrenal cortex
	Follicle-stimulating hormone (FSH)	Initiates growth of ovarian follicle; stimulates secretion of estrogen in females and sperm production in males
	Luteinizing hormone (LH)	Causes ovulation; stimulates secretion of progesterone by corpus luteum; causes secretion of testosterone in testes
	Melanocyte-stimulating hormone (MSH)	Affects skin pigmentation
	Growth hormone (GH)	Influences growth
	Prolactin (lactogenic hormone)	Stimulates breast development and milk production during pregnancy
*Posterior pituitary (neurohypophysis) 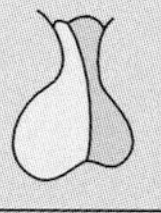	Antidiuretic hormone (ADH)	Influences the absorption of water by kidney tubules
	Oxytocin	Influences uterine contraction
Pineal body	Melatonin	Exact function unknown, affects onset of puberty
	Serotonin	Serves as a precursor to melatonin
Thyroid gland 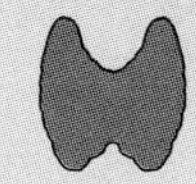	Triiodothyronine (T_3), thyroxine (T_4)	Regulate metabolism
	Calcitonin	Regulates calcium and phosphorus metabolism
Parathyroid glands 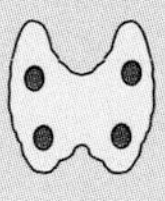	Parathyroid hormone (PTH)	Regulates calcium and phosphorus metabolism
Pancreas (islets of Langerhans) 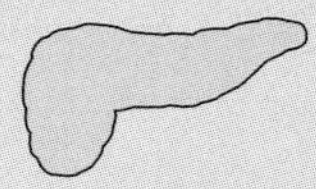	Insulin, glucagon	Regulates carbohydrate/sugar metabolism
Thymus gland 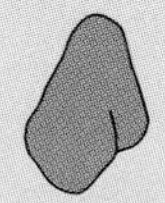	Thymosin	Regulates immune response
Adrenal glands (suprarenal glands) 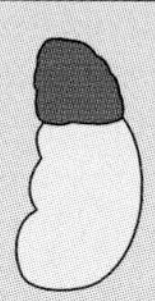	Steroid hormones: glucocorticoids, mineral corticosteroids, androgens	Regulate carbohydrate metabolism and salt and water balance; some effect on sexual characteristics.
	Epinephrine, norepinephrine	Affect sympathetic nervous system in stress response
Ovaries 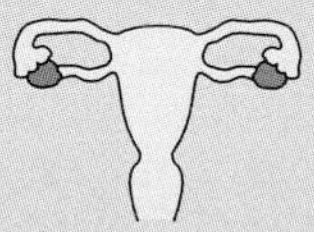	Estrogen, progesterone	Responsible for the development of female secondary sex characteristics, and regulation of reproduction
Testes 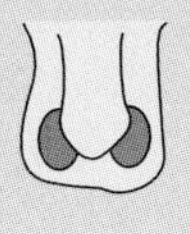	Testosterone	Affects masculinization and reproduction

*Release of hormones in pituitary is controlled by hypothalamus

■ **FIGURE 9-2.** Functions of endocrine glands.

PROGRAMMED REVIEW: COMBINING FORMS

Answers	Review
aden/o -oma adenoma	**9.1** The combining form meaning gland is _____. Put this together with the suffix referring to a tumor, _____, to create the term for a tumor of glandular tissue: _____.
adrenal near enlargement adrenomegaly inflammation adrenalitis	**9.2** The combining forms *adren/o* and *adrenal/o* mean _____ gland. The prefix *ad-* used in these combining forms gives a clue that the gland is to, toward, or _____ the kidney. Using *adren/o* and the suffix *-megaly* meaning _____, the term describing an enlargement of the adrenal gland is _____. Using the combining form *adrenal/o* and *-itis,* meaning _____, the term describing an inflammation of the adrenal gland is _____.
andr/o form pertaining to andromorphous	**9.3** The combining form meaning male is _____. Linked to *morph/o,* the combining form meaning _____, and *-ous,* the suffix meaning _____ _____, the term pertaining to male form or appearance is _____.
secrete within endocrine	**9.4** The combining form *crin/o* means to _____. Recall that the prefix *endo-* means _____. Thus, the medical term for the _____ system refers to secreting within. The endocrine system secretes hormones and other substances from ductless glands.
dips/o many condition of polydipsia	**9.5** The combining form meaning thirst is _____. Recall that the prefix *poly-* means _____ (or excessive), and the suffix *-ia* means a _____ _____. Thus, the term for a condition of excessive thirst is _____.
glyc/o production	**9.6** The two combining terms for sugar are *gluc/o* and _____. The suffix *-genic* pertains to origin or _____. The term for something giving rise to or producing glucose (a form of

glucogenic	sugar) is therefore _____. From the combining form
hyper-	*glyc/o* and the prefix _____, meaning too much or excessive, and
blood	the suffix *-emia*, referring to a _____ condition, comes the term
glucose (or sugar)	hyperglycemia, which refers to too much _____ in the blood.

hormon/o	**9.7** The combining form for hormone is _____, from a
	Greek word meaning "an urging on" (a hormone is a substance that
adjective	urges an action to occur). Hormonal is the _____ form.

	9.8 The two combining forms meaning ketone bodies are *ket/o* and
keton/o	_____. Ketone bodies are chemical substances resulting from
ur/o	metabolism. Recall that the combining form for urine is _____, and
condition of	the suffix *-ia* means a _____ _____. Therefore, the term
ketonuria	for a condition of ketone bodies in the urine is _____.

pancreat/o	**9.9** The combining form meaning the pancreas is _____.
-itis	Recall that the suffix for inflammation is _____. The term for in-
pancreatitis	flammation of the pancreas is _____. Excision of
pancreatectomy	the pancreas is termed _____.

thymus	**9.10** The combining form *thym/o* means the _____ gland. A
thymoma	tumor of thymic tissue is a _____.

	9.11 The two combining forms meaning thyroid gland are
thyr/o, thyroid/o	_____ and _____. The Greek term at the origin of
	these combining forms means *shield*, and the thyroid gland is so named
shield	because it is resembles a _____. The suffix *-ic* means
pertaining to	_____ _____. Combined with *tox/o*, a combining form
poison, thyroid	meaning _____, and *thyr/o,* meaning _____
gland	_____, the term pertaining to poison of the thyroid gland is
thyrotoxic	_____. Thyroiditis describes an
inflammation, thyroid	_____ of the _____ gland.

SELF-INSTRUCTION: ANATOMICAL TERMS

Study the following:

Gland or Hormone	Location or Function
adrenal glands *ă-drē′năl* **suprarenal glands** *sū′pră-rē′năl*	located on the superior surface of each kidney; the adrenal cortex secretes steroid hormones, and the adrenal medulla secretes epinephrine and nor epinephrine

steroid hormones
stēr′oyd
 glucocorticoids
 glūkō-kōr′ti-koydz
 mineral
  corticosteroids
 min′er-ăl
  kōr′ti-kō-stēr′oydz
 androgens
 an′drō-jenz
	regulate carbohydrate metabolism and salt and water balance; have some effect on sexual characteristics

epinephrine *ep′i-nef′rin* **norepinephrine** *nōr′ep-i-nef′rin*	affect sympathetic nervous system in stress response
ovaries *ō′vă-rēz*	located on both sides of the uterus in the female pelvis, secreting estrogen and progesterone
estrogen *es′trō-jen* **progesterone** *prō-jes′ter-ōn*	responsible for the development of female secondary sex characteristics and regulation of reproduction
pancreas (islets of Langerhans) *pan′krē-as*	located behind the stomach in front of the first and second lumbar vertebrae, secreting insulin and glucagons
insulin *in′sŭ-lin* **glucagons** *glū′kă-gon*	regulate carbohydrate and sugar metabolism
parathyroid glands *par-ă-thī′royd*	two paired glands located on the posterior aspect of the thyroid gland in the neck, secreting parathyroid hormone (PTH)
parathyroid hormone (PTH)	regulates calcium and phosphorus metabolism
pineal gland *pin′ē-ăl*	located in the center of the brain, secreting melatonin and serotonin
melatonin *mel-ă-tōn′in*	exact function unknown; affects onset of puberty

serotonin	a neurotransmitter that serves as the precursor to melatonin
pituitary gland *pi-tū'i-tār-ē* **(hypophysis)** *hī-pof'i-sis*	located at the base of the brain; the anterior pituitary secretes thyroid-stimulating hormone, adrenocorticotrophic hormone, follicle-stimulating hormone, luteinizing hormone, melanocyte-stimulating hormone, growth hormone, and prolactin; the posterior pituitary releases antidiuretic hormone and oxytocin
anterior pituitary (adenohypophysis) *ad'ĕ-nō-hī-pof'i-sis*	
thyroid-stimulating hormone (TSH)	stimulates secretion from thyroid gland
adrenocorticotrophic hormone (ACTH) *ă-drē'nō-kōr'ti-kō-trō'fik*	stimulates secretion from adrenal cortex
follicle-stimulating hormone (FSH) *fol'i-kl*	initiates growth of ovarian follicle; stimulates secretion of estrogen in females and sperm production in males
luteinizing hormone (LH) *lū'tē-ĭ-nīz-ing*	causes ovulation; stimulates secretion of progesterone by corpus luteum; causes secretion of testosterone in testes
melanocyte-stimulating hormone (MSH) *mel'ă-nō-sīt*	affects skin pigmentation
growth hormone (GH)	influences growth
prolactin (lactogenic hormone) *prō-lak'tin*	stimulates breast development and milk production during pregnancy
posterior pituitary (neurohypophysis) *nūr'ō-hī-pof'i-sis*	
antidiuretic hormone (ADH) *an'tē-dī-yū-ret'ik*	influences the absorption of water by kidney tubules

oxytocin *ok-sē-tō'sin*	influences uterine contraction
testes *tes'tēz*	located on both sides within the scrotum in the male, secreting testosterone
testosterone *tes-tos'tĕ-rōn*	affects masculinization and reproduction
thymus gland *thī'mŭs*	
thymosin *thī'mō-sin*	regulates immune response
thyroid gland	located in front of the neck, secreting triiodothyronine (T_3), thyroxine (T_4), and calcitonin
triiodothyronine **(T_3)** *trī-ī'ō-dō-thī'rō-nēn*	regulate metabolism
thyroxine (T_4) *thī-rok'sēn*	
calcitonin *kal-si-tō'nin*	regulates calcium and phosphorus metabolism

PROGRAMMED REVIEW: ANATOMICAL TERMS

Answers	Review
adrenal above	**9.12** The suprarenal, or _____ glands are located above the kidneys. The term renal refers to the kidneys, and *supra-* means _____. These glands secrete steroid hormones and other hormones.
corticoids steroids male	**9.13** Steroid hormones have several functions, including an effect on sexual characteristics. They include gluco_____ and mineral cortico_____. Androgens are steroids that stimulate development of _____ sex characteristics.
suprarenal norepinephrine nervous	**9.14** Also secreted by the adrenal, or _____ glands are epinephrine and _____, which are hormones that affect the _____ system in a stress response of the body. For example, epinephrine, also called adrenaline, stimulates the heart and breathing rates.

endocrine

secrete

progesterone

female

9.15 The ovaries in women are both reproductive and _____ organs because they both produce eggs for reproduction and _____ hormones. The hormones secreted by the two ovaries are estrogen and _____, which stimulate development of _____ sex characteristics and help regulate reproduction.

pancreas

glucagon

gluc/o

9.16 The islets of Langerhans are groups of cells in the _____, an organ located behind the stomach. The pancreas secretes insulin and _____, which help regulate carbohydrate/sugar metabolism. The condition of diabetes mellitus involves abnormal utilization of insulin. The term glucagon is made from the combining form for sugar: _____.

alongside of

parathyroid

parathyroid

9.17 Recall that the prefix *para-* means _____ ____. Located alongside of the thyroid glands in the neck are the _____ glands. They secrete _____ hormone (PTH), which regulates calcium and phosphorus metabolism.

pineal

serotonin

melatonin

9.18 Located in the center of the brain is the _____ gland, which secretes the neurotransmitter _____. Also secreted by the pineal is the substance _____, whose exact function is unknown but which affects the onset of puberty.

hypophysis

below

anterior

posterior

9.19 The pituitary gland, located at the base of the brain, secretes a long list of hormones. It is also called the _____, a term using the prefix *hypo-* meaning _____ (or deficient), as it hangs below the hypothalamus part of the brain. The front subdivision of the pituitary gland is called the _____ pituitary, or the adenohypophysis. The rear subdivision is called the _____ pituitary, or the neurohypophysis.

thyroid

corticotrophic

follicle

hormone

9.20 The anterior pituitary secretes seven hormones, often identified by their abbreviations. TSH is _____ -stimulating hormone. ACTH is adreno_____ hormone. FSH is _____-stimulating hormone. LH is luteinizing _____.

growth

stimulating

before, prolactin

9.21 Also secreted by the anterior pituitary are _____ hormone (GH) and melanocyte-_____ hormone (MSH). The hormone that stimulates breast development and milk during pregnancy (from the combining form *lact/o* meaning milk, and the prefix *pro-* meaning _____) is called _____.

neurohypophysis

antidiuretic

promotes

9.22 The posterior pituitary, also called the _____, secretes two hormones. ADH, or _____ hormone, influences the absorption of water in the kidney. (Note that diuretic drugs stimulate the body to excrete water, and thus the term antidiuretic would involve an action that _____ retention of water.)

oxytocin

9.23 The other hormone secreted by the posterior pituitary is _____, which stimulates uterine contractions during labor (childbirth).

testes

testosterone

testis

9.24 In males, located on both sides within the scrotum, are the _____, two glands that secrete a hormone that affects masculinization and reproduction: _____. The singular of testes is _____. The testes are also called the testicles.

thymus

9.25 Located in the mediastinal cavity above and anterior to the heart is the _____ gland, secreting thymosin, which regulates the immune response.

thyroid thyroxine calcitonin	**9.26** From the combining form *thyr/o*, the _____ gland is located in front of the neck and secretes three hormones. Triiodothyronine (T_3) and _____ (T_4) help regulate metabolism. The third hormone, which regulates calcium metabolism, and which is from the same combining form as calcium, is _____.

SELF-INSTRUCTION: SYMPTOMATIC TERMS

Study the following:

Term	Meaning
exophthalmos *ek-sof-thal'mos* **exophthalmus** (*see* Fig. 9-7B)	protrusion of one or both eyeballs, often because of thyroid dysfunction or a tumor behind the eyeball
glucosuria *glū-kō-sū're̅-ă* **glycosuria** *glã-ko-su're-_a*	glucose (sugar) in the urine
hirsutism *her'sū-tizm*	shaggy; an excessive growth of hair, especially in unusual places (e.g., a woman with a beard)
hypercalcemia *hī'per-kal-se̅'me̅-ă*	an abnormally high level of calcium in the blood
hypocalcemia *hī'pō-kal-se̅'me̅-ă*	an abnormally low level of calcium in the blood
hyperglycemia *hī'per-glī-se̅'me̅-ă*	high blood sugar
hypoglycemia *hī'pō-glī-se̅'me̅-ă*	low blood sugar
hyperkalemia *hī'per-kă-le̅'me̅-ă*	an abnormally high level of potassium in the blood (kalium = potassium)
hypokalemia *hī'pō-ka-le̅'me̅-ă*	deficient level of potassium in the blood
hypersecretion *hī'per-se-kre̅'shŭn*	abnormally increased secretion
hyposecretion *hī'pō-se-kre̅'shŭn*	decreased secretion

ketosis *kē-tō′sis* **ketoacidosis** *kē-tō-as-i-dō′sis* **diabetic ketoacidosis** **(DKA)**	presence of an abnormal amount of ketone bodies (acetone, betahydroxybutyric acid, and acetoacetic acid) in the blood and urine indicating an abnormal use of carbohydrates, such as in uncontrolled diabetes and starvation (keto = alter)
metabolism *mĕ-tab′ō-lizm*	all chemical processes in the body that result in growth, generation of energy, elimination of waste, and other body functions
polydipsia *pol-ē-dip′sē-ă*	excessive thirst
polyuria *pol-ē-yū′rē-ă*	excessive urination

PROGRAMMED REVIEW: SYMPTOMATIC TERMS

Answers	Review
away exophthalmos (exophthalmus)	**9.27** One of the combining forms for eye is *ophthalm/o*. Recall that the prefix *ex-* means _____ or out. The term for the condition in which one or both eyeballs protrude out is _____, usually because of a thyroid dysfunction.
hirsutism condition of	**9.28** From the Latin word meaning shaggy (hirsutus), this term for an excessive growth of hair in an unusual place is _____. The suffix *-ism* means _____ _____.
metabolism after	**9.29** Using the same suffix as above, although not in this case for a medical condition, the term for all chemical processes in the body involving growth and energy is _____. The prefix *meta-* means beyond, _____, or change. In this case, metabolism refers to changes occurring in those chemical processes.
urine condition of glucosuria	**9.30** Recall that the combining form *ur/o* means _____ and the suffix *-ia* means _____ _____. The condition of glucose (sugar) in the urine is termed _____ or glycosuria.

many

polyuria

9.31   The prefix *poly-* means _____. The condition in which one urinates excessively many times is _____.

polydipsia

9.32   Using the same prefix and suffix as above, the term for the condition of excessive thirst is _____.

hyper-

hypo-

hypersecretion

hyposecretion

9.33   The most common prefix meaning above or excessive is _____. The opposite prefix meaning below or deficient is _____. These prefixes are used in many symptomatic terms related to levels of secretions and substances in the blood, influenced by endocrine functions. Abnormally increased secretion is _____, whereas abnormally decreased secretion is _____.

-emia

hypercalcemia

hypocalcemia

9.34   Recall that the suffix for blood condition is _____. An abnormally high blood level of calcium is _____, whereas an abnormally low blood level of calcium is _____.

hypoglycemia

hyperglycemia

9.35   An abnormally low level of blood sugar is _____, whereas an abnormally high blood sugar level is _____.

hypokalemia

hyperkalemia

9.36   From the Latin root kalium for potassium, an abnormally low blood level of potassium is _____, whereas an abnormally high blood level of potassium is _____.

increase

ketosis

keto, ketoacidosis

9.37   The suffix *-osis* means condition or _____. The condition of an increased presence of ketone bodies is _____, or _____acidosis. DKA refers to diabetic _____.

SELF-INSTRUCTION: DIAGNOSTIC TERMS

Study the following:

Term	Meaning
ADRENAL GLANDS	
Cushing syndrome (Fig. 9-3)	a collection of signs and symptoms caused by an excessive level of cortisol hormone from any cause, such as a result of excessive production by the adrenal gland (often as a result of tumor), or more commonly as a side effect of treatment with glucocorticoid (steroid) hormones such as prednisone for asthma, rheumatoid arthritis, lupus, or other inflammatory diseases; symptoms include upper body obesity, facial puffiness (moon-shaped appearance), hyperglycemia, weakness, thin, and easily bruised skin with stria (stretch marks), hypertension, and osteoporosis
adrenal virilism *ă-drē'năl vir'i-lizm*	excessive output of the adrenal secretion of androgen (male sex hormone) in adult women caused by tumor or hyperplasia; evidenced by amenorrhea (absence of menstruation), acne, hirsutism, and deepening of the voice (virilis = masculine)
PANCREAS *Pan'krē-as*	
diabetes mellitus (DM) *dī-ă-bē'tēz mel'i-tŭs*	metabolic disorder caused by the absence or insufficient production of insulin secreted by the pancreas resulting in hyperglycemia and glycosuria (diabetes = passing through; mellitus = sugar)
insulin	a hormone secreted by the beta cells of the Islets of Langerhans of the pancreas responsible for regulating the metabolism of glucose (insulin = island)
Type 1 diabetes mellitus	diabetes in which there is no beta cell production of insulin, and the patient is dependent on insulin for survival
Type 2 diabetes mellitus	diabetes in which either the body does not produce enough insulin, or there is insulin resistance (a defective use of the insulin that is produced); the patient usually is not dependent on insulin for survival

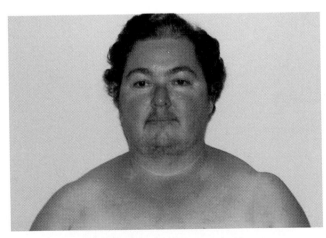

FIGURE 9-3. Cushing syndrome.

hyperinsulinism *hī′per-in′sū-lin-izm*	condition resulting from an excessive amount of insulin in the blood that draws sugar out of the bloodstream, resulting in hypoglycemia, fainting, and convulsions; often caused by an overdose of insulin or by a tumor of the pancreas
pancreatitis *pan′krē-ă-tī′tis*	inflammation of the pancreas

PARATHYROID GLANDS
par-ă-thī′royd

hyperparathyroidism *hī′per-par-ă-thī′royd-izm*	hypersecretion of the parathyroid glands, usually caused by a tumor
hypoparathyroidism *hī′pō-par-ă-thī′royd-izm*	hyposecretion of the parathyroid glands

PITUITARY GLAND (HYPOPHYSIS)	a gland that secretes hormones that regulate the function of other glands, such as the thyroid gland, adrenal glands, ovaries, and testicles; considered the master gland
acromegaly (Fig. 9-4) *ak-rō-meg′ă-lē*	disease characterized by enlarged features, especially the face and hands, caused by hypersecretion of the pituitary growth hormone after puberty, when normal bone growth has stopped; most often caused by a pituitary tumor
pituitary dwarfism (Fig. 9-5) *dwōrf′izm*	condition of congenital hyposecretion of growth hormone slowing growth and causing short yet proportionate stature (not affecting intelligence), often treated during childhood with growth hormone; other forms of dwarfism are most often caused by gene defects
pituitary gigantism *jī′gan-tizm*	condition of hypersecretion of growth hormone during childhood bone development that leads to an abnormal overgrowth of bone, especially of the long bones; most often caused by a pituitary tumor

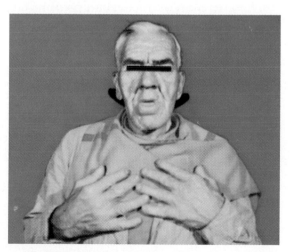

FIGURE 9-4. Enlarged hands and facial features in patients with acromegaly.

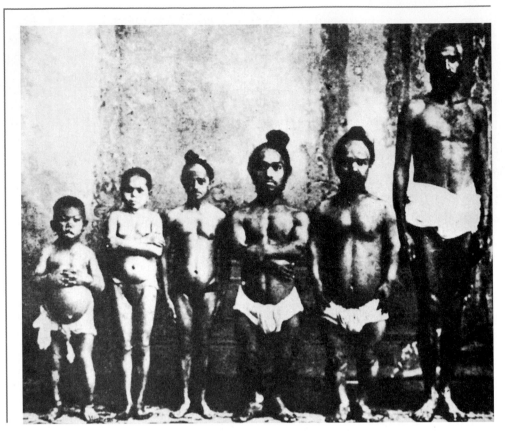

■ **FIGURE 9-5.** Normal male (extreme right) and three types of dwarfism. On the extreme left is a child who has not grown because of congenital absence of the thyroid gland (cretin). The next pair of dwarfs have entirely normal proportions but are half average size. The next pair to the right show disproportionately short extremities but average size trunk and head.

THYROID GLAND

goiter (Fig. 9-6A) *goy'ter*	enlargement of the thyroid gland caused by thyroid dysfunction, tumor, lack of iodine in the diet, or inflammation (goiter = throat)
hyperthyroidism (Fig. 9-6A, B) *hī-per-thī'royd-izm* **Graves disease** *Grāvz di-zēz'* **thyrotoxicosis** *thī'rō-tok-si-kō'sis*	condition of hypersecretion of the thyroid gland characterized by protrusion of the eyeball (exophthalmos), tachycardia, goiter, and tumor
hypothyroidism (Table 9-1) *hī'pō-thī'royd-izm*	condition of hyposecretion of the thyroid gland causing low thyroid levels in the blood that result in sluggishness, slow pulse, and often obesity
myxedema *mik-se-dē'mă*	advanced hypothyroidism in adults characterized by sluggishness, slow pulse, puffiness in hands and face, and dry skin (myx = mucous)
cretinism (*see* Fig. 9-5) *krē'tin-izm*	condition of congenital hypothyroidism in children that results in a lack of mental development and dwarfed physical stature

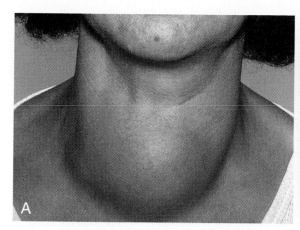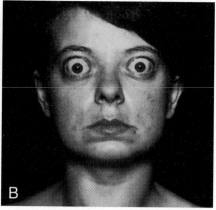

FIGURE 9-6. Hyperthyroidism. **A.** Patient with goiter. **B.** Patient with exophthalmos.

TABLE 9-1.   COMPARISON OF SYMPTOMS: HYPERTHYROIDISM VERSUS HYPOTHYROIDISM

Hyperthyroidism	Hypothyroidism
Restless, nervous, irritable, fine tremor, insomnia	Lethargic, poor memory, slow, expressionless
Fine, silky hair with hair loss	Dry, brittle hair with hair loss
Skin: warm, moist	Skin: pale, cold, dry, scaling
Increased perspiration	Decreased perspiration
Fast heart rate (tachycardia)	Slow heart rate (bradycardia)
Weight loss	Weight gain
Protrusion of eyeball (exophthalmos)	Edema of face and eyelids
Absence of menses (amenorrhea)	Heavy menses (menorrhagia)
Diffuse goiter	Thick tongue, slow speech

PROGRAMMED REVIEW: DIAGNOSTIC TERMS

Answers	Review
inflammation	**9.38** Recall that the suffix *-itis* means _____.
pancreatitis	Inflammation of the pancreas is _____.
	9.39 Most endocrine problems involve excessive or deficient secretion of hormones or the body's use of those hormones. The condition caused by the absence or insufficient production of insulin secreted by the pancreas resulting in hyperglycemia (_____ blood sugar) and glyco-
high	
sugar, diabetes mellitus	suria (_____ in the urine) is _____ _____

1, no insulin 2 resistance	(DM). The patient with type ___ diabetes mellitus produces _____ insulin and is thereby dependent on _____ for survival. Patients with type ___ diabetes mellitus produce insulin, but not enough, or there is insulin _____ (a defective use of the insulin that is produced).
hyper- condition of hyperinsulinism hypoglycemia	**9.40** Recall that the prefix for excessive is _____ and the suffix -*ism* refers to a _____ _____. The condition of having excessive insulin is _____. This condition results in low blood sugar, called _____.
hypoparathyroidism hyperparathyroidism	**9.41** The terms for diagnostic conditions are formed from the combining form for the gland's name with the prefixes for deficient or excessive, referring to the gland's secretion. The condition of hyposecretion of the parathyroid glands is _____, and hypersecretion of these glands is _____.
hypothyroidism hyperthyroidism Graves, toxicosis	**9.42** Similarly, hyposecretion of the thyroid gland is _____, and hypersecretion of the thyroid gland is _____. Hyperthyroidism is also called _____ disease, or thyro_____.
cretinism	**9.43** Congenital hypothyroidism in children, characterized by reduced stature and poor mental development, is called _____.
myxedema	**9.44** The term edema refers to a swollen body area caused by fluid retention. This root is used in the term for a form of advanced hypothyroidism in adults that involves swollen hands and face along with other symptoms: _____.
goiter	**9.45** The Latin word guttur means throat. The condition of an enlarged thyroid gland caused by thyroid dysfunction, tumor, or other causes, characterized by a swollen throat appearance, is _____.

9.46 Cortisol is a hormone secreted by the adrenal gland. Excessive levels of cortisol, caused by tumor or as a side effect of treatment with steroid hormones, cause a collection of signs and symptoms known as _____ syndrome.

Cushing

9.47 The adrenal glands also secrete a male sex hormone named from the combining form for male: _____. This hormone is called _____. Hypersecretion of androgen in adult women causes a condition named in part from the Latin word for masculine (virilis). This condition is _____ _____.

andr/o

androgen

adrenal virilism

9.48 Recall that the pituitary gland produces a number of hormones, including growth hormone. The condition of congenital hyposecretion of growth hormone, marked by small but proportionate stature, is pituitary _____.

dwarfism

9.49 The combining form *acr/o* refers to the extremities. Recall that the suffix *-megaly* means _____. The condition characterized by enlarged hands (and face) resulting from pituitary hypersecretion of growth hormone after puberty, when normal bone growth has stopped, is termed _____. The condition of hypersecretion of pituitary growth hormone during childhood bone development that leads to an abnormal overgrowth of bone, especially of the long bones, is _____ _____. Acromegaly occurs in adulthood, and gigantism occurs in _____. Each is a result of _____secretion of pituitary growth hormone, most often caused by a _____.

enlargement

acromegaly

pituitary gigantism

childhood, hyper

tumor

SELF-INSTRUCTION: DIAGNOSTIC TESTS AND PROCEDURES

Study the following:

Test or Procedure	Explanation
LABORATORY TESTING	
blood sugar (BS) **blood glucose**	measurement of the level of sugar (glucose) in the blood
fasting blood sugar (FBS)	measurement of blood sugar level after fasting (not eating) for 12 hours
postprandial blood sugar (PPBS)	measurement of blood sugar level after a meal (commonly 2 hours later)
glucose tolerance test (GTT)	measurement of the body's ability to metabolize carbohydrates by administering a prescribed amount of glucose after a fasting period, then measuring blood and urine for glucose levels every hour thereafter for 4 to 6 hours
glycohemoglobin *glī-kō-hē-mō-glō'bin*	a molecule (fraction) in hemoglobin that rises in the blood as a result of an increased level of blood sugar; a common blood test used in diagnosing and treating diabetes
electrolytes *ē-lek'tro-lītz*	measurement of the level of specific ions (sodium, potassium, CO_2, and chloride) in the blood; electrolyte balance is essential for normal metabolism
thyroid function study	measurement of thyroid hormone levels in blood plasma to determine efficiency of glandular secretions, including T_3, T_4, and TSH
urine sugar and ketone studies *kē'tōn*	chemical tests to determine the presence of sugar or ketone bodies in urine; used as a screen for diabetes

IMAGING PROCEDURES

computed tomography (CT)	CT of the head is used to obtain a transverse (horizontal) view of the pituitary gland
magnetic resonance imaging (MRI)	nonionizing images of magnetic resonance are useful in identifying abnormalities of the pituitary, pancreas, adrenal, and thyroid glands
sonography	sonographic images are used to identify endocrine pathology, such as with thyroid ultrasound
thyroid uptake and image (Fig. 9-7)	nuclear image produced by a scan of the thyroid to visualize the radioactive accumulation of previously injected isotopes to detect thyroid nodules or tumors

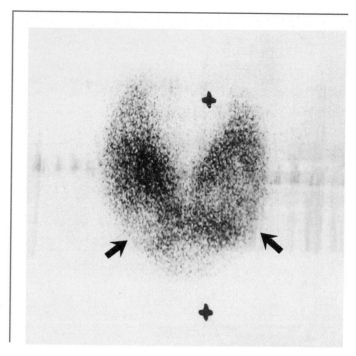

■ **FIGURE 9-7.** Thyroid uptake and image detecting presence of multiple nodules *(arrows)*.

PROGRAMMED REVIEW: DIAGNOSTIC TESTS AND PROCEDURES

Answers	Review
glucose	**9.50** Several laboratory tests are used to diagnose problems in the endocrine system. Because diabetes is a serious and common disorder, blood sugar levels are particularly important for diagnostic purposes. The measurement of the level of sugar (glucose) in the blood is simply called a blood sugar (BS) or blood _____.
fasting blood sugar	**9.51** A measurement of blood sugar level after a 12-hour fast is called _____ _____ _____ (FBS).
post- postprandial blood sugar	**9.52** The prefix for after or behind is _____. The Latin word prandium means a meal. The medical adjective formed from these two parts is used to refer to a blood sugar test made about 2 hours after a meal, termed a _____ _____ _____ (PPBS).
	9.53 A more complex blood sugar test measures the body's ability to metabolize carbohydrates. Glucose is administered after a fasting pe-

glucose tolerance test	riod, and blood and urine glucose levels are measured hourly thereafter to determine how well the body tolerates this glucose. This is called a _____ _____ _____ (GTT).
glycohemoglobin	**9.54** Another type of blood sugar test examines the effect of blood sugar on hemoglobin, called a _____.
electrolytes	**9.55** The Greek word lytos means soluble—as in any substance that dissolves in water or blood. Some ions when dissolved conduct electricity. These substances are called electrolytes. The measurement of the level of specific ions such as sodium and potassium is simply called _____.
thyroid function	**9.56** The laboratory study that measures thyroid hormone levels in the blood to determine how well the thyroid is functioning is called a _____ _____ study.
urine sugar, ketone	**9.57** Chemical measurements of sugar and ketones in the urine, used as a screen for diabetes, are _____ _____ and _____ studies.
computed tomography	**9.58** In addition to these laboratory tests, several imaging procedures are used to diagnose endocrine disorders. The type of x-ray imaging using a computer to create a transverse view, such as of the pituitary gland, is called _____ _____ (CT).
magnetic resonance imaging	**9.59** Nonionizing images using _____ _____ _____ (MRI) can identify abnormalities in several glands.
son/o recording sonography	**9.60** Recall that the combining form meaning sound is _____. The suffix -*graphy* refers to the process of _____. The imaging modality using very high sound frequencies to record images of endocrine glands is _____.

9.61   A test of the thyroid involves injection of radioactive isotopes that are taken up in the thyroid, leading to production of a nuclear image. This is called _____ _____ and _____.

thyroid uptake, image

SELF-INSTRUCTION: OPERATIVE TERMS

Study the following:

Term	Meaning
adrenalectomy *ă-drē-năl-ek′tō-mē*	excision of adrenal gland
hypophysectomy *hī′pof-i-sek′tō-mē*	excision of pituitary gland
pancreatectomy *pan′krē-ă-tek′tō-mē*	excision of pancreas
parathyroidectomy *pa′ră-thī-roy-dek′tō-mē*	excision of parathyroid gland
thymectomy *thī-mek′tō-mē*	excision of thymus gland
thyroidectomy *thī′roy-dek′tō-mē*	excision of thyroid gland

PROGRAMMED REVIEW: OPERATIVE TERMS

Answers	Review
excision adrenalectomy	**9.62** Recall that the suffix *-ectomy* means _____. The excision of the adrenal gland is an _____.
pancreatectomy	**9.63** The excision of the pancreas is a _____.
thyroidectomy	**9.64** The excision of the thyroid gland is a _____.
parathyroid	**9.65** A parathyroidectomy is the excision of the _____ gland.
thymectomy	**9.66** The excision of the thymus gland is a _____.

hypophysis	**9.67** Recall that the pituitary gland is also called the
	_____. That combining form is used in the term for
hypophysectomy	excision of the pituitary gland: _____.

SELF-INSTRUCTION: THERAPEUTIC TERMS

Study the following:

Term	Meaning
radioiodine therapy _rā′dē-ō-ī′ō-dīn_	use of radioactive iodine to treat disease, such as to eradicate thyroid tumor cells; treatment is administered in a nuclear medicine facility

COMMON THERAPEUTIC DRUG CLASSIFICATIONS

antihypoglycemic _an′tē-hī′pō-glī-sē′mik_	a drug that raises blood glucose
hormone replacement therapy (HRT) _hōr′mōn_	treatment with a hormone to correct a hormone deficiency (e.g., estrogen, testosterone, and thyroid)
hypoglycemic **antihyperglycemic** _hī′pō-glī′sē′mik_ _an′tē-hī′per-glī′sē′mik_	a drug that lowers blood glucose (e.g., insulin)

PROGRAMMED REVIEW: THERAPEUTIC TERMS

Answers	Review
	9.68 Because the thyroid gland absorbs iodine, when radioactive iodine is administered into the body, it becomes localized in the thyroid where it can kill thyroid tumor cells. This is called
radioiodine	_____ therapy and is administered in a
nuclear	_____ medicine facility.
	9.69 Drug classifications are often named by their action against some process or condition in the body. The prefix meaning against is
anti-, -emia	_____. The suffix for a blood condition is _____. Recall that the
hypoglycemia	condition of low blood glucose is termed _____.
	A drug that works against this condition by raising the blood glucose
antihypoglycemic	level is an _____ drug.

9.70   Recall that the condition of high blood sugar is called

hyperglycemia

_____. A drug that works against this condi-

tion by lowering the blood glucose level is an

antihyperglycemic

_____ drug. Another term for this is

hypoglycemic

a _____ drug.

9.71   A patient with a deficiency of a particular hormone may be

treated by administration of that hormone to replace what is missing.

hormone

This treatment is referred to as _____

replacement therapy

_____ _____ (HRT).

Practice Exercises

For the following terms, on the lines below the term, write out the indicated word parts:
prefixes, combining forms, roots, and suffixes. Then define the word.

For example:
parathyroid

<u>para/thyr/oid</u>
  P   R   S

DEFINITION: alongside of/thyroid gland/resembling

1. adenitis

_____ / _____
  R   S

DEFINITION: _____

2. hyperglycemia

_____ / _____ / _____
      P   R   S

DEFINITION: _____

3. thyrotoxicosis

_____ / _____ / _____
      CF   R   S

DEFINITION: _____

4. polydipsia

_____ / _____ / _____
P   R   S

DEFINITION: _____

5. hormonal

_____ / _____
R   S

DEFINITION: _____

6. ketosis

_____ / _____
R   S

DEFINITION: _____

7. polyuria

_____ / _____ / _____
P   R   S

DEFINITION: _____

8. endocrine

_____ / _____ / _____
P   R   S

DEFINITION: _____

9. thyroptosis

_____ / _____
CF   S

DEFINITION: _____

10. thymoma

_____ / _____
R   S

DEFINITION: _____

11. acromegaly

_____ / _____
CF   S

DEFINITION: _____

12. android

_____ / _____
R   S

DEFINITION: _____

13. adrenotrophic

_____ / _____ / _____
        CF   R   S

DEFINITION: _____

14. pancreatogenic

_____ / _____ / _____
        CF   R   S

DEFINITION: _____

15. glycosuria

_____ / _____ / _____
     R   R   S

DEFINITION: _____

Write the correct medical term for each of the following:

16. hypothyroidism in adults _____

17. congenital hypothyroidism _____

18. another name for Graves disease _____

19. condition resulting from hypersecretion of the adrenal cortex causing obesity, hyperglycemia, and weakness _____

20. disease characterized by enlarged features caused by hypersecretion of the pituitary
hormone _____

21. enlargement of thyroid gland _____

22. protrusion of eyeball _____

23. condition of congenital hyposecretion of growth hormone _____

24. a deficient level of potassium in the blood

_____

25. nuclear image of the thyroid _____

26. condition of congenital hypersecretion of the growth hormone

_____

Match the following terms with their meanings:

27. congenital hypothyroidism _____

28. polydipsia _____

29. hyperthyroidism _____

30. hypophysis _____

31. thyromegaly _____

32. adult hypothyroidism _____

33. adrenal virilism _____

34. type 2 diabetes _____

35. pituitary hypersecretion _____

36. type 1 diabetes _____

a. gigantism

b. hirsutism

c. goiter

d. depends on insulin

e. cretinism

f. pituitary

g. does not usually depend on insulin

h. excessive thirst

i. myxedema

j. thyrotoxicosis

Complete the medical term by writing the missing part:

37. poly_____ia = excessive thirst

38. _____secretion = abnormally increased secretion

39. _____glycemia = low blood sugar

40. glucos_____ = sugar in the urine

41. _____secretion = decreased secretion

42. _____glycemia = high blood sugar

43. _____graphy = ultrasound imaging

Write the full medical term for the following abbreviations:

44. BS _____

45. HRT _____

46. FBS _____

47. DM _____

48. PPBS _____

49. GTT _____

50. DKA _____

Write in the missing words on the blank line in the illustration:

THE ENDOCRINE SYSTEM

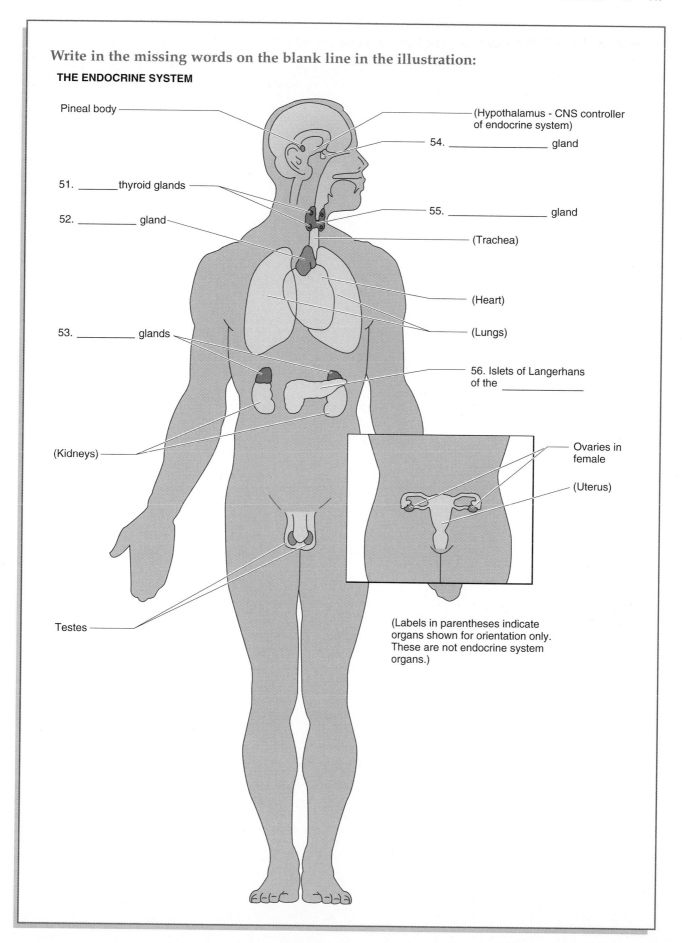

Pineal body

(Hypothalamus - CNS controller of endocrine system)

54. _____ gland

51. _____ thyroid glands

52. _____ gland

55. _____ gland

(Trachea)

(Heart)

(Lungs)

53. _____ glands

56. Islets of Langerhans of the _____

(Kidneys)

Ovaries in female

(Uterus)

Testes

(Labels in parentheses indicate organs shown for orientation only. These are not endocrine system organs.)

For each of the following, circle the meaning that corresponds to the combining form given:

57. **adren/o**	male	extremity	adrenal gland
58. **thyr/o**	nourishment	shield	chest
59. **crin/o**	blue	cell	secrete
60. **gluc/o**	stomach	sugar	pancreas
61. **dips/o**	thirst	ketones	secrete
62. **thym/o**	shield	hormone	thymus gland
63. **hormon/o**	development	urging on	ketones
64. **aden/o**	male	extremity	gland

For each of the following, circle the correct spelling of the term:

65. hirsutism	hirsuitism	hirsitism
66. exopthalmos	exopthamamos	exophthalmos
67. myexedema	mixedema	myxedema
68. goiter	goyter	goitir
69. androgenius	androgenous	andreogenous
70. virillism	virilism	viralism
71. epinephrine	epinefrine	epineprine
72. hypoglicemic	hypoglicemic	hypoglycemic

Give the noun that was used to form the following adjectives.

73. _____ acromegalic

74. _____ exophthalmic

75. _____ metabolic

76. _____ diabetic

77. _____ hypoglycemic

Medical Record Analyses

MEDICAL RECORD 9-1

S: This is a 27 y.o. ♀ c̄ a known Hx of diabetes seen in the ER with nausea and vomiting for the past three hours. She has skipped two doses of her insulin because BS levels monitored at home have been low. She is now experiencing a cephalalgia similar to what she has had in the past before coma.

O: T 35.5° C, P 90, R 20, BP 126/68
Lab blood studies: sodium 130, potassium 4.1, CO_2 9, chloride 102, glucose 296

A: Diabetic ketoacidosis

P: Admit to ICU: give 10 units insulin IV; measure BS 1° p̄ insulin given, then q 4 h; check urine for sugar and ketosis q void; repeat electrolytes in a.m.

1. What is the CC?
   a. nausea, vomiting, and headache
   b. nausea, vomiting, and dizziness
   c. nausea, vomiting, and high blood pressure
   d. nausea, vomiting, and ringing in the ears
   e. nausea, vomiting, and unconsciousness

2. What is the diagnosis?
   a. hyperglycemia
   b. hypoglycemia
   c. type 1 DM with presence of ketone bodies in the blood
   d. type 2 DM without the presence of ketone bodies in the blood
   e. combination of hyperglycemia and glucosuria

3. As an inpatient, where was treatment provided?
   a. neuropsychiatric facility
   b. coronary care facility
   c. emergency room
   d. recovery room
   e. critical care facility

4. Which of the following are electrolytes?
   1. sodium 2. potassium 3. chloride
   4. glucose
   a. only 1, 2, and 3 are correct
   b. only 1 and 3 are correct
   c. only 2 and 4 are correct
   d. only 4 is correct
   e. all are correct

5. Why were the blood electrolyte studies performed?
   a. to examine the electrical impulses of the brain
   b. to measure the level of ions in the blood in evaluation of metabolism
   c. to measure hormone levels and determine glandular efficiency
   d. to visualize the accumulation of radioactive isotopes to eliminate the presence of tumor
   e. to measure the level of glucose in the blood

6. How should the insulin be administered?
   a. within the skin
   b. absorption through unbroken skin
   c. within the muscle
   d. within the vein
   e. under the skin

7. How often should the blood glucose be measured?
   a. one hour after insulin administration, then every four hours
   b. once each morning
   c. each time the patient urinates
   d. one hour before insulin administration, then four times a day
   e. one hour before insulin administration, then every four hours thereafter

MEDICAL RECORD 9-2 FOR ADDITIONAL STUDY

CENTRAL MEDICAL CENTER

211 Medical Center Drive • Central City, US 90000-1234 • PHONE: (012) 125-6784 • FAX: (012) 125-9999

THYROID UPTAKE AND IMAGING STUDY

Date of Exam: 5/29/20xx

CLINICAL HISTORY: The patient has more than a six year history of hyperthyroidism which was treated until approximately one year ago with propylthiouracil (PTU). The patient relates some instability in symptomatology during the treatment. She had no previous uptake and imaging study, and radioiodine therapy was never discussed with the patient. She spontaneously discontinued taking the PTU approximately one year ago and has had recurrent symptoms of hyperthyroidism in the last two months.

TECHNIQUE: The patient ingested a capsule containing 200 $\mu Ci^{123}I$ sodium iodide. Uptakes in the neck were measured at 6 and 24 hours. Images of the thyroid were obtained in multiple projections at 6 hours.

FINDINGS: Radioiodine uptake at 6 hours was 37% (normal: 0-15%), and at 24 hours, uptake was 57% (normal: 5-35%). Thyroid images reveal the gland to be diffusely modestly enlarged. Multiple areas of reduced function correlating with palpable nodules are present in both thyroid lobes with the largest nodule being present in the lower poles of both lobes but with the right lobe being somewhat more severely overall affected than the left lobe. No dominant functioning thyroid nodule is evident.

CONCLUSION:

TOXIC MULTINODULAR GOITER

NOTE: Because of the presence of the multiple nodules which are likely on a benign basis, I took the liberty of ordering a thyroid ultrasound as a baseline. This will be separately reported, and it is suggested that the thyroid ultrasound be repeated in six months to one year.

C. Rincon, M.D.

CR:se

D: 5/29/20xx   T: 5/31/20xx

THYROID UPTAKE AND IMAGING STUDY	PT. NAME: NGUYEN, TARA T. ID NO: NM-384023 Sex: F Age: 58 Y DOB: 02/18/xx ATT. PHYS. T. Hutton

MEDICAL RECORD 9-2 FOR ADDITIONAL STUDY

Tara Nguyen had a long history of hyperthyroidism that was managed by pharmacologic treatment for more than 5 years. She was often unhappy with how she felt, however, and decided on her own to stop taking the drug. Two months ago the symptoms of hyperthyroidism recurred, and she sought medical attention.

Read Medical Record 9-2 (page 420) for Ms. Nguyen, and answer the following questions. This record is the report by Dr. Rincon, who analyzed Ms. Nguyen's thyroid uptake and imaging study.

1. Below are medical terms used in this record you have not yet encountered in this text. Underline each where it appears in the record and define below.

   propylthiouracil (PTU) _____

   uptake _____

   baseline (nonmedical term) _____

2. In your own words, not using medical terminology, briefly describe what seems to have been missing in Ms. Nguyen's past medical management.

   _____

   _____

3. In nonmedical terms, explain how the sodium iodide was administered.

   _____

4. In your own words, not using medical terminology, briefly describe Dr. Rincon's diagnosis.

   _____

   _____

   _____

5. What additional test did Dr. Rincon order on his own authority?
   a. thyroid function study
   b. fasting blood sugar
   c. thyroid MRI
   d. thyroid ultrasound

6. Which of the following tests is recommended to be performed in 6 months?
   a. thyroid function study
   b. fasting blood sugar
   c. thyroid MRI
   d. thyroid ultrasound

Answers to Practice Exercises

1. aden/itis
   R   S
   gland/inflammation
2. hyper/glyc/emia
   P   R   S
   above or excessive/sugar/
   blood condition
3. thyro/toxic/osis
   CF   R   S
   thyroid gland (shield)/
   poison/condition or
   increase
4. poly/dips/ia
   P   R   S
   many/thirst/condition of
5. hormon/al
   R   S
   hormone (an urging on)/
   pertaining to
6. ket/osis
   R   S
   ketone bodies/condition or
   increase
7. poly/ur/ia
   P   R   S
   many/urine/condition of
8. endo/crin/e
   P   R   S
   within/to secrete/noun
   marker
9. thyro/ptosis
   CF   S
   thyroid gland (shield)/falling
   or downward displacement
10. thym/oma
    R   S
    thymus gland/tumor
11. acro/megaly
    CF   S
    extremity/enlargement
12. andr/oid
    R   S
    male/resembling

13. adreno/troph/ic
    CF   R   S
    adrenal gland/nourishment
    or development/pertaining
    to
14. pancreato/gen/ic
    CF   R   S
    pancreas/origin or
    production/pertaining to
15. glycos/ur/ia
    R   R   S
    sugar/urine/condition of
16. myxedema
17. cretinism
18. hyperthyroidism or
    thyrotoxicosis
19. Cushing syndrome
20. acromegaly
21. goiter
22. exophthalmos or
    exophthalmus
23. pituitary dwarfism
24. hypokalemia
25. thyroid uptake and image
26. gigantism or pituitary
    gigantism
27. e
28. h
29. j
30. f
31. c
32. i
33. b
34. g
35. a
36. d
37. polydipsia
38. hypersecretion
39. hypoglycemia
40. glucosuria
41. hyposecretion
42. hyperglycemia
43. sonography
44. blood sugar
45. hormone replacement therapy

46. fasting blood sugar
47. diabetes mellitus
48. postprandial blood sugar
49. glucose tolerance test
50. diabetic ketoacidosis
51. para
52. thymus
53. adrenal
54. pituitary
55. thyroid
56. pancreas
57. adrenal gland
58. shield
59. secrete
60. sugar
61. thirst
62. thymus gland
63. urging on
64. gland
65. hirsutism
66. exophthalmos
67. myxedema
68. goiter
69. androgenous
70. virilism
71. epinephrine
72. hypoglycemic
73. acromegaly
74. exophthalmos
75. metabolism
76. diabetes
77. hypoglycemia

Answers to Medical Records Analyses

1. a
2. c
3. e
4. a
5. b
6. d
7. c

CHAPTER 10

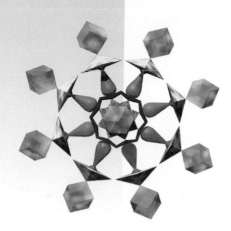

The Eye

Eye Overview

The eyes are the organs of sight that provide three-dimensional vision (Fig. 10-1).

* Light enters the eye through the pupil, the size of which is regulated by the muscles of the iris.
* The lens focuses light rays on the retina, the nerve tissue in the inner posterior part of the eye.
* The rods and cones, the visual receptor neurons in the retina, respond to the light waves.
* Nerve fibers from the rods and cones join in the optic disc, from which the optic nerve carries transmission to the brain.
* Other functions of the eye are performed by protective and lubricating structures.

SELF-INSTRUCTION: COMBINING FORMS

Study the following:

Combining Form	Meaning
aque/o	water
blephar/o	eyelid
conjunctiv/o	conjunctiva (to join together)
corne/o kerat/o	cornea
ir/o irid/o	colored circle, iris
lacrim/o dacry/o	tear

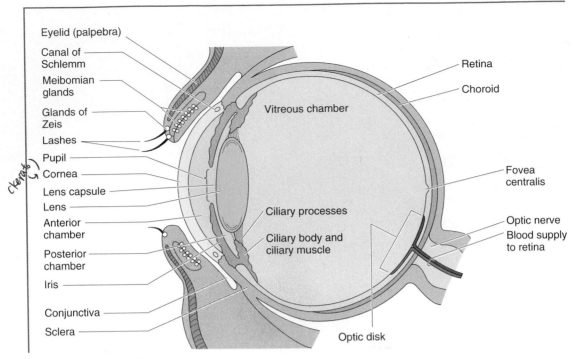

■ FIGURE 10-1. Anatomy of the eye.

ocul/o ophthalm/o opt/o	eye
phac/o phak/o	lens (lentil)
phot/o	light
presby/o	old age
retin/o	retina
scler/o	hard or sclera
vitre/o	glassy
-opia (additional suffix)	condition of vision

PROGRAMMED REVIEW: COMBINING FORMS

Answers	Review
	10.1 The three combining forms meaning eye are *ocul/o*, *opt/o*, and
ophthalm/o	_____. Ophthalmology defines the specialty field re-
study, logist	lated to the _____ of the eye. An ophthalmo_____ is a

eye

physician who specializes in the study and treatment (including surgery) of the _____.

opt/o

measuring

eye

10.2 Optometry is the profession that examines the eyes for vision problems and other disorders. The term is made from another combining form meaning eye, _____. The suffix *-metry* generally refers to a process of _____. Optometrist is the title of this professional who specializes in measuring the _____.

ocul/o

10.3 A third combining form for eye is _____, such as is used in the adjective ocular.

eyelid, blephar/o

inflammation

blepharitis

10.4 A <u>blepharospasm</u> is an involuntary muscular contraction of the _____eyelid_____. The combining form for eyelid is __blephar/o__. For example, because the suffix *-itis* means _____, the term for an inflamed eyelid is _____.

water

10.5 The combining form *aque/o* means _____ in reference to the eye.

cornea

kerat/o

keratoplasty

10.6 *Corne/o* is the Latin combining form used to name the part of the eye called the _____. The second combining form meaning cornea, from the <u>Greek word kera</u> (meaning horn or hard tissue), is __Kerato__. It is used in the term describing the surgical repair or reconstruction of the cornea: _____.

lacrim/o

dacryo<u>cyst</u>itis

dacry/o

10.7 As often happens, there are two combining forms for tears, one based on a Latin word and one on a Greek word. The lacrimal gland (tear gland) comes from this combining form: __lacrim/o__. The term dacryo<u>cyst</u> means the lacrimal sac (cyst = sac), where tears are collected before they flow to the nose. Inflammation of the lacrimal sac therefore is __dacryo cystitis__. The second combining form for tears is __dacry/o__.

10.8 The Greek word phakos means lentil or anything shaped like a

lentil, and thus was used for the lens of the eye because it looks like a

lentil

phac/o, phak/o

_____lentil_____. As sometimes happens, two spellings evolved for this

combining form: ___phac/o___ and ___phak/o___. Recall that the suffix

dissolution

-_lysis_ means breaking down or ___dissolution___. Phacolysis is

breaking down

therefore the ___breaking___ ___down___ of the lens. A phakoma is a

lens

tumorlike condition of the ___lens___.

phot/o

10.9 The combining form meaning light is _____. An abnormal

photophobia

fear or sensitivity to light is _____.

vision

10.10 The suffix -_opia_ refers to condition of ___vision___. Since the

old

combining form _presby/o_ means ___old___ age, the term presbyopia refers

condition

to a vision ___condition___ common in old age.

10.11 Many combining forms are very similar to the terms that ex-

press their meaning. For example, the combining form meaning the con-

junctiva is _conjunctiv/o_. The combining form for the sclera is

scler/o, retino/o

___scler/o___. The combining form meaning retina is ___retin/o___,

and the combining form referring to the vitreous (glassy substance) of

vitre/o

the eye is ___vitre/o___.

10.12 Similarly, one of the two combining forms for the iris of the eye

ir/o

is ___ir/o___. It is used to form iritis, which means an

inflammation

_____ of the iris. The second combining form is

used to form irid_ectomy_, which is an excision of a portion of the iris.

irid/o

That combining form is _____. Recall that the suffix -_ectomy_

excision

means ___excision___.

SELF-INSTRUCTION: ANATOMICAL TERMS

Study the following:

Term	Meaning
anterior chamber	fluid-filled space between cornea and iris
aqueous humor *ak′wē-ŭs hy′ūmer*	watery liquid secreted at the ciliary body that fills the anterior and posterior chambers of the eye and provides nourishment for the cornea, iris, and lens (humor = fluid)
canal of Schlemm	duct in anterior chamber that carries filtered aqueous humor to the veins and bloodstream
choroid *kō′royd*	vascular layer beneath the sclera that provides nourishment to outer portion of the retina
ciliary body *sil′ē-ar-ē*	ring of muscle behind the peripheral iris that controls the focusing shape of the lens
ciliary muscle	smooth muscle portion of the ciliary body, which contracts to assist in near vision capability
ciliary processes	epithelial tissue folds on the inner surface of the ciliary body that secrete aqueous humor
conjunctiva *kon-jŭnk-tī′vă*	mucous membrane that lines the eyelids and outer surface of the eyeball
cornea *kōr′n-ē-ă*	transparent, anterior part of the eyeball covering the iris, pupil, and anterior chamber that functions to refract (bend) light to focus a visual image
eyelid (palpebra) *pal-pē′bră*	movable protective fold that opens and closes, covering the eye
fovea centralis *fō′vē-ă sen-trā′lis*	pinpoint depression in the center of the macula lutea that is the site of sharpest vision (fovea = pit)
fundus (base) *fŭn′dŭs*	interior surface of the eyeball including the retina, optic disc, macula, and posterior pole (curvature at the back of the eye)
glands of Zeis	oil glands surrounding the eyelashes
meibomian glands *mī-bō′mē-an*	oil glands located along the rim of the eyelids
iris *ī′ris*	colored circle; colored part of the eye located behind the cornea that contracts and dilates to regulate light passing through the pupil
lacrimal gland (Fig. 10-2) *lak′ri-măl*	gland located in the upper outer region above the eyeball that secretes tears
lacrimal ducts	tubes that carry tears to the lacrimal sac

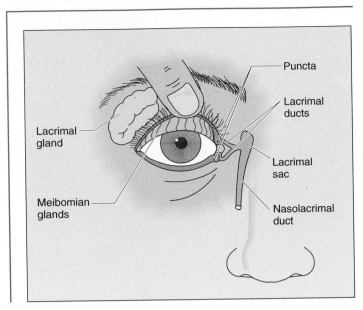

Puncta

Lacrimal
ducts

Lacrimal
gland

Lacrimal
sac

Meibomian
glands

Nasolacrimal
duct

■ **FIGURE 10-2.** Lacrimal apparatus.

lacrimal sac	structure that collects tears before emptying into nasolacrimal duct
lens	transparent structure behind the pupil that bends and focuses light rays on the retina
lens capsule	capsule that encloses the lens
macula lutea (macula) (See later Fig. 10-8B)	central region of the retina responsible for central vision; yellow pigment provides its color (lutea = yellow)
nasolacrimal duct *nā-zō-lak′ri-măl*	passageway for tears from the lacrimal sac into the nose
optic disc (See later Fig. 10.8B) *op′tik*	exit site of retinal nerve fibers
optic nerve	nerve responsible for carrying impulses for the sense of sight from the retina to the brain
posterior chamber	space between the back of the iris and the front of the vitreous chamber filled with aqueous humor
pupil *pyū′pĭl*	black circular opening in the center of the iris through which light passes as it enters the eye
retina (See later Fig. 10-8B) *ret′i-nă*	innermost layer that perceives and transmits light to the optic nerve
cones	cone-shaped cells within the retina that are color sensitive and respond to bright light
rods	rod-shaped cells within the retina that respond to dim light

sclera *sklēr'ă*	tough, fibrous, white outer coat extending from the cornea to the optic nerve
trabecular meshwork *tră-bek'yū-lăr*	mesh-like structure in the anterior chamber that filters the aqueous humor as it flows into the canal of Schlemm
vitreous *vit'rē-ŭs*	jelly-like mass filling the inner chamber between the lens and retina that gives bulk to the eye

PROGRAMMED REVIEW: ANATOMICAL TERMS

Answers	Review

10.13   Let's look at the anatomy of the eye in the approximate order of structures involved as light waves enter the eye and result in nerve transmissions to the brain. Light first passes through a transparent outer covering over the iris, pupil, and anterior chamber called the

cornea   _cornea_ .

10.14   The _anterior_ chamber is a fluid-filled space between

anterior

front   the cornea and iris. It is called anterior because it is the _front_

fluid chamber in the eye. The fluid within the anterior chamber is

aqueous   _aqueous_ humor. Recall that the combining form *aque/o* means

water   _____. This watery fluid is carried to the veins through the

canal   _canal_ of Schlemm. As the aqueous humor flows into this canal, it

trabecular   is filtered by a meshlike structure called the _trabecular_

meshwork.

10.15   The light waves then pass through the black circular opening in

pupil, iris   the center of the iris called the _pupil_ . The _iris_ surrounding

the pupil is the colored part of the eye that contracts and dilates to regu-

light   late the amount of _light_ that passes through the pupil.

10.16   Between the back of the iris and the upper and lower sections of

posterior   the lens and vitreous chamber is the _posterior_ chamber,

humor   which is also filled with aqueous _humor_ . It is called the posterior

chamber, behind (back of)   _chamber_ because it is _____ the anterior camber.

lens

capsule

10.17 Light waves passing through the pupil and anterior chamber reach the ___lens___, a transparent structure that focuses the light rays on the retina. The lens is enclosed in a structure called the lens _____.

ciliary

ciliary muscle

10.18 Tiny muscles control the shape of the lens, allowing it to change its focus for near and far vision. The ring of muscle around the lens, behind the iris, is called the ___ciliary___ body, and its smooth muscle portion is called ___ciliary___ ___muscle___.

processes

posterior

Schlemm

10.19 Tissue folds on the inner surface of the ciliary body, called ciliary ___processes___, secrete aqueous humor, which fills the anterior and ___post.___ chambers and drains through the canal of ___Schlemm___.

vitreous

glassy

10.20 Light waves focused by the lens now pass through the ___vitreous___ chamber on the way to the retina. The vitreous is a jellylike mass that fills this inner chamber and gives bulk to the eye. Recall that the combining form *vitre/o* means ___glassy___, referring to the vitreous of the eye.

retina

rods

bright, rods

10.21 The light waves passing through the vitreous chamber, then strike the ___retina___, the innermost layer at the back of the eye, which contains visual receptor neurons that respond to light. These special cells are the _____ and cones. The cones respond to _____ light, and the _____ respond to dim light. These neuron reactions are transmitted to the optic nerve and then to the brain.

macula lutea

fovea centralis

10.22 The central region of the retina, which has a yellow color (lutea = yellow), is the ___macula___ ___lutea___. At the center of the macular lutea is a pinpoint depression, which is the site of sharpest vision, called the ___fovea___ ___centralis___ (fovea = pit)

10.23 The entire interior surface of the eyeball, including the retina, optic disc, and macula, is termed the ___*fundus*___. The layer behind the retina that provides nourishment to the retina is called the ___*choroid*___.

fundus

choroid

10.24 Nerve fibers from the retina come together at the optic ___*disk*___, the site where the nerves exit the eye. The ___*optic*___ nerve then carries the nerve impulses to the brain to create the sense of sight.

disk, optic

10.25 The tough outer layer of the eye extending from the cornea around the retina to the optic nerve is the ___*sclera*___.

sclera

10.26 Additional eye structures help protect the eye from the environment. The medical term for eyelid is ___*palpebra*___. The plural of this term is ___*palpebrae*___. The palpebrae can close over the eye.

palpebra

palpebrae

10.27 The oil glands located along the rim of the eyelids are called the ___*meibomian*___ glands. Other oil glands surrounding the eyelashes are called glands of ___*Zeis*___.

meibomian

Zeis

10.28 The mucous membrane that lines the eyelids and outer surface of the eyeball is the ___*conjunctiva*___, from the combining form *conjunctiv/o*. Because this is the outermost structure of the eye, it is easily irritated by foreign substances, causing an inflammation called ___*conjunctivitis*___.

conjunctiva

conjunctivitis

10.29 There are two combining forms meaning tear or tears: *dacry/o* is Greek, and ___*lacrim/o*___ is Latin. Note that the Latin form is used to name the anatomy related to tears. For example, the glands that secrete tears, located in the upper outer region above the eyeball, are called the ___*lacrimal glands*___.

lacrim/o

lacrimal glands

ducts, sac	**10.30** The tiny tubes that carry tears away from the eye are the lacrimal _____. These ducts carry tears to the lacrimal _____, which collects tears before emptying into the nasolacrimal duct.
nasolacrimal nose	**10.31** Tears from the lacrimal sac reach the nose through the _____ duct. The combining form *nas/o* means _____.

SELF-INSTRUCTION: SYMPTOMATIC TERMS

Study the following:

Term	Meaning
asthenopia *as-thĕ-nō′pē-ă*	eyestrain (asthenia = weak condition)
blepharospasm *blef′ă-rō-spazm*	involuntary contraction of the muscles surrounding the eye causing uncontrolled blinking and lid squeezing
diplopia *di-plō′pē-ă*	double vision
exophthalmos *ek-sof-thal′mos* **exophthalmus**	abnormal protrusion of one or both eyeballs
lacrimation *lak-ri-mā′shŭn*	secretion of tears
nystagmus *nis-tag′mŭs*	involuntary rapid oscillating movement of the eyeball (nystagmos = a nodding)
photophobia *fō-tō-fō′be-ă*	extreme sensitivity to, and discomfort from, light
scotoma *skō-tō′mă*	blind spot in vision (skotos = darkness)

PROGRAMMED REVIEW: SYMPTOMATIC TERMS

Answers	Review
vision diplopia	**10.32** Recall that the suffix *-opia* means condition of ___vision___. The combining form *dipl/o* means double. The condition of having double vision is termed ___diplopia___.

asthenopia

10.33   Based on the Greek word <u>asthenia</u>, which means <u>weakness</u>, the condition of eyestrain (weak vision) is ___*asthenopia*___.

phot/o

10.34   Recall that the combining form meaning light is ___*phot/o*___.
Extreme sensitivity to, and discomfort from, light is termed

photophobia

___*p*___.

blephar/o

10.35   Again, the combining form for eyelid is ___*blephar/o*___.
The term for a <u>sudden involuntary contraction of the muscles around</u>

blepharospasm

the eyelid is ___*blepharospasm*___.

ophthalm/o, out

10.36   The three combining forms for eye are *ocul/o, opt/o,* and
___*ophthalm/o*___. The prefix *ex-* means ___*out*___ or away. Using
this last combining form, the term for the condition in which the eye-

exophthalmos
exophthalmus

balls protrude out is termed ___*exophthalmos*___ or
___*exophthalmus*___ (alternate spellings).

tear

process

lacrimation

10.37   *Lacrim/o* is a combining form meaning ___*tear*___. The suffix
-ation refers to a ___*process*___. The term for the process of secreting
tears is called ___*lacrimation*___.

10.38   The Greek word nystagmos means a nodding, such as the
movement of the head up and down or sideways. The condition of
rapid oscillation of the eyeballs is ___*nystagmus*___.

nystagmus

10.39   The medical term for a <u>visual blind (dark) spot</u> comes from the
Greek word that means darkness. The blind spot is called a

scotoma

___*scotoma*___.

SELF-INSTRUCTION: DIAGNOSTIC TERMS

Study the following:

Term	Meaning
refractive errors rē-frak'tiv	defects in the bending of light as it enters the eye, causing an improper focus on the retina
astigmatism ă-stig'mă-tizm	distorted vision caused by an oblong or cylindrical curvature of the lens or cornea that prevents light rays from coming to a single focus on the retina (stigma = point)
hyperopia (Fig. 10-3A and B) hī-per-ō'pē-ă	farsightedness; difficulty seeing close objects when light rays are focused on a point behind the retina
myopia (Fig. 10-3A and C) mī-ō'pē-ă	nearsightedness; difficulty seeing distant objects when light rays are focused on a point in front of the retina
presbyopia prez-bē-ō'pē-ă	impaired vision caused by old age or loss of accommodation
accommodation ă-kom'ŏ-dā'shŭn	ability of the eye to adjust focus on near objects
aphakia ă-fā'kē-ă	absence of the lens, usually after cataract extraction
blepharitis blef'ă-rī'tis	inflammation of the eyelid
blepharochalasis blef'ă-rō-kal'ă-sis **dermatochalasis** der'mă-tō-kal'ă-sis	baggy eyelid; overabundance and loss of elasticity of skin on the upper eyelid causing a fold of skin to hang down over the edge of the eyelid when the eyes are open (chalasis = a slackening)
blepharoptosis blef'ă-rop'tō-sis **ptosis**	drooping of the eyelid, usually caused by paralysis
chalazion (Fig. 10-4) sha-lā'zē-on	chronic nodular inflammation of a meibomian gland, usually the result of a blocked duct (chalaza = hailstone)

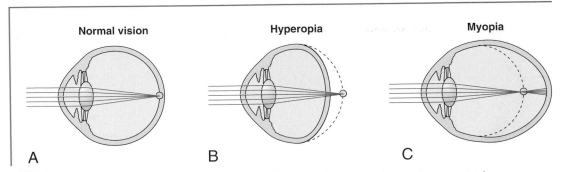

■ **FIGURE 10-3.** **A.** Proper focus of light rays on retina. **B.** Light rays are focused on a point behind the retina in hyperopia. **C.** Light rays are focused at a point in front of the retina in myopia.

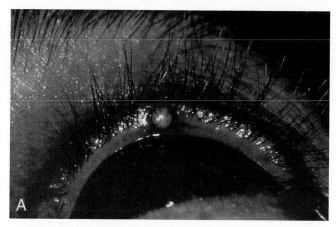

FIGURE 10-4. Upper-lid chalazion.

cataract (Fig. 10-5) *kat'ă-rakt*	opaque clouding of the lens causing decreased vision
conjunctivitis *kon-jŭnk-ti-vī'tis*	pinkeye; inflammation of the conjunctiva
dacryoadenitis *dak'rē-ō-ad-ĕ-nī'tis*	inflammation of the lacrimal gland
dacryocystitis *dak'rē-ō'sis-tī'tis*	inflammation of the tear sac
diabetic retinopathy (See Fig. 10-8C) *dī-ă-bet'ik ret-i-nop'ă-thē*	disease of the retina in diabetics characterized by capillary leakage, bleeding, and new vessel formation (neovascularization) leading to scarring and loss of vision
ectropion (Fig. 10.6A) ek-trō'pē-on	outward turning of the rim of the eyelid (tropo = turning)
entropion (Fig. 10-6B) en-trō'pē-on	inward turning of the rim of the eyelid
epiphora *ē-pif'ō-ră*	abnormal overflow of tears caused by blockage of the lacrimal duct (epi= upon; phero = to bear)
glaucoma *glaw-kō'mă*	a group of diseases of the eye characterized by increased intraocular pressure that results in damage to the optic nerve, producing defects in vision
hordeolum *hōr-dē'ō-lŭm*	a sty; an acute infection of a sebaceous gland of the eyelid (hordeum = barley)
iritis *ī-rī'tis*	inflammation of the iris
keratitis *ker-ă-tī'tis*	inflammation of the cornea

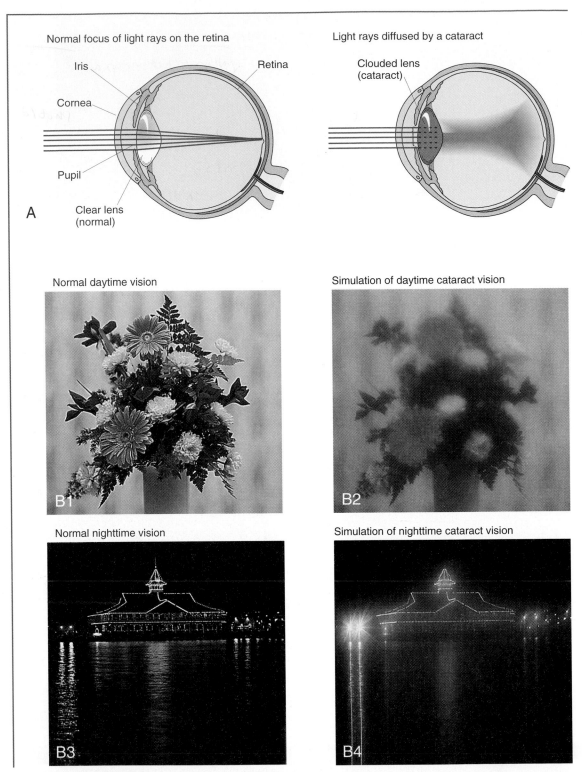

■ **FIGURE 10-5.** Cataract. **A.** Normal light focus compared with light focus interference caused by cataract. **B.** Simulation of cataract vision.

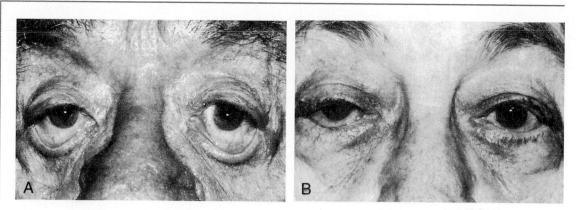

■ **FIGURE 10-6.** Eyelid abnormalities. **A.** Severe, bilateral, lower-lid ectropion. **B.** Lower-lid entropion causing lashes to rub on cornea.

macular degeneration *mak'yū-lăr* *dē-jen-er-ā'shŭn*	breakdown or thinning of the tissues in the macula, resulting in partial or complete loss of central vision
pseudophakia *sū-dō-fak'ē-ă*	an eye in which the natural lens is replaced with an artificial lens implant (pseudo = false)
pterygium (Fig. 10-7) *tĕ-rij'ē-ŭm*	a fibrous, wing-shaped growth of conjunctival tissue that extends onto the cornea, developing most commonly from prolonged exposure to ultraviolet light
retinal detachment *ret-i-nal*	separation of the retina from underlying epithelium, disrupting vision and resulting in blindness if not repaired surgically
retinitis *ret-i-nī'tis*	inflammation of the retina
strabismus *stra-biz'mŭs* **heterotropia** *het'er-ō-trō'pē-ă*	a condition of eye misalignment caused by intraocular muscle imbalance (strabismus = a squinting; hetero = other)
esotropia *es-ō-trō'pē-ă*	right or left eye deviates inward toward nose (eso = inward; tropo = turning)
exotropia *ek-sō-trō'pē-ă*	right or left eye deviates outward away from nose (exo = out; tropo = turning)

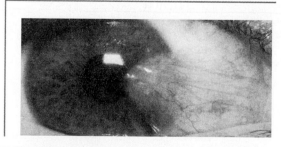

■ **FIGURE 10-7.** Pterygium caused by ultraviolet exposure and drying.

scleritis sklĕ-rī′tis	inflammation of the sclera
trichiasis trĭ-kī′ă-sis	misdirected eyelashes that rub on conjunctiva or cornea

PROGRAMMED REVIEW: DIAGNOSTIC TERMS

Answers   **Review**

inflammation

blepharitis

conjunctivitis

10.40 Recall that the suffix *-itis* means _____.
Inflammation of the eyelid is therefore termed _____.
Inflammation of the conjunctiva is _____ (or pinkeye).

kerat/o

keratitis

10.41 In addition to *corne/o,* a combining form that means cornea, is
_____. The term for inflammation of the cornea uses this second form: _____.

ir/o

iritis

10.42 The two combining forms for iris of the eye are *irid/o* and
_____. The latter is used to make the term for inflammation of the iris:
_____.

retinitis

scleritis

10.43 Inflammation of the retina is termed _____. Inflammation of the sclera is _____.

dacry/o

dacryocyst

dacryocystitis

10.44 The two combining forms for tears are *lacrim/o* and
_____. The combining form *cyst/o* means a sac. Using the latter form for tears, the tear sac is termed the _____. Inflammation of the tear sac is _____.

inflammation, lacrimal (tear)

10.45 The combining form *aden/o* means gland. Thus, the dacryoadenitis means _____ of the _____ gland.

refractive

10.46 Conditions in which the eye incorrectly focuses light on the retina are called _____ errors. Recall that the suffix

vision

beyond

hyperopia

myopia

-*opia* means a condition of ___vision___. The prefix *hyper-* means excessive or _____. The condition of farsightedness occurs when the light rays from near objects focus beyond the retina. This is called ___hyperopia___. The opposite condition of nearsightedness is called ___myopia___.

presby/o

presbyopia

accommodation

10.47 The combining form meaning old age is ___presby/o___. The visual condition of impaired vision caused by old age is called ___presbyopia___. This happens because of a loss of accommodation. The ability of the eye to adjust focus on near objects is ___accommodation___.

blepharochalasis

dermatochalasis

10.48 The Greek word chalasis means a slackening, such as with baggy skin. The term for a baggy eyelid (using the combining form for eyelid) is ___blepharochalasis___. The combining form *dermat/o* means skin. Another term for baggy eyelid uses that combining form: ___dermato chalasis___.

downward

blepharoptosis

10.49 Recall that the suffix *-ptosis* means a falling or ___downward___ displacement. The term for a drooping of the eyelid is ___blepharoptosis___. This is usually caused by paralysis.

chalazion

chalazia

10.50 From the Greek word for a small hailstone (chalazion), which it may resemble in appearance, comes the term for a chronic nodular inflammation of a meibomian gland: ___chalazion___. The plural of chalazion is ___chalazia___.

cataract

10.51 The clouding of the lens that causes decreased vision is called a ___cataract___.

condition of

disease

10.52 The combining form *path/o* means disease, and the suffix *-y* means process of or ___condition___ ___of___. Thus, *-pathy* refers to a condition of ___disease___. A retinal disease condition in diabetics

retinopathy

caused by problems with the capillaries is called diabetic
___retinopathy___.

10.53 The Greek word tropo means turning. The prefix *ec-* means

out

away or ___out___. The condition of the eyelid rim turning outward is

ectropion

called ___ectropion___. The prefix *en-*, however, means

within

___within___ or inward. The condition of the rim of the eyelid turning

entropion

in is called ___entropion___.

10.54 If the lacrimal duct becomes blocked, tears that might otherwise
flow to the lacrimal sac overflow. The term for this condition begins

upon

with the prefix *epi-*, which means ___upon___. The tears flow upon and
out of the outer surface of the eye. This condition is called

epiphora

___epiphora___.

10.55 The group of diseases characterized by increased intraocular
pressure resulting in damage to the ocular nerve, causing visual defects,

glaucoma

is ___glaucoma___.

10.56 Recall that the combining forms for lens are *phac/o* and

phak/o

___phak___. The latter spelling along with the prefix *pseudo-* (false),

condition of

and the suffix *-ia* meaning ___condition___ ___of___, forms the term

pseudophakia

for an implanted artificial lens: ___pseudophakia___.

10.57 From the Greek work strabismos, meaning a squinting, comes

strabismus

this term for a condition of eye misalignment: ___strabismus___.
Recall that the word root *tropo* means a turning, and *-ia* means

condition of

___condition___ ___of___. The combining form *heter/o* means the
other. Another term for strabismus is named for the appearance of one

heterotropia

eye turning toward the other: ___heterotropia___. If the eye
turns inward (eso = inward) toward the nose, this is called

esotropia

___esotropia___. If the eye turns outward (exo = outward), this is

exotropia

called ___exotropia___.

macular degeneration

10.58   A breakdown of tissues in the macula that causes a loss of central vision is called _Macular_ _degeneration_.

detachment

10.59   Separation of the retina from the underlying tissue, usually requiring surgical repair, is called retinal _detachment_.

hordeolum

10.60   The Latin word hordeolus means <u>a little barley grain</u>, which is similar in appearance to a sty, an acute infection of a sebaceous gland of the eyelid. The medical term for a (sty) is _hordeolum_.

pterygium

ultraviolet

10.61   The combining form *pteryg/o* means wing-shaped. <u>A triangular, or wing-shaped, fibrous growth</u> of conjunctival tissue extending onto the cornea is called _pterygium_. Pterygia are most commonly caused by prolonged exposure to _UV_ light.

presence

trichiasis

10.62   Recall that the suffix *-iasis* means formation or _presence_ of. The combining form *trich/o* means (hair). The <u>presence of misdirected eyelashes that rub on the conjunctiva or cornea</u> is called _trichiasis_.

SELF-INSTRUCTION: DIAGNOSTIC TESTS AND PROCEDURES

Study the following:

Test or Procedure	Explanation
distance visual acuity	a measure of the ability to see the details and shape of identifiable objects from a specified distance, usually from <u>20 feet (6 meters)</u>; normal distance visual acuity is 20/20 (6/6)
fluorescein angiography *flūr-es′ē-in an-jē-og′ră-fē*	visualization and photography of retinal and choroidal vessels made as fluorescein dye, which is injected into a vein, circulates through the eye
ophthalmoscopy (Fig. 10-8) *of-thal-mos′kō-pē*	use of an ophthalmoscope to view the interior of the eye
slit lamp biomicroscopy (Fig. 10-9) *bi′ō-mi-kros′kŏ-pē*	use of a tabletop microscope used to examine the eye, especially the cornea, lens, fluids, and membranes

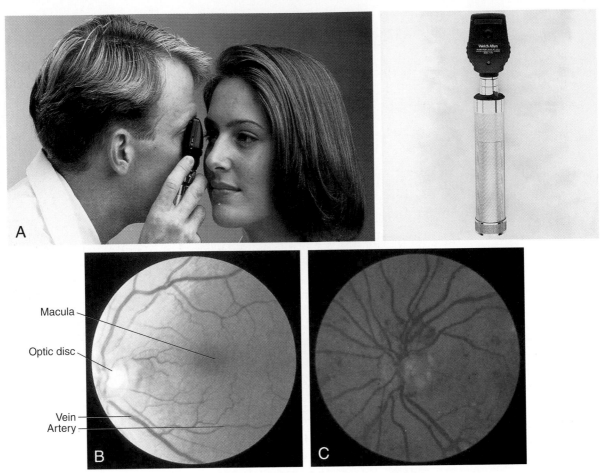

Macula

Optic disc

Vein
Artery

FIGURE 10-8. A. Doctor performing ophthalmoscopy using ophthalmoscope. **B.** Normal retina. **C.** Neovascularization of blood vessels seen in diabetic retinopathy.

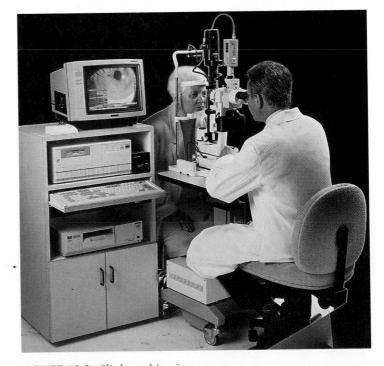

FIGURE 10-9. Slit-lamp biomicroscope.

sonography sŏ-nog′ră-fē	use of high-frequency sound waves to detect pathology within the eye, such as foreign bodies or detached retina
tonometry tō-nom′ĕ-trē	use of a tonometer to measure intraocular pressure, which is elevated in glaucoma

PROGRAMMED REVIEW: DIAGNOSTIC TESTS AND PROCEDURES

Answers   **Review**

ophthalm/o

10.63   Again, the three combining forms meaning eye are *ocul/o*, *opt/o*, and _____. The last one is used with the suffix that means process of examination to make this term for the use of an ophthalmoscope to view the interior of the eye:

ophthalmoscopy

_____

10.64   The diagnostic test that measures the ability to see objects at a specified distance, usually from 20 feet (6 meters), is called distance

visual acuity, normal

_____ _____. 20/20 (6/6) represents _____ distance visual acuity.

10.65   Angiography, which is radiography of blood vessels after injection of a contrast medium, is used in many body areas. The procedure

fluorescein

used with the eye is called _____ angiography, so named for the fluorescein dye that is injected into a vein to circulate through the eye.

10.66   The use of high-frequency sound waves to make an image for

sonography

detecting pathology in the eye is called _____, or ul-

recording

trasound. The suffix *-graphy* means process of _____.

10.67   A tonometer measures intraocular pressure as a test for glau-

tonometry

coma. This procedure is called _____tonometry_____. The suffix *-metry*

process

means _____process_____ of measuring.

| biomicroscopy | **10.68** A special microscope is used to examine eye structures. This procedure is called slit lamp _____. |

SELF-INSTRUCTION: OPERATIVE TERMS

Study the following:

Term	Meaning
blepharoplasty *blef′ă-ro-plast-tē*	surgical repair of an eyelid
cataract extraction *kat′ă-rakt ek-strak′shŭn*	excision of a cloudy lens from the eye
cryoretinopexy *krī-ō-ret′i-nō-pek-se* **cryopexy**	use of intense cold to seal a hole or tear in the retina; used to treat retinal detachment
dacryocystectomy *dak′rē-ō-sis-tek′tō-mē*	excision of a lacrimal sac
enucleation *ē-nū-klē-ā′shŭn*	excision of an eyeball
iridectomy *ir′i-dek′tō-mē*	excision of a portion of iris tissue
iridotomy *ir-i-dot′ō-mē*	incision into the iris (usually with a laser) to allow for drainage of aqueous humor from the posterior to anterior chamber; used to treat a type of glaucoma
keratoplasty *ker′ă-tō-plas-tē*	corneal transplant
laser surgery	use of a laser to make incisions or destroy tissues (used to create fluid passages or obliterate tumors, aneurysms, etc.)
laser-assisted in situ keratomileusis (LASIK)	a technique using the excimer laser to reshape the surface of the cornea to correct refractive errors such as myopia, hyperopia, and astigmatism (smileusis = carving)
intraocular lens (IOL) implant *in′tră-ok′yū-lăr*	implantation of an artificial lens to replace a defective natural lens (e.g., after cataract extraction)
phacoemulsification *fak′ō-ē-mŭl-si-fi-kā′shŭn*	use of ultrasound to shatter and break up a cataract with aspiration and removal

PROGRAMMED REVIEW: OPERATIVE TERMS

Answers	Review

Answers

-plasty

blepharoplasty

-pexy

cryoretinopexy

cataract

intraocular lens implant

within

lacrimal

-ectomy

dacryocystectomy

iridectomy

-tomy

iridotomy

enucleation

kerat/o

Review

10.69   Recall that the suffix for surgical repair or reconstruction is

_____. The surgical repair of an eyelid is termed

_____.

10.70   The combining form *cry/o* means cold. Recall that the operative suffix meaning <u>suspension or fixation</u> is ___*pexy*___. The operative procedure using intense cold to seal a hole in the retina is called

_____*cryoretinopexy*_____, or simply cryopexy.

10.71   When a cloudy lens is excised from the eye, this is called

____*cataract*____ extraction. After the lens has been excised, an artificial lens may be implanted in a procedure called

_____ _____ _____ (IOL). The prefix *intra-* means ___*within*___.

10.72   Recall that dacryocyst means ___*lacrimal*___ sac. The surgical suffix for excision is ___*-ectomy*___. Therefore, the term for excision of a lacrimal sac is ___*dacryocystectomy*___.

10.73   The excision of a portion of iris tissue is ___*iridectomy*___.

10.74   The surgical suffix meaning <u>incision</u> is ___"*tomy*"___. An incision <u>into the iris</u> to allow for <u>draining from the posterior chamber</u> is called an ___*iridotomy*___.

10.75   The Latin word <u>enucleo</u> means to <u>remove the kernel</u>, such as the kernel of a nut. The medical term for <u>removing an entire structure, such as the eyeball</u> (or a tumor), without rupturing it is ___*enucleation*___.

10.76   The two combining forms referring to the cornea are *corne/o* and ___*kerat/o*___, which also can mean hard. Combining the latter with keratoplasty

the suffix for surgical repair or reconstruction yields this term for

corneal transplant: _____.

laser

surgery

in situ

keratomileusis

10.77   Lasers are used in many operative techniques to make

incisions or destroy tissues. This is generally called _____

_____. A special technique using a laser to reshape

the surface of the cornea is termed laser-assisted _____ _____

_____ (LASIK).

phacoemulsification

10.78   The term emulsification refers to breaking up a substance and

distributing it through another substance, generally a liquid. A surgical

procedure uses ultrasound to shatter and break up a cataract such that

after emulsification it can be removed by aspiration. This procedure is

called _____.

SELF-INSTRUCTION: THERAPEUTIC TERMS

Study the following:

Term	Meaning
contact lens	a small, plastic, curved disc with optical correction that fits over the cornea; used to correct refractive errors
eye instillation	introduction of a medicated solution in the eye usually administered by drop (gt) or drops (gtt) in the affected eye or eyes: OD (oculus dexter) right eye OS (oculus sinister) left eye OU (oculi unitas) both eyes
eye irrigation	washing of the eye with water or other fluid (like saline)

COMMON THERAPEUTIC DRUG CLASSIFICATIONS

antibiotic ophthalmic solution an′tē-bī-ot′ik of-thal′mik	antimicrobial agent in solution; used to treat bacterial infections (such as conjunctivitis and corneal ulcers)
mydriatic (dilation of pupil) mi-drē-at′ik	an agent that causes dilation of the pupil (used for certain eye examinations)
miotic mī-ot′ik	an agent that causes the pupil to contract (mio = less)

PROGRAMMED REVIEW: THERAPEUTIC TERMS

Answers	Review

Answers

contact lens

instillation, drop

gtt

right, left

both

irrigation

antibiotic

ophthalmic

mydriatic

miotic

Review

10.79   The plastic lens that the user fits over the cornea to correct re-fractive errors is called a _____ _____.

10.80   Introduction of a medicated solution in the eye is called an eye _____, usually administered by _____ (gt) or drops (_____) in the affected eye or eyes: OD is the abbreviation for the _____ eye, OS is the _____ eye, and OU refers to _____ eyes. Washing the eye with water or other fluid is called eye _____.

10.81   A solution composed of an antimicrobial agent in a fluid for treatment of bacterial eye infections is called an _____ _____ solution.

10.82   The term mydriasis means dilation of the pupil. A therapeutic drug that causes dilation of the pupil for eye examination is called a _____.

10.83   In contrast, miosis means contraction of the pupil. A therapeutic drug that causes the pupil to contract is called a _____.

Practice Exercises

For the following terms, on the lines below the term, write out the indicated word parts: prefixes, combining forms, roots, and suffixes. Then define the word.

Example:
epikeratophakia

epi/kerato/phak/ia
P   CF   R   S

DEFINITION: upon/cornea/lens/condition of

1. blepharoptosis

   eyelid / falling or downward
   CF   S

   DEFINITION: falling or downward of eyelid.

2. iridotomy

   iris / incision
   CF   S

   DEFINITION: incision of iris

3. ophthalmology

   eye / study of
   CF   S

   DEFINITION: study of eye

4. vitrectomy

   glassy / excision
   R   S

   DEFINITION: _____

5. dacryolithiasis

   tear / stone / formation or presence of
   CF   R   S

   DEFINITION: _____

6. lacrimal

   tear / pertaining to
   R   S

   DEFINITION: _____

7. photophobia

   light / sensitivity / condition of
   CF   R   S

   DEFINITION: _____

8. keratoplasty

_____ / _____
  CF   S

DEFINITION: _____

9. aqueous

_____ / _____
  R   S

DEFINITION: _____

10. iritis

_____ / _____
  R   S

DEFINITION: _____

11. corneal

_____ / _____
  R   S

DEFINITION: _____

12. phacolysis

_____ / _____
  CF   S

DEFINITION: _____

13. retinopathy

_____ / _____ / _____
  CF   R   S

DEFINITION: _____

14. ocular

_____ / _____
  R   S

DEFINITION: _____

15. conjunctivitis

_____ / _____
  R   S

DEFINITION: _____

16. presbyopia

_____ / _____
  R   S

DEFINITION: _____

17. optometry

___ / _____
  CF   S

DEFINITION: _____

18. aphakia

___ / _____ / _____
  P   R   S

DEFINITION: _____

19. hyperopia

___ / _____
  P   S

DEFINITION: _____

20. scleromalacia

___ / _____
  CF   S

DEFINITION: _____

Match the following terms for refractive disorders with their meanings:

21. myopia _____   a. old age loss of accommodation

22. strabismus _____   b. nearsightedness

23. presbyopia _____   c. farsightedness

24. astigmatism _____   d. crossed eyes

25. hyperopia _____   e. distorted vision

Complete the following medical term by writing the missing part:

26. _____itis = inflammation of the cornea

27. _____phobia = extreme sensitivity to light

28. dacryo_____ectomy = excision of a tear sac

29. _____ophthalmos = protrusion of the eyeball

30. _____chalasis = baggy eyelids

Briefly define the following medical terms:

31. entropion _____

32. diplopia _____

33. tonometer _____

34. ectropion _____

35. scotoma _____

Write the correct medical term for each of the following:

36. pinkeye _____

37. inflammation of the eyelid _____

38. eyestrain _____

39. an agent that causes dilation of the pupil _____

40. absence of the lens of the eye _____

41. sty; acute infection of a meibomian gland of the eyelid

_____

42. clouding of the lens causing decreased vision _____

43. breakdown or thinning of the tissues in the macula, resulting in partial or complete loss of central vision

_____

44. involuntary contraction of the muscles surrounding the eye

_____

45. an involuntary, rapid oscillating movement of the eyeball

_____

For each of the following, circle the combining form that corresponds to the meaning given:

46. **eye**	or/o	opt/o	ot/o
47. **old age**	presby/o	scler/o	phas/o
48. **glassy**	aque/o	vitre/o	hydr/o
49. **light**	phon/o	phot/o	opt/o
50. **hard or sclera**	corne/o	vitre/o	scler/o
51. **lens (lentil)**	phac/o	scler/o	conjunctiv/o
52. **colored circle**	chrom/o	irid/o	corne/o
53. **tear**	dacry/o	hydr/o	aque/o
54. **eyelid**	ocul/o	ophthalm/o	blephar/o
55. **water**	aque/o	hidr/o	vitre/o

Write in the missing words on lines in the illustration of the eye's anatomy;

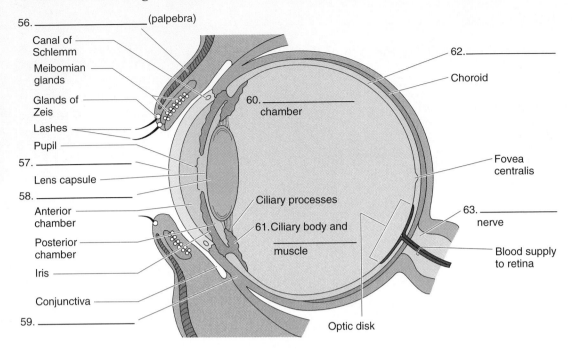

56. _____ (palpebra)

Canal of Schlemm

Meibomian glands

Glands of Zeis

Lashes

Pupil

57. _____

Lens capsule

58. _____

Anterior chamber

Posterior chamber

Iris

Conjunctiva

59. _____

60. _____ chamber

61. Ciliary body and _____ muscle

Ciliary processes

Optic disk

62. _____

Choroid

Fovea centralis

63. _____ nerve

Blood supply to retina

For each of the following, circle the correct spelling of the term:

64. asthenopia	assthinopia	asthinopia
65. terigium	pterygium	pteregium
66. horadeolum	hordeolum	hordeaolum
67. nistagmis	nystagmis	nystagmus
68. chalazeon	shalazion	chalazion
69. mydriatic	midriatic	myadriatic
70. skotoma	scotoma	schotoma
71. epiphora	epifora	epifhora
72. dakryeocyst	dacryocyst	dacreyocyst
73. opthalmoscope	ofthalmoscope	ophthalmoscope

Give the noun that was used to form the following adjectives.

74. conjunctival _____

75. myopic _____

76. scleral _____

77. macular _____

78. exophthalmic _____

Medical Record Analyses

MEDICAL RECORD 10-1

S: This 51 y/o ♀ c/o a growth in the corner of her right eye that is dry and irritated. She has had the feeling that there was "something in the eye" for about four months before actually noticing the growth three weeks ago. She wears contacts to correct farsightedness, but has recently switched to eyeglasses because of the discomfort. She is active physically and loves tennis and water sports, but does not frequently wear sunglasses.

O: Inspection of the right eye reveals an inflamed, raised, whitish, triangular wedge of fibrovascular tissue, whose base lies within the interpalpebral conjunctiva and whose apex encroaches the cornea. A photo documentation is made and included in the chart.

A: INFLAMED PTERYGIUM, RIGHT EYE

P: 1) The patient is advised that the pterygium is not dangerous, but further growth could interfere with vision and warrant surgical excision. She was counseled on the importance of wearing UV blocking sunglasses and advised to avoid smoky or dusty areas as much as possible.
2) RX: fluorometholone, 0.1% suspension, 1 gt q 4 h OD during the day for inflammation; OTC artificial tears solution, prn dryness/irritation
3) RTO in 3 months for slit lamp evaluation, or sooner if symptoms persist.

1. Describe the refractive error noted in the subjective information.
   a. eyestrain
   b. inflammation of the cornea
   c. difficulty seeing distant objects
   d. difficulty seeing close objects
   e. blind spot in vision

2. Which action on the part of the patient likely contributed to the condition?
   a. wearing contact lenses
   b. removing contact lenses
   c. playing tennis
   d. not routinely wearing sunglasses
   e. strenuous physical activity

3. Which ophthalmologic procedure is included in the plan?
   a. use of laser to reshape the surface of the cornea
   b. use of an ophthalmoscope to view the interior of the eye
   c. use of a tabletop microscope to examine the eye, especially the cornea
   d. implantation of an artificial lens
   e. use of a tonometer to measure intraocular pressure

4. How should the fluorometholone be administered?
   a. one drop every four hours
   b. four drops in the eye every morning
   c. one drop every day for four days
   d. as needed during the day
   e. one drop every other day for four days

5. When should the patient instill the artificial tears?
   a. every day
   b. every night
   c. during the day
   d. only as needed
   e. when feeling the need to cry

6. What caused the ptergygium?
   a. misdirected eyelashes that rub on conjunctiva or cornea
   b. intraocular muscle imbalance
   c. separation of the retina from underlying epithelium
   d. abnormal overflow of tears
   e. ultraviolet exposure and drying

7. What was the patient told about the pterygium?
   a. it is cancerous
   b. it is not cancerous
   c. it must be removed
   d. both a and c

MEDICAL RECORD 10-2 FOR ADDITIONAL STUDY

CENTRAL MEDICAL GROUP, INC.
Department of Ophthalmology
201 Medical Center Drive • Central City, US 90000-1234 • PHONE: (012) 125-8888 • FAX: (012) 125-3434

HISTORY

HISTORY OF PRESENT ILLNESS:
This 57-year-old female complains of progressive loss of vision in the right eye over the last two years which has been diagnosed as a cataract. The patient recently underwent cataract surgery in the left eye and is currently scheduled for surgery in the right eye due to her decreased vision.

PAST MEDICAL HISTORY:
The patient has had the normal childhood diseases and has essential hypertension and hypothyroidism.

SURGERIES:
Appendectomy 40 years ago. Tonsillectomy and adenoidectomy as a child. Cataract surgery in the left eye with a posterior chamber lens implant in 199x.

ALLERGIES:
None.

MEDICATIONS:
Propranolol 80 mg b.i.d. Hydrochlorothiazide 50 mg b.i.d. Clonidine, 0.1 mg, 2 tablets p.o. t.i.d. Synthroid 0.1 mg q.d. Slow-K 2 tablets p.o. q.d.

PHYSICAL EXAMINATION

VITAL SIGNS:
WEIGHT: 135 lb. BLOOD PRESSURE: 180/100.

HEENT:
HEAD, EARS, EYES, NOSE, THROAT: Normal.

EYES: Best corrected visual acuity in the right eye is counting fingers at two feet and 20/50 in the left eye. Pinhole vision in the left eye is 20/30. Slit lamp examination reveals normal lids, conjunctivae, and sclerae. Corneas are clear. Anterior chambers are clear and deep. Irides are within normal limits in the right eye. Evaluation of the lens reveals a 4+ posterior subcapsular plaquing with 3-4+ nuclear sclerosis, and in the left eye, there is a posterior chamber lens that is in place with posterior lens capsular plaquing. Intraocular pressure: OD: 18. OS: 17. Fundus examination in the right eye was severely hindered due to the dense cataract. However, evaluation of the posterior pole in the right eye was within normal limits.

(continued)

HISTORY AND PHYSICAL Page 1	PT. NAME: AQUERO,CASSANDRE D. ID NO: 008654 ATT PHYS: O. TRAN, M.D.

CENTRAL MEDICAL GROUP, INC.
Department of Ophthalmology
201 Medical Center Drive • Central City, US 90000-1234 • PHONE: (012) 125-8888 • FAX: (012) 125-3434

PHYSICAL EXAMINATION

CHEST:
Clear to percussion and auscultation. The breasts were normal, and the lungs were clear.

PELVIC/RECTAL:
Within normal limits.

EXTREMITIES:
Within normal limits.

NEUROLOGICAL:
Within normal limits.

IMPRESSION:
1)   Cataract, right eye.
2)   Pseudophakia, left eye.
3)   Essential hypertension.
4)   Hypothyroidism.

RISKS/BENEFITS:
The patient is aware of the alternatives, risks, benefits, and possible complications of the procedure that include hemorrhage, infection, loss of vision, reoperation, retinal detachment, macular edema; and the patient still desires to undergo the procedure.

PLAN:
Extracapsular cataract extraction with posterior chamber lens implant under local anesthesia using a +21 diopter posterior chamber lens with the ultraviolet filter. Preoperative medication will consist of the patient's morning dose of Inderal, 80 mg; Hydrochlorothiazide, 50 mg; Clonidine, 0.2 mg; and Diamox, 250 mg with ¼ glass of water at approximately 10 a.m. on the day of surgery. The patient was also instructed to take Maxitrol, 1 gt OD, q 3 h starting 24 hours prior to the procedure, while awake.

O. Tran, M.D.

OT:mk
D: 10/19/20xx   T: 10/20/20xx

HISTORY AND PHYSICAL	PT. NAME:	AQUERO, CASSANDRE D.
Page 2	ID NO:	008654
	ATT PHYS:	O. TRAN, M.D.

MEDICAL RECORD 10-2 FOR ADDITIONAL STUDY

Not long ago, Cassandre Aquero had cataract surgery for her left eye and is now losing vision in her right eye because of another cataract. She is consulting an ophthalmologist, Dr. Oanh Tran, about surgery on the right eye.

Read Medical Record 10-2 (pages 454-455) for Ms. Aquero and answer the following questions. This record shows the history and physical examination written by Dr. Tran in planning for her surgery.

1. The following are medical terms used in this record that you have not yet encountered in this text. Underline each where it appears in the record, and define below.

   appendectomy _____

   irides _____

2. In your own words, briefly describe Ms. Aquero's current complaint and diagnosis noted under "History of Present Illness."

   _____

   _____

   _____

3. Describe, in lay language, the two medical conditions Ms. Aquero has in addition to her current problem and past surgeries.

   _____

   _____

   _____

4. Which of the following findings on physical examination is related to her general medical condition in addition to her eye problems?
   a. rales on auscultation
   b. disoriented consciousness
   c. BP 180/100
   d. weight 135 lb.

5. The planned operation involves several risks that the patient has accepted in the hopes of regaining good eyesight. Which of the following was *not* mentioned by Dr. Tran as a risk?
   a. hypertensive crisis
   b. retinal detachment
   c. edema of the macula
   d. bleeding

6. The preoperative nursing staff will ensure that Ms. Aquero receives five medications before surgery. Translate the instructions for these:

   a. _____

   b. _____

   c. _____

   d. _____

   e. _____

7. In your own words, not using medical terminology, briefly describe what will occur in the surgery.

_____

_____

_____

Answers to Practice Exercises

1. blepharo/ptosis
   CF   S
   eyelid/falling or downward displacement
2. irido/tomy
   CF   S
   iris/incision
3. ophthalmo/logy
   CF   S
   eye/study of
4. vitr/ectomy
   R   S
   glassy/excision (removal)
5. dacryo/lith/iasis
   CF   R   S
   tear/stone/formation or presence of
6. lacrim/al
   R   S
   tear/pertaining to
7. photo/phob/ia
   CF   R   S
   light/sensitivity/condition of
8. kerato/plasty
   CF   S
   cornea/surgical repair or reconstruction
9. aque/ous
   R   S
   water/pertaining to
10. ir/itis
    R   S
    iris/inflammation
11. corne/al
    R   S
    cornea/pertaining to

12. phaco/lysis
    CF   S
    lens (lentil)/breaking down or dissolution
13. retino/path/y
    CF   R   S
    retina/disease/condition or process of
14. ocul/ar
    R   S
    eye/pertaining to
15. conjunctiv/itis
    R   S
    conjunctiva (to join together)/inflammation
16. presby/opia
    R   S
    old age/condition of vision
17. opto/metry
    CF   S
    eye/process of measuring
18. a/phak/ia
    P   R   S
    without/lens (lentil)/condition or process of
19. hyper/opia
    P   S
    above or excessive/condition of vision
20. sclero/malacia
    CF   S
    sclera/softening
21. b
22. d
23. a
24. e
25. c
26. keratitis
27. photophobia
28. dacryocystectomy

29. exophthalmos
30. blepharochalasis or dermatochalasis
31. inward turn of rim of the eyelid
32. double vision
33. instrument to measure intraocular pressure
34. outward turn of rim of the eyelid
35. blind spot in vision
36. conjunctivitis
37. blepharitis
38. asthenopia
39. mydriatic
40. aphakia
41. hordeolum
42. cataract
43. macular degeneration
44. blepharospasm
45. nystagmus
46. opt/o
47. presby/o
48. vitre/o
49. phot/o
50. scler/o
51. phac/o
52. irid/o
53. dacry/o
54. blephar/o
55. aque/o
56. eyelid
57. cornea
58. lens
59. sclera
60. vitreous
61. ciliary
62. retina
63. optic

64. asthenopia
65. pterygium
66. hordeolum
67. nystagmus
68. chalazion
69. mydriatic
70. scotoma

71. epiphora
72. dacryocyst
73. ophthalmoscope
74. conjunctiva
75. myopia
76. sclera
77. macula
78. exophthalmos or
    exophthalmus

Answers to Medical Records Analyses

1. d
2. d
3. c
4. a
5. d
6. e
7. b

CHAPTER 11

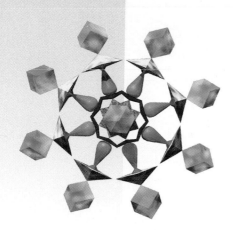

The Ear

Overview of the Ear

The three divisions of the ear function to provide the sense of hearing (Fig. 11-1):

❋ The external ear, from the pinna or auricle, gathers sounds, which funnel through the external auditory canal.

❋ Sounds reach the tympanum, or eardrum, in the middle ear, which transmits sound vibrations to the auditory ossicles (the malleus, incus, and stapes) and to the oval window, which stimulates the auditory fluids in the inner ear. In the middle ear, the eustachian tube connects with the throat to maintain equal air pressure.

❋ The inner ear receives sound vibrations and passes them through intricate intercommunicating tubes and chambers to the organ of Corti. This stimulates nerve fibers and generates impulses to the brain for processing.

The labyrinth of the inner ear also helps to maintain the body's equilibrium by stimulating nerve impulses resulting from movement or changes in position.

SELF-INSTRUCTION: COMBINING FORMS

Study the following:

Combining Form	Meaning
acous/o **audi/o**	hearing
aer/o	air or gas
aur/i **ot/o**	ear
cerumin/ o	wax

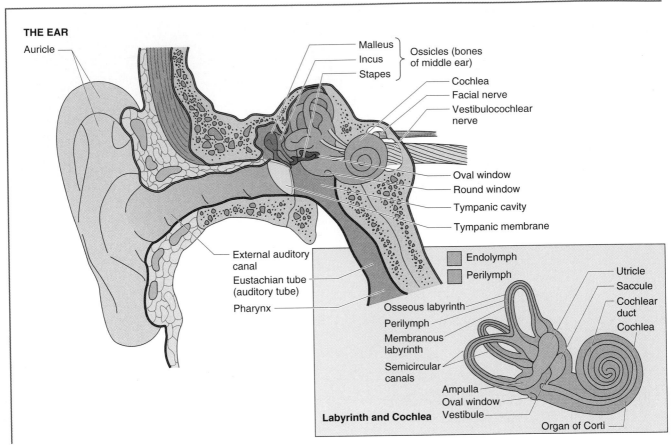

■ **FIGURE 11-1.** Anatomy of the ear.

salping/o	eustachian tube or uterine tube
tympan/o **myring/o**	eardrum
-acusis (additional suffix)	hearing condition

PROGRAMMED REVIEW: COMBINING FORMS

| **Answers** | **Review** |

11.1   The two combining forms for hearing are used in many everyday words in addition to medical terms. People speak of the acoustics of a room, for example, and audible noises. These two combining forms are

acous/o, audi/o

_____acous/o_____ and ___audi/o___. Related to the combining form *acous/o*

-acusis

is the suffix for hearing condition: ___-acusis___. The term presbyacu-sis, for example, means hearing loss caused by old age. Recall that the

-metry	suffix meaning process of measuring is ___*metry*___ . The medical process of measuring hearing, using the other combining form, is there-
audiometry	fore ___*audio metry*___ .

11.2 The combining form for air or gas is ___*aer/o*___ . This combining form is used in many medical terms. An aerobe, for example, is a microbe that lives in the presence of air, whereas a microbe that lives without air (formed with the prefix meaning without) is an

aer/o	
anaerobe	___*anaerobe*___ .

11.3 The two combining forms for ear are *aur/i* and ___*ot/o*___ . Medical study of the ear is called otology. The physician who specializes in the study and treatment of the ear is an ___*otologist*___ . Otology is a subspecialty of otorhinolaryngology (otolaryngology), involving study and treatment of the ___*ear*___ , nose, and throat, more commonly known as ENT.

ot/o	
otologist	
ear	

11.4 The other combining form meaning ear is ___*aur/i*___ . The auricle, for example, is the outer, visible part of the ear.

aur/i	

11.5 The combining form referring to earwax comes from the Latin word cera, meaning wax. That combining form is ___*cerumin/o*___ . Recall that the suffix meaning condition or increase is ___*-osis*___ , and therefore the term for a condition of excessive earwax is

cerumin/o	
-osis	
ceruminosis	___*ceruminosis*___ .

11.6 The combining form for the eustachian tube (or uterine tube) comes from the Greek word salpinx, meaning trumpet. That combining form is ___*salping/o*___ . Using the common suffix for inflammation, the medical term for <u>inflammation of the eustachian tube in the ear or uterine tube</u> is ___*salpingitis*___ . The context in which the term is used is key to knowing which meaning is appropriate.

salping/o	
salpingitis	

11.7 A kind of drum used in symphony orchestras is called a tympany, from the Greek word for drum. The combining form for the

tympan/o

eardrum is _____*tympan/o*_____. Recall that the suffix for surgical incision

-tomy

is _____*tomy*_____. An incision into the eardrum is therefore called a

tympanotomy

_____*tympano tomy*_____.

11.8 A second combining form for eardrum comes from the Latin word for drum membrane: <u>myringa</u>. That combining form is

myring/o

_____*myring/o*_____. Recall that the suffix for surgical <u>excision</u> is

-ectomy

_____*-ectomy*_____. The medical term for the excision of the eardrum, using

myringectomy

that suffix and combining form, is _____*The myring ectomy*_____.

SELF-INSTRUCTION: ANATOMICAL TERMS

Study the following:

Term	Meaning
external ear	
pinna *pin'ă*	auricle (little ear); projected part of the external ear (pinna = feather)
external auditory canal	external passage for sounds collected from the pinna to the tympanum
cerumen *sĕ-rū'men*	a waxy substance secreted by glands located throughout the external canal
middle ear	
tympanic membrane (TM) (Fig. 11.2) *tim-pan'ik mem'brān*	eardrum; drumlike structure that receives sound collected in the external auditory canal and amplifies it through the middle ear
malleus *mal'ē-ŭs*	hammer; first of the three auditory ossicles of the middle ear
incus *ing'kŭs*	anvil; middle of the three auditory ossicles of the middle ear
stapes *stā'pēz*	stirrup; last of the three auditory ossicles of the middle ear

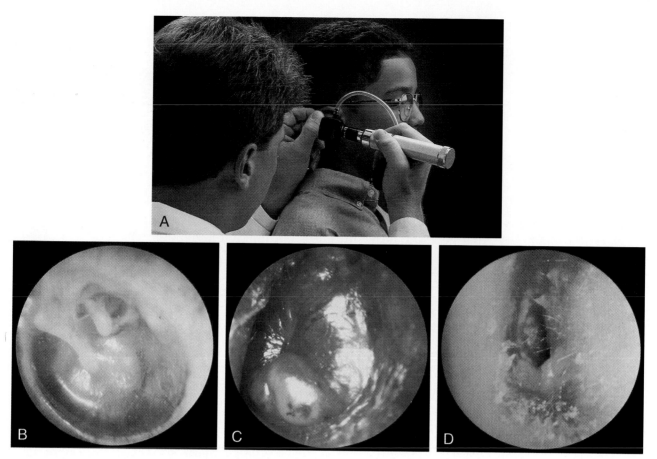

FIGURE 11-2. A. Doctor examining patient using otoscope. **B.** Normal tympanic membrane. **C.** Otitis media. **D.** Otitis externa.

eustachian tube *yū-stā′shŭn* **auditory tube**	tube connecting the middle ear to the pharynx (throat)
oval window	membrane that covers the opening between the middle ear and inner ear
inner ear	structures and liquids that relay sound waves to the auditory nerve fibers on a path to the brain for interpretation of sound
labyrinth *lab′i-rinth*	maze; inner ear consisting of bony and membranous passages
cochlea *kok′lē-ă*	coiled tubular structure of the inner ear that contains the organ of Corti (cochlea = snail)
perilymph *per′i-limf*	fluid that fills the bony labyrinth of the inner ear
endolymph *en′dō-limf*	fluid within the cochlear duct of the inner ear

organ of Corti	organ located in the cochlea; contains receptors (hair cells) that receive vibrations and generate nerve impulses for hearing
vestibule *ves'ti-būl*	middle part of the inner ear in front of the semilunar canals and behind the cochlea that contains the utricle and the saccule
utricle *ū'tri-kl*	larger of two sacs within the membranous labyrinth of the vestibule in the inner ear (uter = leather bag)
saccule *sak'yūl*	smaller of two sacs within the membranous labyrinth of the vestibule in the inner ear (sacculus = small bag)
semicircular canals *sem'ē-sir'kyū-lăr kă-nalz'*	three canals within the inner ear that contain specialized receptor cells that generate nerve impulses with body movement

PROGRAMMED REVIEW: ANATOMICAL TERMS

Answers	Review
pinna, pinnae	**11.9** The outer, projecting part of the external ear is called the auricle or ___pinna___. The plural form of this term is ___pinnae___. The adjective form is pinnal.
external auditory cerumen	**11.10** Sound waves travel from the pinna through the _____ _____ canal toward the eardrum. Glands along this canal secrete a waxy substance called ___cerumen___.
tympanum	**11.11** The tympanic membrane, or ___tympanum___, is the beginning of the middle ear. Also called the eardrum, this structure amplifies sounds into the middle ear.
bones malleus incus stapes	**11.12** The middle ear has three ossicles, which are small ___malleus___ *bone*. These are named because of their shapes. The first, named for its hammer shape, is the ___malleus___. The malleus receives sound vibrations from the tympanum and transmits them to the anvil-shaped bone called the ___incus___, which transmits them to the stirrup-shaped bone called the ___stapes___. The stapes transfers the vibrations on to the inner ear.

11.13   It is necessary to equalize air pressures outside the body and in the middle ear. The tube connecting the middle ear to the throat (pharynx) is the _____ tube (named for an Italian anatomist named Eustachio). This is sometimes also called the auditory tube.

eustachian

11.14   The opening between the middle ear and the inner ear is covered with a membrane called the _____ _____, so named for its shape as a rounded window covering this opening. The stapes transmits sound vibration to the oval window and thus into the _____ ear.

oval window

inner

11.15   Inside the inner ear is a network of interconnecting tubes and chambers that looks like a maze, called the __labyrinth_____.

labyrinth

11.16   The combining form _lymph/o_ refers to clear liquid. The prefix _peri-_ means around, and the prefix _endo-_ means _____. The fluid around the cochlea in the inner ear is called __peri lymph_____, and the fluid within the cochlear duct is called __endo lymph_____. The coiled, snail-shaped structure containing the organ of Corti is the __cochlea_____.

within

perilymph

endolymph

cochlea

11.17   Nerve receptors are located inside the __organ___ of ___Corti__. This organ generates nervous impulses for hearing.

organ of

Corti

11.18   The middle part of the inner ear that contains the utricle and saccule is the ___vestibule_____. Recall that the suffix _-ule_ means __small_____. The larger of two sacs in the vestibule is the __utricle_____, and the smaller sac is the __saccule_____.

vestibule

small

utricle, saccule

11.19   The labyrinth structures in partially circular shapes that generate nerve impulse with body movement are called __semicircular_____ __canals__. These nerve receptors help maintain the body's balance and equilibrium.

semicircular canals

SELF-INSTRUCTION: SYMPTOMATIC TERMS

Study the following:

Term	Meaning
anacusis *an'ă-kū'sis*	total hearing loss
otalgia *ō-tal'jē-ă* **otodynia** *ō-tō-din'ē-ă*	earache
otorrhagia *ō-tō-rā'jē-ă*	bleeding from the ear
otorrhea *ō-tō-rē'ă*	purulent drainage from the ear
paracusis *par'ă-kū'sis*	impaired hearing
tinnitus *ti-nī'tŭs*	a jingling; ringing or buzzing in the ear
vertigo *ver'ti-gō*	a turning round; dizziness

PROGRAMMED REVIEW: SYMPTOMATIC TERMS

Answers	Review
hearing hearing condition	**11.20** Recall that *acous/o* means _____, and the suffix *-acusis* refers to a _____ _____.
without anacusis	**11.21** Recall that the prefix *an-* means _____. Thus, the term for being without hearing, or having total hearing loss, is _____.
abnormal paracusis	**11.22** Recall that the prefix *para-* means alongside of or _____. The term for abnormal or impaired hearing is therefore _____.
ear pain otalgia	**11.23** The combining form *ot/o* means _____. Recall that the suffix *-algia* means _____. Thus, the term for ear pain, or an earache, is _____.

bleeding (to burst forth) otorrhagia	**11.24** The suffix *-rrhagia* means _____. The term for bleeding from the ear is _____.
-rrhea otorrhea	**11.25** Recall that the symptomatic suffix meaning discharge is ___rrhea___. The term for a <u>purulent drainage (discharge)</u> from the ear is ___otorrhea___.
tinnitus	**11.26** The Latin word tinnitus means to jingle. The symptom of hear- ing a jingling, ringing, or buzzing sound in the ear is ___tinnitus___.
vertigo	**11.27** The Latin word vertigo means dizziness or turning around. The symptom of feeling that one is turning around, or feeling dizzy, is called _____.

SELF-INSTRUCTION: DIAGNOSTIC TERMS

Study the following:

Term	Meaning
otitis externa (Fig. 11-2D) *ō-tī′tis eks-ter′nă*	inflammation of the external auditory canal
cerumen impaction *sĕ-rū′men im-pak′shŭn*	excessive buildup of wax in ear, often reducing hearing acuity, espe- cially in elderly persons
myringitis *mir-in-jī′tis* **tympanitis** *tim-pă-nī′tis*	inflammation of the eardrum
otitis media (Fig. 11-2C) *ō-tī′tis mē′dē-ă*	inflammation of the <u>middle ear</u>
aerotitis media *ār-o-tī′tis mē′dē-ă*	inflammation of the middle ear from changes in atmospheric pressure; often occurs in frequent air travel
eustachian **obstruction** *yū-stā′shŭn* *ob-strŭk′shŭn*	blockage of the eustachian tube usually as a result of infection, as in otitis media

labyrinthitis *lab'ĭ-rin-thī'tis*	inflammation of the labyrinth (inner ear)
otosclerosis *ō'tō-sklē-rō'sis*	hardening of the bony tissue in the ear
deafness *def'nes*	general term for partial or complete hearing loss
conductive hearing loss *kon-dŭk'tiv*	hearing impairment caused by interference with sound or vibratory energy in the external canal, middle ear, or ossicles
sensorineural hearing loss *sen'sōr-i-nū'răl*	hearing impairment caused by lesions or dysfunction of the cochlea or auditory nerve
presbyacusis *prez'bē-ă-kū'sis* **presbycusis** *prez-bē-kū'sis*	hearing impairment in old age

PROGRAMMED REVIEW: DIAGNOSTIC TERMS

Answers	Review
-itis	**11.28** Recall that the suffix for inflammation is _–itis_. Using the two different combining forms meaning eardrum, two terms for an inflamed tympanic membrane are ___myringitis___ and
myringitis	
tympanitis	___tympanitis___.
	11.29 There are three different types of otitis, depending on whether the inflammation is in the external ear, middle ear, or inner ear.
otitis	Inflammation of the external auditory canal is termed ___otitis___
externa	___externa___, and inflammation of the middle ear is termed
otitis media, inflammation	___otitis___ ___media___. Otitis interna, or _____ of the inner ear, is more commonly known as inflammation of the
labyrinthitis	labyrinth, or ___labyrinthitis___.
	11.30 Using the combining forms for both air and ear, the term for inflammation of the middle ear due to changes in atmospheric pressure is
aerotitis media	_____ _____.

11.31   Ear wax can build up in the external auditory canal and become impacted. This condition of excessive earwax is called _____

_____.

cerumen

impaction

11.32   The general term for partial or complete hearing loss is

_____, often called hearing impairment or hearing disabled. Hearing loss can be caused by mechanical <u>factors that interfere</u> <u>with transmission of sound vibrations through the external and middle</u> ear. This is called _____ *conductive* _____ hearing loss. The term for a hearing loss caused by <u>dysfunction of the cochlea</u> or <u>auditory nerve</u> is formed from combining forms referring to the <u>senses</u> and <u>nerves</u>:

_____ *Sensorineural* _____ hearing loss.

deafness

conductive

sensorineural

11.33   A middle ear infection such as <u>otitis media</u> may cause a blockage of the <u>eustachian tube</u> called an _____ *eustachian*

obstruction _____. This condition is common in young children when the tube is small and easily obstructed.

eustachian

obstruction

11.34   The combining for *scler/o* means hard. Recall that the suffix *-osis* means condition or _____ *increase* _____. The medical term for the hardening (increased hardness) of bony tissue in the ear is therefore

_____ *otosclerosis* _____.

increase

otosclerosis

11.35   The suffix *-acusis* means _____ *hearing* _____ *condition* _____.
Because the combining form *presby/o* means old age, the term for <u>hearing impairment in old age</u> is _____. This term has a shortened form: _____ *presbycusis* _____.

hearing condition

presbyacusis

presbycusis

SELF-INSTRUCTION: DIAGNOSTIC TESTS AND PROCEDURES

Study the following:

Test or Procedure	Explanation
audiometry *aw-de-om'_e-tre*	process of measuring hearing
audiometer *aw-dē-om'ĕ-ter*	instrument to measure hearing
audiogram *aw'dē-ō-gram*	record of hearing measurement
audiologist *aw-dē-ol'ō-jist*	the health professional who specializes in the study of hearing impairments
auditory acuity testing (Fig. 11-3) *aw'di-tōr-ē ă-kyū'i-tē*	physical assessment of hearing; useful in differentiating between conductive and sensorineural hearing loss
tuning fork	two-pronged, forklike instrument that vibrates when struck; used to test hearing, especially bone conduction
otoscopy (See Fig. 11-2) *ō-tos'kŏ-pē*	use of an otoscope to examine the external auditory canal and tympanic membrane
tympanometry *tim'pă-nom'ĕ-trē*	measurement of the conductibility of the tympanic membrane and ossicles of the middle ear by monitoring the response to external airflow pressures

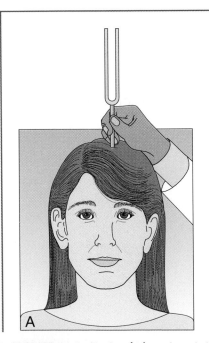
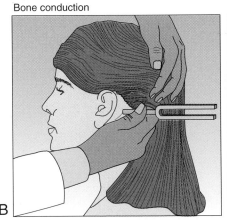
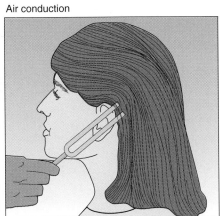

Bone conduction

Air conduction

A

B

■ **FIGURE 11-3.** Tuning fork testing. **A.** Webber test. **B.** Rinne test.

PROGRAMMED REVIEW: DIAGNOSTIC TESTS AND PROCEDURES

Answers	Review
-metry audiometry	**11.36** Recall that the suffix referring to process of measuring is _____. Thus, the term for the process of measuring hearing acuity is _____.
-meter audiometer	**11.37** The suffix for an instrument for measuring is _____. Thus, the term for an instrument that measures hearing is _____.
-gram audiogram	**11.38** The suffix for a record is _____. Thus, the term for a record of hearing measurement is _____.
-logist audiologist	**11.39** The suffix for someone who specializes in the study or treatment of a certain subject area is _____. Thus, the term for a health professional who specializes in the study of hearing impairments is an _____.
-metry tympanometry	**11.40** Again, the suffix for the process of measuring is _____. The measuring of the conductibility of the tympanic membrane is called _____. This test can be used to help diagnose someone with hearing loss.
auditory acuity middle, sensorineural	**11.41** A physical assessment of hearing that differentiates between conductive and sensorineural hearing loss is called _____ _____ testing. A conductive hearing loss is usually caused in the external or _____ ear, whereas a _____ hearing loss involves a problem in the cochlea or auditory nerve.
tuning fork bone	**11.42** The vibrating device that is used in acuity testing is a _____ _____. One test uses it to assess the conduction of vibration through _____.

ot/o	**11.43** The combining forms meaning ear are *aur/i* and _____. The latter form is used with the suffix referring to a process of examination to form this medical term for using an otoscope to examine the external auditory canal and tympanic membrane: _____. The tympanic membrane is also called the _____ or eardrum.
otoscopy	
tympanum	

SELF-INSTRUCTION: OPERATIVE TERMS

Study the following:

Term	Meaning
microsurgery *mī-krō-ser′jer-ē*	surgery with the use of a microscope used in delicate tissue such as the ear
myringotomy *mir-ing-got′ŏ-mē*	incision into the eardrum, most often for insertion of a small polyethylene (PE) tube to keep the canal open and prevent fluid buildup, such as occurs in otitis media
otoplasty *ō′tō-plas-tē*	surgical repair of the external ear
stapedectomy *stā-pĕ-dek′tō-mē*	excision of the stapes to correct otosclerosis
tympanoplasty *tim′p_a-no-plas-te*	vein graft of a scarred tympanic membrane to improve sound conduction

PROGRAMMED REVIEW: OPERATIVE TERMS

Answers	Review
-plasty otoplasty	**11.44** Recall that the suffix for surgical repair or reconstruction is __-plasty__. A surgeon might repair the external ear after trauma, for example. This is called an __otoplasty__.
tympanoplasty	**11.45** A surgical repair of the tympanic membrane is a __tympano plasty__. This may include a graft to a scarred membrane to improve sound conduction.
microsurgery	**11.46** Many of the ear's internal structures are small and delicate, and surgery must be performed using a microscope. This is called __mi_____.

11.47 Small children often have middle ear infections, called
otitis _media_. To drain fluids from the middle ear, small
tubes are often inserted into the eardrum after a surgical incision
through the eardrum. Recall that the suffix for incision is _-otomy_.
This procedure is called a _myringotomy_.

otitis media

-tomy

myringotomy

11.48 The suffix meaning excision is _-ectomy_. For the condition
of hardening of the bony tissue of the ear, _otosclerosis_,
the stapes may be excised to correct the hearing problem. This procedure is called a _stapedectomy_. The stapes is the last of
the three auditory _____ in the _____ ear.

-ectomy

otosclerosis

stapedectomy

ossicles (bones), middle

SELF-INSTRUCTION: THERAPEUTIC TERMS

Study the following:

Term	Meaning
ear lavage _lă-vahzh'_	irrigation of the external ear canal, often to remove excessive buildup of cerumen

ear instillation
in-sti-lā'shŭn
	introduction of a medicated solution into the external canal, usually administered by drop (gt) or drops (gtt) in the affected ear or ears:
	    AD (auris dextra) right ear
	    AS (auris sinistra) left ear
	    AU (aures unitas) both ears

COMMON THERAPEUTIC DRUG CLASSIFICATIONS

antibiotic _an'tē-bī-ot'ik_	drug that inhibits the growth of or destroys microorganisms; used to treat diseases caused by bacteria (e.g., otitis media)
antihistamine _an-tē-his'tă-men_	drug that blocks the effects of histamine
histamine _his'tă-men_	a regulatory body substance released in allergic reactions, causing swelling and inflammation of tissues; seen in hay fever and urticaria (hives)
anti-inflammatory _an'tē-in-flam'ă-tō-rē_	a drug that reduces inflammation
decongestant _dē-kon-jes'tant_	a drug that reduces congestion and swelling of membranes, such as those of the nose and eustachian tube in an infection

PROGRAMMED REVIEW: THERAPEUTIC TERMS

Answers	Review

11.49 The Latin term lavo means to wash. The process by which a cavity or organ is washed out by irrigating it with water or other fluid is called lavage. The external ear canal is often irrigated to remove buildup of cerumen in a process called ear _____. An excessive buildup of earwax is called _____ _____.

Answers: lavage; cerumen impaction

11.50 The administration of a medicated solution into the ear's external canal is an ear _____, usually introduced by _____ (gt) or drops _____ in the affected ear or ears: AS is the abbreviation for the _____ ear, AD is the _____ ear, and AU refers to _____ ears.

Answers: instillation; drop, gtt; left, right; both

11.51 A substance in the body that is released in allergic reactions and that causes swelling and inflammation of tissues is _____. A drug that acts to inhibit the effects of histamine is an _____. The prefix *anti-* means _____ or opposed to.

Answers: histamine; antihistamine; against

11.52 Similarly, a drug that reduces inflammation is an _____.

Answers: anti-inflammatory

11.53 The same prefix joined with the combining form for life (*bio*) denotes a drug class that acts to kill or inhibit microbial life. This drug is an _____.

Answers: antibiotic

11.54 The prefix *de-* means from, down, or _____. A drug that is given to reduce congestion, such as may occur in the eustachian tube in an infection, is a _____.

Answers: not; decongestant

THE EAR ■ 475

Practice Exercises

For the following terms, on the lines below the term, write out the indicated word parts: prefixes, combining forms, roots, and suffixes. Then define the word.

For example:
macrotia

$$\frac{macr/ot/ia}{P \quad R \quad S}$$

DEFINITION: large or long/ear/condition of

1. aerotitis

————————— / ————————— / ———
      R   R   S

DEFINITION: _____

2. otorrhea

——— / ———————
  CF   S uffix

DEFINITION: _____

3. myringoplasty

——— / ———————
  CF   S

DEFINITION: _____

4. acoustic

——— / ———————
  R   S

DEFINITION: _____

5. otogenous

————————— / ————————— / ———
    CF   R   S

DEFINITION: _____

6. ceruminolysis

——— / ———————
  CF   S

DEFINITION: _____

7. salpingoscope

——— / ———————
  CF   S

DEFINITION: _____

8. anacusis

———— / ————————
  P   S

DEFINITION: ————————————————————————————

9. audiometry

———— / ————————
  CF   S

DEFINITION: ————————————————————————————

10. tympanocentesis

———— / ————————
  CF   S

DEFINITION: ————————————————————————————

11. otodynia

———— / ————————
  CF   S

DEFINITION: ————————————————————————————

12. auricle

———— / ————————
  R   S

DEFINITION: ————————————————————————————

13. myringotomy

———— / ————————
  CF   S

DEFINITION: ————————————————————————————

14. ceruminosis

———— / ————————
  R   S

DEFINITION: ————————————————————————————

15. audiology

———— / ————————
  CF   S

DEFINITION: ————————————————————————————

Complete the medical term by writing the missing part:

16. oto_____osis = condition of hardening of the bony tissue of the ear

17. aero_____media = inflammation of the middle ear caused by changes in atmospheric pressure

18. _____logist = person who specializes in the study of hearing impairments

19. _____tomy = incision into the eardrum for the insertion of tubes

20. _____scope = instrument used to view the ear canal and tympanum

Write the correct medical term for each of the following:

21. inflammation of labyrinth _____

22. dizziness _____

23. bleeding from the ear _____

24. impaired hearing _____

25. hearing impairment of old age _____

26. ringing in the ear _____

27. excision of stapes to correct otosclerosis _____

28. excessive buildup of earwax _____

29. earache _____

30. the study of hearing _____

31. The introduction of a medicated solution into the external canal is called ear instillation.

Irrigation of the external ear canal is called ear _____

For each of the following, circle the combining form that corresponds to the meaning given:

32. **eardrum**	salping/o	ot/o	myring/o
33. **hearing**	ot/o	audi/o	angi/o
34. **wax**	cerumin/o	crin/o	scler/o
35. **eustachian tube**	tympan/o	myring/o	salping/o
36. **ear**	rhin/o	ot/o	or/o
37. **air**	acr/o	aur/i	aer/o

Write in the missing words on lines in the illustration:

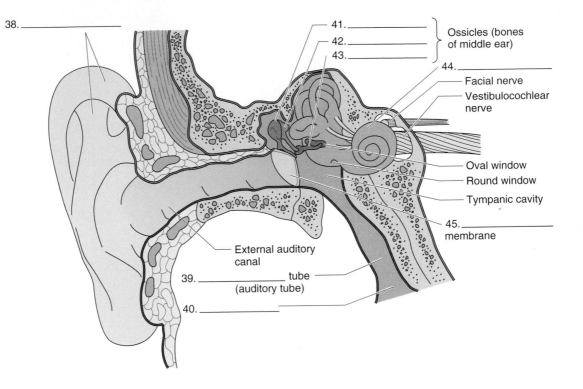

38. _____

41. _____ ⎫ Ossicles (bones
42. _____ ⎬ of middle ear)
43. _____ ⎭

44. _____
— Facial nerve
— Vestibulocochlear
  nerve

— Oval window
— Round window
— Tympanic cavity

45. _____
membrane

— External auditory
  canal

39. _____ tube
(auditory tube)

40. _____

For each of the following, circle the correct spelling of the term:

46. aerotitus	aerotitis	airotitis
47. cerumen	ceramen	ceruman
48. myrimogotomy	mirongotomy	myringotomy
49. anacusis	annacusis	anakusis
50. vertigo	vertago	verttigo
51. antihestamine	antihistamine	antehistamine
52. tinnitis	tinitus	tinnitus
53. stapedectomy	stapesectomy	stapedecktomy
54. defness	deafnass	deafness
55. eustation	eustachian	euhstation

Medical Record Analyses

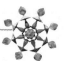

MEDICAL RECORD 11-1

Progress Note

S: This 21 y.o white male c/o a clogged Ⓡ ear c̄ increasing tinnitus. He has had a slight pharyngitis and nasal congestion × 7 d.

O: On PE there was moist infectious debris in the Ⓡ ear that was suctioned clear. The Ⓡ tympanum was dull and thickened. The Ⓛ external ear was clear and the tympanic membrane intact.

A: otitis media Ⓡ ear

P: *(1)* keep ears dry; *(2)* Rx PenVeek 250 mg #24 ʈ q.i.d. p.c. and h.s.; *(3)* RTO in 10 d for follow-up (f/u)

1. Summarize the subjective information:
   a. patient complains of clogged, ringing ears, sore throat, and stuffy nose
   b. patient has a clogged right ear, sore throat, stuffy nose, and dizziness
   c. patient's right eardrum is thick and dull and clogged with infectious matter, causing dizziness
   d. patient complains of a sore throat, stuffy nose, and a clogged right ear that is buzzing
   e. patient has a sore throat, stuffy nose, and purulent drainage from the right ear

2. What was the assessment?
   a. clogged right ear, sore throat, and stuffy nose
   b. inflammation of right middle ear
   c. inflammation of right external ear canal
   d. blockage of eustachian tube
   e. inflammation of right eardrum

3. When should the patient take the prescribed medication?
   a. twice in 24 hours
   b. before meals
   c. at bedtime
   d. four times a day
   e. every four hours

4. Which is true of the plan?
   a. patient should return to the office immediately if a fever develops
   b. patient is given ear drops and advised not to get ears wet fo 10 days
   c. doctor wants to examine the patient again in 10 days
   d. patient is given an antibiotic and advised to increase fluid intake
   e. if not better in 10 days, patient will be referred to a otolaryngologist

MEDICAL RECORD 11-2 FOR ADDITIONAL STUDY

CENTRAL MEDICAL CENTER

211 Medical Center Drive • Central City, US 90000-1234 • PHONE: (012) 125-6784 • FAX: (012) 125-9999

HISTORY

DATE OF ADMISSION: August 28, 20xx

HISTORY OF PRESENT ILLNESS: The patient is a 4-year-old white male with recurrent ear infections and ear congestion nonresponsive to antibiotic and decongestant therapy over the past 12 months. The patient also has a history of nasal obstruction and nasal speech. The patient is being admitted for myringotomy, polyethylene tubes, and examination of the nasopharynx and adenoidectomy. The patient has also seen other doctors who have recommended surgery, including Dr. Feldman and Dr. Saunders.

PAST MEDICAL HISTORY: Medications: None. Allergies: None. Hospitalizations: None. Surgeries: None. Childhood Diseases: Normal.

FAMILY HISTORY: No cancer or diabetes, although the patient's grandparents have a history of adult-onset diabetes.

SOCIAL HISTORY: Normal development except for speech.

REVIEW OF SYSTEMS: CARDIOVASCULAR: No hypertension and no heart murmurs. PULMONARY: No croup or asthma. GASTROINTESTINAL: No hepatitis. RENAL: Negative. ENDOCRINE: No diabetes. MUSCULOSKELETAL: No joint disease. HEMATOLOGIC: `No anemia or bleeding tendencies.

(continued)

R. Baird, M.D.

RB:nn

D: 8/28/20xx
T: 8/29/20xx

HISTORY AND PHYSICAL Page 1	PT. NAME: BALL, HANK F.
	ID NO: OP-372201
	ROOM: OPS
	ADM. DATE: August 28, 20xx
	ATT. PHYS: R. BAIRD, M.D.

MEDICAL RECORD 11-2 FOR ADDITIONAL STUDY

CENTRAL MEDICAL CENTER

211 Medical Center Drive • Central City, US 90000-1234 • PHONE: (012) 125-6784 • FAX: (012) 125-9999

PHYSICAL EXAMINATION

GENERAL: The patient is alert and afebrile.

HEENT: TMs are dull and slightly retracted; there is decreased mobility. There is dull light reflex bilaterally. No sinus tenderness on percussion of the maxillary or frontal sinuses; there are swollen turbinates on nasal examination. The oropharynx shows hypertrophic tonsils, and there are hypertrophic adenoids on examination of the nasopharynx.

CHEST: LUNGS: Clear to percussion and auscultation. HEART: Pulse: 88 and regular. There are no murmurs, gallops, or rubs. ABDOMEN: There are no masses or tenderness. No hepatosplenomegaly was noted. There was no costovertebral angle (CVA) tenderness.

BACK: Supple. There are no masses or tenderness. There is mild anterior cervical adenopathy.

RECTAL/GENITALIA: Deferred.

EXTREMITIES: There was no peripheral edema, and there were no ecchymoses.

IMPRESSION: CHRONIC OTITIS MEDIA WITH EFFUSION, NASAL SPEECH, AND NASAL OBSTRUCTION SECONDARY TO ADENOID HYPERTROPHY.

PLAN: The patient is to be admitted as an outpatient for adenoidectomy, myringotomy, and polyethylene (PE) tubes as noted above. The surgery and potential risks and complications have been discussed with the grandfather and mother as well as the possible need for further repeat myringotomy and PE tubes.

R. Baird, M.D.

RB:nn

D: 8/28/20xx
T: 8/29/20xx

HISTORY AND PHYSICAL Page 2	PT. NAME: BALL, HANK F. ID NO: OP-372201 ROOM NO: OPS ADM. DATE: August 28, 20xx ATT. PHYS: R. BAIRD, M.D.

MEDICAL RECORD 11-2 FOR ADDITIONAL STUDY

CENTRAL MEDICAL CENTER

211 Medical Center Drive • Central City, US 90000-1234 • PHONE: (012) 125-6784 • FAX: (012) 125-9999

OPERATIVE REPORT

DATE OF OPERATION: August 28, 20xx

PREOPERATIVE DIAGNOSIS: Chronic otitis media with effusion bilaterally and nasal obstruction with chronic adenoiditis and adenoid hypertrophy.

POSTOPERATIVE DIAGNOSIS: Chronic otitis media with effusion bilaterally and adenoid hypertrophy and chronic adenoiditis.

OPERATION PERFORMED: Bilateral myringotomy and tubes with adenoidectomy.

SURGEON: R. Baird, M.D.

ANESTHESIOLOGIST: F. Kodama, M.D.

PROCEDURE AND FINDINGS: After general anesthesia induction and oral intubation, the patient's ears were prepped and draped in the usual manner for microscopic myringotomy surgery. A myringotomy in the right ear was carried out following debridement of cerumen. Incision of the circumferential inferior anterior quadrant was carried out. Mucoid material was aspirated from the middle ear. A Shepard polyethylene tube was placed in position without difficulty. Cotton dressing was applied to the ear. The left ear was examined. A similar dull, nonmobile TM was noted. An inferior anterior myringotomy was carried out again, and thick mucoid material was aspirated. A Shepard polyethylene tube was inserted again in the left ear. Cotton dressing was applied to the ear canal. The patient was repositioned in the Rose's position for examination of the nasopharynx which was carried out with a palate retractor, McIvor mouth gag, tongue retractor, and was stabilized with the Mayo stand. The marked adenoid hypertrophy was noted, and the adenoidectomy was carried out with curette technique. The patient tolerated the procedure well, and following extubation, he was sent back to the recovery room in satisfactory postoperative condition.

FINAL DIAGNOSIS: Chronic otitis media with effusion bilaterally, with chronic adenoiditis, adenoid hypertrophy, and nasal obstruction.

R. Baird, M.D.

RB:as
D: 8/28/20xx   T: 8/29/20xx

OPERATIVE REPORT Page 1	PT. NAME: BALL, HANK F. ID NO: OP-372201 ROOM NO: OPS ATT. PHYS: R. BAIRD, M.D.

MEDICAL RECORD 11-2 FOR ADDITIONAL STUDY

Hank Ball, a preschooler, has had recurrent ear infections for one year that his doctor has not been able to treat successfully with antibiotics and other drugs. His preschool teacher also identified nasal speech patterns that his doctor later confirmed were related to his medical problems. After seeing several doctors who recommended surgery, Hank's parents have admitted him to Central Medical Center.

   Read Medical Record 11-2 (pages 480 to 482) for Hank Ball, and answer the following questions. These records are the history and physical examination before surgery and the subsequent operative report, both dictated by Dr. Baird, the surgeon.

1. Below are medical terms used in this record you have not yet encountered in this text. Underline each where it appears in the record and define below.

   hepatosplenomegaly _____

   turbinates _____

   extubation _____

2. In the left column, list the patient's 3 medical problems noted in the HPI; in the right column, write the diagnosis that pertains to each.

Medical Problem	Diagnosis
a. _____	
_____	_____
b. _____	
_____	_____
c. _____	

3. In your own words, explain how Hank's social history is related to his medical history.

   _____

   _____

   _____

4. Under the "Review of Systems," were any additional medical symptoms or problems identified? If so, list below.

   _____

   _____

5. What does it mean that at the time of the examination Hank was afebrile?

   _____

   _____

6. Carefully read the physical examination. Mark the body areas or systems in which Dr. Baird found any abnormalities.

_____ general   _____ back

_____ HEENT   _____ rectal/genitalia

_____ chest   _____ extremities

7. List the surgical procedures identified under "Plan," and briefly describe them in your own words, not using medical terminology.

a. _____

_____

_____

_____

b. _____

_____

_____

_____

c. _____

_____

_____

_____

8. In your own words, not using medical terminology, briefly describe oral intubation.

_____

_____

_____

9. Put the following operative actions in correct order by numbering them 1 to 11:

_____ removal of adenoids

_____ incision in right eardrum

_____ PE tube placement in right tympanum

_____ repositioning in Rose's position

_____ incision in left eardrum

_____ aspiration of right middle ear

_____ extubation

_____ removal of wax in right ear

_____ nasopharynx examination

_____ polyethylene tube placement in left tympanum

_____ intubation

10. In your own words, not using medical terminology, briefly describe the condition of Hank's adenoids before adenoidectomy.

_____

_____

Answers to Practice Exercises

1. aer/ot/itis
   R   R   S
   air or gas/ear/inflammation
2. oto/rrhea
   CF   S
   ear/discharge
3. myringo/plasty
   CF   S
   eardrum/surgical repair or reconstruction
4. acous/tic
   R   S
   hearing/pertaining to
5. oto/gen/ous
   CF R   S
   ear/origin or production/pertaining to
6. cerumino/lysis
   CF   S
   wax/breaking down or dissolution
7. salpingo/scope
   CF   S
   eustachian tube/instrument for examination
8. an/acusis
   P   S
   without/hearing condition
9. audio/metry
   CF   S
   hearing/process of measuring

10. tympano/centesis
    CF   S
    eardrum/puncture for aspiration
11. oto/dynia
    CF   S
    ear/pain
12. aur/icle
    R   S
    ear/small
13. myringo/tomy
    CF   S
    eardrum/incision
14. cerumin/osis
    R   S
    wax/condition or increase
15. audio/logy
    CF   S
    hearing/study of
16. otosclerosis
17. aerotitis media
18. audiologist
19. myringotomy
20. otoscope
21. labyrinthitis
22. vertigo
23. otorrhagia
24. paracusis
25. presbycusis
26. tinnitus
27. stapedectomy
28. cerumen impaction
29. otalgia
30. audiology
31. lavage

32. myring/o
33. audi/o
34. cerumin/o
35. salping/o
36. ot/o
37. aer/o
38 auricle
39. eustachian
40. pharynx
41. malleus
42. incus
43. stapes
44. cochlea
45. tympanic
46. aerotitis
47. cerumen
48. myringotomy
49. anacusis
50. vertigo
51. antihistamine
52. tinnitus
53. stapedectomy
54. deafness
55. eustachian

Answers to Medical Records Analyses

1. d
2. b
3. d
4. c

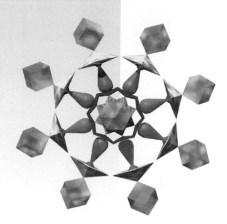

CHAPTER 12

Gastrointestinal System

Gastrointestinal System Overview

The gastrointestinal (GI) system has three functions:

* Digestion is the process of breaking down food by chewing, swallowing, and mixing in digestive juices to convert some of the food into absorbable molecules

* Absorption is the passage of digested food molecules through the walls of the intestines into the bloodstream to be carried to body cells.

* Excretion is the elimination of nonabsorbable nutrients and waste products from the body.

SELF-INSTRUCTION: COMBINING FORMS

Study the following:

Combining Form	Meaning
abdomin/o **celi/o** **lapar/o**	abdomen
an/o	anus
appendic/o	appendix
bil/i **chol/e**	bile
bucc/o	cheek
cheil/o	lip
col/o **colon/o**	colon

cyst/o	bladder or sac
dent/i	teeth
doch/o	duct
duoden/o	duodenum
enter/o	small intestine
esophag/o	esophagus
gastr/o	stomach
gingiv/o	gum
gloss/o lingu/o	tongue
hepat/o hepatic/o	liver
herni/o	hernia
ile/o	ileum
inguin/o	groin
jejun/o	jejunum (empty)
lith/o	stone
or/o stomat/o	mouth
pancreat/o	pancreas
peritone/o	peritoneum
phag/o	eat or swallow
proct/o	anus and rectum
pylor/o	pylorus (gatekeeper)
rect/o	rectum
sial/o	saliva
sigmoid/o	sigmoid colon (resembles s)
steat/o	fat
-emesis (additional suffix)	vomiting

PROGRAMMED REVIEW: COMBINING FORMS

Answers	Review

Answers

gastr/o

enter/o

GI

pertaining to, adjective

duodenal

herni/o

hernia

ile/o

ileostomy

jejun/o

inflammation

jejunitis

pancreat/o

pancreatitis

an/o

anal, rectum

rectal

Review

12.1 A gastroenterologist specializes in the gastrointestinal tract. This term is made from the combining forms for stomach and intestine. The combining form meaning stomach is _____. The combining form meaning small intestine is _____. The abbreviation for gastrointestinal is ____.

12.2 Many combining forms related to the gastrointestinal system are similar to the words in English for their meaning. For example, the combining form for duodenum is *duoden/o*. Recall that the suffix *-al*, meaning _____ ____, makes an _____ ending. The adjective form of duodenum is _____.

12.3 Other combining forms similar to their meaning are as follows. The combining form meaning hernia is _____. For example, a herniorrhaphy is suturing a repaired _____.

12.4 The combining form for ileum is _____. For example, the surgical creation of an opening for the ileum is _____.

12.5 The combining form for the jejunum is _____. Recall that the suffix *-itis* means _____. Inflammation of the jejunum is _____.

12.6 The combining form for pancreas is _____. Inflammation of the pancreas is _____.

12.7 The combining form for anus is _____. The common adjective form is _____. *Rect/o*, the combining form for _____, is derived from the Latin word rectus, meaning straight. The common adjective form is _____. The rectum was so named for its straight passage from the lower bowel to the anus. The combining form refer-

proct/o anus, rectum	ring to the anus and rectum is _____. A proctological examination involves the study of the _____ and _____.
appendic/o appendicitis	**12.8** The combining form for appendix is _____. Inflammation of the appendix is _____.
peritone/o examination peritoneoscopy	**12.9** The combining form for peritoneum is _____. Recall that the suffix *-scopy* means process of _____ with an instrument. The use of a peritoneoscope to examine the peritoneum is called _____.
pylor/o adjective pertaining to pyloric	**12.10** The combining form for pylorus is _____. Recall that the suffix *-ic* is an _____ ending meaning _____ _____. The adjective form of pylorus is _____.
sigmoid/o sigmoidoscopy	**12.11** The combining form for sigmoid colon is _____. The process of examining the sigmoid colon with a sigmoidoscope is called _____.
esophag/o pertaining to adjective esophageal	**12.12** The combining form for esophagus is _____. Recall that the suffix *-eal*, meaning _____ _____, makes an _____ ending. The adjective form of esophagus is _____.
puncture abdominocentesis celi/o, lapar/o	**12.13** In many other cases, there are two or more combining forms with the same meaning. One combining form meaning abdomen is *abdomin/o*. Recall that the suffix *-centesis* means a _____ for aspiration. A puncture of the abdomen for aspiration of an abdominal fluid is _____. Two other combining forms for abdomen are _____ and _____, as in the terms celiocentesis and laparoscopy.

col/o

colon, colon/o

12.14   There are two combining forms for colon. An inflammation of the colon is termed colitis, made with the combining form _____. The second form is used in the term colonoscopy, which is examination of the _____. That form is _____.

bil/i

presence

stone

bile

chol/e

12.15   There are two combining forms for bile. The term referring to the production of bile is biligenic, made from the combining form _____. The second combining form is used to make the term cholelithiasis. Recall that the suffix *-iasis* means formation of or _____ of, and the combining form *lith/o* means _____. Therefore, the term cholelithiasis refers to the presence of a stone in the gallbladder or _____ ducts. This combining form for bile is _____.

gloss/o

under

lingu/o

12.16   There are two combining forms for tongue. An inflammation of the tongue is glossitis. The combining form used to make that term is __gloss__. The other combining form is used in the term sublingual, which means _____ the tongue. This second combining form is _____.

or/o

condition

condition

stomat/o

12.17   There are two combining forms for mouth. One is used in the common adjective form oral. That combining form is or/o. The other is used, for example, in the term stomatosis, which refers to any ___condition___ of the oral cavity. Recall that the suffix *-osis* means increase or ___condition___. The combining form used in this term is ___stomat/o___.

enlargement

hepat/o

incision

hepatic/o

12.18   There are two combining forms meaning liver, which are similar. The term hepatomegaly, which means an _____ of the liver, is made from the combining form _____. The other is used to make the term hepaticotomy, which refers to an _____ into the liver. That combining form is _____.

bucc/o	**12.19** The adjective buccal pertains to the cheek. The combining form for cheek is _bucc/o_ .
repair cheil/o	**12.20** Recall that the suffix -*plasty* refers to surgical _repair_ or reconstruction. The term cheiloplasty means repair of the lip. The combining form for lip is _____.
chol/e doch/o	**12.21** A choledochotomy is an incision into a bile duct. The combining form for bile used here is _____. The combining form meaning duct is _____.
dent/i	**12.22** The adjective dental refers to the teeth. The combining form used to make this word is _____.
bile, bladder	**12.23** A cholecystectomy is excision of the gallbladder. Chol/e means _____, and *cyst/o* means _____ or sac. Put together, these two combining forms refer to the gallbladder, which holds bile.
gum(s) gingiv/o	**12.24** Gingivitis is inflammation of the _____. The combining form meaning gum is _gingiv/o_ .
sial/o	**12.25** A sialolith is a stone of the salivary gland or duct. The combining form for saliva is _sial_ .
inguin/o	**12.26** The adjective inguinal pertains to the groin. The combining form meaning groin is _____.
condition of without phag/o	**12.27** The term aphagia means the condition of being unable to eat. Recall that the suffix -*ia* means _____ _____, and the prefix *a*- means _____. The combining form meaning to eat or to swallow is _____.
dissolution steat/o	**12.28** Recall that the suffix -*lysis* means breaking down or _____. The term steatolysis refers to the breaking down of fat in digestion. The combining form for fat is _____.

blood	**12.29** The term hematemesis refers to the vomiting of blood (*hemat/o* is the combining form for _____). The suffix meaning vomiting is
-emesis	_____.

SELF-INSTRUCTION: ANATOMICAL TERMS (FIG. 12-1)

Study the following:

Term	Meaning
oral cavity mouth	cavity that receives food for digestion
salivary glands *sal'i-vār-ē*	three pairs of exocrine glands in the mouth that secrete saliva: the parotid, submandibular (submaxillary), and sublingual glands
cheeks	lateral walls of the mouth
lips	fleshy structures surrounding the mouth
palate *pal'ăt*	structure that forms the roof of the mouth, divided into the hard and soft palate
uvula *yū'vyū-lă*	small projection hanging from the back middle edge of the soft palate
tongue	muscular structure of the floor of the mouth covered by mucous membrane and held down by a bandlike membrane known as the frenulum
gums	tissue covering the processes of the jaws
teeth	hard bony projections in the jaws for masticating (chewing) food
pharynx *far'ingks*	throat; passageway for food traveling to the esophagus and air traveling to the larynx
esophagus *ē-sof'ă-gŭs*	muscular tube that moves food from the pharynx to the stomach
stomach *stŭm'ŭk*	saclike organ that chemically mixes and prepares food received from the esophagus
cardiac sphincter *kar'dē-ak sfingk'ter*	opening from the esophagus to the stomach (sphincter = band)
pyloric sphincter *pī-lōr'ik sfingk'ter*	opening from the stomach into the duodenum
small intestine *in-tes'tin*	tubular structure that digests food received from the stomach
duodenum *dū-ō-dē'nŭm*	first portion of the small intestine

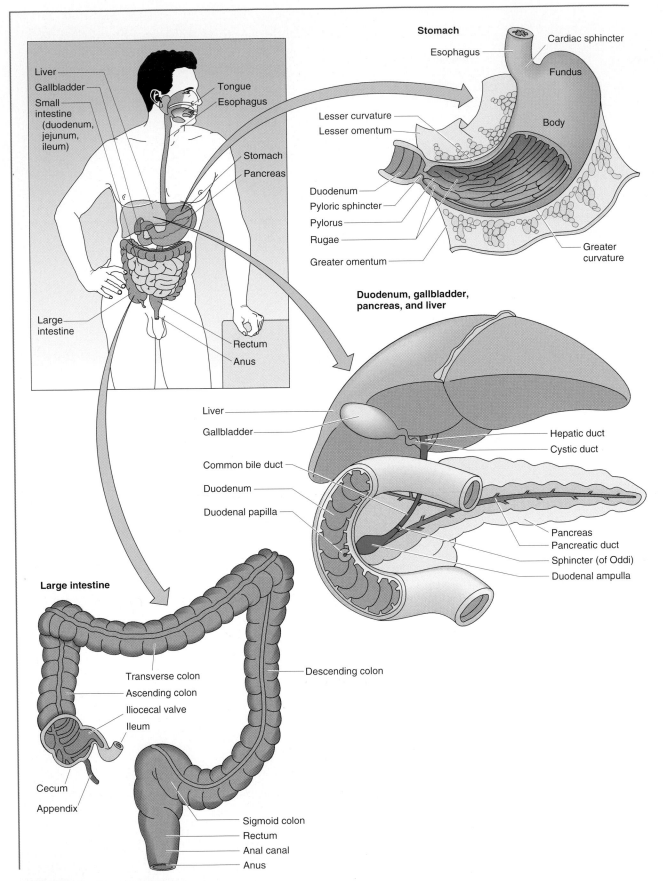

■ **FIGURE 12-1.** Gastrointestinal system.

jejunum *jĕ-jū′nŭm*	second portion of the small intestine
ileum *il′ē-ŭm*	third portion of the small intestine
large intestine	larger tubular structure that receives the liquid waste products of digestion, reabsorbs water and minerals, and forms and stores feces for defecation
cecum *se′kŭm*	first part of the large intestine
vermiform appendix *ver′mi-fōrm ă-pen′diks*	wormlike projection of lymphatic tissue hanging off the cecum with no digestive function; may help resist infection (vermi = worm)
colon *kō′lon*	portions of the large intestine extending from the cecum to the rectum, identified by direction or shape
ascending colon *as-send′ing*	portion of colon that extends upward from the cecum
transverse colon *trans-vers′*	portion of colon that extends across from the ascending cecum
descending colon *dē-send′ing*	portion of colon that extends down from the transverse colon
sigmoid colon *sig′moyd*	portion of colon (resembling an S) that terminates at the rectum
rectum *rek′tŭm*	distal (end) portion of the large intestine
rectal ampulla *rek′tăl am-pūl′lă*	dilated portion of the rectum just above the anal canal
anus *a′nŭs*	opening of the rectum to the outside of the body
feces *fē′sēz*	waste formed by absorption of water in the large intestine; usually solid
defecation *def-ĕ-kā′shŭn*	evacuation of feces from the rectum
peritoneum *per′i-tō-ne′ŭm*	membrane surrounding the entire abdominal cavity, consisting of the parietal layer (lining the abdominal wall) and visceral layer (covering each organ in the abdomen)
peritoneal cavity *per-i-tō-nē′ăl*	space between the parietal and visceral peritoneum
omentum *ō-men′tŭm*	an extension of the peritoneum attached to the stomach and connecting it with other abdominal organs

liver	organ in the upper right quadrant that produces bile, which is secreted into the duodenum during digestion
gallbladder *gawl′blad-er*	receptacle that stores and concentrates the bile produced in the liver
pancreas *pan′krē-as*	gland that secretes pancreatic juice into the duodenum, where it mixes with bile to digest food
biliary ducts *bil′ē-ār-ē*	ducts that convey bile; include the hepatic, cystic, and common bile ducts

PROGRAMMED REVIEW: ANATOMICAL TERMS

Answers	Review

12.30   Let's trace the anatomy of the gastrointestinal system from be-

ginning to end. Food is taken in at the _____ cavity, or mouth,

oral

where the digestive process begins as food is chewed and saliva from

the _____ glands is mixed with the food. Structures of the

salivary

mouth include the cheeks, lips, tongue, teeth, and gums. The roof of the

mouth, or _____, is divided into the hard and soft palate. The

palate

small tissue projection hanging from the back edge of the soft palate is

the ___*uvula*___.

uvula

12.31   Chewed food then passes through the throat to the esophagus

and then to the stomach. The medical term for the throat is the

_____. From the pharynx the food reaches the

pharynx

_____, which is a muscular tube descending to the

esophagus

stomach. At the bottom of the esophagus is the _____

cardiac

sphincter, the opening from the esophagus to the _____.

stomach

12.32   The saclike organ that mixes and prepares food received from

the esophagus is the _____. From the stomach, food moves

stomach

next to the small intestine through the _____ sphincter.

pyloric

12.33   The small intestine does most of the digestive work. It has three

segments. The first, connected to the stomach at the pyloric

sphincter, duodenum	_____, is the _____. After the duodenum
jejunum	comes the second portion, the _____. After the jejunum
ileum	comes the third portion, the _____. From the ileum, the food passes into the large intestine.

12.34 Other organs produce substances to help the small intestine digest food. Bile is produced in the _____ and conveyed through

liver

_____ ducts to the gallbladder. The _____

biliary, gallbladder

stores and concentrates the bile produced in the liver, which is then

conveyed to the first portion of the small intestine, called the

duodenum

_____.

12.35 Pancreatic juice is also secreted into the duodenum from the

gland where it is produced, the _____. This also assists in

pancreas

digestion.

12.36 After leaving the small intestine, the digested food enters the

large

_____ intestine, where water and minerals are reabsorbed, and

wastes are formed into feces for defecation. The first part of the large in-

cecum

testine is called the _____. Hanging from the cecum is a projec-

tion of tissue with no known digestive function, called the vermiform

appendix

_____.

colon

12.37 The next part of the large intestine, the _____, is identi-

fied in four sections named for their direction or shape. The portion of

the colon extending upward from the cecum is the

ascending

_____ colon. The portion that extends from the ascend-

transverse

ing portion across the body is the _____ colon. The por-

tion extending down from the transverse colon is the

descending

_____ colon. The S-shaped portion at the end of the

sigmoid

descending colon is the _____ colon. The sigmoid colon ter-

rectum

minates at the _____, the end of the large intestine.

ampulla

anus

feces

defecation

12.38 The dilated portion of the rectum just above the anal canal is the rectal _____. Feces leave the body through the opening of the rectum, the _____. The waste formed in the large intestine is called _____. The evacuation of feces from the rectum is called _____.

peritoneum

abdominal

peritoneal

peritoneum

12.39 Surrounding the entire abdominal cavity is a membrane called the _____. The peritoneum lines not only the _____ cavity (the parietal layer) but also each organ in the abdomen (visceral layer). The space between the parietal and visceral peritoneum is the _____ cavity. The omentum is an extension of the _____ attached to the stomach and connecting it with other abdominal organs.

Anatomical and Clinical Divisions of the Abdomen

Anatomical and clinical divisions of the abdomen provide reference points to describe abdominal locations. There are nine specific anatomical divisions and four general clinical divisions (Figs. 12-2–12-4). All references are based on the *patient's* right or left.

SELF-INSTRUCTION: ANATOMICAL DIVISIONS (FIG. 12-2)

Study the following:

Region	Location
hypochondriac regions *hī-pō-kon'drē-ak*	upper lateral regions beneath the ribs
epigastric region *ep-i-gas'trik*	upper middle region below the sternum
lumbar regions *lŭm'bar*	middle lateral regions
umbilical region *ŭm-bil'i-kăl*	region of the navel
inguinal regions *ing'gwi-năl*	lower lateral groin regions
hypogastric region *hī-pō-gas'trik*	region below the navel

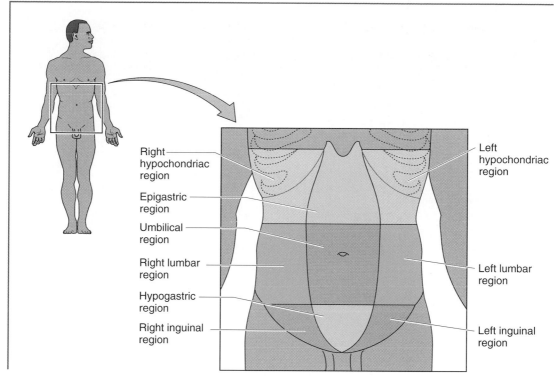

■ FIGURE 12-2. Anatomic divisions of the abdomen.

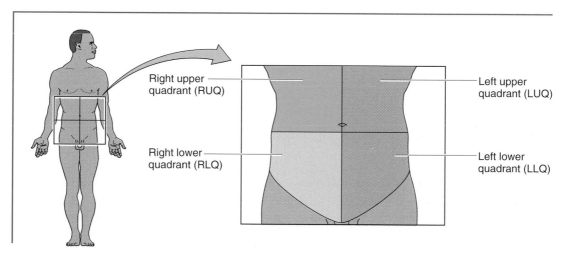

■ FIGURE 12-3. Clinical divisions of the abdomen.

PROGRAMMED REVIEW: ANATOMICAL DIVISIONS

Answers	Review

12.40 The abdomen is divided into several anatomical regions for reference purposes. Recall that the prefix *hypo-* means _____ or deficient. The upper lateral regions beneath the ribs (chondro = cartilaginous) are the _____ regions.

below

hypochondriac

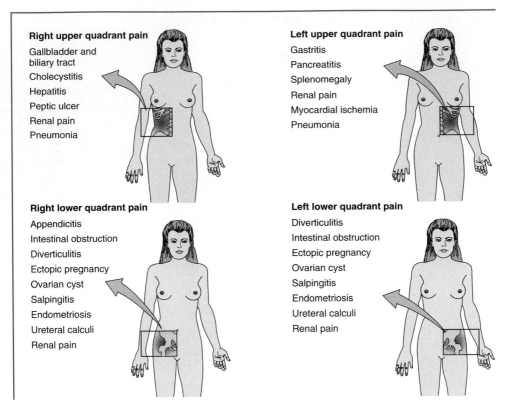

Right upper quadrant pain

Gallbladder and
biliary tract

Cholecystitis

Hepatitis

Peptic ulcer

Renal pain

Pneumonia

Left upper quadrant pain

Gastritis

Pancreatitis

Splenomegaly

Renal pain

Myocardial ischemia

Pneumonia

Right lower quadrant pain

Appendicitis

Intestinal obstruction

Diverticulitis

Ectopic pregnancy

Ovarian cyst

Salpingitis

Endometriosis

Ureteral calculi

Renal pain

Left lower quadrant pain

Diverticulitis

Intestinal obstruction

Ectopic pregnancy

Ovarian cyst

Salpingitis

Endometriosis

Ureteral calculi

Renal pain

■ **FIGURE 12-4.** Common sites of abdominal pain characteristic of various conditions.

upon gastr/o epigastric	**12.41** The prefix *epi-* means _____. The combining form meaning stomach is _____. Thus, the name for the upper middle region below the sternum and lying approximately upon the stomach is the _____ region.
lumbar	**12.42** The middle lateral areas of the abdomen, to each side of the lumbar spine, are the _____ regions.
umbilical	**12.43** The medical term for the navel is the umbilicus. The anatomical area in the region of the navel is the _____ region.
inguin/o inguinal	**12.44** The combining form for groin is _____. The lower lateral groin regions are the _____ regions.
hypo- gastr/o hypogastric	**12.45** The prefix for below is _____, and the combining form for stomach is _____. Thus, the area below the navel, approximately below the stomach, is the _____ region.

SELF-INSTRUCTION: SYMPTOMATIC TERMS

Study the following:

Term	Meaning
anorexia *an-ō-rek′sē-ă*	loss of appetite (orexia = appetite)
aphagia *ă-fā′jē-ă*	inability to swallow
ascites (Fig. 12-5) *ă-sī′tēz*	an accumulation of fluid in the peritoneal cavity (ascos = bag)
buccal *bŭk′ăl*	in the cheek
diarrhea *dī-ă-rē′ă*	frequent loose or liquid stools

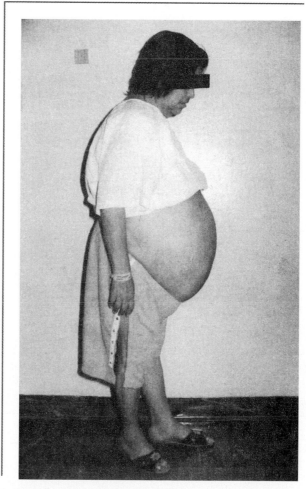

■ **FIGURE 12-5.** Side view of patient showing massive ascites and distention of abdomen.

constipation *kon-sti-pā'shŭn*	infrequent or incomplete bowel movements characterized by hardened, dry stool that is difficult to pass (constipo = to press together)
dyspepsia *dis-pep'sē-ă*	indigestion (pepsis = digestion)
dysphagia *dis-fā'jē-ă*	difficulty in swallowing
eructation *ē-rŭk-tā'shŭn*	belch
flatulence *flat'yū-lens*	gas in the stomach or intestines (flatus = a blowing)
halitosis *hal-i-tō'sis*	bad breath (halitus = breath)
hematochezia *hē'mă-tō-kē'zē-ă*	red blood in stool (chezo = defecate)
hematemesis *hē-mă-tem'ă-sis*	vomiting blood
hepatomegaly *hep'ă-tō-meg'ă-lē*	enlargement of the liver
hyperbilirubinemia *hī'per-bil'i-rū-bi-nē'mē-ă*	excessive level of bilirubin (bile pigment) in the blood
icterus *ik'ter-ŭs* **jaundice** *jawn'dis*	yellow discoloration of the skin, sclera (white of the eye), and other tissues caused by excessive bilirubin in the blood (jaundice = yellow)
melena *me-lē'nă*	dark colored, tarry stool caused by old blood
nausea *naw'zē-ă*	feeling of sick in the stomach
steatorrhea *ste'ă-tō-rē'ă*	feces containing fat
sublingual *sŭb-ling'gwăl* **hypoglossal** *hī-pō-glos'ăl*	under the tongue

PROGRAMMED REVIEW: SYMPTOMATIC TERMS

Answers	Review
condition of	**12.46** Recall that the suffix -*ia* means _____ ____.
without	The prefix *a*- means _____. Again, the combining form
phag/o	meaning to eat or swallow is _____. Therefore, the term for the
	condition of being unable to swallow (without swallowing) is
aphagia	_____.
faulty	**12.47** The prefix *dys*- means painful, difficult, or _____. The
	term for the condition of having difficulty swallowing is therefore
dysphagia	_____.
anorexia	**12.48** The condition of loss of (or without) appetite (orexia = appetite) is _____.
dyspepsia	**12.49** The condition of indigestion, or painful digestion (pepsis = digestion), is _____.
adjective	**12.50** The suffix -*al* is an _____ ending meaning
pertaining to	_____ ____. The combining form meaning cheek is
bucc/o, buccal	_____. The adjective form pertaining to the cheek is _____.
ascites	**12.51** Formed from the root ascos (meaning bag), the term for an accumulation of fluid in the peritoneal cavity is _____.
eructation	**12.52** From the Latin word eructo comes this term for belch: _____.
flatulence	**12.53** From the Latin word flatus (meaning a blowing) comes this term for gas in the stomach or intestines: _____.
condition	**12.54** The suffix -*osis* means increase or _____. The
halitosis	condition of having bad breath is called _____.

-emesis hematemesis	**12.55** A combining form for blood is *hemat/o*. Again, the suffix meaning vomiting is _____. The term for vomiting blood is _____.
hematochezia	**12.56** Formed from the root word chezo (defecate) comes this term for the condition of having red blood in the stool: _____
hepat/o, -megaly hepatomegaly	**12.57** The two combining forms for liver are *hepatic/o* and _____. Recall that the suffix for enlargement is _____. Using the latter combining form for liver, the term for enlargement of the liver is _____.
-emia excessive hyperbilirubinemia	**12.58** Recall that the suffix meaning blood condition is _____. The prefix *hyper-* means above or _____. The condition of having excessive bilirubin in the blood is _____
icterus	**12.59** When there is excessive bilirubin in the blood, the skin is discolored yellow. This is called jaundice or _____.
melena	**12.60** From the Greek word melaina (meaning black) comes this term for dark colored, tarry stool caused by old blood: _____.
nausea	**12.61** From a Greek word originally referring to seasickness comes this term for feeling sick in the stomach: _____.
steat/o discharge steatorrhea	**12.62** Again, the combining form for fat is _____. Recall that the suffix *-rrhea* means _____. The term for fat in the feces (a discharge of fat) is _____.
lingu/o, below or under sublingual	**12.63** The two combining forms for tongue are *gloss/o* and _____. The prefix *sub-* means _____. Made with the latter combining form, the term for under the tongue is _____.
through discharge	**12.64** Formed from the prefix *dia-*, meaning across or _____, and the suffix *rrhea-*, meaning _____, the term describ-

| diarrhea | ing frequent, loose or liquid stool is _____. In contrast, the term describing hardened, dry stool that is difficult to pass is |
| constipation | _____. |

SELF-INSTRUCTION: DIAGNOSTIC TERMS

Study the following:

Term	Meaning
stomatitis *stō-mă-tī′tis*	inflammation of the mouth
sialoadenitis *sī′ă-lō-ad-ĕ-nī′tis*	inflammation of a salivary gland
parotiditis *pă-rot-i-dī′tis* **parotitis** *par-ō-tī′tis*	inflammation of the parotid gland, also called mumps
cheilitis *kī-lī′tis*	inflammation of the lip
glossitis *glo-sī′tis*	inflammation of the tongue
ankyloglossia *ang′ki-lō-glos′ē-ă*	a defect of the tongue characterized by a short, thick frenulum (*ankyl/o* = crooked or stiff)
gingivitis *jin-ji-vī′tis*	inflammation of the gums
esophageal varices (Fig. 12-6) *ē-sof′ă-jē′ăl*	swollen, twisted veins in the esophagus that are especially susceptible to ulceration and hemorrhage
esophagitis *ē-sof-ă-jī′tis*	inflammation of the esophagus
gastritis (Fig. 12-6) *gas-trī′tis*	inflammation of the stomach
gastroesophageal reflux disease (GERD) *gas′trō-ē-sof′ă-jē′ăl rē′flŭks di-zēz′*	a backflow of contents of the stomach into the esophagus, often resulting from abnormal function of the lower esophageal sphincter, causing burning pain in the esophagus
pyloric stenosis *pī-lōr′ik ste-nō′sis*	a narrowed condition of the pylorus

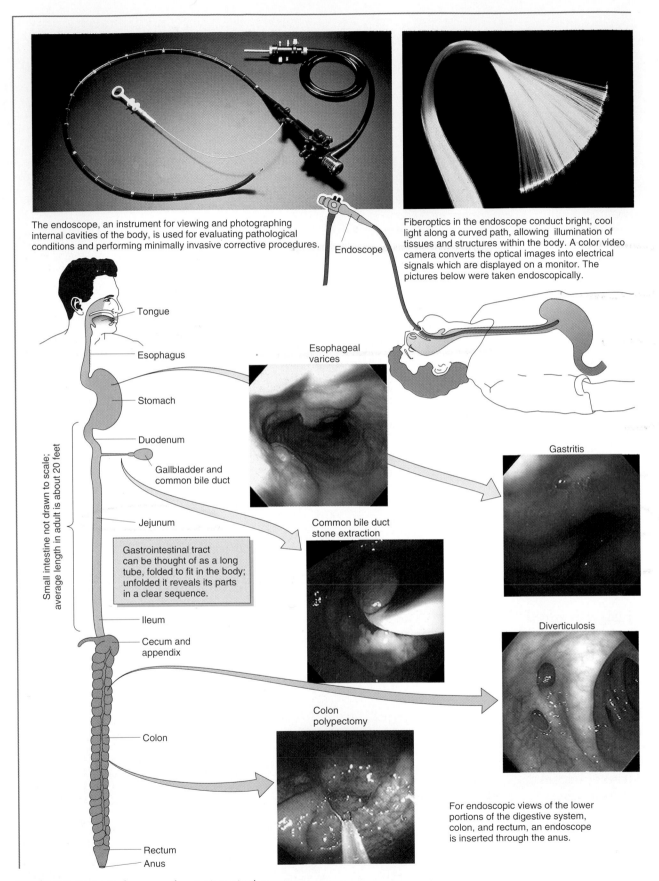

The endoscope, an instrument for viewing and photographing internal cavities of the body, is used for evaluating pathological conditions and performing minimally invasive corrective procedures.

Endoscope

Fiberoptics in the endoscope conduct bright, cool light along a curved path, allowing illumination of tissues and structures within the body. A color video camera converts the optical images into electrical signals which are displayed on a monitor. The pictures below were taken endoscopically.

Tongue

Esophagus

Stomach

Duodenum

Gallbladder and common bile duct

Jejunum

Ileum

Cecum and appendix

Colon

Rectum

Anus

Small intestine not drawn to scale; average length in adult is about 20 feet

Gastrointestinal tract can be thought of as a long tube, folded to fit in the body; unfolded it reveals its parts in a clear sequence.

Esophageal varices

Gastritis

Common bile duct stone extraction

Diverticulosis

Colon polypectomy

For endoscopic views of the lower portions of the digestive system, colon, and rectum, an endoscope is inserted through the anus.

■ **FIGURE 12-6.** Endoscopy of gastrointestinal system.

Term	Definition
peptic ulcer disease (PUD) *pep'tik ŭl'ser di-zēz'*	a sore on the mucous membrane of the stomach, duodenum, or any other part of the gastrointestinal system exposed to gastric juices; commonly caused by infection with *Helicobacter pylori* bacteria (pept/o = to digest)
gastric ulcer *gas'trik*	ulcer located in the stomach
duodenal ulcer *dū'ō-dē'năl*	ulcer located in the duodenum
gastroenteritis *gas'trō-en-ter-ā'tis*	inflammation of stomach and small intestine
enteritis *en-ter-ī'tis*	inflammation of small intestine
ileitis *il-ē-ī'tis*	inflammation of the lower portion of the small intestine
colitis *kō-lī'tis*	inflammation of the colon (large intestine)
ulcerative colitis *ŭl'ser-ă-tiv*	chronic inflammation of the colon along with ulcerations
diverticulum *dī-ver-tik'yū-lŭm*	an abnormal side pocket in the gastrointestinal tract usually related to lack of dietary fiber
diverticulosis (Fig. 12-6) *dī'ver-tik-yū-lō'sis*	presence of diverticula in the gastrointestinal tract, especially the bowel
diverticulitis *dī'ver-tik-yū-lī'tis*	inflammation of diverticula
dysentery *dis'en-tār-ē*	inflammation of the intestine characterized by frequent, bloody stools, most often caused by bacteria or protozoa (e.g., amebic dysentery)
appendicitis *ă-pen-di-sī'tis*	inflammation of the appendix
hernia *her'nē-ă*	protrusion of a part from its normal location
hiatal hernia (*see* Fig. 12-13) *hī-ā'tăl*	protrusion of part of the stomach upward through the opening in the diaphragm
inguinal hernia *ing'gwi-năl*	protrusion of a loop of the intestine through layers of the abdominal wall in the inguinal region
incarcerated hernia *in-kar'ser-ā-ted*	hernia that is swollen and fixed within a sac, causing an obstruction
strangulated hernia *strang'gyū-lā-ted*	hernia that is constricted, cut off from circulation, and likely to become gangrenous

umbilical hernia *ŭm-bil'i-kăl*	protrusion of the intestine through a weakness in the abdominal wall around the umbilicus (navel)
intussusception (Fig.12-7) *in'tŭs-sŭ-sep'shŭn*	prolapse of one part of the intestine into the lumen of the adjoining part (intus = within; suscipiens = to take up)
volvulus (Fig. 12-8) *vol'vū-lŭs*	twisting of the bowel on itself, causing obstruction (volvo = to roll)
polyposis (Fig. 12-6) *pol'i-pō'sis*	multiple polyps in the intestine and rectum with a high potential for becoming malignant
polyp *pol'ip*	tumor on a stalk
proctitis *prok-tī'tis*	inflammation of the rectum and anus
anal fistula (Fig. 12-9) *a'n_al fis'tyu-l_a*	an abnormal tubelike passageway from the anus that may connect with the rectum (fistula = pipe)
hemorrhoid *hem'ŏ-royd*	swollen, twisted vein (varicosity) in the anal region (haimorrhois = a vein likely to bleed)

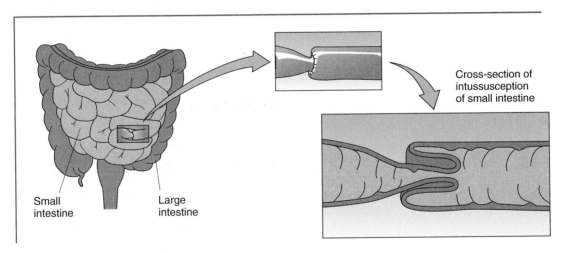

Cross-section of intussusception of small intestine

Small intestine

Large intestine

■ **FIGURE 12-7.** Intussusception.

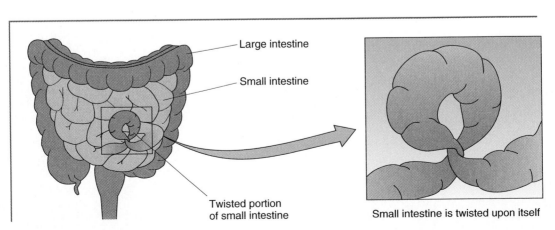

Large intestine

Small intestine

Twisted portion of small intestine

Small intestine is twisted upon itself

■ **FIGURE 12-8.** Volvulus.

peritonitis *per'i-tē-nī'tis*	inflammation of the peritoneum
hepatitis *hep-ă-tī'tis*	inflammation of the liver
hepatitis A	infectious inflammation of the liver caused by the hepatitis A virus (HAV), usually transmitted orally through fecal contamination of food or water
hepatitis B	inflammation of the liver caused by the hepatitis B virus (HBV), which is transmitted sexually or by exposure to contaminated blood or body fluids
hepatitis C	inflammation of the liver caused by the hepatitis C virus (HCV), transmitted by exposure to infected blood (rarely contracted sexually)
cirrhosis *sir-rō'sis*	chronic disease characterized by degeneration of liver tissue most often caused by alcoholism or a nutritional deficiency (cirrho = yellow)
cholangitis *kō-lan-jī'tis*	inflammation of the bile ducts
cholecystitis *kō'lē-sis-tī'tis*	inflammation of the gallbladder
cholelithiasis (Fig. 12-10) *kō'lē-li-thī'ă-sis*	presence of stones in the gallbladder or bile ducts
choledocholithiasis (Fig. 12-6 and 12-10) *kō-led'ō-kō-lith-ī'ă-sis*	presence of stones in the common bile duct
pancreatitis *pan'krē-ă-tī'tis*	inflammation of the pancreas

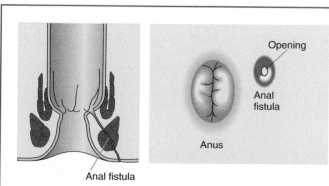

■ **FIGURE 12-9.** Anal fistula.

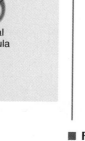

■ **FIGURE 12-10.** Sites of gallstones.

PROGRAMMED REVIEW: DIAGNOSTIC TERMS

Answers	Review

-itis

12.65 The suffix for inflammation is _____. Many parts of the gastrointestinal system can become inflamed, and thus there are many diagnostic terms for inflammation of different organs. The two combining

stomat/o

forms for mouth are (or/o) and ___Stomat/o___. Made with the latter,

stomatitis

the term for inflammation of the mouth is ___Stomatitis___.

sial/o

12.66 The combining form for saliva is ___sial/o___. Using that combining form along with *aden/o*, meaning gland, the term for inflamma-

sialoadenitis

tion of a salivary gland is ___Sialoadenitis___. Inflamma-

parotiditis or parotitis

tion of the parotid gland is called ___parotiditis___ (also mumps).

cheil/o

12.67 The combining form meaning (lip) is ___cheil/o___. Inflamma-

cheilitis

tion of the lip is ___cheilitis___.

12.68 The two combining forms for tongue are *lingu/o* and

gloss/o

___gloss/o___. Using the latter, the term for inflammation of the

glossitis

tongue is ___glossitis___. The combining form for gums is

gingiv/o

___gingiv/o___, and the term for inflammation of the gums is

gingivitis

___gingivitis___.

esophag/o

12.69 The combining form for esophagus is _____, and

esophagitis

the term for inflammation of the esophagus is _____.

gastr/o

The combining form for stomach is _____, and the term for in-

gastritis

flammation of the stomach is _____.

enter/o

12.70 The combining form for small intestine is _____, and

enteritis

the term for inflammation of the small intestine is _____. Inflammation of both the stomach and the small intestine is

gastroenteritis

_____.

ile/o

12.71 The combining form for the ileum is _____, and inflamma-

ileitis

tion of the ileum (lower portion of small intestine) is _____.

col/o

The two combining forms for the colon are *colon/o* and _____. Made from the latter form, the term for inflammation of the colon is

colitis

_____. When this occurs chronically along with ulcerations,

ulcerative colitis

it is called _____ _____.

12.72   Recall that the suffix *-osis* means increase or

condition of

_____ ____. The condition of having diverticula (abnormal little pockets) in the gastrointestinal tract is called

diverticulosis

_____. If the diverticula are inflamed, this

diverticulitis

is called _____.

appendic/o

12.73   The combining form for the appendix is _____,

appendicitis

and inflammation of the appendix is termed _____.

peritone/o

The combining form for the peritoneum is _____, and

peritonitis

inflammation of the peritoneum is _____.

12.74   The combining form referring to the anus and rectum is

proct/o

_____. It is used in the term for inflammation of the rectum

proctitis

and anus: _____.

gallbladder

12.75   *Cholecyst/o* refers to the _____. Inflammation of the gallbladder is termed _____.

cholecystitis

Formed from *chol/e* (bile) and *angi/o* (vessels), together referring to bile ducts, the term for inflammation of the bile ducts is

cholangitis

_____.

pancreat/o

12.76   The combining form for pancreas is _____. Inflammation of the pancreas is _____.

pancreatitis

12.77   The two combining forms for liver are hepatic/o and

hepat/o

_____. Made from the latter, the term for inflammation of the

hepatitis

liver is _____. The several types of hepatitis are named

A

after the viruses that cause them. Hepatitis __ is transmitted orally

fecal, B	through _____ contamination of food or water. Hepatitis ___ is
sexually	transmitted _____ or by exposure to contaminated
blood, C	_____ or body fluids. Hepatitis ___ is transmitted primarily
blood	through exposure to infected _____.
condition	**12.78** Again, the suffix *-osis* refers to an increase or _____. The chronic liver condition that causes yellowing (cirrho = yellow) of
cirrhosis	tissues is _____. It is usually caused by alcoholism or a nutritional deficiency.
polyposis	**12.79** The condition of having multiple polyps (stalked tumors) in the intestine is called _____.
pyloric stenosis	**12.80** Stenosis refers to a narrowed condition of an organ. A narrowing of the pylorus is termed _____ _____.
condition of	**12.81** The combining form *ankyl/o* means (crooked) or (stiff.) Recall that the suffix (*-ia*) means a _condition of_ ___. The two combining
gloss/o	forms for tongue are <u>lingu/o</u> and _gloss/o_. Made from the latter, the term for a condition of a <u>tongue defect with a (stiff,</u> short (frenulum) is
ankyloglossia	_ankylo glossia_.
esophageal	**12.82** Varices are swollen, twisted veins. When they occur in the esophagus, this condition is called _____
varices	_____.
gastroesophageal	**12.83** Reflux is a backflow. When stomach contents flow back into the esophagus, this is called _____
reflux disease	_____ _____ (GERD).
	12.84 An ulcer is a sore on the skin or a mucous membrane. The disease characterized by ulcer formation on the mucous membrane of the stomach, duodenum, or any other part of the GI system exposed to gas-
peptic ulcer disease	tric juices is called _____ _____ _____.

gastric	(PUD). An ulcer located in the stomach is called a _____ ulcer, and an ulcer in the duodenum is called a _____ ulcer.
duodenal	

12.85 The prefix *dys-* means painful, difficult, or faulty. The

enter/o

combining form for small intestine is _____. The suffix *-y*

condition of (process of)

means _____ _____. The condition of a painful inflammation of the intestine (usually caused by bacteria or protozoa) is

dysentery

called _____.

12.86 The protrusion of a part from its normal location is termed a

hernia

_____. Hernias are often named according to the location of
the protrusion. The protrusion of a part of the stomach upward through

hiatal

the opening in the diaphragm (hiatus) is called a _____ hernia.
Protrusion of a loop of intestine through the abdominal wall in the in-

inguinal

guinal region is an _____ hernia. Protrusion of the intestine through a weakness in the abdominal wall around the umbilicus is

umbilical

called an _____ hernia.

12.87 A hernia that is swollen and becomes fixed within a sac is an

incarcerated

_____ hernia. A hernia that becomes constricted

strangulated

and cut off from circulation is a _____ hernia.

12.88 A section of intestine may prolapse into the lumen of an adjoin-

intussusception

ing section, causing an _____. If a section of intestine twists upon itself, an obstruction may result; this condi-

volvulus

tion is called _____ (volvo = to roll).

12.89 A fistula (fistula = pipe) is an abnormal connection. A fistula

anal fistula

from the anus to the rectum is called an _____ _____.

12.90 *Hem/o* is a combining form referring to blood. A swollen,
twisted vein in the anal region liable to bleed is called a

hemorrhoid

_____.

bile	**12.91** The combining form *chol/e* means _____. The combining form for stone is _____. The suffix for formation of or presence of is _____. Therefore, the term for the presence of stones in the gallbladder or bile ducts is _____.
lith/o	
-iasis	
cholelithiasis	
choledocholithiasis	**12.92** The combining forms *chol/e* and *doch/o* together refer to the common bile duct. The term for the presence of stones in the common bile duct is _____.

SELF-INSTRUCTION: DIAGNOSTIC TESTS AND PROCEDURES

Study the following:

Test or Procedure	Explanation
biopsy (Bx) *bī'op-sē*	removal and microscopic study of tissue
incisional Bx *in-sizh'ŭn-ăl*	removal of a portion of a lesion for pathologic examination
excisional Bx *ek-sizh'ŭn-ăl*	removal of an entire lesion for pathologic examination
endoscopy (Fig. 12-6) *en-dos'kŏ-pē*	examination within a body cavity with a flexible endoscope for diagnosis or treatment; used in the gastrointestinal tract to detect abnormalities and perform procedures such as biopsy, excision of lesions, dilations of narrowed areas, and removal of swallowed objects
esophagoscopy *ē-sof-ă-gos'kŏ-pē*	examination of the esophagus with an esophagoscope
gastroscopy *gas-tros'kŏ-pē*	examination of the stomach with a gastroscope
upper gastrointestinal endoscopy (Fig. 12-6)	examination of the lining of the esophagus, stomach, and duodenum with a flexible endoscope; also called esophagogastroduodenoscopy (EGD) or panendoscopy
endoscopic retrograde cholangiopancreatography (ERCP) *en-dos'kŏp'ik ret'rō-grād kō-lan'jē-ō-pan-krē-ă-tog'ră-fē*	endoscopic procedure including x-ray fluoroscopy to examine the ducts of the liver, gallbladder, and pancreas (biliary ducts)

laparoscopy (Fig. 12-11) *lap-ă-ros'kŏ-pē*	examination of the abdominal cavity with a laparoscope, often including interventional surgical procedures
peritoneoscopy *per'i-tō-nē-os'kŏ-pē*	examination of the peritoneal cavity with a peritoneoscope, often performed to examine the liver and obtain a biopsy specimen
colonoscopy (Fig. 12-6) *kō-lon-os'kŏ-pē*	examination of the colon using a flexible colonoscope
sigmoidoscopy *sig'moy-dos'kŏ-pē*	examination of the sigmoid colon with a rigid or flexible sigmoidoscope
proctoscopy *prok-tos'kŏ-pē*	examination of the rectum and anus with a proctoscope
magnetic resonance imaging (MRI)	nonionizing imaging technique for visualizing the abdominal cavity to identify disease or deformity in the gastrointestinal tract
radiography (Fig. 12-12) *rā'dē-og'ră-fē*	x-ray imaging used to detect a condition or anomaly within the gastrointestinal tract
upper GI series (Fig. 12-13)	x-ray of the esophagus, stomach, and duodenum after the patient has swallowed a contrast medium (barium is most commonly used)
barium swallow *ba're-ŭm*	x-ray of the esophagus only, often used to locate swallowed objects
fluoroscopy *flū r-os'kŏ-pe*	x-ray using a fluorescent screen to visualize structures in motion (such as during a barium swallow)
small bowel series	x-ray examination of the small intestine, generally done in conjunction with an upper GI series

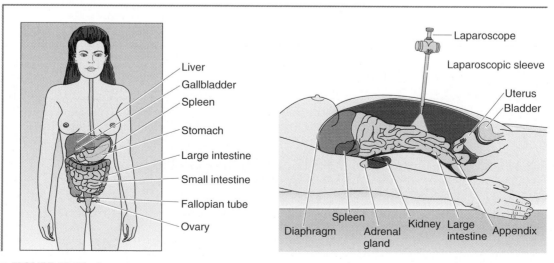

■ **FIGURE 12-11.** Laparoscopy.

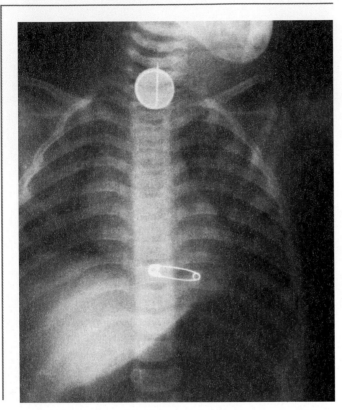

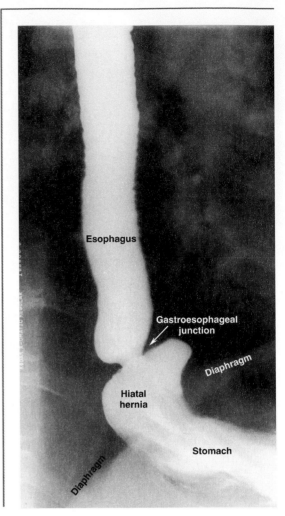

◼ **FIGURE 12-12.** Radiograph showing two impacted foreign bodies in a child 2 1/2 years old. The child ingested a safety pin and an ornamental pin. Endoscopic removal was required.

◼ **FIGURE 12-13.** Upper gastrointestinal radiograph showing hiatal hernia.

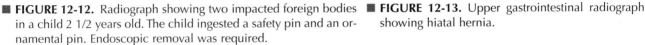

lower GI series barium enema *en'ĕ-mă*	x-ray of the colon after administration of an enema containing a contrast medium
computed tomography (CT) of abdomen (See Fig. 2-12 in Chapter 2) *tō-mogră-fē*	cross-sectional x-ray of the abdomen used to identify a condition or anomaly within the gastrointestinal tract
cholangiogram *kō-lan'jē-ō-gram*	x-ray of the bile ducts, often performed during surgery
cholecystogram *kō-lē-sis'tō-gram*	x-ray of the gallbladder taken after oral ingestion of iodine

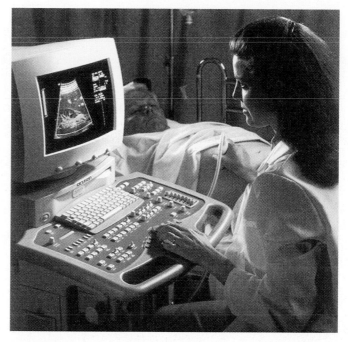

FIGURE 12-14. Abdominal sonography.

sonography *sō-nog′ră-fē*	ultrasound imaging
abdominal sonogram (See Fig. 12-14) *son′ō-gram*	ultrasound image of the abdomen to detect disease or deformity in organs and vascular structures (e.g., liver, pancreas, gallbladder, spleen, aorta)
endoscopic sonography	an endoscopic procedure using a sonographic transducer within an endoscope to examine a body cavity and make sonographic images of structures and tissues
stool culture and sensitivity (C&S)	isolation of a stool specimen in a culture medium to identify disease-causing organisms; if organisms are present, the drugs to which they are sensitive are listed
stool occult blood study	a chemical test of a stool specimen to detect the presence of blood; positive findings indicate bleeding in the GI tract

PROGRAMMED REVIEW: DIAGNOSTIC TESTS AND PROCEDURES

Answers	Review
	12.93 Recall that the suffix for the process of examination is
-scopy, within	_____. The prefix *endo-* means _____. The general term
endoscope	for a scope used to examine within the body is _____.

endoscopy

The process of examination using this instrument is

_____.

esophagoscopy

12.94   Many specialized kinds of endoscopes have been developed to examine different structures within the gastrointestinal tract. Examination of the esophagus, for example, uses an esophagoscope. This examination is called _____.

gastroscopy

peritoneoscopy

colonoscopy

sigmoidoscopy

12.95   Examination of the stomach with a special scope is called _____. Examination of the peritoneal cavity with a special scope is called _____. Examination of the colon with a special scope is called _____. Examination of the sigmoid colon with a special scope is called

_____.

proct/o

proctoscopy

12.96   Recall that the combining form for the anus and rectum is _____. The term for examination of the rectum and anus with a special scope is _____.

lapar/o

laparoscopy

12.97   Recall that the three combining forms for abdomen are *abdomin/o, celi/o,* and _____. Built from the last of these, the term for examination of the abdominal cavity with a special scope is _____.

esophagogastroduodenoscopy

12.98   Upper gastrointestinal endoscopy includes examination of the whole upper part of the gastrointestinal tract—the esophagus, stomach, and duodenum—using a flexible endoscope. The technical term, using the combining forms for esophagus, stomach, and duodenum, is _____ (EGD) or panendoscopy.

biopsy

12.99   Tissue samples can be taken of gastrointestinal organs through the endoscope during the examination. The removal and microscopic study of such tissue samples is called _____. Incisional biopsy

portion	removes a _____ of a lesion for examination, whereas removal of the entire lesion for examination is called an
excisional	_____ biopsy.

12.100 Another endoscopic procedure is performed under x-ray fluoroscopy to examine the ducts of the liver, gallbladder, and pancreas. Abbreviated ERCP, this procedure is called _____

endoscopic retrograde

cholangiopancreatography

_____ _____.

12. 101 The nonionizing imaging technique used in many body systems is used also in the gastrointestinal system to visualize the abdominal cavity. Abbreviated MRI, this procedure is _____

magnetic

resonance imaging

_____ _____.

12.102 Recall that the suffix meaning process of recording is

-graphy

radiography

_____. The general term for recording an x-ray image is

_____.

12.103 Several specialized radiographic procedures are performed to

gastrointestinal

image the _____ (GI) tract. An x-ray of

the esophagus after the patient swallows a barium contrast medium is

swallow

called a barium _____ . A series of x-rays taken of the upper

part of the gastrointestinal tract, from the esophagus to the duodenum,

upper GI

after the patient swallows barium is called an _____ _____

series

_____.

12.104 Bowel is another term for intestine. The x-ray examination of

small

the small intestine (using the term bowel) is called a _____

bowel series

_____ _____.

12.105 Barium contrast can also be introduced into the lower gastrointestinal tract through an enema. An x-ray made of the colon after a barium enema is called either simply a barium enema or a _____

lower

GI

_____ series.

record

cholangiogram

cholecystogram

12.106 The suffix *-gram* means _____. Built from the combining form referring to bile ducts, an x-ray record of bile ducts is called a _____. Built from the combining form referring to the gallbladder, an x-ray of the gallbladder is called a _____.

fluoroscopy

12.107 The type of x-ray examination using a fluorescent screen to visualize structures in motion is called _____.

computed tomography

12.108 Computer cross-sectional x-rays of the abdomen are made with _____ _____ (CT) of the abdomen.

recording

sonography

abdominal

sonogram

endoscopic sonography

12.109 The suffix *-graphy* means process of _____. Another term for ultrasound imaging is _____. An ultrasound image of the abdomen is termed an _____ _____. When the sonographic transducer is placed inside an endoscope for examining a body cavity with ultrasound, this is called _____ _____.

stool culture

sensitivity

12.110 Stool specimens can be diagnostically examined to detect pathology. Isolation of a stool specimen in a culture medium to grow and identify microorganisms and determine drugs to which they are sensitive is called a _____ _____ and _____ (C&S).

occult blood

12.111 Occult means hidden or not obvious. A chemical test of a stool specimen to detect unseen blood and thereby bleeding in the GI tract is called a stool _____ _____ study.

SELF-INSTRUCTION: OPERATIVE TERMS

Study the following:

Term	Meaning
cheiloplasty *kī'lō-plas-tē*	repair of the lip
glossectomy *glo-sek'tō-mē*	excision of the tongue
glossorrhaphy *glo-sōr'ă-fē*	suture of the tongue
esophagoplasty *ē-sof'ă-gō-plas-tē*	repair of the esophagus
gastrectomy *gas-trek'tō-mē*	partial or complete removal of the stomach
gastric resection *gas'trik rē-sek'shŭn*	partial removal and repair of the stomach
gastroenterostomy *gas'trō-en-ter-os'tō-mē*	formation of an artificial opening between the stomach and small intestine; often performed at the time of a gastrectomy to route food from the remainder of the stomach to the intestine (also performed to repair a perforated duodenal ulcer)
abdominocentesis *ab-dom'i-nō-sen-tē'sis* **paracentesis** *par'ă-sen-tē'sis*	puncture of the abdomen for aspiration of fluid; e.g., fluid accumulated in ascites
laparotomy *lap'ă-rot'ō-mē*	incision into the abdomen
laparoscopic surgery *lap'ă-rō-skō-pik*	abdominal surgery using a laparoscope
herniorrhaphy *her'nō-ōr'ă-fē* **hernioplasty** *her'nē-ō-plas-tē*	repair of a hernia
colostomy (Fig. 12-15) *kō-los'tō-mē*	creation of an opening in the colon through the abdominal wall to create an abdominal anus allowing stool to bypass a diseased portion of the colon; performed to treat ulcerative colitis, cancer, or obstructions
anastomosis *ă-nas'tō-mō'sis*	union of two hollow vessels, a technique of bowel surgery
ileostomy *il'ē-os'tō-mē*	surgical creation of an opening on the abdomen to which the end of the ileum is attached, providing a passageway for ileal discharges, performed after removal of the colon such as to treat chronic inflammatory bowel diseases such as ulcerative colitis

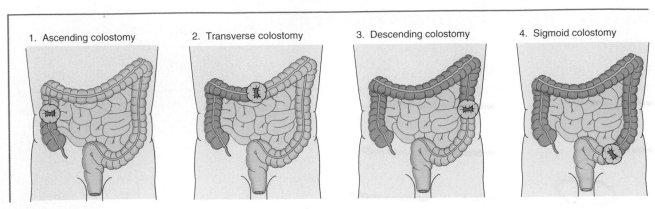

■ **FIGURE 12-15.** Common colostomy sites.

appendectomy *ap-pen-dek'tō-mē*	excision of a diseased appendix
incidental appendectomy	removal of the appendix during abdominal surgery for another procedure (e.g., a hysterectomy)
polypectomy *pol-i-pek'tō-mē*	excision of polyps
proctoplasty *prok'tō-plas-tē*	repair of the anus and rectum
anal fistulectomy *fis-tyū-lek'tō-mē*	excision of an anal fistula
hemorrhoidectomy *hem'ō-roy-dek'tō-mē*	excision of hemorrhoids
hepatic lobectomy *he-pat'ik lō-bek'tō-mē*	excision of a lobe of the liver
cholecystectomy *kō'lē-sis-tek'tō-mē*	excision of the gallbladder
laparoscopic cholecystectomy *lap'ă-rō-skŏp'ik*	excision of the gallbladder through a laparoscope
cholelithotomy *kōlē-li-thot'ō-mē*	an incision for removal of gallstones
choledocholithotomy *kō-led'ō-kō-li-thot'ō-mē*	incision of the common bile duct for extraction of gallstones
pancreatectomy *pan'krē-ă-tek'tō-mē*	excision of the pancreas

PROGRAMMED REVIEW: OPERATIVE TERMS

Answers	Review

gastr/o	**12.112** Recall that the combining form for stomach is _____.
-ectomy	The suffix for excision is _____. The surgical excision of part or
gastrectomy	all of the stomach is _____.

hemorrhoidectomy	**12.113** Excision of hemorrhoids is termed _____.

pancreat/o	**12.114** The combining form for pancreas is _____.
pancreatectomy	Surgical excision of the pancreas is termed _____.

	12.115 The two combining forms for tongue are *lingu/o* and
gloss/o	_gloss_____. Made from the latter, the term for surgical excision of
glossectomy	the tongue is _____.

cholecystectomy	**12.116** Excision of the gallbladder is termed _____.
	When performed through a laparoscope, it is called
laparoscopic	_____ cholecystectomy.

	12.117 Excision of a lobe of the liver is termed a hepatic
lobectomy	_____.

appendic/o	**12.118** The combining form for appendix is _____.
appendectomy	Surgical excision of the appendix is termed _____.
	(Note the "ic" in the combining form is removed to prevent the un-
	wieldy "ic-ec" sound.) If the appendix is removed during another ab-
	dominal surgery, such as an abdominal hysterectomy (excision of the
incidental	uterus), this is called an _____ appendectomy.

	12.119 The procedure of surgical excision of polyps is termed
polypectomy	_____.

anal	**12.120** Excision of an anal fistula is termed an _____
fistulectomy	_____.

-plasty

cheiloplasty

esophagoplasty

hernioplasty

proctoplasty

12.121 Recall that the suffix for surgical repair or reconstruction is _____. Surgical repair of the lip is termed _____. Repair of the esophagus is _____. Repair of a hernia is _____. Repair of the anus and rectum is _____.

-rrhaphy

glossorrhaphy

herniorrhaphy

12.122 Recall that the suffix meaning suture is _____. Suture of the tongue is therefore _____. Surgical repair and suture of a hernia is _____.

gastric resection

12.123 Resection typically involves less tissue removal than full excision. The procedure of partial removal and repair of the stomach is called _____ _____.

opening

colostomy

ileostomy

12.124 Recall that the operative suffix *-stomy* means creation of an _____. The surgical creation of an opening in the colon through the abdominal wall allowing stool to bypass a diseased portion of the colon is called a _____. The creation of an opening for the end of ileum to exit from the abdomen after removal of the colon is called an _____.

gastroenterostomy

12.125 The term for the creation of an artificial opening between the stomach and small intestine is built from the combining forms for both the stomach and intestine. This procedure is called a _____.

-tomy

lapar/o

laparotomy

12.126 The operative suffix meaning incision is _____. Recall that the three combining forms meaning abdomen are *adomin/o, celi/o,* and _____. Formed from the last of these, the term for an incision into the abdomen is _____.

12.127 The term for an incision made to remove gallstones is made from the combining forms for bile and stone. This procedure is a

cholelithotomy

_____.

12.128 The term for an incision made into the common bile duct to remove gallstones is made from the combining forms for bile duct and

choledocholithotomy

stone. This procedure is a _____.

12.129 Recall that the suffix meaning puncture for aspiration is

-centesis

_____. The three combining forms meaning abdomen are

abdomin/o

celi/o, lapar/o, and _____. Made from the last of these, the

term for puncture of the abdomen for the aspiration of a fluid is

abdominocentesis

_____. Another general term for aspi-

paracentesis

ration of fluid from any cavity is _____.

12.130 The term for the operative procedure in which two hollow ves-

anastomosis

sels are joined is _____. This technique is some-

times used in bowel surgery.

12.131 A general term for abdominal surgery carried out using a

laparoscopic

laparoscope is _____ surgery.

SELF-INSTRUCTION: THERAPEUTIC TERMS

Study the following:

Term	Meaning
gastric lavage _gas'trik l_a-vahzh'_	oral insertion of a tube into the stomach for examination and treatment, such as to remove blood clots from the stomach or monitor bleeding (lavage = to wash)
nasogastric (NG) intubation _nā-zō-gas'trik in-tū-bā'shŭn_	insertion of a tube through the nose into the stomach for various purposes, such as to obtain a gastric fluid specimen for analysis

COMMON THERAPEUTIC DRUG CLASSIFICATIONS

antacid *ant-as'id*	drug that neutralizes stomach acid
antiemetic *an'tē-ĕ-met'ik*	drug that prevents or stops vomiting
antispasmodic *an'tē-spaz-mod'ik*	drug that decreases motility in gastrointestinal tract to arrest spasm or diarrhea
cathartic *kă-thar'tik*	drug that causes movement of the bowels; also called a laxative

PROGRAMMED REVIEW: THERAPEUTIC TERMS

Answers	Review
gastric lavage	**12.132** The word lavage means to wash. The therapeutic procedure in which a tube is inserted into the stomach from the mouth to remove fluids such as blood clots is termed _____ _____.
nasogastric, intubation	**12.133** A tube can be inserted through the nose to the stomach for purposes such as obtaining a gastric fluid specimen for analysis. This is called _____ (NG) _____.
anti-	**12.134** Therapeutic drug classifications are often named for their actions, often their actions against some process or condition. The common prefix meaning against is _____.
adjective, pertaining to antiemetic	**12.135** Recall that *-emesis* means vomiting. The suffix *-ic* is used to make an _____ ending, meaning _____ _____, often used for a drug class. Therefore, a drug that prevents or stops vomiting (against vomiting) is an _____.
antispasmodic	**12.136** Similarly, a drug to stop spasms (of the gastrointestinal tract) is an _____.
antacid	**12.137** A drug that works against excess stomach acid by neutralizing it is an _____. (Note that in this case, the *-ic* ending is not used.)

12.138 The Greek word katharsis means purification—by purging. A drug that purges the large intestine by stimulating a bowel movement is

cathartic

a _____, also called a laxative.

Practice Exercises

For the following terms, on the lines below the term, write out the indicated word parts: prefixes, combining forms, roots, and suffixes. Then define the word.For example:

Example:
sublingual

$$\frac{sub/lingu/al}{P \quad R \quad S}$$

DEFINITION: below or under/tongue/pertaining to

1. transabdominal

   _____ / _____ / _____
   P   R   S

   DEFINITION: _____

2. hepaticotomy

   _____ / _____
   CF   S

   DEFINITION: _____

3. sialolithotomy

   _____ / _____ / _____
   CF   CF   S

   DEFINITION: _____

4. glossorrhaphy

   _____ / _____
   CF   S

   DEFINITION: _____

5. hematemesis

   _____ / _____
   R   S

   DEFINITION: _____

6. cheilostomatoplasty

_____ / _____ / _____
  CF   CF   S

DEFINITION: _____

7. appendicitis

_____ / _____
  R   S

DEFINITION: _____

8. celiotomy

_____ / _____
  CF   S

DEFINITION: _____

9. cholangiogram

_____ / _____ / _____
  R   CF   S

DEFINITION: _____

10. colonoscopy

_____ / _____
  CF   S

DEFINITION: _____

11. anorectal

_____ / _____ / _____
  CF   R   S

DEFINITION: _____

12. enterocolitis

_____ / _____ / _____
  CF   R   S

DEFINITION: _____

13. orolingual

_____ / _____ / _____
  CF   R   S

DEFINITION: _____

14. proctosigmoidoscopy

_____ / _____ / _____
  CF   CF   S

DEFINITION: _____

15. laparoscope

    _____ / _____
      CF   S

DEFINITION: _____

16. dysphagia

    _____ / _____ / _____
       P   R   S

DEFINITION: _____

17. pancreatoduodenostomy

    _____ / _____ / _____
      CF   CF   S

DEFINITION: _____

18. hernioplasty

    _____ / _____
      CF   S

DEFINITION: _____

19. biliary

    _____ / _____
      R   S

DEFINITION: _____

20. gastroesophageal

    _____ / _____ / _____
      CF   R   S

DEFINITION: _____

21. choledochotomy

    _____ / _____ / _____
      CF   CF   S

DEFINITION: _____

22. steatorrhea

    _____ / _____
      CF   S

DEFINITION: _____

23. dentalgia

    _____ / _____
      R   S

DEFINITION: _____

24. pylorospasm

_____ / _____
   CF   S

DEFINITION: _____

25. hepatotoxic

_____ / _____ / _____
   CF   R   S

DEFINITION: _____

26. ileojejunitis

_____ / _____ / _____
   CF   R   S

DEFINITION: _____

27. peritoneocentesis

_____ / _____
   CF   S

DEFINITION: _____

28. buccogingival

_____ / _____ / _____
   CF   R   S

DEFINITION: _____

29. cholecystectomy

_____ / _____ / _____
   CF   R   S

DEFINITION: _____

30. perirectal

_____ / _____ / _____
   P   R   S

DEFINITION: _____

Write the correct medical term for each of the following:

31. inflammation of the stomach _____

32. loss of appetite _____

33. inability to swallow _____

34. in the cheek _____

35. gas in the stomach or intestines _____

36. rupture or protrusion of a part from its normal location _____

37. black tarry stool _____

38. belch _____

39. instrument used to examine the rectum _____

40. inflammation of the large intestine _____

41. x-ray image of the esophagus only _____

42. accumulation of fluid in the peritoneal cavity _____

43. inflammation of the gallbladder _____

44. feces containing fat _____

45. presence of inflamed abnormal side pockets in gastrointestinal tract

_____

46. peptic ulcer located in the stomach _____

47. enlargement of the liver _____

48. a tongue-tie condition _____

Complete the medical term by writing the missing part or word:

49. hemi_____ectomy = removal of half of the stomach

50. _____itis = inflammation of the appendix

51. _____rrhaphy = suture of the lip

52. cholelitho_____ = crushing of gallstones

53. _____plasty = surgical repair of the mouth

54. chol_____gram = x-ray of bile ducts (vessels)

55. _____bilirubin_____ = excessive level of

bilirubin in the blood

56. gastric _____ = partial removal and repair of the stomach

57. diverticul_____ = the presence of diverticula

Name the anatomical divisions of the abdomen:

58. lower lateral groin regions _____

59. upper lateral regions beneath ribs _____

60. upper middle region below the sternum _____

61. region below the navel _____

62. middle lateral regions _____

63. region of the navel _____

Name the clinical divisions of the abdomen:

64. _____

65. _____

66. _____

67. _____

Match the following terms with the appropriate term on the right:

68. cathartic _____   a. cholelithotomy

69. herniorrhaphy _____   b. barium swallow

70. appendicitis _____   c. oro

71. lower GI series _____   d. appendectomy

72. icterus _____   e. colostomy

73. chole _____   f. hernioplasty

74. abdominocentesis _____   g. bili

75. parotitis _____   h. barium enema

76. procto _____   i. mumps

77. upper GI series _____   j. paracentesis

78. ulcerative colitis _____ k. jaundice

79. cholelithiasis _____   l. recto

80. stomato _____   m. laxative

An endoscope is an instrument used to examine within the body. Name the specific type of endoscope used to examine the following body parts:

81. abdomen _____

82. anus _____

83. stomach _____

84. colon _____

85. peritoneal cavity _____

86. esophagus _____

87. Which type of hernia is swollen and fixed within a sac, causing obstruction?

_____

88. Which type of biopsy involves the removal of an entire growth? _____

Write the full medical term for the following abbreviations:

89. NG tube _____

90. ERCP _____

91. GERD _____

92. LUQ _____

93. GI _____

94. MRI _____

95. EGD _____

For each of the following, circle the combining form that corresponds to the meaning given:

96. **abdomen**	gastr/o	lapar/o	stomat/o
97. **tongue**	gloss/o	proct/o	gingiv/o
98. **small intestine**	col/o	appendic/o	enter/o
99. **teeth**	dent/i	chol/e	lingu/o
100. **stomach**	lapar/o	stomat/o	gastr/o
101. **cheek**	bucc/o	or/o	proct/o
102. **bile**	col/o	celi/o	chol/e
103. **mouth**	gastr/o	stomat/o	lapar/o
104. **liver**	hepat/o	nephr/o	ren/o
105. **eat**	phas/o	phag/o	gloss/o
106. **stone**	scler/o	steat/o	lith/o
107. **rectum**	an/o	proct/o	col/o

Write in the term components related to each of the gastrointestinal organs on the lines provided in the following illustration.

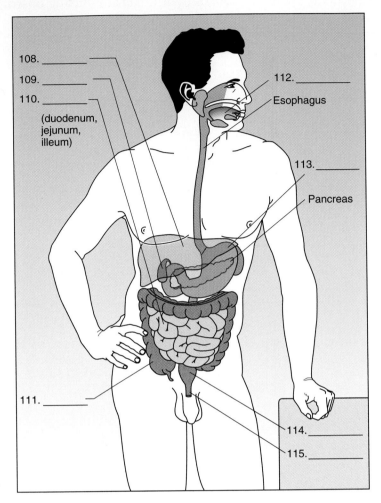

108. _____

109. _____

110. _____
(duodenum,
jejunum,
illeum)

111. _____

112. _____

Esophagus

113. _____

Pancreas

114. _____

115. _____

For each of the following, circle the correct spelling of the term:

116. anorexia   annorexia   anorrexia

117. asites   ascitis   ascites

118. hematochesia   hemochezia   hematochezia

119. icterus   ickterus   icteris

120. ankleoglossia   ankyloglosia   ankyloglossia

121. volvulis   volvulus   volvolus

122. cirhosis   cirrhosus   cirrhosis

123. glossectomy   glozectomy   glosectomy

124. hernniorhaphy   herniorraphy   herniorrhaphy

125. hemorroidectomy   hemroidectomy   hemorrhoidectomy

126. anteacid   anacid   antacid

127. antiemetic	antemetic	antaemetic
128. cathartik	cathartic	catarthic
129. melena	melenna	melana

Give the noun that was used to form the following adjectives.

130. fecal _____

131. icteric _____

132. ileal _____

133. endoscopic _____

134. hemorrhoidal _____

135. pancreatic _____

Medical Record Analyses

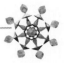

MEDICAL RECORD 12-1

S: This is a 36 y.o. ♂ with a complaint of abdominal pain. He describes having lifted a 75# beam yesterday at work. He noticed a sharp pain in his navel but continued to work. The pain intensified as the day went on and persisted through last night and today. He claims his navel now bulges forward. He denies fever, chills, dysphagia, anorexia, or vomiting.
PMH: No hospitalizations or surgeries
Meds: none
Allergies: NKDA

O: T 97.5°F, P 87, R 18, BP 128/86
WDWN male in moderate distress secondary to abdominal pain. Upon palpation, the abdomen is soft with spasm of the muscles in the periumbilical region, and there is an obvious bulge in the umbilicus. The omentum is also palapable. There is no hepatosplenomegaly.

A: Incarcerated umbilical hernia

P: Admit for STAT umbilical hernia repair

1. Summarize the subjective information:
   a. pain in stomach
   b. pain in abdomen
   c. pain in the groin area
   d. generalized abdominal pain with chills and fever
   e. stomach pain and has difficulty swallowing

2. What kind of an appetite does the patient have?
   a. normal
   b. increased
   c. decreased

3. What is the condition of the patient's liver?
   a. not stated
   b. enlarged
   c. not enlarged
   d. inflamed
   e. ruptured

4. What were the objective findings
   a. involuntary contraction of the muscles around the navel
   b. pouching of the muscles under the navel
   c. contraction of abdominal muscles and enlargement of the spleen
   d. protrusion of the navel and enlargement of the liver
   e. pouching of the stomach and omentum

5. Which of the following best describes the diagnosis?
   a. portion of the bowel has protruded through the abdominal wall and has been cut off from circulation
   b. prolapse of one part of the intestine into the lumen of the adjoining part
   c. portion of the intestine has protruded through a weakness in the abdominal wall around the navel and is swollen and fixed in a sac
   d. portion of the bowel has twisted on itself causing obstruction
   e. inflammation of the stomach and small intestine

6. Which of the following medical terms describes the planned surgery?
   a. laparotomy
   b. gastroenterostomy
   c. hernioplasty
   d. ileostomy
   e. abdominocentesis

MEDICAL RECORD 12-2 FOR ADDITIONAL STUDY

CENTRAL MEDICAL CENTER

211 Medical Center Drive • Central City, US 90000-1234 • PHONE: (012) 125-6784 • FAX: (012) 125-9999

CONSULTATION

REASON FOR CONSULTATION:

This 77-year-old female presented herself to the emergency room with a one week history of rather severe nausea and vomiting and also diarrhea and epigastric pain; she was sent by Dr. Shigeda, her family practitioner. The most troubling symptom for her is the vomiting and nausea because she vomits everything she drinks and eats. The epigastric pains are tolerable. The diarrhea also has somewhat improved. The patient's bowel movements usually are normal without history of black or bloody stools. Her appetite has been down markedly, and she has lost at least two to three pounds in the last several days. Her urination is normal. She does not drink or smoke. Her last admission was about a month ago after a fall.

MEDICATIONS: Prednisone, 10 mg, 1 q.i.d.; Naprosyn, 250 mg, 1 q noc; Voltaren 1 q d; penicillamine t.i.d.; and Mylanta and Tylenol p.r.n.

ALLERGIES: Demerol which gives her severe confusion lasting for days.

PAST MEDICAL HISTORY/REVIEW OF SYSTEMS:

The patient has reading glasses. There is no history of cephalalgia, diplopia, or tinnitus. There is no history of thyroid disease. CARDIOPULMONARY: There is no history of angina, dyspnea, hemoptysis, emphysema, hypertension, or heart murmurs. GASTROINTESTINAL: The patient had peptic ulcer disease about 20 years ago, nonbleeding, and does not remember whether it was gastric or duodenal. It was healed by diet and antacids. There has been no recurrence since. There is no history of gallbladder disease, hepatitis, pancreatitis, or colitis. However, years ago, she was told she had diverticulosis. GENITOURINARY: She is Gravida III Para III (3 pregnancies and 3 live births). Her last menstrual period was some 25 years ago. There is no history of dysuria, hematuria, or nephrolithiasis. MUSCULOSKELETAL: The patient has had severe rheumatoid arthritis for about 20 years and has been in treatment with Dr. Clemons. The disease is relatively well controlled with the above-mentioned medications. She had a right hip replacement in 20xx and left knee arthroscopy. NEUROMUSCULAR: There is no history of loss of consciousness or seizure disorder. PSYCHIATRIC REVIEW: Negative.

FAMILY HISTORY:

All siblings and parents died of old age.

SOCIAL HISTORY:

The patient is a widow. She lives with her daughter.

(continued)

CONSULTATION Page 1 October 19, 20xx	PT. NAME: HILLMAN, KATHLEEN E. ID NO: IP-990960 ROOM NO: 508 ATT. PHYS: R. FLAGSTONE, M.D.

MEDICAL RECORD 12-2 FOR ADDITIONAL STUDY (CONTINUED)

CENTRAL MEDICAL CENTER

211 Medical Center Drive • Central City, US 90000-1234 • PHONE: (012) 125-6784 • FAX: (012) 125-9999

CONSULTATION

PHYSICAL EXAMINATION:

GENERAL: The patient appeared to be in moderate to severe distress, appearing pale, chronically ill, with dehydration.

VITAL SIGNS: Blood pressure, lying: 100/70. Blood pressure, sitting: 90/65. Temperature: 98°C. Pulse: 80; went to 100 on sitting up. Respirations: 12.

HEENT: Head: Normocephalic. Eyes: Pupils equal, round, reactive to light and accommodation. No scleral icterus. Fundi benign. Ears, nose throat, and mouth were unremarkable.

NECK: Supple. No lymphadenopathy. No thyromegaly.

CHEST: Chest, costovertebral angle, and back were nontender.

LUNGS: Clear to percussion and auscultation.

HEART: There was an irregular rate, possibly atrial fibrillation, with a II/VI systolic ejection-type murmur mostly along the left sternal border.

ABDOMEN: Soft. There was moderate epigastric tenderness. There was no hepatospleno-megaly, no guarding, no rebound tenderness, no masses, no ascites, no abdominal bruits.

VAGINAL EXAMINATION: Refused.

RECTAL EXAMINATION: Good sphincter tone. Light brown, semiformed stool in the rectal ampulla which was occult blood negative.

EXTREMITIES: No edema. No varicose veins. Good peripheral pulses. No clubbing. No palmar erythema. There were, however, brownish changes of chronic stasis dermatitis.

SKIN: The skin showed 10-15% dehydration without jaundice. There were multiple ecchymoses secondary to the patient's prednisone.

(continued)

CONSULTATION Page 2 October 19, 20xx	PT. NAME: HILLMAN, KATHLEEN E. ID NO: IP-990960 ROOM NO: 508 ATT. PHYS: R. FLAGSTONE, M.D.

MEDICAL RECORD 12-2 FOR ADDITIONAL STUDY (CONTINUED)

CENTRAL MEDICAL CENTER

211 Medical Center Drive • Central City, US 90000-1234 • PHONE: (012) 125-6784 • FAX: (012) 125-9999

CONSULTATION

INITIAL IMPRESSION:

1. SEVERE NAUSEA AND VOMITING, INTRACTABLE, WITH DEHYDRATION, PROBABLY SECONDARY TO MEDICATION-INDUCED GASTRITIS OR POSSIBLE RECURRENT PEPTIC ULCER DISEASE

2. R/O POSSIBLE PANCREATITIS SECONDARY TO PREDNISONE OR PENICILLAMINE.

3. R/O POSSIBLE VIRAL GASTROENTERITIS, THOUGH LESS LIKELY.

SECONDARY DIAGNOSES:

1. HISTORY OF LONGSTANDING, ADVANCED RHEUMATOID ARTHRITIS WITH LEFT KNEE SURGERY AND RIGHT HIP REPLACEMENT.

2. HISTORY OF DIVERTICULOSIS AND PREVIOUS PEPTIC ULCER DISEASE.

PLAN:

The patient will be admitted at least for a 23-hour hold and is then to be re-evaluated and will receive fluid volume replacement and potassium replacement; she will have her electrolytes checked, as well as her blood count, and will also be placed on Zantac intravenously. She will then have a gastroscopy in the morning. Her stools will also be checked, if they are still loose, for further occult blood, ova and parasites, and a possible culture and sensitivity.

R. Flagstone, M.D.

RF:ti

D: 10/19/20xx
T: 10/20/20xx

CONSULTATION
Page 3
October 19, 20xx

PT. NAME: HILLMAN, KATHLEEN E.
ID NO: IP-990960
ROOM NO: 508
ATT. PHYS: R. FLAGSTONE, M.D.

MEDICAL RECORD 12-2 FOR ADDITIONAL STUDY

At age 77, Kathleen Hillman has been in fairly good health. However, one week ago she developed what she called "stomach problems" that led to frequent vomiting. She refused to seek medical help at first, until her daughter coaxed her into calling her family practitioner, Dr. Shigeda. Once she learned how serious Ms. Hillman's problem had become, Dr. Shigeda urged her to go to the emergency room immediately.

Read Medical Record 12-2 (pages 537–539) for Kathleen Hillman, and answer the following questions. This record is the consultation report dictated by Dr. Flagstone after he examined her in the emergency room at Central Medical Center.

1. Below are medical terms used in this record that you have not yet encountered in this text. Underline each where it appears in the record, and define below.

    rebound tenderness _____

    abdominal guarding _____

    dehydration _____

    stasis dermatitis _____

    intractable _____

2. What was Ms. Hillman's complaint that led her to call Dr. Shigeda, who then sent her to the emergency room at Central Medical Center?

    _____

3. According to Dr. Flagstone's initial impression, which factor in Ms. Hillman's present history might be a cause of her gastrointestinal symptoms?
    a. her drinking
    b. stress from living with her daughter
    c. her allergies
    d. her arthritis medications

4. Describe the two previous operations Ms. Hillman has had involving the musculoskeletal system:

    _____

    _____

    _____

5. Using nonmedical language, explain what Ms. Hillman does not remember exactly about her gastrointestinal history two decades ago.

    _____

    _____

    _____

6. Check all of the findings below that Dr. Flagstone noted in the physical examination of Ms. Hillman:

    _____ dehydration

_____ pulse 98

_____ icterus in the whites of eyes

_____ chronic stasis dermatitis

_____ varicose veins

_____ irregular heart rate

_____ vaginal infection

_____ possible atrial fibrillation

_____ parotitis

_____ yellowing of skin

_____ multiple ecchymoses

_____ clear lungs

7. Does Ms. Hillman have blood in her stool? Write the phrase from the medical record that indicates this.

_____

8. In your own words, explain the initial diagnoses, including the possibilities to eliminate:

a. _____

b. _____

c. _____

9. Dr. Flagstone's plan calls for administering medications, checking tests, and performing a procedure. Fill in the details below.

Administered to Ms. Hillman

a. _____

b. _____

c. _____

Check Ms. Hillman's

d. _____

e. _____

f. _____

Perform

g. _____

10. In your own words, describe stool culture and sensitivity.

_____

_____

Answers to Practice Exercises

1. trans/abdomin/al
   P   R   S
   across or through/
   abdomen/pertaining to
2. hepatico/tomy
   CF   S
   liver/incision
3. sialo/litho/tomy
   CF   CF   S
   saliva/stone/incision
4. glosso/rrhaphy
   CF   S
   tongue/suture
5. hemat/emesis
   R   S
   blood/vomiting
6. cheilo/stomato/plasty
   CF   CF   S
   lip/mouth/surgical repair
   or reconstruction
7. appendic/itis
   R   S
   appendix/inflammation
8. celio/tomy
   CF   S
   abdomen/incision
9. chol/angio/gram
   R   CF   S
   bile/vessel/record
10. colono/scopy
    CF   S
    colon/process of
    examination
11. ano/rect/al
    CF   R   S
    anus/rectum/pertaining to
12. entero/col/itis
    CF   R   S
    small intestine/colon/
    inflammation
13. oro/lingu/al
    CF   R   S
    mouth/tongue/pertaining to
14. procto/sigmoido/scopy
    CF   CF   S
    anus and rectum/sigmoid
    colon/process of
    examination
15. laparo/scope
    CF   S
    abdomen/instrument for
    examination

16. dys/phag/ia
    P   R   S
    painful, difficulty or faulty/
    eat or swallow/condition
    of
17. pancreato/duodeno/stomy
    CF   CF   S
    pancreas/duodenum/
    creation of an opening
18. hernio/plasty
    CF   S
    hernia/surgical repair or
    reconstruction
19. bil/iary
    R   S
    bile/pertaining to
20. gastro/esophage/al
    CF   R   S
    stomach/esophagus/
    pertaining to
21. chole/docho/tomy
    CF   CF   S
    bile/duct/incision
22. steato/rrhea
    CF   S
    fat/discharge
23. dent/algia
    R   S
    teeth/pain
24. pyloro/spasm
    CF   S
    pylorus (gatekeeper)
25. hepato/tox/ic
    CF   R   S
    liver/poison/pertaining to
26. ileo/jejun/itis
    CF   R   S
    ileum/jejunum/
    inflammation
27. peritoneo/centesis
    CF   S
    peritoneum/puncture for
    aspiration
28. bucco/gingiv/al
    CF   R   S
    cheek/gum/pertaining to
29. chole/cyst/ectomy
    CF   R   S
    bile/bladder or sac/excision
    (removal)
30. peri/rect/al
    P   R   S
    around/rectum/pertaining to
31. gastritis
32. anorexia
33. aphagia
34. buccal

35. flatulence
36. hernia
37. melena
38. eructation
39. anoscope or proctoscope
40. colitis
41. barium swallow
42. ascites
43. cholecystitis
44. steatorrhea
45. diverticulitis
46. gastric ulcer
47. hepatomegaly
48. ankyloglossia
49. hemigastrectomy
50. appendicitis
51. cheilorrhaphy
52. cholelithotomy
53. stomatoplasty
54. cholangiogram
55. hyperbilirubinemia
56. gastric resection
57. diverticulosis
58. inguinal regions
59. hypochondriac regions
60. epigastric region
61. hypogastric region
62. lumbar regions
63. umbilical region
64. right upper quadrant (RUQ)
65. left upper quadrant (LUQ)
66. right lower quadrant (RLQ)
67. left lower quadrant (LLQ)
68. m
69. f
70. d
71. h
72. k
73. g
74. j
75. i
76. l
77. b
78. e
79. a
80. c
81. laparoscope
82. anoscope or proctoscope
83. gastroscope
84. sigmoidoscope or colono-
    scope
85. peritoneoscope
86. esophagoscope
87. incarcerated
88. excisional biopsy
89. nasogastric tube

90. endoscopic retrograde cholangiopancreatography
91. gastroesophageal reflux disease
92. left upper quadrant
93. gastrointestinal
94. magnetic resonance imaging
95. esophagogastroduodenoscopy
96. lapar/o
97. gloss/o
98. enter/o
99. dent/i
100. gastr/o
101. bucc/o
102. chol/e
103. stomat/o
104. hepat/o
105. phag/o
106. lith/o

107. proct/o
108. hepat/o or hepatic/o
109. cholecyst
110. enter/o
111. col/o or colon/o
112. gloss/o or lingu/o
113. gastr/o
114. proct/o or rect/o
115. an/o
116. anorexia
117. ascites
118. hematochezia
119. icterus
120. ankyloglossia
121. volvulus
122. cirrhosis
123. glossectomy
124. herniorrhaphy
125. hemorrhoidectomy
126. antacid

127. antiemetic
128. cathartic
129. melena
130. feces
131. icterus
132. ileum
133. endoscopy
134. hemorrhoid
135. pancreas

Answers to Medical Records Analyses

1. b
2. a
3. c
4. a
5. c
6. c

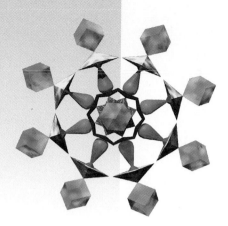

CHAPTER 13

Urinary System

Urinary System Overview

The urinary system is the organs and structures involved in the secretion and elimination of urine (Fig. 13-1):

* The kidneys filter the blood and secrete water and nitrogenous wastes in urine.
* The kidneys regulate the blood's levels of critical elements, such as water, sodium, and potassium.
* The ureters carry the urine from the kidney.
* The urinary bladder holds urine until it is expelled.

SELF-INSTRUCTION: COMBINING FORMS

Study the following:

Combining Form	Meaning
albumin/o	protein
bacteri/o	bacteria
cyst/o vesic/o	bladder or sac
dips/o	thirst
glomerul/o	glomerulus (little ball)
gluc/o glyc/o	sugar
ket/o keton/o	ketone bodies

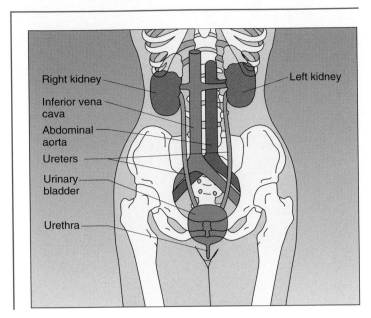

■ FIGURE 13-1. Urinary system.

lith/o	stone
meat/o	opening
nephr/o **ren/o**	kidney
pyel/o	basin
py/o	pus
ureter/o	ureter
urethr/o	urethra
ur/o **urin/o**	urine

PROGRAMMED REVIEW: COMBINING FORMS

Answers	Review
	13.1 The combining form meaning protein comes from the Latin term for egg white: albumen. That combining form is _____. Recall that the suffix *-oid* means _____. Therefore, the term _____ means resembling albumin, referring to any protein.
albumin/o	
resembling	
albuminoid	

bacteri/o

against

pertaining to

antibacterial

13.2 The combining form meaning bacteria is _____. Using the prefix *anti-* meaning _____, and the suffix *-al* meaning _____ _____, an agent such as a soap that kills bacteria is an _____.

bladder

-scope

cystoscope

13.3 The combining form *cyst/o* means sac or _____. Using the suffix referring to an instrument for examination, _____, the term for the special kind of endoscope used to examine the bladder is _____.

vesic/o

-tomy

vesicotomy (or cystotomy)

13.4 Another combining form meaning bladder or sac is _____ (from the Latin word vesica, meaning bladder). Using the operative suffix for incision, _____, the term for an incision into the bladder is _____.

dips/o, many

condition of

polydipsia

13.5 The combining form meaning thirst (from the Greek word dipsa for thirst) is _____ Recall that the suffix *poly-* means _____. The suffix *-ia* refers to a _____ _____. Thus, the term for excessive thirst (the need to drink many times) is _____.

ur/o

-logist

urologist

urin/o

13.6 The combining form for urine is _____. Recall that the suffix for a specialist in the study of a particular area is _____. Therefore, a physician who specializes in conditions of the urinary system is a _____. A second combining form for urine, used to form the adjective urinary, is _____.

gluc/o

urine

condition of

sugar

13.7 The two combining terms for sugar are *glyc/o* and _____. Glucose is a form of sugar found in the blood and used for energy. Because the combining form *ur/o* means _____ and the suffix *-ia* means a _____ _____, the term glycosuria therefore refers to a condition of _____ in the urine.

glomerul/o

13.8 The combining form that means glomerulus (a little ball-shaped cluster of capillaries in the kidney) is _____.The plural

glomeruli

of glomerulus is _____. Because each nephron in the kidney has a glomerulus, each kidney has as many as one million glomeruli.

keton/o

ur/o

condition of

ketonuria

13.9 The two combining forms meaning ketone bodies are *ket/o* and _____. Ketone bodies are chemical substances resulting from metabolism. Recall that the combining form for urine is _____, and the suffix *-ia* means _____ _____. Therefore, the term for a condition of ketone bodies in the urine is _____.

increase

ketosis

13.10 Recall that the suffix *-osis* means condition or _____. The term for the condition of increased ketone bodies in the body is therefore _____.

lith/o

lithiasis

13.11 The combining form meaning stone is _____ (from the Greek word for stone, lithos). The suffix meaning formation of, or presence of, is *-iasis.* Therefore, the term for the formation of any stone is _____.

ureter/o

ureterolithiasis

13.12 Two similar words refer to different urinary system structures that carry urine. The ureters carry urine from the kidney to the bladder. The urethra carries urine from the bladder to the outside of the body. The combining form for ureter is _____. The condition of having a stone form in the ureter is _____.

urethr/o

-algia, -dynia

urethralgia, urethrodynia

13.13 The combining form for urethra is _____. Recall that there are two suffixes that mean pain: _____ and _____. Each suffix is used to form synonyms meaning pain in the urethra: _____ or _____.

meat/o

urine

13.14 The combining form that means opening is _____ (from the Latin word meatus). The urethral meatus is the structure from which _____ leaves the body.

ren/o	**13.15** Two different combining forms refer to the kidneys: *nephr/o* and _____. As often happens, these two forms come from Greek and Latin roots, both meaning the kidneys. Recall that the suffix *-osis* refers
condition	to an increase or a _____; it is combined with the first combining form to make this term for a kidney condition:
nephrosis	_____. The second form combines with the common suffix *-al* to create this common adjective referring to the kidney:
renal	_____.
py/o	**13.16** The Greek word pyon is the origin of this combining form referring to pus: _____. It is combined with *nephr/o* and the suffix for inflammation to create this term for suppurative (forming pus) inflamma-
pyonephritis	tion of the kidney: _____.
pyel/o	**13.17** The combining form meaning basin is _____. This combining form also can refer to pelvis, although usually it refers to the renal pelvis, a basinlike portion of the ureter within the kidney. Recall that
-plasty	the suffix for surgical repair or reconstruction is _____. Thus, a
pyeloplasty	surgical repair of the renal pelvis is called a _____.

SELF-INSTRUCTION: ANATOMICAL TERMS

Study the following:

Term	Meaning
kidneys (Fig. 13-2) *kid'nēz*	two structures located on each side of the lumbar region that filter blood and secrete impurities, forming urine
cortex *kōr'teks*	outer part of the kidney (cortex = bark)
hilum *hī'lŭm*	indented opening in the kidney where vessels enter and leave
medulla *me-dūl'ă*	inner part of the kidney
calices (calyces) *kal'i-sēz*	ducts that carry urine from the nephrons to the renal pelvis (kalyx = cup of a flower)

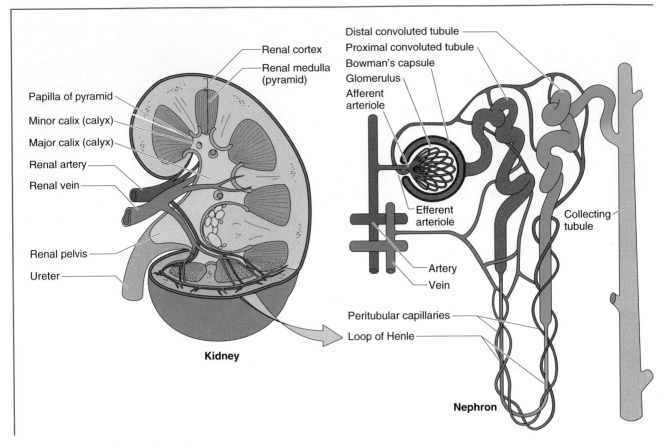

■ **FIGURE 13-2.** Kidney and nephron.

nephron *nef'ron*	microscopic functional units of the kidney, comprised of kidney cells and capillaries, each capable of forming urine
glomerulus *glō-măr'yū-lŭs*	little ball-shaped cluster of capillaries located at the top of each nephron
Bowman's capsule *bō-mĕnz kap'sūl*	the top part of the nephron that encloses the glomerulus
renal tubule *rē'năl tū'byūl*	the stem portion of the nephron
ureter *ū-rē'ter*	the tube that carries urine from the kidney to the bladder
renal pelvis *rē'năl pel'vis*	the basinlike portion of the ureter within the kidney
ureteropelvic junction *yū'rē'ter-ō-pel'vik*	point of connection between the renal pelvis and ureter
urinary bladder *yūr'i-nār-ē*	sac that holds the urine

urethra *yū-rē'thră*	single canal that carries urine to the outside of the body
urethral meatus *mē-ā'tŭs*	opening in the urethra to the outside of the body
urine *yūr'in*	fluid produced by the kidneys, containing water and waste products
urea *yū-rē'ă*	waste product formed in the liver, filtered out of the blood by the kidneys, and excreted in urine
creatinine *krē-at'i-nēn*	waste product of muscle metabolism, filtered out of the blood by the kidneys and excreted in urine

PROGRAMMED REVIEW: ANATOMICAL TERMS

Answers	Review
kidneys cortex medulla medullae	**13.18** The two structures to the sides of the lumbar region that filter flood to remove wastes are the _____. The outer part of the kidney is called the _____ (from a word originally meaning bark, as tree bark is the outer part of a tree trunk). The inner part, where the urine is collected, is called the _____. (Note that this same term, meaning middle, is used to refer to the middle part of several body structures.) The plural of medulla is _____.
hilum	**13.19** The indented opening in the kidney where vessels enter and leave is the _____.
nephrons glomerulus capsule renal tubule kidney	**13.20** Inside the cortex of the kidneys are the microscopic functional units that form urine, called _____. At the top of each nephron is a ball-shaped cluster of capillaries, called a _____ that carries blood to and away from each nephron. Enclosing each glomerulus is a structure called Bowman's _____. From the Bowman's capsule, the urine flows through the _____ _____. Recall that the adjective renal refers generally to the _____.

urine urea creatinine	**13.21** The fluid secreted by the nephrons that contains water and waste products is _____. The waste product formed in the liver but filtered from the blood in the kidneys is _____. A second waste product filtered from the blood in the kidneys is a product of muscle metabolism: _____.
calices (calyces) calix (calyx)	**13.22** The urine flows through the renal tubules from each nephron through a system of ducts called _____. The singular form of this term is _____. The calices (calyces) carry the urine to the renal pelvis, the basinlike portion of the ureter within the kidney.
renal pelvis ureteropelvic	**13.23** The basinlike portion of the ureter collecting urine from the calyces is the _____ _____. The point of connection between the renal pelvis and the ureter is the _____ junction.
ureter hilum	**13.24** From the renal pelvis, urine moves through the _____ to the bladder, a sac that holds the urine before its excretion. Each kidney has one ureter, which exits the kidney at the same point where arteries and veins enter it, at the _____ of the kidney.
bladder urethra	**13.25** The sac that holds urine is the urinary _____. From the bladder, the urine exits through a canal called the _____.
urethral meatus	**13.26** Formed from the combining forms meaning urethra and opening, the opening from the urethra to the outside of the body, through which urine leaves the body, is the _____ _____.

SELF-INSTRUCTION: SYMPTOMATIC TERMS

Study the following:

Term	Meaning
albuminuria *al-byū-mi-nū′rē-ă* **proteinuria** *prō-tē-nū′rē-ă*	presence of albumin in the urine, such as occurs in renal disease or in normal urine after heavy exercise

anuria *an-yū′rē-ă*	absence of urine formation
anuresis *an-yū-rē′sis*	inability to pass urine
bacteriuria *bak-tēr-ē-ū′rē-ă*	presence of bacteria in the urine
dysuria *dis-yū′rē-ă*	painful urination
enuresis *en-yū-rē′sis*	involuntary discharge of urine, usually referring to a lack of bladder control
nocturnal enuresis *nok-ter′năl*	bedwetting during sleep
hematuria (Fig. 13-3) *hē-mă-tū′rē-ă*	presence of blood in the urine
incontinence *in-kon′ti-nens*	involuntary discharge of urine or feces
urinary stress incontinence	involuntary discharge of urine with coughing, sneezing, or strained exercise
ketonuria *kē-tō-nū′rē-ă*	presence of ketone bodies in the urine
ketone bodies *kē′tōn* **ketone compounds**	acetone, beta-hydroxybutyric acid, and acetoacetic acid are products of metabolism that appear in the urine from the body's abnormal use of carbohydrates, such as occurs in uncontrolled diabetes or starvation
nocturia *nok-tū′rē-ă*	urination at night

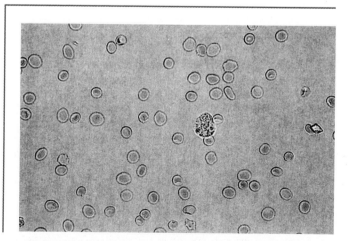

■ **FIGURE 13-3.** Hematuria. Microscopic urine showing a large number of red blood cells. One lone white blood cell is present in the center of the field.

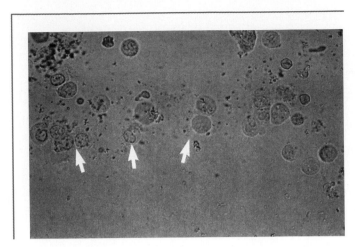

■ **FIGURE 13-4.** Pyuria. Microscopic urine showing the presence of white blood cells *(arrows)*.

oliguria *ol-i-gŭ′rē-ă*	scanty production of urine
pyuria (Fig. 13-4) *pī-yŭ′rē-ă*	presence of white cells in the urine, usually indicating infection
urinary retention *yŭr′i-nār-ē rē-ten′shŭn*	retention of urine caused by an inability to void (urinate) naturally because of spasm or obstruction

PROGRAMMED REVIEW: SYMPTOMATIC TERMS

Answers	Review
urine condition of bacteriuria	**13.27** Ur/o is a combining form for _____. The suffix *-ia* refers to a _____ _____. Many symptomatic terms end in *-uria*, referring to the presence of abnormal amounts of a substance in the urine. For example, the presence of bacteria in the urine is _____.
hematuria	**13.28** A combining form meaning blood is *hemat/o*. The presence of blood in the urine is _____.
py/o pyuria	**13.29** The combining form for pus is _____. Pus consists mostly of white blood cells that fight infection. The presence of white blood cells in the urine is therefore termed _____, which often indicates a urinary tract infection (UTI).

albumin/o

albuminuria

13.30   The combining form meaning protein is _____.
The presence of protein in the urine is therefore termed
_____. Another term for this is proteinuria.

13.31   The ending -*uria* is used with other urinary conditions, not just
those indicating the presence of some substance in the urine. The prefix
an- means _____; therefore, the term for absence of urine

without

anuria

formation (i.e., being without urine) is _____. Another term
modified by -*uria* describes excessive voluntary urination at night:

nocturia

_____.

13.32   Uresis is a term synonymous with urination. Modified by the
prefix meaning without, it forms the term for the inability to pass urine:

anuresis

enuresis

nocturnal

_____. The term referring to an involuntary discharge of
urine is _____, using the prefix *en*-. An involuntary discharge of urine during sleep is called _____ enuresis
(bedwetting).

13.33   Recall that the prefix *dys*- means faulty, difficult or

painful

dysuria

_____. The term for a condition of painful urination is
_____.

deficient

oliguria

13.34   Recall that *oligo*- is a prefix meaning few or _____.
Therefore, the term for a condition of scanty (deficient) production of
urine is _____. (Remember that the final vowel is occasionally dropped from the prefix when joined with a root beginning
with a vowel.)

urine

incontinence

stress

13.35   Enuresis, again, is the involuntary discharge of _____.
The general term for involuntary discharge of urine or feces is
_____. When this occurs during the stress of
coughing, sneezing, or exercise, it is called urinary _____
incontinence.

urine

13.36 Urinary retention is the retention of _____ caused by an inability to void (urinate) naturally because of spasm, an obstruction, or other factors.

ketone

13.37 The combining form *ket/o* means _____ bodies or ketone compounds. These are metabolic products that may appear in the urine because of abnormal use of carbohydrates. The condition in which

ketonuria

ketone bodies appear in the urine is called _____.

SELF-INSTRUCTION: DIAGNOSTIC TERMS

Study the following:

Term	Meaning
glomerulonephritis *glō-mār′yū-lō-nef-rī′tis*	form of nephritis involving the glomerulus
hydronephrosis (Fig. 13-5) *hī′drō-ne-frō′sis*	pooling of urine in dilated areas of the renal pelvis and calices of one or both kidneys caused by an obstructed outflow of urine
nephritis *ne-frī′tis*	inflammation of the kidney

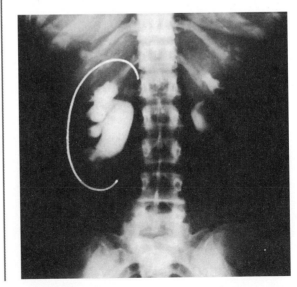

■ **FIGURE 13-5.** Hydronephrosis. Collection of contrast media in the kidney displays an extraordinary amount of material, which indicates right-sided hydronephrosis caused by obstruction in the ureter.

pyelonephritis *pī′ĕ-lō-ne-frī′tis*	inflammation of the renal pelvis
nephrosis *ne-frō′sis*	degenerative disease of the renal tubules
nephrolithiasis *nef′rō-li-thī′ă-sis*	presence of a renal stone or stones
cystitis *sis-tī′tis*	inflammation of the bladder
urethritis *yū-rē-thrī′tis*	inflammation of the urethra
urethrocystitis *yū-rē′thrō-sis-tī′tis*	inflammation of the urethra and bladder
urethral stenosis *yū-rē′thrăl ste-nō′sis*	narrowed condition of the urethra
urinary tract infection (UTI)	invasion of pathogenic organisms (commonly bacteria) in the urinary tract, especially the urethra and bladder; symptoms include dysuria, urinary frequency, and malaise
uremia *yū-rē′mē-ă* **azotemia** *az-ō-tē′mē-ă*	excess of urea and other nitrogenous waste in the blood caused by kidney failure

PROGRAMMED REVIEW: DIAGNOSTIC TERMS

Answers	Review
-itis nephr/o nephritis glomerulonephritis	**13.38** Recall that the suffix meaning inflammation is _____. Many diagnostic terms are formed using this suffix added to the combining forms for anatomical structures. In addition to the combining form *ren/o*, another combining form meaning kidney is _____. Using that form, the term for inflammation of the kidney is _____. A form of nephritis involving the glomerulus is called _____.
cyst/o cystitis	**13.39** In addition to the combining form *vesic/o*, another combining form for the bladder is _____. Using that form, the term for inflammation of the bladder is _____.

urethritis

13.40 Inflammation of the urethra is termed _____.

urethrocystitis

13.41 Inflammation of both the urethra and the bladder is

_____.

pyel/o

renal

pelvis

13.42 Recall that the combining form meaning basin is _____.
The basinlike portion of the ureter is called the _____

_____. Therefore, that combining form is used in this

term for inflammation of the renal pelvis area of the kidney:

pyelonephritis

_____.

condition

nephrosis

13.43 Recall that the suffix *-osis* means an increase or

_____. That suffix is used to make a term

for degenerative disease of the kidney (specifically, the renal

tubules), called _____.

condition

hydronephrosis

13.44 A combining form meaning water (or watery fluid) is *hydr/o.*
Recall that the suffix *-osis* means _____ or increase. The

term referring to a condition of urine pooling in the renal pelvis caused

by an outflow obstruction is _____.

lith/o

-iasis

nephrolithiasis

13.45 Recall that the combining form for stone is _____. The

suffix for formation of or presence of is _____. These word parts

along with *nephr/o* create the term for the presence of stones in the kid-

ney: _____.

urethral stenosis

13.46 A general medical term for the condition of a narrowed struc-

ture is stenosis. A narrowed condition of the urethra is called

_____ _____.

urinary tract infection

13.47 The invasion of pathogenic bacteria in urinary structures is

called a _____ _____ _____, or UTI.

-emia	**13.48** Recall that the suffix for a blood condition is _____. Using the combining form for urine (in this case, referring to urea and waste products normally excreted in urine), the condition of nitrogenous
uremia	wastes in the blood because of kidney failure is _____. A syn-
azotemia	onym for uremia is _____, made with the prefix *azo-*, which refers to a nitrogen molecule.

SELF-INSTRUCTION: DIAGNOSTIC TESTS AND PROCEDURES

Study the following:

Test or Procedure	Explanation
cystoscopy (Fig. 13-6) *sis-tos′kŏ-pē*	examination of the bladder using a rigid or flexible cystoscope
kidney biopsy (Bx) **renal biopsy**	removal of kidney tissue for pathologic examination
radiography *rā′dē-og′ră-fē*	x-ray studies commonly used in urology

intravenous
      pyelogram (IVP)
      (Fig. 13-5)
      in′tră-vē′nŭs
        pī′el-ō-gram
    intravenous
      urogram (Fig. 13-7)
	x-rays of the urinary tract taken after an iodine contrast medium is injected into the bloodstream; the contrast passes through the kidney and may reveal an obstruction, evidence of trauma, and so on

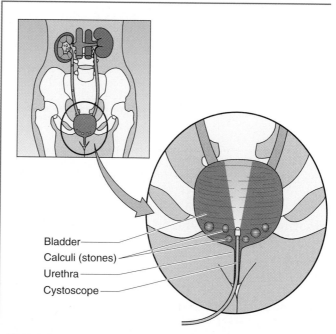

Bladder

Calculi (stones)

Urethra

Cystoscope

■ **FIGURE 13-6.** Cystoscopy.

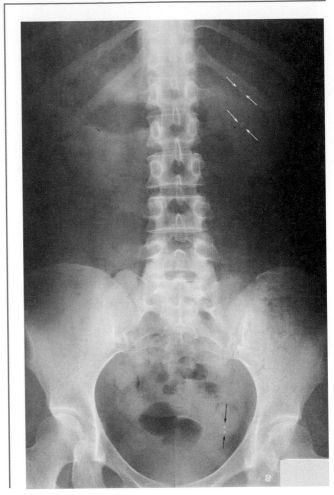

■ **FIGURE 13-7.** Kidney, ureter, bladder (KUB) showing kidney stones in ureters and bladder *(arrows)*.

kidney, ureter, bladder (KUB)	abdominal x-ray of kidney, ureter, and bladder typically used as a scout film before doing an IVP
scout film	plain x-ray taken to detect any obvious pathology before further imaging (e.g., a KUB before an IVP)
renal angiogram *an'jē-ō-gram* **(arteriogram)**	x-ray of the renal artery made after injecting contrast material into a catheter in the artery
retrograde pyelogram (RP) *ret'rō-grād*	x-ray of the ureters, bladder, and kidney taken after contrast medium is administered backward through a small catheter through a cystoscope to detect the presence of stones, obstruction, and so on
voiding (urinating) cystourethrogram (VCU or VCUG) *sis-tō-yū-rēth'rō-gram*	x-ray of the bladder and urethra taken during urination
abdominal sonogram *son'ō-gram*	ultrasound image of the urinary tract, including the kidney and bladder

CENTRAL MEDICAL CENTER

211 Medical Center Drive • Central City, US 90000-1234 • PHONE: (012) 125-6784 • FAX: (012) 125-9999

11//02/20xx
13:49

NAME : TEST, PATIENT   LOC: TEST   DOB: 2/2/XX   AGE: 38Y
MR#   :   TEST-221   SEX: M
ACCT #   :   H111111111

M63560 COLL: 11/2/20xx 13:24   REC: 11/2/20xx   13:25

URINE BASIC
Color	STRAW		
Appearance	CLEAR		
Specific Gravity	1.010	[1.003 - 1.035]	
pH	5.5	[5.0 - 9.0]	
Protein	NEG	[0 - 10]	MG/DL
Glucose	NEG	[NEG]	
Ketones	NEG	[NEG]	
Bilirubin	NEG	[NEG]	
Urine Occult Blood	NEG	[NEG]	
Nitrites	NEG		

URINE MICROSCOPIC
Epithelial Cells	3 to 4	/HPF
WBCs	0 to 1	/HPF
RBCs	0	/HPF
Bacteria	0	
Mucous Threads	0	

TEST, PATIENT   TEST-221   END OF REPORT   PAGE 1
11/02/20xx   13:49   INTERIM REPORT
INTERIM REPORT COMPLETED

FIGURE 13-8. Sample urinalysis report.

LABORATORY TESTING

urinalysis (UA) (Fig. 13-8) *yū-ri-nal'i-sis*	physical, chemical, and microscopic examination of urine
specific gravity (SpGr)	measure of the concentration or dilution of urine
pH	measure of the acidity or alkalinity of urine
glucose (sugar) *glū'kōs*	chemical test used to detect sugar in the urine; used most often to screen for diabetes
albumin (alb) *al-byu'min* **protein**	chemical test used to detect the presence of albumin in the urine

ketones	chemical test used to detect the presence of ketone bodies in the urine; positive test indicates fats are being used by the body instead of carbohydrates, which occurs in starvation or in an uncontrolled diabetic state
occult blood, urine	chemical test for the presence of hidden blood in the urine resulting from red blood cell hemolysis; indicates bleeding in the kidneys (occult = hidden)
bilirubin *bil-i-rū'bin*	chemical test used to detect bilirubin in the urine; seen in gallbladder and liver disease
urobilinogen *yūr-ō-bī-lin'ō-jen*	chemical test used to detect bile pigment in the urine—increased amounts seen in gallbladder and liver disease
nitrite	chemical test to determine the presence of bacteria in the urine
microscopic **findings** (Figs. 13-3 and 13-4) *mī-krō-skop'ik*	microscopic identification of abnormal constituents present in the urine (e.g., red blood cells, white blood cells, and casts); reported per high or low power field (hpf or lpf)
urine culture and **sensitivity (C&S)**	isolation of a urine specimen in a culture medium to propagate the growth of microorganisms; organisms that grow in the culture are identified along with drugs to which they are sensitive
blood urea nitrogen (BUN) *yū-rē'ă nī'trō-jen*	blood test to determine the level of urea in the blood; a high BUN indicates the kidney's inability to excrete urea
creatinine, serum *krē-at'i-nēn sēr'ŭm*	test to determine the level of creatinine in the blood, useful in assessing kidney function
creatinine, urine	test to determine the level of creatinine in the urine
creatinine clearance **testing**	measurements of the level of creatinine in the blood and a 24-hour urine specimen to determine the rate that creatinine is "cleared" from the blood by the kidneys

PROGRAMMED REVIEW: DIAGNOSTIC TESTS AND PROCEDURES

Answers	Review
	13.49 Recall that the two combining forms for bladder are *cyst/o* and
vesic/o	_____. The first of these, combined with the suffix for process of examination with an instrument, forms the term for examination of
cystoscopy	the bladder with a special scope: _____.

13.50 The general term for removal of any body tissue for pathologic examination is _____, abbreviated Bx. The removal of kidney tissue is called a kidney biopsy or _____ biopsy.

biopsy

renal

13.51 Recall that the suffix *-graphy* means the process of _____ (such as an image). The process of making x-ray studies of internal body structures, such as the urinary tract, is termed _____.

recording

radiography

13.52 A plain x-ray taken to detect any obvious pathology before further imaging is called a _____ film. An abdominal x-ray of the kidney, ureter, and bladder (called a _____) is often made as a scout film before additional images using a contrast medium.

scout

KUB

13.53 Recall that the suffix *-gram* means a _____. The combining form *pyel/o* means basin, referring to the basinlike portion of the ureter in the kidney known as the _____ _____. These components are used to name the type of x-ray made of the urinary tract after contrast iodine is injected into the bloodstream to reveal obstruction, trauma, or other problems in the kidney: _____ _____ (IVP). The other term for this x-ray, using the combining form for urine, is intravenous _____. Recall that the prefix *intra-* means _____, referring in this case to the contrast medium administered within a vein.

record

renal pelvis

intravenous pyelogram

urogram, within

13.54 The term angiogram comes from the combining form *angi/o,* meaning _____; angiograms are x-rays taken of blood vessels in many parts of the body. The general term describing an x-ray of the renal artery made after a contrast medium is injected into it is therefore called a _____ _____. The specific term uses the combining for artery: renal _____ .

vessel

renal angiogram

arteriogram

13.55 The type of x-ray of urinary structures taken after a contrast medium is sent up (backward) through a catheter is called a

retrograde pyelogram	_____ _____ (RP). The word retro-grade refers to the insertion of the medium in a direction against the usual flow (of urine in this case).
urinate voiding cystourethrogram	**13.56**　To void means to _____. An x-ray of the bladder and urethra (using the combining forms for both) taken during urination is called a _____ _____ (VCU or VCUG).
abdominal sonogram	**13.57**　Ultrasound is also used to image the urinary tract. An ultrasound image of the abdomen showing the kidneys and bladder is called an _____ _____.
urinalysis	**13.58**　Many different laboratory tests are conducted on the urine to aid in diagnosing urinary system conditions. The term for a full set of physical, chemical, and microscopic examinations of urine is _____ (UA).
specific gravity	**13.59**　The measurement of the concentration of urine, showing the kidney's ability to concentrate or dilute urine, is _____ _____ (SpGr).
pH	**13.60**　The measurement of the acidity or alkalinity of any fluid is called its ____. The urinalysis includes urine pH.
glucose	**13.61**　Sugar in the blood or urine is called _____. When detected in the urine, glucose may be an indication of diabetes.
albumin/o albumin	**13.62**　Recall that the combining form meaning protein is _____. The test in the urinalysis that detects the presence of protein in the urine is called an _____ or protein test.
ketones	**13.63**　The test to detect the presence of ketone bodies in the urine is simply called _____.

breaking down

urine occult

blood

bilirubin

urobilinogen

liver

bacteriuria

nitrite

microscopic findings

urine culture, sensitivity

creatinine

urine creatinine

13.64   Recall that the suffix *-lysis* means dissolution or

_____ _____. Hemolysis occurs when the intact membranes of red blood cells break down. The cells, once intact, are now hidden. The presence of free-flowing hemoglobin, the pigment normally contained within red blood cells, is a clue to their hidden state. The chemical test of urine to determine the presence of these once intact and now hidden blood cells is _____ _____ _____.

13.65   Bilirubin is a component of bile, which is secreted by the liver and is not normally present in urine. The urinalysis chemical test for its presence in urine is simply called _____.

13.66   The chemical test for the presence of a bile pigment in the urine is _____. Increased amounts of urobilinogen are seen in gallbladder and _____ disease.

13.67   The presence of bacteria in the urine is termed _____. Nitrite is a waste product produced by bacteria. The chemical test to determine the presence of this waste product in urine, thereby indicating bacteriuria, is simply called _____.

13.68   Urine is examined under a microscope to identify abnormal constituents, such as blood cells. The results of this examination are called _____ _____.

13.69   The isolation of a urine specimen in a culture medium to grow microorganisms and identify drugs to which they are sensitive is called a _____ _____ and _____ (C&S).

13.70   Recall that a waste product of muscle metabolism is _____. The test that determines the level of creatinine in the urine is _____ _____.

serum creatinine

13.71 Blood tests (serum tests) also help diagnose problems in the urinary system. The test to determine the level of creatinine in the blood is _____ _____. Measurements taken in the blood and in a 24-hour urine specimen determine the rate that creatinine is cleared by the kidneys; this is called _____

creatinine

clearance

_____ testing.

blood urea

13.72 BUN is the abbreviation for _____ _____

nitrogen

_____, a blood test to determine the level of urea in the blood, which may indicate a kidney disorder.

SELF-INSTRUCTION: OPERATIVE TERMS

Study the following:

Term	Meaning
urologic endoscopic surgery (Fig. 13-9) *yū-rō-loj'ik*	use of specialized endoscopes (e.g., resectoscope) within the urinary tract to perform various surgical procedures such as resection of a tumor, repair of an obstruction, stone retrieval, placement of a stent, and so on
resectoscope *rē-sek'tō-skōp*	urologic endoscope inserted through the urethra to resect (cut and remove) lesions of the bladder, urethra, or prostate
intracorporeal lithotripsy (Fig. 13-10) *in'tră-kōr-pō'rē-ăl ē-lek'trō-hī-dro'lik lith'ō-trip-sē*	method of destroying stones within the urinary tract using electrical energy discharges transmitted to a probe within a flexible endoscope; most commonly used to pulverize bladder stones

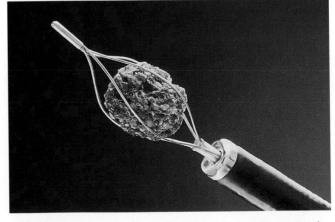

FIGURE 13-9. Stone basket used in kidney stone retrieval.

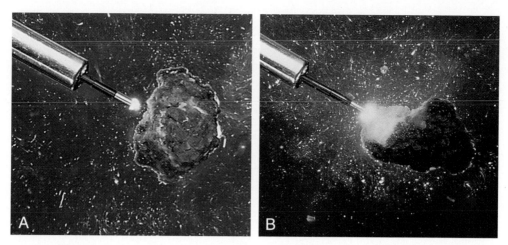

FIGURE 13-10. Simulation of the pulverizing of stones performed by intracorporeal

nephrotomy *ne-frot'ō-mē*	incision into the kidney
nephrorrhaphy *nef-rōr'ă-fē*	suture of an injured kidney
nephrolithotomy *nef'rō-li-thot'ō-mē*	incision into the kidney for the removal of stones
nephrectomy *ne-frek'tō-mē*	excision of a kidney
pyeloplasty *pī'e-lō-plas-tē*	surgical reconstruction of the renal pelvis
stent placement (Fig. 13-11)	use of a device (stent) to hold open vessels or tubes (e.g., an obstructed ureter)

Before

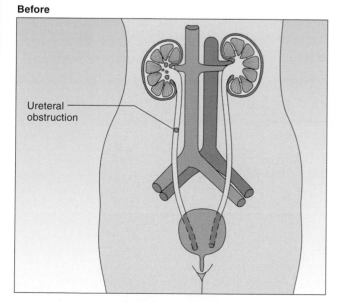

Ureteral obstruction

After

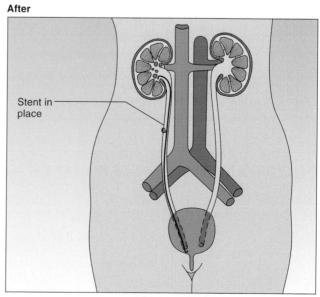

Stent in place

■ **FIGURE 13-11.** Placement of a double-J stent to relieve ureteral obstruction.

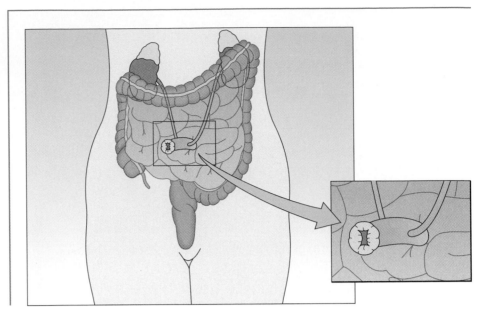

■ **FIGURE 13-12.** Urostomy: ileal conduit.

kidney transplantation **renal transplantation**	transfer of a kidney from the body of one person (donor) to another
urinary diversion	creation of a temporary or permanent diversion of the urinary tract to provide a new passage through which urine exits the body; used to treat defects or disease such as bladder cancer

common types:
  noncontinent ileal
    conduit
    (Fig. 13-12)
    non-kon'ti-nent
    il'ē-ăl kon'dū-it
	removal of a portion of the ileum to use as a conduit to which the ureters are attached at one end; the other end is brought through an opening (stoma) created in the abdomen—urine drains continually into an external appliance (bag)

continent urostomy
    kon'ti-nent
    yu-ros'tō-mē
	an internal reservoir (pouch) constructed from a segment of intestine which diverts urine through an opening (stoma) that is brought through the abdominal wall—a valve is created internally to prevent leakage and the patient empties the pouch by catheterization

orthotopic bladder **neobladder**	bladder constructed from portions of intestine connected to the urethra, allowing "natural" voiding

PROGRAMMED REVIEW: OPERATIVE TERMS

Answers	Review
-tomy	**13.73** Recall that the suffix meaning incision is _____. The term
nephrotomy	for an incision into the kidney is therefore _____.
lith/o	The combining form meaning stone is _____. An incision into the

kidney to remove a stone (using the combining forms for both kidney and stone) is therefore _____.

nephrolithotomy	

13.74 The suffix *-ectomy* means _____. Therefore, the excision of a kidney is _____.

excision or removal	
nephrectomy	

13.75 The suffix referring to surgical repair or reconstruction is _____. Therefore, the term for surgical reconstruction of the renal pelvis (using the combining form meaning basin, for this basinlike structure) is _____.

-plasty	
pyeloplasty	

13.76 Recall that the suffix for suturing is _____. The procedure of suturing an injured kidney is therefore called _____.

-rrhaphy	
nephrorrhaphy	

13.77 The suffix referring to the surgical creation of an opening is _____. In some conditions, a surgeon may have to make a diversion in the urinary tract for urine to exit the body through a new opening. This surgery is called a _____ (using the combining form for urine).

-stomy	
urostomy	

13.78 Urologic endoscopic surgery uses a specialized endoscope called a _____ to resect tumors or perform other surgical procedures within the urinary tract. A device that is surgically placed to hold open a vessel or tube is called a _____. Urologic stent placement is also performed through the _____scope.

resectoscope	
stent	
resecto	

13.79 Stones within the urinary tract may be destroyed by the transmission of electrical energy through an endoscope. The prefix *intra-* means _____, and *corpor/o* combined with *-eal* pertains to the body; thus, this process performed within the body is also termed _____. The suffix *-tripsy* means crushing; thus, the crushing of a stone is termed _____.

within	
intracorporeal	
lithotripsy	

These two terms form the name for the procedure of electrically destroying stones within the urinary tract, usually in the bladder:

intracorporeal lithotripsy

_____ _____.

13.80 In cases in which the patient has two diseased kidneys, a kidney from a donor may be surgically implanted in the patient. This procedure is called _____ _____.

kidney (or renal)

transplantation

13.81 When cystectomy, or removal of the _____, is required because of disease or defect, it is necessary to create a new passage for urine to exit the body. One method, which uses a portion of the ileum as a conduit diverting urine from the ureters to the outside of the body, is called an _____ _____. Continent refers to the ability to hold or retain urine. This method is considered non_____ because urine cannot be held and drains continually into a bag.

bladder

ileal conduit

continent

13.82 The internal reservoir constructed of intestine that diverts urine to a stoma on the abdomen with a valve attachment to allow catheter draining is called _____. Because the reservoir is capable of retaining urine, the procedure is called _____ urostomy.

urostomy

continent

13.83 Construction of a new bladder, or _____bladder, provides a straight connection to the urethra, allowing for a more natural voiding or _____. Neobladder is also called a _____ bladder, a term formed from the combination of _orth/o_, meaning straight, normal or _____, _top/o_, meaning place, and _–ic_, meaning _____ _____.

neo

urination

orthotopic

correct

pertaining to

SELF-INSTRUCTION: THERAPEUTIC TERMS

Study the following:

Term	Meaning
extracorporeal shock wave lithotripsy (ESWL) *eks′tră-kōr-pō′rē-ăl lith′ō-trip-sē*	procedure using ultrasound outside the body to bombard and disintegrate a stone within; most commonly used to treat urinary stones above the bladder
kidney dialysis *dī-al′i-sis*	methods of filtering impurities from the blood, replacing the function of one or both kidneys lost in renal failure
hemodialysis *hē-mō-dī-al′i-sis*	method of removing impurities by pumping the patient's blood through a dialyzer, the specialized filter of the artificial kidney machine (hemodialyzer)
peritoneal dialysis *per-i-tō-n′eăl*	method of removing impurities using the peritoneum as the filter; a catheter inserted in the peritoneal cavity delivers cleansing fluid (dialysate) that is washed in and out in cycles

COMMON THERAPEUTIC DRUG CLASSIFICATIONS

analgesic *an-ăl-jē′zik*	drug that relieves pain
antibiotic *an′tē-bī-ot′ik*	drug that kills or inhibits the growth of microorganisms
antispasmodic *an′tē-spaz-mod′ik*	drug that relieves spasm
diuretic *dī-yū-ret′ik*	drug that increases the secretion of urine

PROGRAMMED REVIEW: THERAPEUTIC TERMS

Answers	Review
body	**13.84** Recall that intracorporeal pertains to within the _____. The
outside	prefix *extra-*, however, means _____. Therefore, the term for
extracorporeal	outside the body is _____. The procedure
	using the shock waves of ultrasound from outside the body to break up
extracorporeal	urinary stones is termed _____
shock wave lithotripsy	_____ _____ _____ (ESWL).

kidney dialysis

13.85   Dialysis is a general medical term meaning filtration. This process of filtering impurities from the blood in patients who have renal failure is called _____ _____. The combining form for blood is *hem/o,* used to create the term for the process of pumping a patient's blood through an artificial kidney machine:

hemodialysis

_____.

13.86   Another method for removing impurities uses the patient's peritoneum (an abdominal cavity) for a filtering bath, called

peritoneal dialysis

_____ _____.

against

13.87   Recall that the prefix *anti-* means _____ or opposed to. Drug classes are commonly named for their actions, such as acting against some thing or process. A drug that acts to prevent or relieve a

antispasmodic

spasm is an _____. The same prefix joined with the combining form for life (bio) denotes a drug class that acts to

antibiotic

kill or inhibit microbial life. This drug is an _____.

without

13.88   The Greek word algesis means sensation of pain. Recall that the prefix *an-* means _____. A type of drug that relieves pain is

analgesic

termed an _____.

diuretic

13.89   A drug that increases the secretion of urine is called a _____. Other common substances, such as coffee and alcohol, also have diuretic effects.

Practice Exercises

For the following terms, on the lines below the term, write out the indicated word parts: prefixes, combining forms, roots, and suffixes. Then define the word.

Example:

pericystitis

<u>peri/cyst/itis</u>
   P   R   S

DEFINITION: around/bladder or sac/inflammation

1. pyuria

————— / ————— / —————
    R   R   S

DEFINITION: _____

2. bacteriosis

————— / —————
    R   S

DEFINITION: _____

3. transurethral

————— / ————— / —————
    P   R   S

DEFINITION: _____

4. urogram

————— / —————
    CF   S

DEFINITION: _____

5. urethrocystitis

————— / ————— / —————
    CF   R   S

DEFINITION: _____

6. nephroptosis

————— / —————
    CF   S

DEFINITION: _____

7. polydipsia

————— / ————— / —————
    P   R   S

DEFINITION: _____

8. glomerulosclerosis

_____ / _____ / _____
    CF   R   S

DEFINITION: _____

9. pyonephritis

_____ / _____ / _____
    CF   R   S

DEFINITION: _____

10. urinal

_____ / _____
    R   S

DEFINITION: _____

11. ureterovesicostomy

_____ / _____ / _____
    CF   CF   S

DEFINITION: _____

12. glycorrhea

_____ / _____
    CF   S

DEFINITION: _____

13. meatorrhaphy

_____ / _____
    CF   S

DEFINITION: _____

14. pyelonephrosis

_____ / _____ / _____
    CF   R   S

DEFINITION: _____

15. cystoscopy

_____ / _____
    CF   S

DEFINITION: _____

16. suprarenal

_____ / _____ / _____
    P   R   S

DEFINITION: _____

17. nephrolithiasis

_____ / _____ / _____
    CF   R   S

DEFINITION: _____

18. urethrostenosis

_____ / _____ / _____
    CF   R   S

DEFINITION: _____

19. albuminuria

_____ / _____ / _____
    R   R   S

DEFINITION: _____

20. ketosis

_____ / _____
    R   S

DEFINITION: _____

Identify the medical term for the following:

21. inflammation of the bladder _____

22. urinating at night _____

23. involuntary discharge of urine _____

24. suture of a torn kidney _____

25. degenerative disease of the kidney without inflammation _____

26. protein in urine _____

27. narrowed condition of the urethra _____

28. incision into the kidney _____

29. cytology study of kidney tissue _____

30. physical, chemical, and microscopic study of urine

_____

Complete the following:

31. _____scopy = examination of the bladder

32. urethral _____osis = a narrowed condition of the urethra

33. extracorporeal shock wave _____ = procedure for disintegration of stones

34. _____scope = urologic endoscope used to cut and remove lesions

35. _____uria = scanty urination

36. _____uria = painful or difficult urination

37. _____uria = presence of infection in urine

38. _____uria = blood in the urine

39. _____uresis = no output of urine

40. _____uresis = involuntary discharge of urine

41. _____ incontinence = involuntary discharge of urine when coughing or sneezing

42. _____blood = hidden blood

Give the appropriate abbreviation for the following:

43. _____ kidney x-ray taken after contrast medium is sent "backward" through a cystoscope

44. _____ cytology study of kidney tissue

45. _____ physical, chemical, and microscopic study of urine

Match the following:

46. sugar _____   a. cysto

47. proteinuria _____   b. ketones

48. uremia _____   c. renal Bx

49. reno _____   d. albuminuria

50. vesico _____   e. nephro

51. ketonuria _____   f. urination

52. diuretic _____   g. azotemia

53. kidney biopsy _____   h. gluco

Define the following abbreviations:

54. C&S _____

55. VCU _____

56. alb _____

57. IVP _____

58. ESWL _____

59. KUB _____

60. SpGr _____

61. UTI _____

62. RP _____

For each of the following, circle the combining form that corresponds to the meaning given:

63. **urine**	hydr/o	ur/o	ren/o
64. **thirst**	dips/o	crin/o	hidr/o
65. **pus**	pyel/o	py/o	albumin/o
66. **bladder**	cyt/o	vesic/o	nephr/o
67. **protein**	albumin/o	lip/o	bacteri/o
68. **kidney**	hepat/o	cyst/o	nephr/o
69. **opening**	or/o	meat/o	orth/o
70. **basin**	meat/o	vesic/o	pyel/o
71. **stone**	scler/o	lip/o	lith/o

Write in the missing words on lines in the following illustration of the urinary anatomy

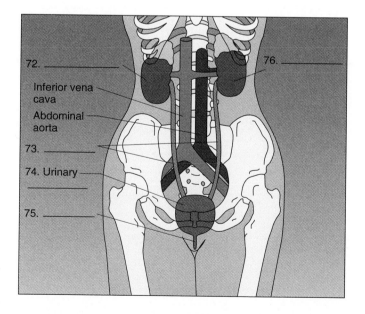

72. _____

Inferior vena cava

Abdominal aorta

73. _____

74. Urinary _____

75. _____

76. _____

For each of the following, circle the correct spelling of the term:

77. cystascope   cystoskope   cystoscope

78. pyleogram   pyelogram   pielogram

79. oliguria   oleguria   oligouria

80. hydronefrosis   hidronephrosis   hydronephrosis

81. azootemia   azothemia   azotemia

82. urinalysis   urinelysis   uranalysis

83. glowmerular   glomerular   glomarular

84. nefrectomy   nephrecktomy   nephrectomy

85. diuretic   dyuretic   diuretik

86. hemadialysis   hemodialysis   hemidialysis

Give the noun that was used to form the following adjectives.

87. urinary   _____

88. glomerular   _____

89. meatal   _____

90. uremic   _____

91. urethral   _____

92. nephrotic   _____

Medical Record Analyses

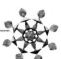

MEDICAL RECORD 13-1

Chart Note

S   This 70 y.o. female has had polyuria, nocturia, and dysuria × 2-3 days. She had a similar infection 6 months ago and was treated with Macrobid, 50 mg, qid × 3d. She has occasional stress incontinence with hard sneezing.

O   The patient is afebrile. UA shows a trace of leukocytes and blood

A   R/O recurrent UTI

P   C&S
    Cipro 500 mg tab po bid pending culture
    pt instructed to ↑ fluid intake and call for culture results in 48 h

1. What is the patient's CC?
   a. the presence of red and white blood cells in her urine
   b. a urinary tract infection
   c. pain when she urinates with the need to go often, even at night
   d. urinary tract infection

2. What were the objective findings?
   a. culture showed leukocytes and blood in the urine
   b. urinalysis indicated red and white blood cells present in urine
   c. bladder infection
   d. return of bladder infection

3. What was the doctor's impression?
   a. there were leukocytes and blood in the patient's urine
   b. the patient has pain when she urinates with the need to go often, even at night
   c. the patient has a bladder infection
   d. the patient may have another bladder infection

4. Which medical terms describe the UA findings?
   a. pyuria and hematuria
   b. dysuria and enuresis
   c. bacteriuria and hematuria
   d. bacteriuria and nocturia

5. To what does C&S refer?
   a. a condition of urinary stress
   b. the isolation of microorganisms in the urine
   c. inflammation of the bladder
   d. physical, chemical, and microscopic study of urine

6. How should the Cipro be administered?
   a. two, by mouth every day
   b. one, by mouth two times a day
   c. one, by mouth three times a day
   d. one, by mouth four times a day

7. Was the patient's temperature elevated?
   a. yes
   b. no
   c. nothing is stated about the patient's temperature

MEDICAL RECORD 13-2 FOR ADDITIONAL STUDY

CENTRAL MEDICAL CENTER

211 Medical Center Drive • Central City, US 90000-1234 • PHONE: (012) 125-6784 • FAX: (012) 125-9999

DISCHARGE SUMMARY

DATE OF ADMISSION: 10/25/20xx DATE OF DISCHARGE: 10/29/20xx

ADMITTING DIAGNOSIS:
Left ureteropelvic junction obstruction.

DISCHARGE DIAGNOSIS:
Left ureteropelvic junction obstruction.

PROCEDURE PERFORMED:
Left dismembered pyeloplasty and placement of stent.

BRIEF SUMMARY:
The patient is a 19-year-old male who was admitted to the hospital a month ago with left pyelonephritis. He was found to have a left ureteropelvic junction obstruction. The patient was brought to the hospital at this time for repair of the moderately to severely obstructed left kidney. A preoperative urine culture was sterile. The patient underwent the procedure without complication. A double-J stent was placed. The Jackson-Pratt drain was removed on the second postoperative day because of minimal drainage. The patient initially had urinary retention, but this resolved by the third postoperative day. He was doing fine at the time of discharge. His condition on discharge is good.

INSTRUCTIONS TO THE PATIENT:
1) Regular diet. 2) No heavy lifting, straining, or driving an automobile for six weeks from the day of surgery. He should also keep the incision relatively dry this week. 3) Follow up in my office in three weeks. 4) It is anticipated the stent will remain indwelling for six weeks and then will be removed cystoscopically at that time. 5) Discharge medication is Tylenol #3, 1-2 q 4 h p.r.n. pain.

L. Zlatkin, M.D.
L. Zlatkin, M.D.

LZ:mr

D: 10/29/20xx
T: 10/30/20xx

DISCHARGE SUMMARY	PT. NAME: MERCIER, CHARLES F.
	ID NO: IP-392689
	ROOM NO: 444
	ATT. PHYS: L.ZLATKIN, M.D.

MEDICAL RECORD 13-2 FOR ADDITIONAL STUDY (CONTINUED)

CENTRAL MEDICAL CENTER

211 Medical Center Drive • Central City, US 90000-1234 • PHONE: (012) 125-6784 • FAX: (012) 125-9999

OPERATIVE REPORT

DATE: December 7, 20xx

PREOPERATIVE DIAGNOSIS: Congenital left ureteropelvic junction obstruction status post pyeloplasty. Indwelling left ureteral stent.

POSTOPERATIVE DIAGNOSIS: Congenital left ureteropelvic junction obstruction status post pyeloplasty. Indwelling left ureteral stent, removed

OPERATION: Cystoscopy, removal of left ureteral stent, and left retrograde pyelogram.

PROCEDURE: The patient was identified, was placed on the operating table, and was administered a general anesthetic. He was placed in the lithotomy position, and a KUB was obtained. The genitalia were prepped and draped in a sterile fashion. After reviewing the KUB, it was noted at this time that the position of the stent was normal. Cystoscopy was performed with a #22 French cystoscope. The stent was identified coming from the left ureteral orifice, and the end was grasped with forceps and removed through the cystoscope. A #8 French cone-tipped ureteral catheter was then placed in the left ureteral orifice and passed to 10 cm. Then, 20 cm^3 of contrast was injected into a left collecting system. A film was exposed, and this showed patency without extravasation at the left ureteropelvic junction. There was some filling of calyces and partial filling of the dilated renal pelvis. A drainage film was subsequently obtained showing complete emptying of the pelvis and partial emptying of the mid and distal ureters. Dilated calyces were noted in the kidney. The patient was allowed to awaken and was returned to the recovery room in satisfactory condition. There were no intraoperative complications. He had no bleeding. The patient did receive 1 gm Ancef one-half hour prior to the onset of the procedure.

L. Zlatkin, M.D.

LZ:mr
D: 12/07/20xx
T: 12/08/20xx

OPERATIVE REPORT	PT. NAME:	MERCIER, CHARLES F.
	ID NO:	OP-912689
	ROOM NO:	ASC
	ATT. PHYS:	L.ZLATKIN, M.D.

MEDICAL RECORD 13-2 FOR ADDITIONAL STUDY

Charles Mercier had urination problems and abdominal pain when he saw his doctor, who referred him to Central Medical Center for a possible kidney infection. Dr. Zlatkin performed surgery, and Mr. Mercier was soon doing fine and was discharged. As planned, he later returned for surgical removal of a device that had been temporarily placed during the first surgery.

Read Medical Record 13-2 (pages 580-581) Mr. Mercier, and answer the following questions. The first record is the discharge summary from the first surgery, dictated by Dr. Zlatkin. The second record is the operative report for Mr. Mercier's return surgery 6 weeks later, also dictated by Dr. Zlatkin.

1. Below are medical terms used in this record that you have not yet encountered in this text. Underline each where it appears in the record, and define below.

   stent (double-J) _____

   drain (Jackson-Pratt) _____

   lithotomy position _____

   ureteral catheter _____

   patency _____

2. In your own words, not using medical terminology, briefly describe the history of Mr. Mercier's medical problems identified in the "Discharge Summary."

   _____

   _____

   _____

3. Put the following events reported in the "Discharge Summary" in chronologic order by numbering them from 1 to 5:

   _____ removal of drain

   _____ reconstruction of renal pelvis

   _____ difficulty with micturition

   _____ urine test for microorganisms

   _____ insertion of stent

4. While at home after the operation, Mr. Mercier is instructed to do two things and *not* do three things. List them below:

   Mr. Mercier should _____

   _____

   Mr. Mercier should not _____

   _____

   _____

5. When Mr. Mercier returned 6 weeks later for follow-up surgery, describe in your own words the preoperative diagnosis:

_____

_____

_____

6. During the second surgery, an endoscopic procedure and two different x-ray procedures were used to visualize internal structures. List and define each procedure, and describe the findings:

Procedure	Definition	Finding
_____	_____	_____
_____	_____	_____
_____	_____	_____

7. The first surgery included insertion of a specialized device, which was then removed in the second surgery. What was this device, and what function did it perform during the time between the two surgeries?

_____

_____

_____

8. In the second surgery, did Mr. Mercier experience any complications? Write the sentence that supports your answer.

_____

_____

Answers to Practice Exercises

1. py/ur/ia
   R R S
   pus/urine/condition of
2. bacteri/osis
   R S
   bacteria/condition or increase
3. trans/urethr/al
   P R S
   across or through/urethra/ pertaining to
4. uro/gram
   CF S
   urine/record
5. urethro/cyst/itis
   CF R S
   urethra/bladder/ inflammation

6. nephro/ptosis
   CF S
   kidney/falling or downward displacement
7. poly/dips/ia
   P R S
   many/thirst/condition of
8. glomerulo/scler/osis
   CF R S
   glomerulus (little ball)/hard/ condition or increase
9. pyo/nephr/itis
   CF R S
   pus/kidney/inflammation
10. urin/al
    R S
    urine/pertaining to
11. uretero/vesico/stomy
    CF CF S
    ureter/bladder/creation of an opening

12. glyco/rrhea
    CF S
    sugar/discharge
13. meato/rrhaphy
    CF S
    opening/suture
14. pyelo/nephr/osis
    CF R S
    basin/kidney/condition or increase
15. cysto/scopy
    CF S
    bladder/process of examination
16. supra/ren/al
    P R S
    above/kidney/pertaining to
17. nephro/lith/iasis
    CF R S
    kidney/stone/formation or presence of

18. urethro/sten/osis
    CF   R   S
    urethra/narrow/condition or increase
19. albumin/ur/ia
    R   R   S
    protein/urine/condition of
20. ket/osis
    R   S
    ketone bodies/condition or increase
21. cystitis
22. nocturia
23. enuresis
24. nephrorrhaphy
25. nephrosis
26. albuminuria or proteinuria
27. urethral stenosis
28. nephrotomy
29. renal or kidney biopsy
30. urinalysis
31. cystoscopy
32. urethral stenosis
33. extracorporeal shock wave lithotripsy
34. resectoscope
35. oliguria
36. dysuria
37. pyuria
38. hematuria
39. anuresis
40. enuresis
41. stress incontinence

42. occult blood
43. RP
44. renal Bx or kidney Bx
45. UA
46. h
47. d
48. g
49. e
50. a
51. b
52. f
53. c
54. culture and sensitivity
55. voiding cystourethrogram
56. albumin or protein
57. intravenous pyelogram
58. extracorporeal shock wave lithotripsy
59. kidney, ureters, bladder
60. specific gravity
61. urinary tract infection
62. retrograde pyelogram
63. ur/o
64. dips/o
65. py/o
66. vesic/o
67. albumin/o
68. nephr/o
69. meat/o
70. pyel/o
71. lith/o
72. right kidney
73. ureters

74. bladder
75. urethra
76. left kidney
77. cystoscope
78. pyelogram
79. oliguria
80. hydronephrosis
81. azotemia
82. urinalysis
83. glomerular
84. nephrectomy
85. diuretic
86. hemodialysis
87. urine
88. glomerulus
89. meatus
90. uremia
91. urethra
92. nephrosis

Answers to Medical Record Analyses

1. c
2. b
3. d
4. a
5. b
6. b
7. b

CHAPTER 14

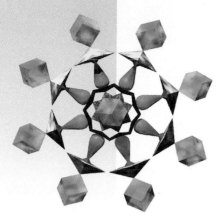

Male Reproductive System

Male Reproductive System Overview

The male reproductive organs have two primary functions:

* Producing *sperm,* the male reproductive cells, and introducing them into the female reproductive tract to fertilize the female ovum
* Secreting hormones necessary for development of secondary sexual characteristics

TERM TIP

Prostate Versus Prostrate
Prostate, a Greek word that literally means to "stand before," describes the gland encircling the male urethra at the base of the bladder. Its spelling is often confused with *prostrate,* which describes helplessness or exhaustion (pro = before; stratus = to strew).

SELF-INSTRUCTION: COMBINING FORMS

Study the following:

Combining Form	Meaning
balan/o	glans penis
epididym/o	epididymis
orch/o **orchi/o** **orchid/o** **test/o**	testis or testicle
perine/o	perineum

prostat/o	prostate
sperm/o spermat/o	sperm (seed)
vas/o	vessel

PROGRAMMED REVIEW: COMBINING FORMS

Answers	Review
	14.1 The combining form meaning glans penis comes from the Greek word balanos, which means acorn. This word was apparently used because the glans has somewhat of an acorn shape. That combining form
balan/o	is _____. Recall that the suffix meaning a surgical repair or re-
-plasty	construction is _____. Thus, the term for surgical reconstruc-
balanoplasty	tion of the glans penis is _____.
	14.2 The Greek word epididymos has an interesting origin: *epi-* means upon, and didymos means twins (referring to the two testicles). The epididymis is a structure on each testicle. The combining form meaning
epididym/o	epididymis is _____. The plural of epididymis is
epididymides	_____. Using the common suffix meaning in-flammation with this combining form, the term for inflammation of the
epididymitis	epididymis is _____.
orch/o, orchi/o	**14.3** Three different combining forms have evolved from the Greek word orchis, meaning testis (testicle): _____, _____, and
orchid/o	_____ (in any order). Having three slightly different forms makes it a little more difficult to know how to form medical terms from them. For example, the term orchitis is from the combining form
orch/o, orchi/o	_____, whereas the term orchiopexy is from _____, and
orchid/o	orchidectomy is from _____.
	14.4 The adjective perineal comes from the combining form
perine/o	_____, referring to the perineum, an anatomic area between the scrotum and the anus in males.

14.5 The Latin term prostata has its origins in a Greek word that means one who stands before. Perhaps the prostate gland was so named because it stands before the opening for sperm leaving the body to exit through the penis. The combining form for prostate

prostat/o, pain

is _____. Recall that the suffix *-algia* means _____. Using this combining form, the term for a painful prostate is

prostatalgia

_____.

14.6 The Greek word sperma means seed, and thus sperm are men's reproductive "seed." The two combining forms for sperm are

sperm/o, spermat/o

_____ and _____. The combining form used to make the term oligospermia (too few sperm in the semen) is

sperm/o

_____. The combining form used to make the adjective form

spermat/o

spermatic is _____.

14.7 The Latin word vas refers to vessel, which includes ducts as well

vas/o

as blood vessels. The combining term for vessel is _____. Recall that

-rrhaphy

the surgical suffix that means suture is _____. Thus, the pro-

vasorrhaphy

cedure of suturing a vessel is a _____.

SELF-INSTRUCTION: ANATOMICAL TERMS (FIG. 14-1)

Study the following:

Term	Meaning
scrotum *skrō′tŭm*	skin-covered pouch in the groin divided into two sacs, each containing a testis and an epididymis
testis (testicle) *tes′tis*	one of the two male reproductive glands, located in the scrotum, that produce sperm and the hormone testosterone
sperm **spermatozoon** *sper′mă-tō-zō′on*	male gamete or sex cell produced in the testes, which unites with the ovum in the female to produce offspring
epididymis *ep-i-did′i-mis*	coiled duct on top and at side of the testis that stores sperm before emission

THE MALE REPRODUCTIVE SYSTEM

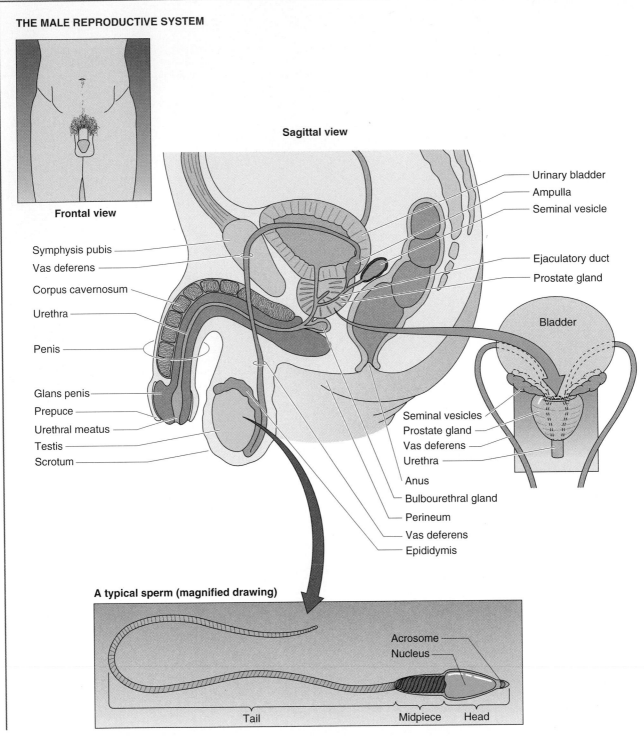

Frontal view

Sagittal view

Symphysis pubis
Vas deferens
Corpus cavernosum
Urethra
Penis
Glans penis
Prepuce
Urethral meatus
Testis
Scrotum

Urinary bladder
Ampulla
Seminal vesicle
Ejaculatory duct
Prostate gland

Bladder

Seminal vesicles
Prostate gland
Vas deferens
Urethra
Anus
Bulbourethral gland
Perineum
Vas deferens
Epididymis

A typical sperm (magnified drawing)

Acrosome
Nucleus

Tail   Midpiece   Head

■ **FIGURE 14-1.** Male reproductive system.

penis *pē′nis*	erectile tissue covered with skin that contains the urethra for urination and ducts for the secretion of seminal fluid (semen)
glans penis *glanz*	bulging structure at the distal end of the penis (glans = acorn)
prepuce *prē′pūs*	foreskin; loose casing covering the glans penis, removed by circumcision

vas deferens *vas def'er-ens*	duct that carries sperm from the epididymis to the ejaculatory duct (vas = vessel; deferens = carrying away)
seminal vesicle *sem'i-năl*	one of two saclike structures behind the bladder and connected to the vas deferens on each side; secretes an alkaline substance into the semen to enable the sperm to live longer
semen *sē'men*	a mixture of the secretions of the testes, seminal vesicles, prostate, and bulbourethral glands discharged from the male urethra during orgasm (semen = seed)
ejaculatory duct *ē-jak'yū-lă-tōr-ē*	duct formed by the union of the vas deferens with the duct of the seminal vesicle; its fluid is carried into the urethra
prostate gland *pros'tāt*	trilobular gland that encircles the urethra just below the bladder, which secretes an alkaline fluid into the semen
bulbourethral glands (Cowper's glands) *bŭl'bō-yū-rē'thrăl*	pair of glands below the prostate with ducts opening into the urethra, which adds a viscid (sticky) fluid to the semen
perineum *per'i-nē'ăm*	external region between the scrotum and anus in a male and between the vulva and anus in a female

PROGRAMMED REVIEW: ANATOMICAL TERMS

Answers	Review
scrotum	**14.8** The testicles (or testes), which produce sperm and testosterone, are enclosed inside the skin-covered pouch called the _____.
testis testes	**14.9** Sperm are produced by each _____ (testicle). The plural of testis is _____.
sperm, spermatozoon	**14.10** Produced by the testes, the male gamete (sex cell) is called _____ or _____.
epididymis epididymides	**14.11** On each testis is a coiled duct that stores the sperm before emission, called an _____. The plural of epididymis is _____.
vas deferens	**14.12** The duct that carries the sperm from the epididymis to the ejaculatory duct is called the _____ _____. Recall that the

vessel	combining form *vas/o* means _____ (or duct). Deferens means "carrying away."
ejaculatory duct	**14.13** From the epididymis, the sperm is carried by the vas deferens to the _____ _____.
semen	**14.14** Various secretions are mixed with the sperm to make the fluid called _____, which is discharged through the male urethra during orgasm. The semen is sometimes called the male "seed."
seminal	**14.15** Connected to the vas deferens on each side is another structure that secretes an alkaline substance into the semen. This is called the _____ vesicle. This alkaline substance enables the sperm to live longer.
prostate	**14.16** The trilobular gland encircling the urethra below the bladder, which also secretes an alkaline substance into the semen, is the _____ gland. Malignancies of this gland, called prostate cancer, are common in men.
bulbourethral, Cowper's	**14.17** Finally, a pair of glands below the prostate with ducts opening into the urethra secrete a viscous fluid into the semen. These are the _____ glands, also called _____ glands.
penis glans prepuce	**14.18** The semen containing sperm and these various secretions exits the body through the urethra, which passes through the skin-covered erectile tissue in the male called the _____. The acorn-shaped end of the penis where semen is ejaculated from the urethra is called the _____ penis. The medical term for foreskin, which covers the glans penis and is removed by circumcision in some men, is the _____.
perineum	**14.19** Between the scrotum and the anus is the external area called the _____.

SELF-INSTRUCTION: SYMPTOMATIC TERMS

Study the following:

Term	Meaning
aspermia *ā-sper′mē-ă*	inability to secrete or ejaculate sperm
azoospermia *ā-zō-ō-sper′mē-ă*	semen without living spermatozoa, a sign of infertility in a male (zoo = life)
oligospermia *ol-i-gō-sper′mē-ă*	scanty production and expulsion of sperm
mucopurulent **discharge** *myū-kō-pū′rū-lent*	drainage of mucus and pus

PROGRAMMED REVIEW: SYMPTOMATIC TERMS

Answers	Review
without condition of aspermia	**14.20** Recall that the prefix *a-* means _____ and the suffix *-ia* means _____ ____. Use the shorter combining form for sperm to create this term for the condition in which one is unable to produce or ejaculate sperm (without sperm): _____
    azoospermia	**14.21** The combining form *zo/o* means life. Joining this with the combining form for sperm and the appropriate prefix and suffix, the term for the condition of semen without living sperm is _____
few (or deficient) oligospermia	**14.22** Recall that the prefix *oligo-* means _____. The condition of deficient production and expulsion of sperm is _____.
   mucopurulent	**14.23** The term purulent refers to pus. The combining form for mucus is *muc/o*. The drainage of mucus and pus is called a _____ discharge.

SELF-INSTRUCTION: DIAGNOSTIC TERMS

Study the following:

Term	Meaning
anorchism *an-ōr′kizm*	absence of one or both testes
balanitis *bal-ă-nī′tis*	inflammation of the glans penis
cryptorchism (Fig. 14-2) *krip-tōr′kizm*	undescended testicle, or failure of a testis to descend into scrotal sac during fetal development; it most often remains lodged in the abdomen or inguinal canal, requiring surgical repair (crypt = to hide)
epididymitis *ep-i-did-i-mī′tis*	inflammation of the epididymis
hydrocele *hī′drō-sēl*	hernia of fluid in the testis or tubes leading from the testis
hypospadias (Fig. 14-3) *hī′pō-spā′dē-ăs*	congenital opening of the male urethra on the undersurface of the penis (spadias = to draw away)
impotence *im′pŏ-tens*	failure to initiate or maintain an erection until ejaculation because of physical or psychological dysfunction (im = not; potis = able)
Peyronie disease *pā-ron′ēz*	disorder characterized by the induration (hardness) of the corpus cavernosum in the penis
benign prostatic hypertrophy/ hyperplasia (BPH) (Fig. 14-4) *bē-nīn′ pros-tat′ik hī-per′trō-fē*	enlargement of the prostate gland that causes urinary obstruction; common in older men

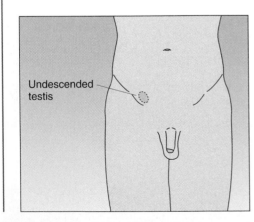

Undescended
testis

■ **FIGURE 14-2.** Cryptorchism.

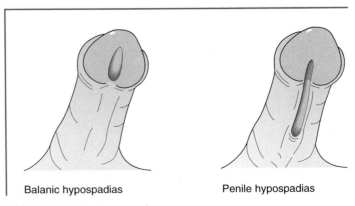

Balanic hypospadias

Penile hypospadias

■ **FIGURE 14-3.** Hypospadias.

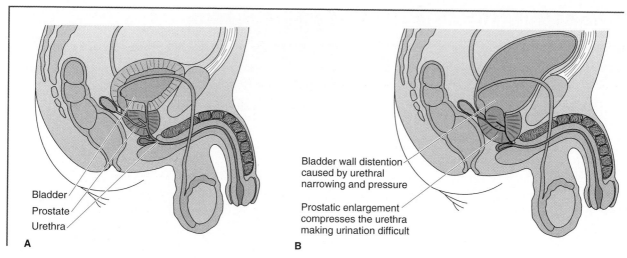

■ **FIGURE 14-4.** **A.** Normal prostate. **B.** Hypertrophic prostate.

prostate cancer	malignancy of the prostate gland
prostatitis *pros-tă-tī′tis*	inflammation of the prostate
seminoma *sem-i-nō′mă*	common type of malignant tumor of the testicle (testicular tumor)
varicocele *var′i-kō-sēl*	enlarged, swollen, herniated veins near the testis (varico = twisted vein)

SEXUALLY TRANSMITTED DISEASE (STD)

Major Bacterial STDs
bak-tēr′ē-ăl

chlamydia *kla-mid′ē-ă*	most common sexually transmitted bacterial infection in North America; often occurs with no symptoms and is treated only after it has spread
gonorrhea *gon-ō-rē′ă*	contagious inflammation of the genital mucous membranes caused by invasion of the gonococcus, *Neisseria gonorrhea*. The term was named for the urethral discharge characteristic of the infection, which was first thought to be a leakage of semen (gono = seed; rrhea = discharge); the genus was named for the Polish dermatologist Albert Neisser.
syphilis (Fig. 14-5) *sif′i-lis*	sexually transmitted infection caused by a spirochete, which may involve any organ or tissue over time; usually manifests first on the skin with the appearance of small, painless red papules that erode and form bloodless ulcers called chancres

Major Viral STDs
vī′răl

hepatitis B virus (HBV) *hep-ă-tī′tis*	virus that causes inflammation of the liver, transmitted through any body fluid, including vaginal secretions, semen, and blood

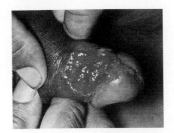

FIGURE 14-5. Syphilitic chancre.

herpes simplex virus type 2 (HSV-2) (*see* Fig. 15.8) *her'pēz*	virus that causes ulcerlike lesions of the genital and anorectal skin and mucosa; after the initial infection, the virus lies dormant in the nerve cell root and may recur at times of stress
human immuno- deficiency virus (HIV) *im'yū-nō-dē-fish'en-sē*	virus that causes acquired immunodeficiency syndrome (AIDS), which permits various opportunistic infections, malignancies, and neurologic diseases; contracted through exposure to contaminated blood or body fluid (e.g., semen or vaginal secretions)
human papilloma virus (HPV) (*see* Fig. 15-9) *papi-lo'm_a* **condyloma acuminatum** *kon-di-lō'mah ă-kyū'mĭ-nāt'ŭm* pl. **condylomata acuminata** *kon-di-lō'mah'tă ă-kyū'mĭ-nātă*	virus transmitted by direct sexual contact that causes an infection that can occur on the skin or mucous membranes of the genitals; on the skin the lesions appear as cauliflowerlike warts, and on mucous membranes they have a flat appearance (also known as venereal or genital warts)

PROGRAMMED REVIEW: DIAGNOSTIC TERMS

Answers	Review
-itis balan/o balanitis	**14.24** Recall that the suffix meaning inflammation is _____. The combining form for glans penis is _____. Inflammation of the glans penis is therefore called _____.
epididymitis	**14.25** Inflammation of the epididymis is called _____.
prostatitis	**14.26** Inflammation of the prostate gland is _____.

condition of

without

testis

anorchism

14.27 Recall that the suffix *-ism* means _____ _____. The prefix *an-* means _____. The combining form *orch/o* means _____. The medical term for the condition in which one or both testes are absent is _____.

condition of

cryptorchism

14.28 The combining form *crypt/o* means hidden. Again, the suffix *-ism* means _____ _____. The condition in which a testicle does not descend during development but remains "hidden" in the abdomen is called _____.

hydrocele

varicocele

14.29 The suffix *-cele* means pouching or hernia. The combining form *hydr/o* refers to water or fluid. A hernia of fluid in the testis or tubes leading from the testis is called a _____. The combining form *varic/o* means a dilated (varicose) vein. A swollen, herniated vein near the testis is called _____.

hypospadias

14.30 The congenital condition in which the urethra opens on the undersurface of the penis is called _____.

impotence

14.31 The failure to have or maintain an erection until ejaculation is called _____.

disease

14.32 A disorder in which the corpus cavernosum of the penis becomes hard is called Peyronie _____.

benign

above or excessive

benign prostatic

hypertrophy

hyperplasia

14.33 The opposite of malignant is _____. Recall that the prefix *hyper-* means _____. Hypertrophy means excessive growth or enlargement of a structure. The nonmalignant enlargement of the prostate gland is called _____ _____ _____ (BPH). Another word for hypertrophy is _____.

prostate

cancer

14.34 Malignancy of the prostate is called _____ _____.

-oma

seminoma

14.35 Recall that the suffix for tumor is _____. The term for a malignant tumor of the testicle uses the root for semen instead of testicle: _____.

chlamydia

14.36 Most sexually transmitted diseases (STDs) are caused by bacteria or viruses. The most common bacterial STD in North America, which often occurs without symptoms, is _____. Like many bacterial diseases, chlamydia gets its name from the Latin genus name for the bacteria: *Chlamydia.*

gonorrhea

14.37 The name for another bacterial STD, whose genus was named for the Polish dermatologist Albert Neisser, was coined in ancient times based on the thought that the urethral discharge characteristic of the infection was a leakage of semen: *Neisseria* _____.

syphilis

14.38 The bacterial STD caused by a spirochete that can over time involve any body tissue or organ is _____.

hepatitis B

14.39 Several viruses also cause STDs. The virus that causes inflammation of the liver, which can be spread through any body fluid, is _____ ___ virus (HBV).

herpes simplex virus

14.40 HSV-2 is the abbreviation for this STD virus, which typically lies dormant after the initial infection but recurs at times of stress: _____ _____ _____ type 2.

human
immunodeficiency virus

14.41 The virus that causes AIDS is _____ _____ _____ (HIV).

papilloma

condylomata, acuminata

14.42 HPV is the abbreviation for human _____ virus, a virus causing an STD characterized by lesions on the skin or mucous membranes. A condyloma is a warty growth; the plural of this term is _____. Condylomata _____ are warty growths in the genital area caused by HPV.

SELF-INSTRUCTION: DIAGNOSTIC TESTS AND PROCEDURES

Study the following:

Test or Procedure	Explanation
biopsy (Bx)	tissue sampling used to identify neoplasia
biopsy of the prostate	needle biopsy of the prostate; often performed using ultrasound guidance
testicular biopsy *tes-tik'yū-lăr*	a biopsy of a testicle
digital rectal exam (DRE)	insertion of a finger into the male rectum to palpate the rectum and prostate
prostate-specific antigen (PSA) **test** *an'ti-jen*	blood test used to screen for prostate cancer; an elevated level of the antigen indicates the possible presence of tumor
urethrogram *yū-rē'thrō-gram*	x-ray of urethra and prostate
semen analysis *sē'men*	the study of semen, including a sperm count with observation of form and motility; usually performed to rule out male infertility
endorectal (transrectal) sonogram of the prostate (Fig. 14-6) *en'dō-rek'tăl trans-rek'tăl*	scan of the prostate made after introducing an ultrasonic transducer into the rectum; also used to guide needle biopsy

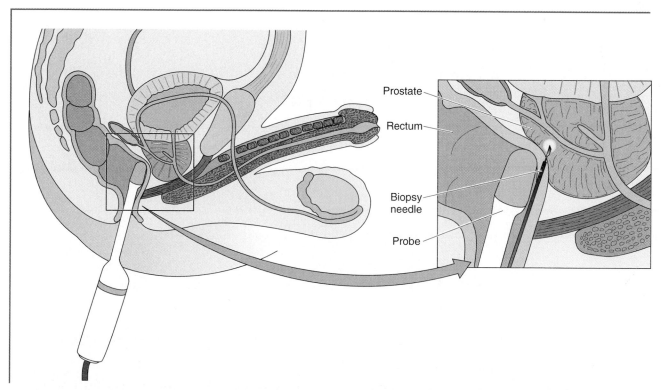

■ **FIGURE 14-6.** Ultrasound and biopsy *(inset)* of prostate.

PROGRAMMED REVIEW: DIAGNOSTIC TESTS AND PROCEDURES

Answers	Review
biopsy testicular	**14.43** The general term for removal of any body tissue for pathologic examination is _____, which is abbreviated Bx. The removal of testicular tissue is called a _____ biopsy.
prostate	**14.44** A needle biopsy of the prostate, often performed with ultrasound guidance, is called a _____ biopsy. This may be performed if prostate cancer is suspected.
prostate specific antigen	**14.45** Prostate cancer often causes the blood level of a specific antigen to become elevated. Thus the _____-_____ _____ (PSA) test may indicate the presence of a prostate tumor.
digital rectal	**14.46** The physical examination procedure involving the physician inserting a finger (digit) into the rectum to palpate the rectum and prostate is called a _____ _____ exam. An enlarged or tender prostate can be detected with this exam.
within endorectal sonogram	**14.47** Recall that the prefix *endo-* means _____. Another type of examination of the prostate involves introducing an ultrasonic transducer within the rectum to produce an _____ (transrectal) _____ of the prostate, which can also be used to guide a needle biopsy.
record urethrogram	**14.48** Recall that the suffix *-gram* means a _____. An x-ray record of the urethra and prostate is called a _____.
semen analysis	**14.49** A study of semen that includes a sperm count and observations of other characteristics of sperm is called a _____ _____. This analysis is often performed to help determine a man's fertility.

SELF-INSTRUCTION: OPERATIVE TERMS

Study the following:

Term	Meaning
circumcision *ser-kŭum-sizh'ŭn*	removal of the foreskin (prepuce), exposing the glans penis
epididymectomy *ep'i-did-i-mek'tō-mē*	removal of an epididymis
orchiectomy *ōr-kē-ek'tō-mē* **orchidectomy** *ōr-ki-dek'tō-mē*	removal of a testicle
orchioplasty *ōr'kē-ō-plas-tē*	repair of a testicle
orchiopexy *ōr'kē-ō-pek'sē*	fixation of an undescended testis in the scrotum
prostatectomy *pros-tă-tek'tō-mē*	excision of the prostate gland
transurethral resection of the prostate (TURP) *trans-yū-rē'thrăl re-sek'shŭn*	removal of prostatic gland tissue through the urethra using a resecto-scope, a specialized urologic endoscope
vasectomy (Fig. 14-7) *va-sek'tō-mē*	removal of a segment of the vas deferens to produce sterility in the male
vasovasostomy *vā'sō-vă-sos'tō-mē*	restoration of the function of the vas deferens to regain fertility after vasectomy

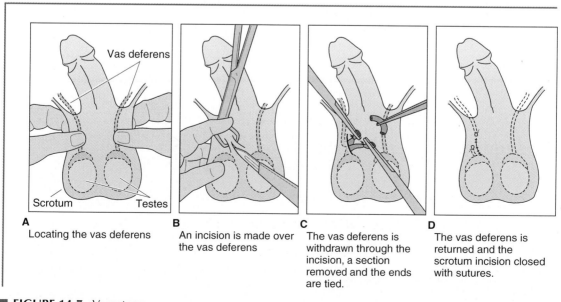

A Locating the vas deferens

B An incision is made over the vas deferens

C The vas deferens is withdrawn through the incision, a section removed and the ends are tied.

D The vas deferens is returned and the scrotum incision closed with sutures.

■ **FIGURE 14-7.** Vasectomy.

PROGRAMMED REVIEW: OPERATIVE TERMS

Answers	Review
excision	**14.50** Recall that the operative suffix *-ectomy* means _____
epididymectomy	or removal. The excision of an epididymis is termed an _____.
orchiectomy	**14.51** The excision of a testicle is called an _____
orchidectomy	or _____.
prostatectomy	**14.52** The surgical removal of the prostate gland is called _____.
vasectomy	**14.53** Excision of part of the vas deferens is called _____. This is done to produce male sterility.
opening	**14.54** In contrast, the operative suffix *-stomy* means to create an _____. The operation performed to restore the function of the vas deferens after a vasectomy, to restore fertility, is called a
vasovasostomy	_____. The combining form *vas/o* is used twice in the term because both free ends of the vas deferens, which was cut in the vasectomy, must be reopened so that they can be reattached together.
repair	**14.55** Recall that the suffix *-plasty* means surgical reconstruction or _____. The surgical repair of a testicle is called
orchioplasty	_____
-pexy	**14.56** The suffix for surgical fixation or suspension is _____. The fixation of an undescended testis in the scrotum is called an
orchiopexy	_____.
around	**14.57** The Latin word root for *-cision* (for example, incision) means to cut. Recall that the prefix *circum-* means _____. The surgical

procedure that cuts the foreskin from around the penis is

circumcision

_____. The medical term for the foreskin is

prepuce

_____.

14.58 Resect is synonymous with excise. A specialized endoscope allows for resection using an instrument through the scope; this is called

through

a resectoscope. Recall that the prefix _trans-_ means across or

_____. The surgical procedure of removal of prostatic gland

transurethral resection

tissue using a resectoscope through the urethra is called a

_____ _____ of the prostate

(TURP).

SELF-INSTRUCTION: THERAPEUTIC TERMS

Study the following:

Term	Meaning
chemotherapy _kem'ō-thār-ă-pē_	treatment of malignancies, infections, and other diseases with chemical agents that destroy selected cells or impair their ability to reproduce
radiation therapy _rā'dē-ā'shŭn_	treatment of neoplastic disease using radiation, usually from a cobalt source, to stop the proliferation of malignant cells
hormone replacement therapy (HRT)	use of a hormone to remedy a deficiency or regulate production (e.g., testosterone)
penile prosthesis _pē'nĭl pros'thē-sis_	implantation of a device designed to provide for erection of the penis; used to treat physical impotence

PROGRAMMED REVIEW: THERAPEUTIC TERMS

Answers	Review

14.59 The combining form referring to chemical agents is _chem/o_. The treatment of malignancies, infections, and other diseases with chemical

chemotherapy

agents that destroy targeted cells is called _____.

14.60 Some kinds of cancer are treated with radiation, which deters the proliferation of malignant cells. This therapy is called

radiation therapy

_____ _____.

hormone

replacement

14.61 If a patient is deficient in the production of a hormone, such as testosterone, treatment may involve administering a replacement hormone to the person. This is called _____ _____ therapy (HRT).

penile prosthesis

14.62 A prosthesis is an artificial substitute for a nonfunctioning or missing body part or organ. A device that is implanted in the penis to provide an erection because the penis cannot become erect naturally is called a _____ _____.

Practice Exercises

For the following terms, on the lines below the term, write out the indicated word parts: prefixes, combining forms, roots, and suffixes. Then define the word.

For example:
synorchism

<u>syn/orch/ism</u>
P   R   S

DEFINITION: together/testis or testicle/condition of

1. oligospermia

_____ / _____ / _____
P   R   S

DEFINITION: _____

2. perineoplasty

_____ / _____
CF   S

DEFINITION: _____

3. testalgia

_____ / _____
R   S

DEFINITION: _____

4. balanic

_____ / _____
R   S

DEFINITION: _____

5. prostatomegaly

_____ / _____
   CF   S

DEFINITION: _____

6. orchidectomy

_____ / _____
   R   S

DEFINITION: _____

7. anorchism

_____ / _____ / ____
   P   R   S

DEFINITION: _____

8. vasectomy

_____ / _____
   R   S

DEFINITION: _____

9. aspermia

_____ / _____ / ____
   P   R   S

DEFINITION: _____

10. prostatorrhea

_____ / _____
   CF   S

DEFINITION: _____

11. balanitis

_____ / _____
   R   S

DEFINITION: _____

12. orchioplasty

_____ / _____
   CF   S

DEFINITION: _____

13. spermatocele

_____ / _____
   CF   S

DEFINITION: _____

14. epididymotomy

_____ / _____
  CF   S

DEFINITION: _____

15. vasovasostomy

_____ / _____ / _____
  CF   CF   S

DEFINITION: _____

Identify the medical term for the following:

16. absence of a testicle _____

17. inflammation of glans penis _____

18. failure to maintain an erection _____

19. enlarged, herniated veins near the testicle _____

20. testicular cancer tumor _____

21. semen without living sperm _____

22. scanty production of sperm _____

23. operative treatment for cryptorchism _____

24. specialized endoscope used to approach the prostate when performing a TURP

_____

25. enlargement of prostate _____

26. fluid hernia in the testis _____

27. removal of a portion of the vas deferens to produce male sterility

_____

28. disorder that causes induration of the corpora cavernosa in the penis

_____

29. removal of foreskin to expose glans penis _____

Complete the following:

30. _____orchism = undescended testicle

31. _____ _____ exam = insertion of a finger into the male rectum to palpate rectum and prostate

32. _____ sonogram of prostate = ultrasound scan of prostate made after introduction of transducer into rectum

33. _____penis = bulging structure at the distal end of the penis

34. _____spermia = inability to secrete or ejaculate semen

Match the following:

35. semen analysis _____   a. orchiopexy

36. testis _____   b. foreskin

37. testo _____   c. sperm morphology

38. BPH _____   d. testes

39. cryptorchism _____   e. TURP

40. prepuce _____   f. orchido

Define the following abbreviations:

41. PSA _____

42. BPH _____

43. TURP _____

44. DRE _____

45. Bx _____

For each of the following, circle the combining form that corresponds to the meaning given:

46. **testis**	prostat/o	epididym/o	orchi/o
47. **perineum**	peritone/o	perine/o	prostat/o
48. **sperm**	test/o	orchi/o	spermat/o
49. **vessel**	aden/o	angin/o	vas/o
50. **glans penis**	prostat/o	orchid/o	balan/o
51. **epididymis**	sperm/o	vas/o	epididym/o

Write in the missing words on lines in the following illustration of male anatomy:

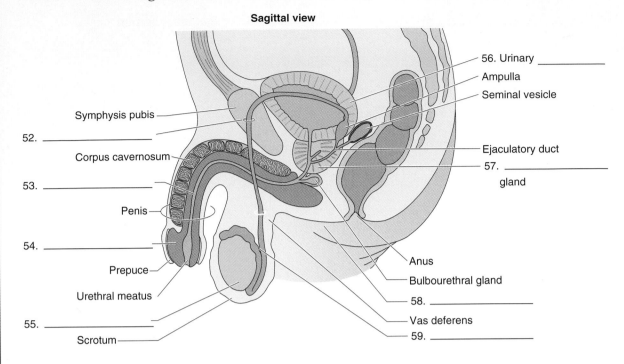

Sagittal view

- 56. Urinary _____
- Ampulla
- Seminal vesicle
- Symphysis pubis
- 52. _____
- Corpus cavernosum
- Ejaculatory duct
- 57. _____
- gland
- 53. _____
- Penis
- 54. _____
- Prepuce
- Anus
- Bulbourethral gland
- Urethral meatus
- 58. _____
- Vas deferens
- 55. _____
- 59. _____
- Scrotum

For each of the following, circle the correct spelling of the term:

60. epididymis	epididymus	epedidimis
61. oligspermia	oligospermia	oligispermia
62. azospermia	asospermia	azoospermia
63. anorches	anorchism	anorschizm
64. balanitis	balanitus	balantis
65. creptorchism	criptorchism	cryptorchism
66. hypospadias	hypospadeas	hypespadias
67. clamidyia	chlamidya	chlamydia
68. syphilis	syphillis	syphyllis

Give the noun that was used to form the following adjectives.

69. prostatic   _____

70. epididymal   _____

71. perineal   _____

72. penile   _____

73. gonorrheal   _____

Medical Record Analyses

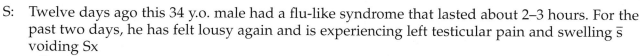

MEDICAL RECORD 14-1

Chart Note

S: Twelve days ago this 34 y.o. male had a flu-like syndrome that lasted about 2–3 hours. For the past two days, he has felt lousy again and is experiencing left testicular pain and swelling s̄ voiding Sx
Allergies: none
PH: negative
Habits: smoking—no
        alcohol—occasional beer
ROS: otherwise negative

O: Slightly small testes bilaterally; tender Ⓛ epididymis; normal circumcised penis
UA: WNL

A: Ⓛ epididymitis

P: Rx: Maxaquin 400 mg #16
Sig: ＃ STAT, then ｉ̇ q.d. × 14 d; return in two weeks for follow-up

1. What was the patient's diagnosis?
   a. testicular pain and swelling
   b. inflammation of the testicle
   c. swollen veins near the testis
   d. inflammation of the coiled duct that stores sperm
   e. fluid hernia in a testicle

2. What was the condition of the patient's penis?
   a. small but normal
   b. prepuce had been excised
   c. inflamed
   d. swollen and tender
   e. not stated

3. What was the Sig: on the prescription?
   a. two every other day for fourteen days
   b. two immediately, then one a day for fourteen days
   c. one immediately, then one a day for fourteen days
   d. one as needed every day for fourteen days
   e. two a day for fourteen days

4. Did the patient have any trouble urinating?
   a. yes
   b. no

5. What was the condition of the right testicle?
   a. inflamed
   b. enlarged
   c. small
   d. normal
   e. had been excised

6. What was the result of the urinalysis?
   a. not stated
   b. normal
   c. not performed because the patient could not void
   d. hematuria
   e. glucosuria

MEDICAL RECORD 14-2 FOR ADDITIONAL STUDY

CENTRAL MEDICAL GROUP, INC.
Department of Urology

201 Medical Center Drive • Central City, US 90000-1234 • PHONE: (012) 125-8888 • FAX: (012) 125-3434

PROGRESS NOTES

PHELPS, LAWRENCE

June 4, 20xx

SUBJECTIVE: This 31-year-old male desires vasectomy for sterility. He and his wife have two children. He states that another pregnancy would put his wife at health risk.

OBJECTIVE: Normal genitalia with single vas bilaterally.

ASSESSMENT: The procedure, goals and risks were thoroughly discussed with the aid of pictures. The vasectomy booklet and consent form were provided to the patient.

PLAN: Schedule bilateral vasectomy.

DL:ti   T:6/7/20xx

J. Derrick, M.D.
J. Derrick, M.D.

June 10, 20xx

PROCEDURE: Bilateral vasectomy.

The patient was placed supine on the table; and the scrotum was shaved, prepped, and draped in the usual fashion. The right testicle was grasped, and the right vas was brought to the skin and was infiltrated with 1% Xylocaine. The vas was freed through a small incision. A segment was resected, and the ends were cauterized and tied with 3-0 silk suture. The skin was closed with 4-0 chromic suture. The same procedure was repeated on the left. There were no complications or bleeding.

PLAN: The patient is discharged to the care of his wife with an Rx for Darvocet-N, 100 mg, 1 q 4 h p.r.n. pain. He has been given a post-vasectomy instruction sheet. He is asked to call if there are any problems. He was also instructed to submit a semen specimen for analysis after 15-20 ejaculations.

DL:ti   T:6/12/20xx

J. Derrick, M.D.
J. Derrick, M.D.

MEDICAL RECORD 14-2 FOR ADDITIONAL STUDY CONTINUED

CENTRAL MEDICAL GROUP, INC.
Department of Urology

201 Medical Center Drive • Central City, US 90000-1234 • PHONE: (012) 125-8888 • FAX: (012) 125-3434

PROGRESS NOTES

PHELPS, LAWRENCE

June 20, 20xx

SUBJECTIVE:	The patient has had pain in the right scrotum since surgery which became worse yesterday with pain in his right back. He states he has had no fevers, nausea, or vomiting.
OBJECTIVE:	1) Mild scrotal ecchymoses inferiorly. Normal testes and epididymides. 2) Small induration at left vasectomy site without tenderness. 3) Exquisitely tender 1.5 cm nodule at right vasectomy site; no induration in upper scrotum or cord.
ASSESSMENT:	Probable small hematoma at right vasectomy site.
PLAN:	Rx: Cipro 500 mg b.i.d. x 5 d Darvocet-N 100 mg q 4 h p.r.n. pain ibuprofen p.r.n. RTO in one week.

DL:ti   T:6/22/20xx

J. Derrick, M.D.
J. Derrick, M.D.

MEDICAL RECORD 14-2 FOR ADDITIONAL STUDY

Larry Phelps, age 31, has been happily married to his wife Nancy for almost five years. They have two children. The second child caused some health problems for Nancy, and her obstetrician recommended that they have no more children because of the risk to her health. After trying different forms of birth control, Nancy and Larry decided that he would have a vasectomy. His doctor referred him to Dr. Jerard Derrick in the urology department at Central Medical Group, Inc.

Read Medical Record 14-2 (pages 608 and 609) for Larry Phelps and answer the following questions. This record is a series of three chart notes written by Dr. Derrick after first meeting with Mr. Phelps to schedule surgery, after the surgery and discharge, and after seeing Mr. Phelps in a follow-up 10 days later.

Write your answers in the spaces provided.

1. Below are medical terms used in this record you have not yet encountered in this text. Underline each where it appears in the record and define below.

    sterility _____

    infiltrated _____

    resect _____

    ejaculation _____

    induration _____

2. The medical record suggests that Mr. Phelps signed which of these before surgery?
    a. last will and testament
    b. consent form
    c. application to sperm bank
    d. none of the above

3. In your own words, not using medical terminology, briefly summarize the procedure Dr. Derrick performed.

    _____

    _____

    _____

4. Complications of the surgery included which of the following:
    a. sterility
    b. fever
    c. nausea and vomiting
    d. bleeding
    e. all of the above
    f. none of the above

5. Translate the instruction for the immediate postoperative medication (how much, how often):

    _____

    _____

    _____

6. Mark any of the following that were symptoms Mr. Phelps reported to Dr. Derrick on his follow-up visit 10 days after surgery?
   a. fever
   b. bleeding
   c. pain in scrotum
   d. impotence
   e. suture loosening

7. Dr. Derrick carefully examined Mr. Phelps in the follow-up visit and noted the following objective findings (mark all that are appropriate):
   a. minor bruising in the scrotum
   b. small area of hard tissue at left vasectomy site
   c. bleeding at left vasectomy site
   d. pain at left vasectomy site
   e. very sore elevated mass at right vasectomy site
   f. bleeding at right vasectomy site
   g. pain at right vasectomy site
   h. hard tissue areas along upper scrotum
   i. black and blue penis

8. In your own words, define the diagnosis Dr. Derrick made in the follow-up visit:

   _____

   _____

   _____

9. Translate Dr. Derrick's medication instructions after the follow-up visit:

Medication	Amount	How Often
_____	_____	_____
_____	_____	_____
_____	_____	_____

Answers to Practice Exercises

1. oligo/sperm/ia
   P   R   S
   few or deficient/sperm/
   condition of

2. perineo/plasty
   CF   S
   perineum/surgical repair or
   reconstruction

3. test/algia
   R   S
   testis or testicle/pain

4. balan/ic
   R   S
   glans penis/pertaining to

5. prostato/megaly
   CF   S
   prostate/enlargement

6. orchid/ectomy
   R   S
   testis or testicle/excision
   (removal)

7. an/orch/ism
   P   R   S
   without/testis or testicle/
   condition of

8. vas/ectomy
   R   S
   vessel/excision (removal)

9. a/sperm/ia
   P   R   S
   without/sperm(seed)/
   condition of

10. prostato/rrhea
    CF   S
    prostate/discharge

11. balan/itis
    R   S
    glans penis/inflammation

12. orchio/plasty
    CF   S
    testis or testicle/surgical
    repair or reconstruction

13. spermato/cele
    CF   S
    sperm(seed)/pouching or
    hernia

14. epididymo/tomy
    CF   S
    epididymis/incision

15. <u>vaso/vaso/stomy</u>
    CF   CF   S
    vessel/vessel/creation of an
    opening
16. anorchism
17. balantis
18. impotence
19. varicocele
20. seminoma
21. azoospermia
22. oligosperma
23. orchiopexy
24. resectoscope
25. benign prostatic hypertro-
    phy/hyperplasia
26. hydrocele
27. vasectomy
28. Peyronie disease
29. circumcision
30. cryptorchism
31. digital rectal exam
32. endorectal or transrectal
    sonogram of prostate
33. glans penis
34. aspermia
35. c

36. d
37. f
38. e
39. a
40. b
41. prostate-specific antigen
42. benign prostatic hypertro-
    phy/hyperplasia
43. transurethral resection of the
    prostate
44. digital rectal exam
45. biopsy
46. orchi/o
47. perine/o
48. spermat/o
49. vas/o
50. balan/o
51. epididym/o
52. vas deferens
53. urethra
54. glans penis
55. testis
56. bladder
57. prostate
58. perineum
59. epididymis

60. epididymis
61. oligospermia
62. azoospermia
63. anorchism
64. balanitis
65. cryptorchism
66. hypospadias
67. chlamydia
68. syphilis
69. prostate
70. epididymis
71. perineum
72. penis
73. gonorrhea

Answers to Medical Records Analyses

1. d
2. b
3. b
4. b
5. c
6. b

CHAPTER 15

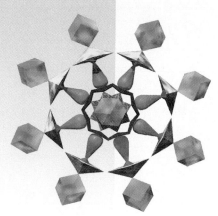

Female Reproductive System

Female Reproductive System Overview

Functions of the female reproductive system:

* Produce and maintain ova
* Provide a place for the implantation and nurturing of the fertilized ovum through the embryo and fetus stages to birth
* Produce some female sex hormones

SELF-INSTRUCTION: COMBINING FORMS

Study the following:

Combining Form	Meaning
cervic/o	neck or cervix
colp/o vagin/o	vagina (sheath)
episi/o vulv/o	vulva (covering)
gynec/o	woman
hyster/o metr/o uter/o	uterus
lact/o	milk
mast/o mamm/o	breast

men/o	menstruation
oophor/o ovari/o	ovary
ov/i ov/o	egg
salping/o	uterine (fallopian) tube (also eustachian tube)
toc/o	labor or birth
-arche (additional suffix)	beginning

PROGRAMMED REVIEW: COMBINING FORMS

Answers	Review
	15.1 The Latin word cervix means neck; the cervix in the female is like a neck between the vagina and the uterus. The combining term for
cervic/o	cervix is _____. The common adjective form, for example, is cervical.
	15.2 There are two combining forms for vagina, as often happens, one from a Latin word and one from a Greek word. The Latin word vagina means sheath (as the vagina sheaths the penis during intercourse); that
vagin/o	combining form is _____. The Greek word kolpos means a hol-
colp/o	low; that combining form is _____. Using the latter, and the suf-
-scope	fix for an instrument of examination, _____, forms the term for a
colposcope	special kind of scope designed to examine the vagina: _____
	15.3 The Greek term episeion, meaning pubic region, is the origin for this combining form for the vulva (the external female genitalia):
episi/o, incision	_____. The operative suffix -*tomy* means _____. An incision made in the perineum to facilitate childbirth, using this
episiotomy	combining form, is an _____.

15.4   A second combining form meaning vulva comes from the Latin word vulva: _____. It is used, for example, to create the common adjective form vulvar.

vulv/o

15.5   A gynecologist is a physician who specializes in the reproductive system of _____. The combining form meaning women is _____.

women

gynec/o

15.6   The uterus is the hollow organ (the womb) where the woman carries the fetus before childbirth. The Latin combining form used to name the uterus is _____. A hysterectomy is surgical removal of the uterus; this term is made from the Greek combining form _____ plus the suffix -*ectomy*, which means _____.

uter/o

hyster/o, excision (removal)

15.7   The Greek word for the uterus, metra, is the origin of a third combining form for uterus: _____. The term metrorrhagia, for example, refers to irregular bleeding from the _____ not occurring during menstruation.

metr/o

uterus

15.8   The suffix -*genic* (a combination of *gen/o* and -*ic*) pertains to origin or _____. It is used to modify the combining form *lact/o*, meaning _____, to form the adjective pertaining to the production of milk: _____.

production

milk

lactogenic

15.9   There are two combining forms meaning breast, again from Greek and Latin roots. Because the suffix -*dynia* means _____, mastodynia means breast pain. The common suffix for a record resulting from an examination technique is _____. Thus, a mammogram is an x-ray of the breast. The two combining forms for breast are _____ and _____.

pain

-gram

mast/o

mamm/o

15.10   From the Greek word men, meaning month, comes the combining form that means _____, which occurs

menstruation

men/o	generally about once a month in the adult female. The combining form is _____. That time later in life when menstruation permanently stops (pauses) is _____.
menopause	

15.11 Once again, the two combining forms for the ovary come from Latin and Greek roots. The adjective ovarian is built from the combining

ovari/o

form _____, from the Latin word for the ovary. The Greek word oophoros means egg-bearing, giving rise to the combining form

oophor/o

_____. Recall that the common suffix for inflammation is

-itis, ovary

_____. Oophoritis is an inflammation of the _____.

egg

15.12 An ovum is the woman's _____, produced in the ovary. The

ov/i, ov/o

two combining forms for egg are very similar: _____ and _____. Ovigenesis is the process of the formation and development of the

ovum (egg)

_____.

15.13 The Greek word salpinx means trumpet or tube. It gives rise to

salping/o

the combining form _____, which refers to the uterine or fallopian tube (which carries the ovum from the ovary to the uterus).

inflammation

Salpingitis is an _____ of the uterine or fallopian tube.

toc/o

15.14 The combining form for birth is _____. Tocophobia, for example, is a morbid fear of childbirth. Recall that the prefix *dys-* means

difficult

faulty, painful or _____, and the suffix *-ia* refers to a

condition of

_____ _____. Therefore, the term for a difficult child-

dystocia

birth is _____.

-arche

15.15 The suffix meaning beginning is _____. Using the com-

menarche

bining form for menstruation, the term for the beginning of menstruation is _____.

SELF-INSTRUCTION: ANATOMICAL TERMS (FIG. 15-1)

Study the following:

Term	Meaning
uterus *ū'ter-ŭs*	womb; pear-shaped organ in the pelvic cavity in which the embryo and fetus develops
fundus *fŭn'dŭs*	upper portion of the uterus above the entry to the uterine tubes
endometrium *en'dō-mē'trē-ŭm*	lining of the uterus, which is shed about every 28 to 30 days in a non pregnant female during menstruation
myometrium *mī'o-mē'trē-ŭm*	muscular wall of the uterus

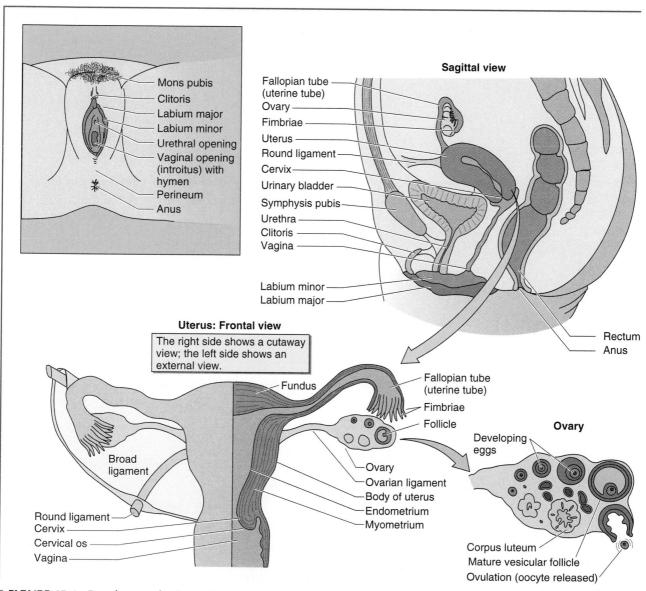

■ **FIGURE 15-1.** Female reproductive system.

uterine or fallopian tubes *yū'ter-in fa-lō'pē-an*	tubes extending from each side of the uterus toward the ovary that provide a passage for ova to the uterus
adnexa *ad-nek'să*	uterine tubes and ovaries (uterine appendages)
right uterine appendage	right tube and ovary
left uterine appendage	left tube and ovary
ovary *ō'vă-rē*	one of two glands located on each side of the pelvic cavity that produce ova and female sex hormones
cervix *ser'viks*	neck of the uterus
cervical os *ser'vĭ-kăl os*	opening of the cervix to the uterus
vagina *vă-jī'nă*	tubular passageway from the cervix to the outside of the body
vulva *vŭl'vă*	external genitalia of the female
labia *lā'bē-ă*	folds of tissue on either side of the vaginal opening, known as the labia majora and labia minora
clitoris *klitō'-ris*	female erectile tissue in the anterior portion of the vulva
hymen *hī'men*	fold of mucous membrane that encircles the entrance to the vagina
introitus *in-trō'i-tŭs*	entrance to the vagina
Bartholin glands	two glands located on either side of the vaginal opening that secrete a lubricant during intercourse
perineum *per'i-nē'ŭm*	region between the vulva and anus
mammary glands (Fig. 15-2) *mam'ă-rē*	two glands in the female breasts capable of producing milk
mammary papilla *pă-pil'ă*	nipple
areola *ă-rē'ō-lă*	dark pigmented area around the nipple

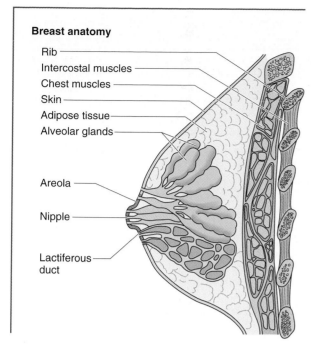

Breast anatomy

- Rib
- Intercostal muscles
- Chest muscles
- Skin
- Adipose tissue
- Alveolar glands
- Areola
- Nipple
- Lactiferous duct

■ **FIGURE 15-2.** Breast.

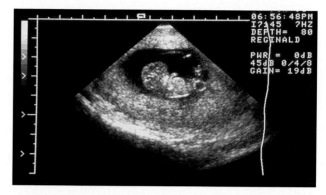

FIGURE 15-3. Two-dimensional sonogram of 8-week embryo.

embryo (Fig. 15-3) *em'brē-ō*	the developing organism from fertilization to the end of the eighth week
fetus (Fig. 15-4) *fē'tŭs*	the developing organism from the ninth week to birth
placenta *plă-sen'tă*	vascular organ that develops in the uterine wall during pregnancy to provide nourishment for the fetus (placenta = cake)

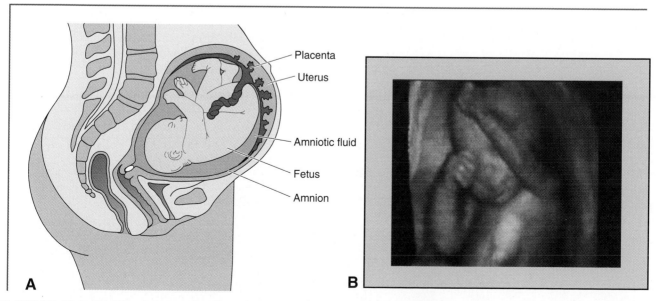

- Placenta
- Uterus
- Amniotic fluid
- Fetus
- Amnion

A

B

■ **FIGURE 15-4. (A)** Fetus in utero. **(B)** Three-dimensional sonogram of fetus "waking

amniotic sac *am-nē-ot'ik*	membranes surrounding the embryo in the uterus, filled with amniotic fluid
amniotic fluid	fluid within the amniotic sac that surrounds and protects the fetus
meconium *mē-kō'nē-ŭm*	intestinal discharges of the fetus that form the first stools in the newborn

PROGRAMMED REVIEW: ANATOMICAL TERMS

Answers	Review

15.16   The external genitalia of the female are collectively called the

vulva

_____ . The region between the vulva in the female (the scrotum

perineum

in the male) and the anus is the _____ .

15.17   The vulva consist of the folds of tissue on either side of the vagi-

labia

nal opening, called the _____ majora and minora, and the female

clitoris

erectile tissue, the _____ . The labia majora are the larger

tissue folds, and within them are the labia minora, smaller folds.

15.18   Inward from the labia, the fold of mucous membrane encircling

hymen

the entrance to the vagina is the _____ .

15.19   The term for the entrance to the vagina is used in medical lan-

guage for the entrance to other hollow organs as well. It comes from the

Latin intro-eo, meaning to go into. This term is _____ .

introitus

Two glands located on either side of the vaginal opening, called

Bartholin

_____ glands, secrete a lubricant during intercourse.

15.20   The vagina is a tubular passageway between the _____

cervix

and the outside of the body, where the penis is inserted during inter-

course. The cervix is the _____ of the uterus. The term for the open-

neck

ing of the cervix to the uterus, using the Latin word os, meaning mouth,

cervical os

is _____ _____ . The term os is used in other anatomical ar-

eas to indicate an opening to a hollow organ or canal.

uterus

fundus

fundi

15.21 The cervix is the neck of the _____ (the womb), where after conception the embryo and fetus develop. The upper part of the uterus, above the uterine tubes, is the _____, from the Latin word fundus referring to the largest part of a sac farthest from the opening. The plural of fundus is _____.

uterus

myometrium

within

endometrium

15.22 The combining form *metr/o* refers to the _____. The suffix *-ium* refers to a structure or tissue. The combining form *my/o* means muscle. Therefore, the term for the muscular wall of the uterus is the _____. Recall that the prefix endo- means _____. Within the uterus is a tissue that forms its lining, which is shed during menstruation, called the _____.

ova

ovaries

ovum

15.23 Human eggs, called _____, are produced in each of the two _____. The ovaries also secrete female sex hormones. The singular of ova is _____.

fallopian

appendage

uterine

adnexa

15.24 The tubes through which the ova move from the ovaries to the uterus are called the _____ or uterine tubes. The right tube and ovary collectively are called the right uterine _____. The left tube and ovary are called the left _____ appendage. The collective term for both uterine appendages is the _____.

uterus

ovum

15.25 Sperm deposited in the vagina during intercourse swim through the cervix into the _____. Sperm may meet an egg, or _____, in the uterus or fallopian tubes, and fertilization may occur.

embryo

endometrium

15.26 If fertilization occurs, the resultant developing organism, called an _____ for the first eight weeks, is implanted in the lining of the uterus, the _____.

placenta

15.27 The vascular (blood-rich) organ that develops in the uterine wall to nourish the embryo and fetus is the _____.

amniotic sac fluid	**15.28** The membrane sac surrounding the embryo is the _____ _____. It is filled with a protective fluid called amniotic _____.
fetus	**15.29** After 8 weeks, the developing organism is no longer called an embryo; instead, it is called a _____.
meconium	**15.30** The first stools of a newborn develop from intestinal discharges of the fetus, called _____.
mamm/o mammary	**15.31** Recall that the two combining forms for breast are *mast/o* and _____. Using an adjective form of the latter, the term for the glands in the female breast that make milk is _____ glands.
nipple	**15.32** The mammary papilla is the _____ of the breast, through which milk flows to the infant.

SELF-INSTRUCTION: GYNECOLOGICAL *(gī′nĕ-kō-lojʹi-kăl)* SYMPTOMATIC TERMS

Study the following:

Term	Meaning
amenorrhea *ă-men-ō-reʹă*	absence of menstruation
dysmenorrhea *dis-men-ōr-eʹă*	painful menstruation
oligomenorrhea *olʹi-gō-men-ō-reʹă*	scanty menstrual period
anovulation *an-ov-yū-lāʹshŭn*	absence of ovulation
dyspareunia *dis-pa-rūʹnē-ă*	painful intercourse (coitus) (dys = painful; para = alongside of; eunia = a lying)
leukorrhea *lū-kō-reʹă*	abnormal white or yellow vaginal discharge
menorrhagia *men-ō-rāʹje-ă*	excessive bleeding at the time of menstruation (menses)

| **metrorrhagia**
mē-trō-rā'jē-ă | bleeding from the uterus at any time other than normal menstruation |
| **oligo-ovulation**
ol'i-gō-ov'yū-lā'shŭn | irregular ovulation |

PROGRAMMED REVIEW: GYNECOLOGICAL SYMPTOMATIC TERMS

Answers	Review
men/o	**15.33** The combining form for menstruation is _____. A number of symptomatic terms for different menstrual conditions are made with this combining form. Recall that the suffix *-rrhea* means
discharge, without	_____. The prefix *a-* means _____. Therefore, the term for being without menstrual discharge (the absence of
amenorrhea	menstruation) is _____.
painful	**15.34** The prefix *dys-* means faulty, difficult, or _____. The term for painful menstruation (menstrual discharge) is
dysmenorrhea	_____.
deficient	**15.35** The prefix *oligo-* means few or _____. The term
oligomenorrhea	for scanty (deficient) menstrual discharge is _____.
oligo-ovulation	**15.36** The same prefix is used in the term for irregular (deficient) ovulation: _____
without anovulation	**15.37** The prefix *an-* means _____. The absence of ovulation, therefore, is termed _____.
blood (bleeding) menorrhagia	**15.38** The suffix *-rrhagia* means to burst forth, usually referring to _____. Excessive bleeding during menstruation is therefore called _____.
uterus metrorrhagia	**15.39** The combining form *metr/o* means _____. Excessive bleeding from the uterus other than in normal menstruation, using this combining form, is called _____.

15.40 The combining form *leuk/o* means white. An abnormal white or yellow discharge (from the vagina) is termed _____.

leukorrhea

15.41 Painful intercourse is called _____ (using the prefix *dys-*, meaning _____).

dyspareunia

painful

SELF-INSTRUCTION: GYNECOLOGICAL DIAGNOSTIC TERMS

Study the following:

Term	Meaning
cervicitis *ser-vi-sī′tis*	inflammation of the cervix
congenital anomalies (irregularities) *kon-jen′i-tăl ă-nom′ă-lēz*	birth defects that cause the abnormal development of an organ or structure (e.g., double uterus or absent vagina)
dermoid cyst *der′moyd sist*	congenital tumor composed of displaced embryonic tissue (teeth, bone, cartilage, and hair) typically found in an ovary; usually benign
displacements of uterus (Fig. 15-5)	displacement of the uterus from its normal position
anteflexion *an-tē-flek′shŭn*	abnormal forward bending of the uterus (ante = before; flexus = bend)
retroflexion *re-trō-flek′shŭn*	abnormal backward bending of the uterus
retroversion *re-trō-ver′zhŭn*	backward turn of the whole uterus; also called tipped uterus
endometriosis *en′dō-mē-trē-ō′sis*	condition characterized by migration of portions of endometrial tissue outside the uterine cavity
endometritis *en′dō-mē-trī′tis*	inflammation of the endometrium
fibroid *fī′broyd* **fibromyoma** *fī′brō-mī-ō′mă* **leiomyoma** *lī′ō-mī-ō′mă*	benign tumor in the uterus composed of smooth muscle and fibrous connective tissue
fistula *fis′tyū-lă*	abnormal passage, such as from one hollow organ to another (fistula = pipe)
rectovaginal fistula *rek-tō-vaj′i-năl*	abnormal opening between the vagina and rectum

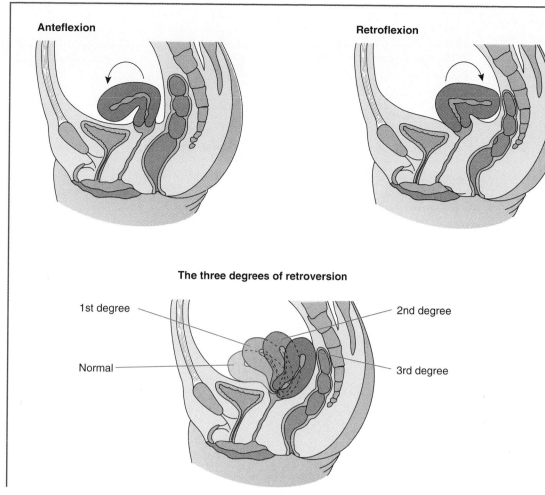

Anteflexion

Retroflexion

The three degrees of retroversion

1st degree

Normal

2nd degree

3rd degree

■ **FIGURE 15-5.** Displacements of the uterus.

vesicovaginal fistula *ves-i-kō-vaj′i-năl*	abnormal opening between the bladder and vagina
cervical neoplasia	abnormal development of cervical tissue cells
cervical intraep- ithelial neoplasia (CIN) *in′tră-ep-i-thē′lē-ăl nē-ō-plā′zē-ă* **cervical dysplasia** *dis-plā′zē-ă*	potentially cancerous abnormality of epithelial tissue of the cervix, graded according to the extent of abnormal cell formation: CIN-1—mild dysplasia CIN-2—moderate dysplasia CIN-3—severe dysplasia
carcinoma in situ (CIS) of the cervix *kar-si-nō′mă in sī′tū*	malignant cell changes of the cervix that are localized without any spread to adjacent structures
menopause *men′ō-pawz*	cessation of menstrual periods caused by lack of ovarian hormones
oophoritis *ō-of-ōr-ī′tis*	inflammation of one or both ovaries

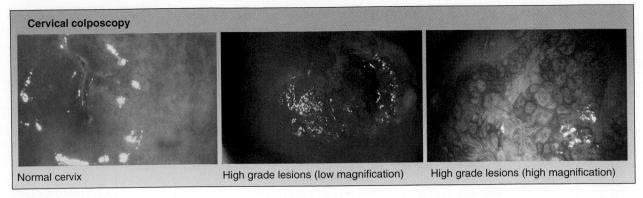

Cervical colposcopy

Normal cervix | High grade lesions (low magnification) | High grade lesions (high magnification)

FIGURE 15-6. Cervical colposcopy.

parovarian cyst *par-ō-var′ē-an*	cyst of the uterine tube (fallopian tube)
pelvic adhesions *pel′vik ad-hē′zhŭnz*	scarring of tissue within the pelvic cavity resulting from endometriosis, infection, or injury
pelvic inflammatory disease (PID)	inflammation of organs in the pelvic cavity; usually includes the fallopian tubes, ovaries, and endometrium; most often caused by bacteria
pelvic floor relaxation (Fig. 15-7)	relaxation of supportive ligaments of the pelvic organs
cystocele *sis′tō-sēl*	pouching of the bladder into the vagina

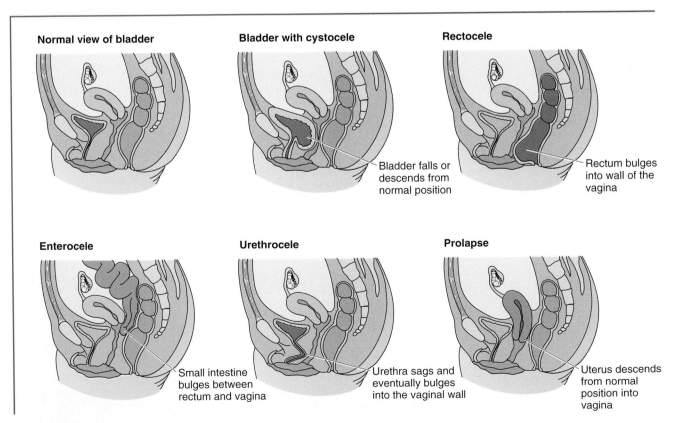

Normal view of bladder

Bladder with cystocele — Bladder falls or descends from normal position

Rectocele — Rectum bulges into wall of the vagina

Enterocele — Small intestine bulges between rectum and vagina

Urethrocele — Urethra sags and eventually bulges into the vaginal wall

Prolapse — Uterus descends from normal position into vagina

■ **FIGURE 15-7.** Pelvic floor relaxation.

rectocele *rek'tō-sēl*	pouching of the rectum into the vagina
enterocele *en'ter-ō-sēl*	pouching sac of peritoneum between the vagina and rectum
urethrocele *yū-rē'thrō-sēl*	pouching of the urethra into the vagina
prolapse *prō-laps'*	descent of the uterus down the vaginal canal
salpingitis *sal-pin-jī'tis*	inflammation of a fallopian tube

PROGRAMMED REVIEW: GYNECOLOGICAL DIAGNOSTIC TERMS

Answers	Review
-itis cervicitis	**15.42** The suffix for inflammation is _____. Inflammation of the cervix is termed _____.
oophor/o oophoritis	**15.43** The two combining forms for the ovaries are *ovari/o* and _____. Using the latter, inflammation of the ovaries is termed _____.
salping/o salpingitis	**15.44** The combining form for fallopian tube (or eustachian tube) is _____. Therefore, inflammation of the fallopian tube is _____.
endometritis	**15.45** Inflammation of the endometrium is _____.
condition endometriosis	**15.46** The suffix *-osis* means increase or _____. Another condition of the endometrium, which involves endometrial tissue migrating outside the uterus, is _____.
anomalies dermoid	**15.47** Birth defects involving abnormal development of a structure are called congenital _____. A congenital tumor composed of displaced embryonic tissue is called a _____ cyst.

15.48   In some women, the uterus is in a somewhat different from normal position in the abdomen. This atypical position is called a

displacement

_____. If it is bent (flexed) forward, the position

anteflexion

is called _____. Retroflexion, however, is an abnormal

backward

mal _____ bending of the uterus. If the whole uterus is

version

tipped or turned backward, it is called retro_____.

15.49   Muscle and connective tissue in the uterus can give rise

-oma

to tumors. The common suffix for a tumor is _____. Combined
with *lei/o,* meaning smooth, and *my/o,* meaning muscle, the term

leiomyoma

_____ refers to a benign smooth muscle tumor, especially of the uterus. A synonymous term uses the combining forms for
muscle and tumor preceded by the combining form *fibr/o* to indicate the

fiber (fibrous), fibromyoma

_____ consistency of the tissue: _____. An additional synonym simply refers to a uterine tumor that resembles fibers:

fibroid

_____.

15.50   An abnormal passage from one organ to another is called a

fistula

_____, from the Latin word fistula (pipe). An abnormal

rectovaginal

opening between the rectum and vagina is a _____
fistula. An abnormal opening between the bladder (*vesic/o*) and the

vesicovaginal

vagina is a _____ fistula.

men/o

15.51   Again, the combining form for menstruation is _____. A
cessation (pause) of menstruation usually occurring in older women is

menopause

called _____.

uterine or fallopian

15.52   A parovarian cyst is a cyst in the _____ tube.

15.53   Scarring of tissue in the pelvic cavity resulting from endometriosis, infection, or injury can cause pelvic tissues to adhere together; this is called _____ _____.

pelvic adhesions

15.54   Inflammation of the pelvic cavity, including the fallopian tubes, ovaries, and endometrium, is called _____ _____ disease (PID).

pelvic

inflammatory

15.55   Neoplasia is a general term describing a new formation of abnormal tissue, which can be benign or malignant. Any new formation of abnormal cervical tissue is called _____ _____. The term describing a condition of faulty formation of tissue with cancerous potential is _____. Cervical dysplasia is also known as _____ _____epithelial neoplasia (CIN) and is classified according to the extent of abnormal cell formation. CIN-1 is _____ dysplasia, CIN-2 is _____ dysplasia, and CIN-3 is _____ _____. Malignant neoplasia of the cervix that is localized without any spread to adjacent structures is called carcinoma _____ _____ (CIS) of the cervix.

cervical neoplasia

dysplasia

cervical intra

mild, moderate

severe dysplasia

in situ

15.56   Pelvic organs are supported with ligaments and other connective tissue. Relaxation of these supportive tissues, called _____ _____ relaxation, may allow anatomical changes or displacements. A descent of the uterus down the vaginal canal is a _____.

pelvic

floor

prolapse

15.57   Recall that the suffix -*cele* means hernia or _____. A pouching of the rectum (*rect/o*) into the vagina is a _____

pouching

rectocele

15.58   A pouching of the urethra (*urethr/o*), the tube that carries urine to outside of the body, into the vagina is a _____.

urethrocele

15.59   *Cyst/o* is a combining form for bladder. A pouching of the bladder into the vagina is a _____.

cystocele

15.60   An enterocele is a _____ing sac of peritoneum between the vagina and rectum.

pouch

SELF-INSTRUCTION: SEXUALLY TRANSMITTED DISEASES

Study the following:

Term	Meaning
MAJOR BACTERIAL STDS	
chlamydia *kla-midē-ă*	most common sexually transmitted bacterial infection in North America, which often occurs with no symptoms and is treated only after it has spread, such as to after causing pelvic inflammatory disease
gonorrhea *gon-ō-rē'ă*	contagious inflammation of the genital mucous membranes caused by invasion of the gonococcus, *Neisseria gonorrhea*. The term was named for the urethral discharge characteristic of the infection, which was first thought to be a leakage of semen (gono = seed; rrhea = discharge); the genus was named for the Polish dermatologist Albert Neisser.
syphilis *sif'i-lis*	infectious disease caused by a spirochete transmitted by direct intimate contact that may involve any organ or tissue over time, usually manifested first on the skin with the appearance of small, painless red papules that erode and form bloodless ulcers called *chancres*
MAJOR VIRAL STDS	
hepatitis B virus **(HBV)** *hep-ă-tī'tis*	virus that causes an inflammation of the liver as a result of transmission through any body fluid, including vaginal secretions, semen, and blood
herpes simplex virus type 2 (HSV-2) **(Fig. 15-8)** *her'pēz*	virus that causes ulcerlike lesions of the genital and anorectal skin and mucosa; after initial infection, the virus lies dormant in the nerve cell root and may recur at times of stress
human immunodeficiency virus (HIV) *im'yū-nō-dē-fish'en-sē*	virus that causes acquired immunodeficiency syndrome (AIDS), permitting various opportunistic infections, malignancies, and neurologic diseases; contracted through exposure to contaminated blood or body fluid (e.g., semen or vaginal secretions)
human papilloma virus (HPV) **(Fig. 15-9)** *pap-i-lō'mă* **condyloma acuminatum** *kon-di-lō'mah* *ă-kyū'mĭ-nāt'ŭm* pl. **condylomata acuminata** *kon-di-lō'mah'tă* *ă-kyū'mĭ-nātă*	virus that causes an infection that can occur on the skin or mucous membranes of the genitals, transmitted by direct sexual contact; on the skin, the lesions appear as cauliflowerlike warts, and on mucous membranes they have a flat appearance (also known as venereal or genital warts)

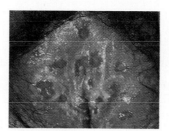

FIGURE 15-8. Herpes simplex virus 2.

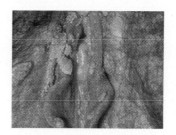

FIGURE 15-9. Condylomata acuminata (genital warts) caused by HPV

vaginitis *vaj-i-nī'tis*	inflammation of the vagina with redness, swelling, and irritation, often caused by a specific organism, such as *Candida* (yeast) or *Trichomonas* (sexually transmitted parasite)
atrophic vaginitis *ă-trof'ik*	thinning of the vagina and loss of moisture because of depletion of estrogen, which causes inflammation of tissue
vaginosis *vaj'i-nō-sis*	infection of the vagina with little or no inflammation, characterized by a milklike discharge and an unpleasant odor; also known as nonspecific vaginitis

PROGRAMMED REVIEW: SEXUALLY TRANSMITTED DISEASES

Answers	Review

15.61 Most sexually transmitted diseases (STDs) are caused by bacteria or viruses. The most common bacterial STD in North America is

chlamydia

_____. Like many bacterial diseases, chlamydia gets its name from the Latin genus name for the bacteria: *Chlamydia*. It may have no symptoms until it spreads, and it can cause pelvic inflammatory disease.

15.62 Another bacterial STD, whose genus was named for the Polish

gonorrhea

dermatologist Albert Neisser, is _____. It causes an inflammation of genital mucous membranes.

15.63 The bacterial STD caused by a spirochete that over time can in-

syphilis

volve any body tissue or organ is _____.

15.64 Several viruses also cause STDs. The virus that causes inflammation of the liver, which can be spread through any body fluid, is

hepatitis B

_____ virus (HBV).

herpes simplex virus	**15.65** HSV-2 is the abbreviation for this STD virus, which typically lies dormant after the initial infection but recurs at times of stress: _____ _____ _____ type 2. It causes ulcer-like lesions on genital and anorectal skin.
human immunodeficiency virus	**15.66** The virus that causes AIDS is _____ _____ _____ (HIV).
papilloma condylomata, acuminata	**15.67** HPV is the abbreviation for human _____ virus, a virus causing an STD characterized by lesions on the skin or mucous membranes. A condyloma is a warty growth; the plural of this term is _____. Condylomata _____ are warty growths in the genital area caused by HPV.
-itis vaginitis atrophic	**15.68** Again, the suffix meaning inflammation is _____. Inflammation of the vagina, often caused by a sexually transmitted organism, is _____. The specific kind of vaginitis involving thinning of the vagina and loss of moisture due to depletion of estrogen is called _____ vaginitis.
condition vaginosis	**15.69** The suffix -osis means increase or simply a _____. A vaginal condition involving infection but little or no inflammation is called _____.

SELF-INSTRUCTION: GYNECOLOGICAL DIAGNOSTIC TERMS: BREASTS

Study the following:

Term	Meaning
adenocarcinoma of the breast *adě′-nō-ka r-si-nō′mă*	malignant tumor of glandular breast tissue
amastia *ă-mas′tē-ă*	absence of a breast

fibrocystic breasts *fī-brō-sishtik*	benign condition of the breast consisting of fibrous and cystic changes that render the tissue more dense; patient feels painful lumps that fluctuate with menstrual periods
gynecomastia *gī'nĕ-kō-mas'tē-ă*	development of mammary glands in the male, caused by altered hormone levels
hypermastia *hī-per-mas'tē-ă* **macromastia** *mak-rō-mas'tē-a*	abnormally large breasts
hypomastia *hī'po-mas'tē-ă* **micromastia** *ī'kro-mas'te-a*	unusually small breasts
mastitis *mas-tī'tis*	inflammation of breast, most commonly in women who are breastfeeding
polymastia *pol-ē-mas'tē-ă*	presence of more than two breasts
polythelia *pol-ē-thē'lē-ă* **supernumerary nipples** *sū-per-nū'mer-ār-ē*	presence of more than one nipple on a breast

PROGRAMMED REVIEW: GYNECOLOGICAL DIAGNOSTIC TERMS: BREASTS

Answers	Review
mast/o condition of without amastia	**15.70** Two combining forms for breast are *mamm/o* and _____. The latter is used more frequently in gynecologic diagnostic terms. Recall that the suffix *-ia* means _____ _____. The prefix *a-* means _____. Thus, the condition of an absence of a breast is _____.
excessive hypermastia large macromastia	**15.71** The prefix *hyper-* means above or _____. The condition of abnormally large breasts is called _____. Recall that the prefix *macro-* means long or _____. It is used to form a synonym for hypermastia: _____.

hypo-	**15.72** The prefix with a meaning opposite to *hyper-* is _____. The
micro-	prefix with a meaning opposite to macro is _____. Therefore, two
hypomastia	other terms for unusually small breasts are _____
micromastia	and _____.

many	**15.73** The prefix *poly-* means _____. The condition of having more
polymastia	than two (many) breasts is termed _____. The suffix
condition of	*-ia* means _____ _____.

woman	**15.74** The combining form *gynec/o* means _____. The condition
	of a man developing mammary glands (as in a woman) is termed
gynecomastia	_____.

-itis	**15.75** Again, the suffix denoting inflammation is _____. An in-
mastitis	flammation of the breast is termed _____.

fibrocystic	**15.76** A benign condition of the breasts consisting of fibrous and cys- tic changes is referred to as _____ breasts.

malignant	**15.77** An adenocarcinoma of the breast is a _____ tumor of glandular breast tissue.

	15.78 The Greek word for nipple is thele. The prefix *poly-* means
many	_____. The condition of having more than one nipple on a breast is
polythelia	called _____. These are also called
numerary	super_____ nipples.

SELF-INSTRUCTION: GYNECOLOGIC DIAGNOSTIC TESTS AND PROCEDURES

Study the following:

Test or Procedure	Explanation
biopsy (Bx) (Fig. 15-10)	removal of tissue for microscopic pathologic examination
aspiration Bx *as-pi-rā′shŭn*	needle draw of tissue or fluid from a cavity for cytological examination; also called needle biopsy

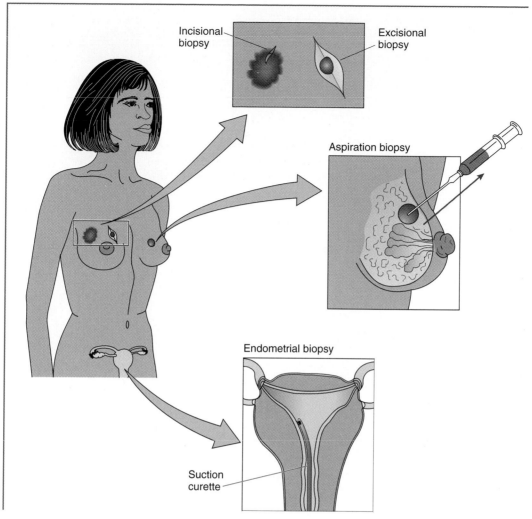

■ **FIGURE 15-10.** Biopsy.

endoscopic Bx *en'dō-skōp'ik*	removal of a specimen for biopsy during an endoscopic procedure (e.g., colposcopy)
excisional Bx *ek-sizh'ŭn-ăl*	removal of an entire lesion for microscopic examination
incisional Bx *in-sizh'ŭn-năl*	removal of a piece of suspicious tissue for microscopic examination (e.g., cervical or endometrial biopsy)
needle biopsy	removal of a core specimen of tissue using a special hollow needle
stereotactic breast Bx *ster'e-ō-tak'tik*	use of x-ray imaging, a specialized stereotactic frame, and a computer to calculate, precisely locate, and direct a needle into a breast lesion for the removal of a core specimen for biopsy
colposcopy (*see* Fig. 15-6) *kol-pos'kŏ-pē*	examination of the vagina and cervix using a colposcope, a specialized microscope used to examine the vagina and cervix, often with a camera attachment for photographs; used to document findings and follow-up treatments

hysteroscopy (Fig. 15-11) *his-ter-os'kŏ-pē*	use of a hysteroscope to examine the intrauterine cavity for assessment of abnormalities (e.g., polyps, fibroids, or anomalies)
magnetic resonance imaging (MRI) *rez'ō-nans*	use of nonionizing images to detect gynecologic conditions (e.g., anomalies of the pelvis or soft tissues of the breast) or to stage tumors arising from the endometrium or cervix
Papanicolaou smear (Pap) *pa-pĕ-nē'kĕ-low*	study of cells collected from the cervix to screen for cancer and other abnormalities
radiography *rā'dē-og'ră-fē*	x-ray imaging
hysterosalpingogram *his'ter-ō-sal-ping-ō-gram*	x-ray of the fallopian tubes after injection of a contrast medium through the cervix; used to determine tubal patency (openness)
mammogram *mam'ō-gram*	low-dose x-ray of breast tissue made to detect neoplasms
pelvic sonography (Fig. 15-12) *sŏ-nog'ră-fē*	ultrasound imaging of the female pelvis
endovaginal sonogram *en'dō-vaj'i-năl* **transvaginal sonogram** *trans-vaj'i-năl son'ō-gram*	ultrasound image of the uterus, tubes, and ovaries made with the ultrasonic transducer within the vagina to detect conditions such as ectopic pregnancy or missed abortion

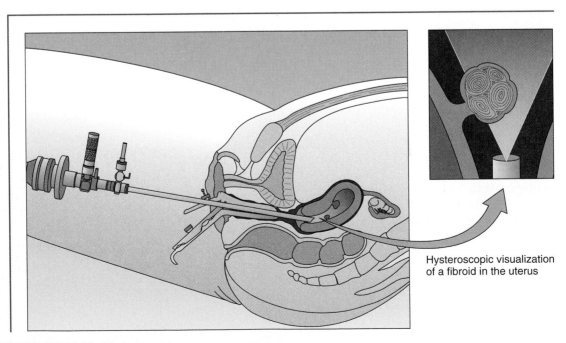

Hysteroscopic visualization of a fibroid in the uterus

■ **FIGURE 15-11.** Hysteroscopy.

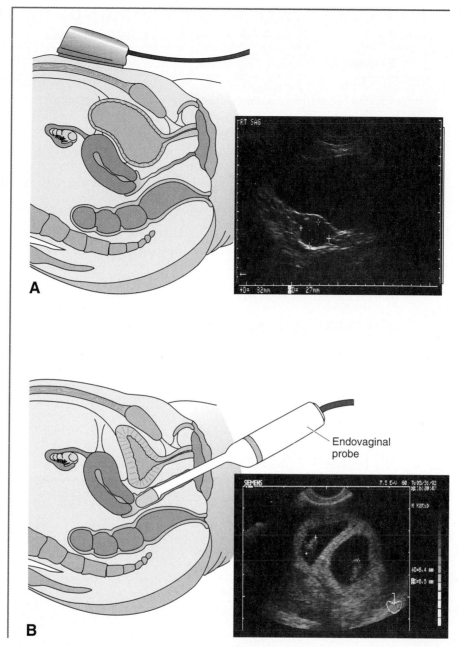

■ **FIGURE 15-12.** Pelvic sonography. **A.** Transabdominal imaging procedure. Inset, simple ovarian cyst. **B.** Transvaginal imaging procedure. *Inset,* twin pregnancies.

hysterosonogram (saline infusion sonogram)	a transvaginal sonographic image made as sterile saline is injected into the uterus; used to assess uterine pathology or determine tubal patency
transabdominal sonogram *trans-ab-dom'i-năl*	ultrasound image of the lower abdomen, including the bladder, uterus, tubes, and ovaries, to detect conditions such as cysts and tumors

PROGRAMMED REVIEW: GYNECOLOGICAL DIAGNOSTIC TESTS AND PROCEDURES

Answers	Review
biopsy	**15.79** The removal of tissue from any part of the body for microscopic pathologic examination is called _____ (Bx). Several forms of biopsies are performed in the female reproductive system. Using a special hollow needle to draw tissue or fluid from a cavity is called an aspiration biopsy or _____ biopsy. If the entire lesion is removed (excised) for examination, this is called an _____ biopsy. Removal of the biopsy specimen during an endoscopic examination is called an _____ biopsy. Cutting out (incising) a small tissue sample for examination is an _____ biopsy.
needle	
excisional	
endoscopic	
incisional	
stereotactic	**15.80** Use of a computer, x-ray imaging, and a specialized stereotactic frame to direct a needle into a breast lesion for removal of a core specimen for biopsy is called a _____ _____ biopsy.
breast	
process	**15.81** Recall that the suffix *-scopy* means _____ of examination with an instrument. The two combining forms for vagina are *vagin/o* and _____. Using the latter form, the term for examination of the vagina using a specialized microscope is called _____.
colp/o	
colposcopy	
hyster/o	**15.82** Recall that the combining forms for uterus are *metr/o, uter/o,* and _____. Using the last form, the term for using a special microscope to examine inside the uterus is called _____.
hysteroscopy	
magnetic resonance	**15.83** Gynecologic conditions are also diagnosed with nonionizing images made with _____ _____ imaging (MRI).
Pap	**15.84** The study of cells collected from the cervix to screen for abnormalities is called a _____ smear, named for Dr. Papanicolaou.

radiography	**15.85** The medical term for x-ray imaging is _____.
record	Recall that the suffix -*gram* means _____. The two combining
mamm/o	forms for breast are *mast/o* and _____. Formed from the latter, the
	x-ray record of breast tissue made to detect neoplasms is a
mammogram	_____.

salping/o	**15.86** The combining form for fallopian tube is _____.
	The medical term for an x-ray of the fallopian tubes after injection
	of a contrast medium uses that combining form as well as *hyster/o*,
uterus	which means _____. This kind of x-ray is called a
hysterosalpingogram	_____.

pelvic	**15.87** Sonography is the imaging modality using ultrasound. Ultrasound imaging of a female's pelvic area is called _____ sonography. Recall that the prefix *endo-* means _____. A sonogram
within	
	made with the ultrasound transducer within the vagina is called an
endovaginal	_____ sonogram. The prefix *trans-* means across or
through	_____. An endovaginal sonogram is also called a
transvaginal	_____ sonogram because the sound waves pass
	through the vagina. An ultrasound image of the whole lower abdomen
transabdominal	is called a _____ sonogram

	15.88 Again, the combining forms for uterus are *metr/o*, *uter/o*, and
hyster/o	_____. A sonogram of the uterus, formed from the last of
	these, which is made as sterile saline is injected into the uterus, is called
hysterosonogram	a _____.

SELF-INSTRUCTION: GYNECOLOGICAL OPERATIVE TERMS

Study the following:

Term	Meaning
adhesiolysis *ad-hē′zē-ōl′i-sis* **adhesiotomy** *ad-hē-sē-otō′-mē*	breaking down or severing of pelvic adhesions

cervical conization *ser'vĭ-kal kō-nī-zā'shŭn*	removal of a cone-shaped portion of the cervix
colporrhaphy *kol-pōrhă-fē*	suture to repair the vagina
anterior repair	repair of a cystocele
posterior repair	repair of a rectocele
A&P repair	anterior and posterior repair of cystocele and rectocele
cryosurgery (Fig. 15-13) *krī-ō-ser'jer-ē*	method of destroying tissue by freezing; used for treating dysplasia and early cancers
dilation and curettage (D&C) (Fig. 15-14) *dī-lā'shŭn* *kyū-rě-tahzh'*	dilation of the cervix and scraping of the endometrium to control bleeding, to obtain tissue for biopsy, or to remove polyps or products of conception
hysterectomy *his-ter-ek'tō-mē*	removal of the uterus
abdominal hysterectomy	removal of the uterus through an incision in the abdomen
vaginal hysterectomy	removal of the uterus through the vagina
total hysterectomy	removal of the uterus and cervix

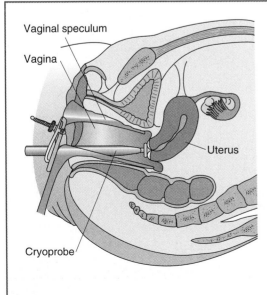
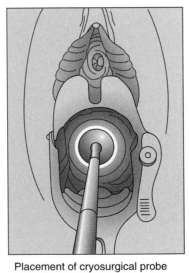
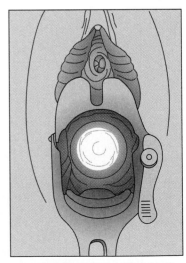
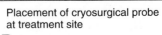

Placement of cryosurgical probe at treatment site

Ice crystals seen immediately after freezing treatment

■ **FIGURE 15-13.** Cryosurgical procedure.

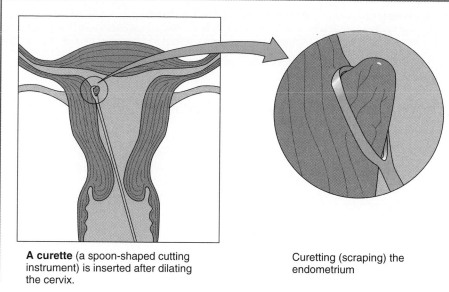

A curette (a spoon-shaped cutting instrument) is inserted after dilating the cervix.

Curetting (scraping) the endometrium

▪ **FIGURE 15-14.** Dilation and curettage.

laparoscopy *lap-ă-ros′kŏ-pē*	inspection of the abdominal or pelvic cavity with a laparoscope, which is an endoscope used to examine the abdominal and pelvic regions
laparoscopic surgery	surgical procedures within the abdominal or pelvic region using a laparoscope
laser surgery *lā′zer*	use of a laser to destroy lesions or dissect or cut tissue, used frequently in gynecology
loop electrosurgical excision procedure (LEEP) **large loop excision of the transformation zone** (LLETZ) (Fig. 15-15)	use of electrosurgical or radio waves transformed through a loop-configured electrosurgical device to treat precancerous cervical lesions by simultaneous excisional biopsy and treatment of affected tissue (e.g., cervical dysplasia or human papilloma virus lesions); note that the transformation zone is the area of the cervix (between the endocervix and ectocervix) where neoplasia (new abnormal cell formation) is most likely to arise

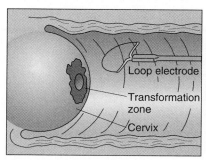
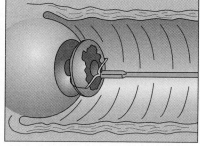
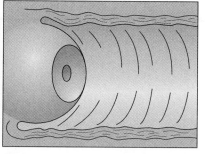

Loop electrode

Transformation zone

Cervix

A **B** **C**

▪ **FIGURE 15-15.** Loop electrosurgical excision procedure (LEEP) or large loop excision of the transformation zone (LLETZ). **A.** electrode approach. **B.** Removal of transformation zone. **C.** Excision site (region between endocervix and ectocervix).

myomectomy *mī-ō-mek′tō-mē*	excision of fibroid tumors
oophorectomy *ō-of-ōr-ek′tō-mē*	excision of an ovary
ovarian cystectomy *ō-var′ē-an sis-tek′tō-mē*	excision of an ovarian cyst
salpingectomy *sal-pin-jek′tō-mē*	excision of a uterine tube
bilateral salpingo-oophorectomy *bi-lat′er-ăl sal-ping′gō-of-ō-rek′tō-mē*	excision of both uterine tubes and ovaries
salpingotomy *sal-pin-jek′tō-mē*	incision into a fallopian tube, often performed to remove an ectopic pregnancy
salpingostomy *sal-ping-gos′tō-mē*	creation of an opening in the fallopian tube to open a blockage
tubal ligation *lī-gā′shŭn*	sterilization of a woman by cutting and tying (ligating) the uterine tubes

PROGRAMMED REVIEW: GYNECOLOGICAL OPERATIVE TERMS

Answers	Review
excision hysterectomy abdominal vaginal total hysterectomy	**15.89** Recall that the suffix *-ectomy* means _____ (or removal). Removal of the uterus is called _____. When performed through an incision in the abdomen, it is called an _____ hysterectomy. When removed through the vagina, it is called a _____ hysterectomy. The total removal of the uterus and cervix is called a _____ _____.
    myomectomy	**15.90** A tumor of muscle tissue is called a myoma. Removal of fibroid tumors from the muscle tissue of the uterus is called _____.
ovary oophorectomy	**15.91** The combining form *oophor/o* means _____. Excision of an ovary is _____.

ovarian	**15.92** Removal of an ovarian cyst is an _____
cystectomy	_____.
salping/o	**15.93** The combining form for fallopian tube is _____.
salpingectomy	Excision of a fallopian tube is _____.
both	**15.94** The prefix *bi-* means two or _____. Thus, the term bilateral
both	generally means on _____ sides. The term for excision of both uter-
bilateral	ine (fallopian) tubes and ovaries is _____
salpingo-oophorectomy	_____-_____.
incision	**15.95** The operative suffix *-tomy* means _____. An inci-
salpingotomy	sion into a fallopian tube is a _____.
	15.96 The surgical suffix *-stomy* means the creation of an
opening	_____. The creation of an opening in the fallopian tube to
salpingostomy	open a blockage is called a _____.
	15.97 Ligation means tying off. The procedure for cutting and tying
tubal ligation	the uterine tubes to cause sterilization is _____ _____.
-tomy	**15.98** The surgical suffix for incision is _____. The breaking
	down or cutting of pelvic adhesions is called adhesiolysis or
adhesiotomy, breaking	_____. The suffix *-lysis* means _____
down	_____ or dissolution.
	15.99 The surgical removal of a cone-shaped portion of the cervix is
cervical conization	called _____ _____.
suture	**15.100** The surgical suffix *-rrhaphy* means _____. The two
colp/o	combining forms for vagina are *vagin/o* and _____. Formed from
	the latter form, a suture to repair the vagina is termed
colporrhaphy	_____. A repair of a cystocele (in the front of the
anterior	vagina) is an _____ repair. The repair of a rectocele (the

posterior repair	back of the vagina) is a _____ _____. Recall
pouching or hernia	that -*cele* means a _____. When both the bladder and rec-tum pouch into the vagina, creating both a cystocele and a rectocele, the
A&P	repair of both is called an _____ repair (anterior and posterior repair).
cryosurgery	**15.101** The combining form *cry/o* means cold. Surgery that destroys tissue by freezing it is called _____. This is used for treating dysplasia and early cancers.
cervix	**15.102** The D&C procedure is performed to control bleeding, to obtain tissue for biopsy, or to remove polyps or the products of conception. The _____ is dilated, and the endometrium is scraped (curet-
dilation, curettage	tage). D&C stands for _____ and _____.
examination	**15.103** Recall that the suffix -*scopy* means process of _____ with a visualizing instrument. The combining form *lapar/o* refers to the abdomen generally. Thus, the examination of the abdominal and pelvic cavity with a special scope
laparoscopy	is called _____. Surgery performed through the
laparoscopic	laparoscope is called _____ surgery.
laser	**15.104** A laser is often used in gynecologic procedures to destroy lesions or cut tissue. This is called _____ surgery.
loop electrosurgical	**15.105** LEEP is a procedure using a loop-shaped device to make an electrosurgical excision of the transformation zone of the cervix; it is used to treat precancerous lesions such as cervical dysplasia. LEEP is an abbreviation for _____ _____
excision	_____ procedure. This procedure is also called LLETZ, or
transformation zone	large loop excision of the _____ _____.

SELF-INSTRUCTION: GYNECOLOGICAL OPERATIVE TERMS: BREASTS

Study the following:

Term	Meaning
lumpectomy *lŭm-pek'tō-mē*	excision of a breast tumor without removing any other tissue or lymph nodes, usually followed by radiation or chemotherapy if the tumor is found to be cancerous
mastectomy (Fig. 15-16) *mas-tek'tō-mē*	removal of a breast
simple mastectomy	removal of an entire breast but with underlying muscle and axillary lymph nodes left intact

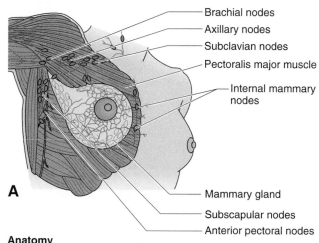

Anatomy
The breast, the underlying muscles, and the lymph nodes are the structures involved in breast cancer surgery. The lymph nodes, which act as barriers against bacteria or tumor cells, are useful in staging breast cancer.

Simple Mastectomy
Only the breast is removed. The underlying muscle and associated lymph nodes are not removed.

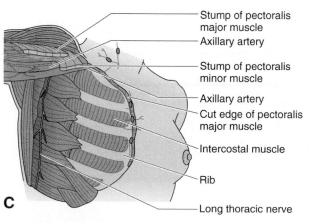

Radical Mastectomy
The breast, pectoralis muscles, and contents of the axilla (including lymph nodes and adipose tissue) are removed.

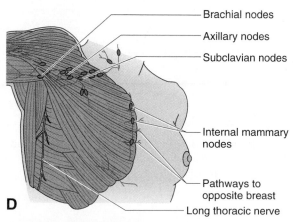

Modified Radical Mastectomy
The breast and lymph nodes of the axilla are removed. Occasionally the pectoralis minor muscle is transected or removed to approach the lymph nodes.

■ **FIGURE 15-16. A.** Anatomy of breast. **B–D.** Mastectomy alternatives.

radical mastectomy	removal of an entire breast along with the underlying chest muscles and axillary lymph nodes
modified radical mastectomy	removal of an entire breast and lymph nodes of the axilla
mammoplasty *mam'ō-plas-tē*	surgical reconstruction of a breast
augmentation mammoplasty (Fig. 15-17)	reconstruction to enlarge the breast, often by inserting an implant
reduction mammoplasty	reconstruction to remove excessive breast tissue
mastopexy *mas'tō-pek-sē*	elevation of pendulous breast tissue

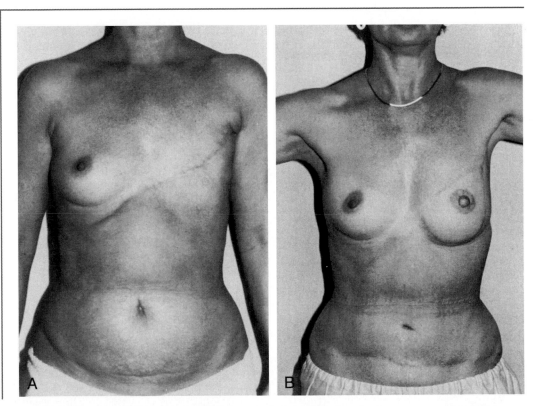

■ **FIGURE 15-17.** Augmentation mammoplasty. **A.** Left modified radical mastectomy in a 53-year-old woman (3 months postoperation). **B.** Same patient 10 months after augmentation mammoplasty.

PROGRAMMED REVIEW: GYNECOLOGICAL OPERATIVE TERMS: BREASTS

Answers	Review
-ectomy	**15.106** The surgical suffix for excision (removal) is _____. The surgical removal of a breast tumor (lump) without removing other
lumpectomy	tissue or lymph nodes is a _____.
	15.107 The combining forms meaning breast are *mamm/o* and
mast/o	_____. Formed from the latter form, the term for surgical re-
mastectomy	moval of a breast is _____. There are several different types of mastectomies, depending on how much tissue is removed to ensure the cancer is excised. Removal of just the breast, leaving under-
simple	lying muscle and axillary lymph nodes intact, is called a _____
radical	mastectomy. A _____ mastectomy involves removal of the breast as well as underlying chest muscles and the axillary lymph
mastectomy	nodes. A modified radical _____ removes the breast and lymph nodes only.
-plasty	**15.108** Recall that the suffix for surgical reconstruction is _____.
mamm/o	The two combining forms meaning breast are _____ and *mast/o*. Using the first of these, the term for surgical reconstruction of the breast
mammoplasty	is _____.
augmentation	**15.109** A mammoplasty performed to enlarge the breast, usually by inserting an implant, is called _____ mammoplasty. A reconstruction performed to remove excessive breast tissue and thereby reduce the size of the breasts is called
reduction mammoplasty	_____ _____.
mast/o	**15.110** In addition to *mamm/o*, the other combining form for breast is _____. The surgical suffix -*pexy* means suspension or
fixation	_____. The procedure to elevate pendulous breast tissue
mastopexy	by fixing tissues higher is a _____.

SELF-INSTRUCTION: THERAPEUTIC TERMS

Study the following:

Term	Meaning
chemotherapy *kem'ō-thār-ă-pē*	treatment of malignancies, infections, and other diseases with chemical agents that destroy selected cells or impair their ability to reproduce
radiation therapy	treatment of neoplastic disease using radiation to deter the proliferation of malignant cells
hormone replacement therapy (HRT)	use of a hormone (e.g., estrogen or progesterone) to replace a deficiency or regulate production
hormonal contraceptives	hormones used to prevent conception by suppressing ovulation
oral contraceptive pill (OCP)	birth control pills
contraceptive injection	injection of the hormone (such as Depo-Provera) into the body
contraceptive implant	insertion of a contraceptive capsule under the skin to provide a continual infusion over an extended time
barrier contraceptives	products that provide a physical barrier to prevent conception (e.g., condoms or diaphragms)
intrauterine device (IUD) *in'tră-yū'ter-in*	contraceptive device inserted into the uterus that prevents implantation of a fertilized egg
spermicidals *sper-mi-sī'dălz*	creams, jellies, lotions, or foams containing agents that kill sperm (cid/o = to kill)

PROGRAMMED REVIEW: THERAPEUTIC TERMS

Answers	Review
	15.111 The combining form referring to chemical agents is *chem/o*. The treatment of malignancies, infections, and other diseases with chemical agents that destroy targeted cells is called _____.
chemotherapy	
	15.112 Some kinds of cancer are treated with radiation, which deters the proliferation of malignant cells. This is called _____
radiation	
therapy	_____.
	15.113 If a woman is deficient in the production of a hormone, such as estrogen, treatment may involve administering a replacement hormone

hormone replacement	to the person. This is called _____ _____ therapy (HRT).
contraceptives against contraceptive contraceptive implant	**15.114** Hormones administered to prevent conception and pregnancy are called hormonal _____. The prefix *contra-* means _____ or opposed to. Oral _____ pills are generally called birth control pills. A hormonal contraceptive that is injected is a _____ injection. Hormonal contraceptives can also be administered in a capsule that is placed under the skin to give a continual infusion; this is called a contraceptive _____.
barrier	**15.115** Contraceptive methods that create a physical block to prevent sperm from reaching the ovum are called _____ contraceptives (such as a condom or diaphragm).
intrauterine within	**15.116** IUD is the abbreviation for _____ device, which is inserted into the uterus to prevent implantation of a fertilized egg. The prefix *intra-* means _____.
spermicidals	**15.117** Contraceptive creams, jellies, lotions, and foams that contain an agent that kills (*cid/o* means to kill) sperm are called _____.

SELF-INSTRUCTION: OBSTETRICAL (*OB-STET′RI-KAL*) (OB) SYMPTOMATIC TERMS

Study the following:

Term	Meaning
gravida (Fig. 15-18) *grav′i-dă*	a pregnant woman
nulligravida *nŭl-i-grav′i-dă*	having never been pregnant

OBSTETRICAL HISTORY ABBREVIATIONS

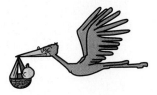

The following abbreviations are used in recording an obstetrical history.

GPA terms:
G   gravida   number of pregnancies
P   para   number of viable birth experiences (may include multiple births)
AB   abortus   abortions
           SAB spontaneous abortion
           TAB therapeutic abortion

Arabic numerals are placed after each abbreviation to indicate the number of pregnancies, viable births or abortions.

Examples:

Obstetric history: G2, P1, AB1. or gravida 2, para 1, abortus 1.
[The patient has been pregnant twice, had one birth experience that resulted in the delivery of at least one viable offspring and had one abortion.]

TPAL terms:
T   term infants
P   premature infants
A   abortions
L   living children

Examples:
Obstetric history: 5 term infants, 0 premature infants, 0 abortions, 5 living children
or Obstetric history: 5-0-0-5.
[The patient has delivered five term infants, no premature infants, no abortion, and has five living children]

Occasionally, combined GPA and TPAL abbreviations are used. For example,

Obstetrical history: gravida 3, 4-0-0-4
[The patient has been pregnant three times, had four term infants, no premature infants, no abortions, and 4 living children. (Numbers indicate one twin birth)]

■ **FIGURE 15-18.** Obstetrical history abbreviations.

primigravida *prī-mi-grav'i-dă*	first pregnancy Note: gravida followed by a number indicates the number of pregnancies (*see* Term Tip)
para (Fig. 15-18) *par'ă*	to bear; a woman who has produced one or more viable (live outside the uterus) offspring
nullipara *nŭl-i-par'ă*	a woman who has not borne a child (nulli = none; para = to bear)
primipara *pri-mip'ă-ră*	first delivery (primi = first; para = to bear)

multipara *mŭl-tip'ă-ră*	a woman who has given birth to two or more children (multi = many; para = to bear) Note: para followed by a number indicates the number of times a pregnancy has resulted in a single or multiple birth (Fig. 15-18)
cervical effacement *ĕ-fās'ment*	progressive obliteration of the endocervical canal during delivery
estimated date of confinement (EDC) *kon-fīn'ment* **estimated date of delivery** EDD	expected date for delivery of the baby, normally 280 days or 40 weeks from last menstrual period (LMP)
meconium staining *mē-kō'nē-ŭm*	presence of meconium in amniotic fluid
ruptured membranes *rŭp'chūrd*	rupture of the amniotic sac, usually at onset of labor
macrosomia *mak-rō-sō'mē-ă*	large-bodied baby commonly seen in diabetic pregnancies (macro = large; soma = body)
polyhydramnios *pol'ē-hī-dram'nē-os*	excessive amniotic fluid

PROGRAMMED REVIEW: OBSTETRICAL SYMPTOMATIC TERMS

Answers	Review
pregnant nulli primigravida, first	**15.118** The obstetrical term gravida refers to a _____ woman. The term for a woman who has never been pregnant is _____-gravida, and a woman in her first pregnancy is a _____. The prefix *primi-* means _____.
para no primipara multipara multiple (many)	**15.119** Similarly, there are several obstetrical terms for women who have borne children, based on the term _____, which means to bear. A nullipara is a woman who has borne ____ children. A woman who has given birth once is _____. A woman who has borne multiple (two or more) children is _____. The prefix *multi-* means _____.

15.120   A pregnant woman is given a date by her obstetrician for her expected due date. In medical language, this date is referred to by two expressions: the _____ _____ of _____ (EDC), or the _____ _____ of _____ (EDD). This calculation is based on the date of the LMP, or _____ _____ _____.

estimated date
confinement, estimated
date, delivery
last menstrual period

15.121   Problems may occur with the amniotic fluid or sac. Recall that the amniotic sac surrounds the embryo and fetus in the woman's _____. The term for the condition of excessive amniotic fluid begins with the prefix *poly-*, which means _____ or much, and uses the combining form meaning water or fluid, *hydr/o*. This condition is called _____.

uterus

many

polyhydramnios

15.122   When the membranes of the amniotic sac break, usually during the labor, this is called _____ membranes.

ruptured

15.123   Recall that the term for intestinal discharges of the fetus is _____. The presence of meconium in the amniotic fluid is called meconium _____.

meconium

staining

15.124   As labor progresses and approaches delivery, the endocervical canal is progressively obliterated in a process known as cervical _____.

effacement

15. 125   Recall that the prefix *macro-* means _____ or long. The term for a large-bodied baby, often occurring in diabetic mothers, is _____.

large

macrosomia

SELF-INSTRUCTION: OBSTETRICAL (OB) DIAGNOSTIC TERMS

Study the following:

Term	Meaning
abortion (AB) *ă-bōr'shŭn*	expulsion of the product of conception before the fetus is viable (able to live outside the uterus)
spontaneous abortion (SAB) *spon-tā'nē-ŭs*	miscarriage; expulsion of products of conception occurring naturally
habitual abortion	spontaneous abortion occurring in three or more consecutive pregnancies
incomplete abortion	incomplete expulsion of products of conception
missed abortion	death of a fetus or embryo within the uterus that is not naturally expelled after death
threatened abortion	bleeding with threat of miscarriage
cephalopelvic disproportion (CPD) *sef'ă-lō-pel'vik*	condition preventing normal delivery through the birth canal; either the baby's head is too large or the birth canal is too small
eclampsia *ek-lamp'sē-ă*	true toxemia of pregnancy characterized by high blood pressure, albuminuria, edema of the legs and feet, severe headaches, dizziness, convulsions, and coma
preeclampsia *prē-ē-klamp'sē-ă* **pregnancy-induced hypertension (PIH)**	toxemia of pregnancy characterized by high blood pressure, albuminuria, edema of the legs and feet, and puffiness of the face, without convulsion or coma
ectopic pregnancy *ek-top'ik*	implantation of the fertilized egg outside the uterine cavity, often in the tube or ovary, or rarely in the abdominal cavity
erythroblastosis fetalis *ĕ-rith'rō-blas-tō'sis fē'tā'lis*	disorder that results from the incompatibility of a fetus with an Rh-positive blood factor and a mother who is Rh negative, causing red blood cell destruction in the fetus; this condition necessitates a blood transfusion to save the fetus
Rh factor	presence, or lack, of antigens on the surface of red blood cells that may cause a reaction between the blood of the mother and fetus, resulting in fetal anemia (which causes erythroblastosis fetalis)
Rh positive	presence of antigens
Rh negative	absence of antigens
hyperemesis gravidarum *cause hī-per-em'ĕ-sis grav-i-dā'rŭm*	severe nausea and vomiting in pregnancy that can cause severe dehydration in the mother and fetus (emesis = vomit)

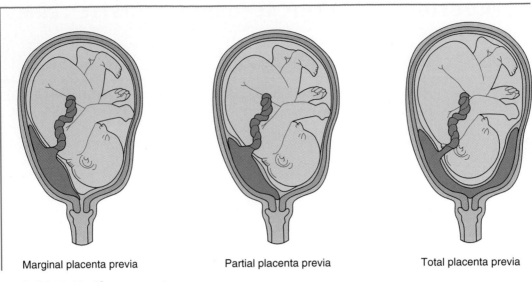

Marginal placenta previa   Partial placenta previa   Total placenta previa

■ **FIGURE 15-19.** Placenta previa.

meconium aspiration *mē-kō'nē-ŭm* *as-pi-rā'shŭn*	fetal aspiration of amniotic fluid containing meconium
placenta previa (Fig. 15-19) *plă-sen'tă prē'vēă*	displaced attachment of the placenta in the lower region of the uterine cavity
abruptio placentae *ab-rŭp'shē-ō pla-sen'tē*	premature detachment of a normally situated placenta

PROGRAMMED REVIEW: OBSTETRICAL DIAGNOSTIC TERMS

Answers	Review
	15.126 The expulsion of the products of conception before fetal viability is called _____. An abortion can occur naturally or therapeutically. A miscarriage, in which the expulsion occurs naturally, is called a _____ abortion (SAB). Spontaneous abortions occurring in three or more consecutive pregnancies are called _____ abortion.
abortion	
spontaneous	
habitual	
	15.127 If the products of conception are not completely expelled, this is called an _____ abortion. If the embryo or fetus dies within the uterus but is not then naturally expelled, this is a
incomplete	

missed

threatened

_____ abortion. Bleeding with the threat of miscarriage is a

_____ abortion.

15.128   The term ectopic comes from a Greek word meaning out of

place. A pregnancy in which the fertilized egg is implanted outside the

ectopic

pregnancy

uterus, such as in the fallopian tube, is called an _____

_____.

15.129   Many women normally experience "morning sickness" early

in pregnancy, but severe nausea and vomiting can cause dehydration.

The word emesis means vomit. Recall that the prefix *hyper-* means

excessive

hyperemesis

gravidarum

above or _____. The term for the condition of severe

nausea and vomiting in pregnancy is _____

_____.

15.130   Eclampsia is a serious condition that can occur in pregnancy,

high

characterized by _____ blood pressure and other symptoms, lead-

ing to convulsions or coma. Recall that the prefix *pre-* means

before

_____. A condition of high blood pressure similar to eclampsia,

but occurring without convulsions or coma, may precede eclampsia. It

preeclampsia, pregnancy-

induced

excessive

is called _____, or _____-

_____ hypertension (PIH). The prefix *hyper-* means

_____ or above.

15.131   Certain antigens may or may not be present on the surface of

Rh

positive

Rh

red blood cells; this is called the ____ factor. The presence of antigens is

designated Rh _____, and the absence of these antigens is

designated ____ negative.

15.132   If the mother's blood is Rh negative and the fetus's blood is Rh

positive, a reaction will occur that causes fetal red blood cell destruc-

tion. Red blood cells are called erythroblasts. Recall that the suffix *-osis*

condition

means increase or _____. The condition that results in

erythroblastosis fetalis	the fetus from this incompatibility of Rh factors is called _____ _____. A blood transfusion is usually necessary to save the fetus.
before placenta previa	**15.133** The term previa comes from a Latin word formed by the combination of *pre-*, meaning _____, and *-via*, meaning the way. If the placenta is attached in an abnormal position low in the uterus, it may obstruct the movement of the fetus out of the uterus at childbirth. This condition of a displaced placenta is called _____ _____.
abruptio placentae	**15.134** An abruption is a tearing away or detachment. The premature detachment of a normally situated placenta is called _____ _____.
amniotic meconium aspiration	**15.135** Recall that meconium staining refers to the presence of meconium in the _____ fluid. If this occurs, the fetus may suck this into its lungs, a condition called _____ _____.
head cephalopelvic	**15.136** Normally, the infant's head passes easily through the birth canal in the mother's pelvis. Recall that the combining form *cephal/o* means _____. If the infant's head is too large or the mother's pelvis too small, a condition of _____ disproportion exists, complicating childbirth.

SELF-INSTRUCTION: OBSTETRICAL DIAGNOSTIC TESTS AND PROCEDURES

Study the following:

Test or Procedure	Explanation
chorionic villus sampling (CVS) (Fig. 15-20) *kō-rē-on'ik vil'us*	sampling of placental tissue for microscopic and chemical examination to detect fetal abnormalities

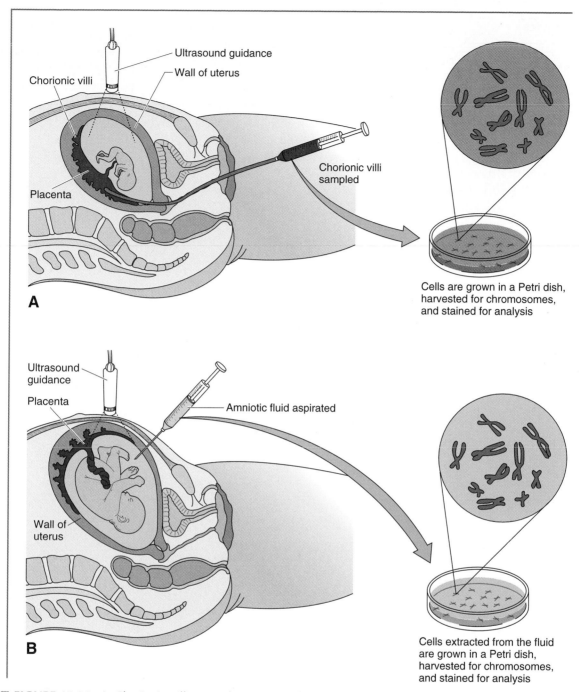

■ **FIGURE 15-20. A.** Chorionic villus sampling (9 to 11 weeks). **B.** Amniocentesis (15 to 18 weeks).

amniocentesis (Fig. 15-20) *am′nē-ō-sen-tē′sis*	aspiration of a small amount of amniotic fluid for analysis of possible fetal abnormalities
fetal monitoring	use of an electronic device for simultaneous recording of fetal heart rate and uterine contractions
pelvimetry *pel-vim′ĕ-trē*	obstetric measurement of the pelvis to evaluate proper conditions for vaginal delivery

pregnancy test	test performed on urine or blood to detect the presence of human chorionic gonadotropin hormone (secreted by the placenta), which indicates pregnancy
endovaginal sonogram transvaginal sonogram (*see* Fig. 15-12)	ultrasound image of the uterus, tubes, and ovaries made after introduction of an ultrasonic transducer within the vagina; useful for detecting pathology (e.g., ectopic pregnancy or missed abortion)
obstetric sonogram (*see* Figs. 2-14 and 15-4)	ultrasound image of the pregnant uterus to determine fetal development

PROGRAMMED REVIEW: OBSTETRICAL DIAGNOSTIC TESTS AND PROCEDURES

Answers	Review
	15.137 Various diagnostic tests are often performed during pregnancy. Recall that the suffix *-centesis* refers to puncture for
aspiration	_____. Puncturing the amniotic sac and aspirating a small amount of amniotic fluid for analysis is called
amniocentesis	_____.
chorionic villus	**15.138** Another fetal sampling procedure is performed with placental tissue to detect fetal abnormalities. This is called _____ _____ sampling (CVS).
fetal monitoring	**15.139** The fetal heart rate and uterine contractions can be monitored with an electronic recording device; this process is called _____ _____.
-metry pelvimetry	**15.140** Recall that the suffix meaning process of measuring is _____. Obstetrical measuring of the pelvis for conditions related to vaginal delivery is called _____.
pregnancy test	**15.141** A woman who suspects she may be pregnant can have a _____ _____ performed with a blood or urine sample to detect whether she is pregnant.

obstetrical	**15.142** An ultrasound image of the pregnant uterus is called an
within	_____ sonogram. Recall that the prefix *endo-* means
endovaginal	_____. A sonogram made with the ultrasound transducer
transvaginal	within the vagina is called an _____ sonogram or a _____ sonogram (trans = through).

SELF-INSTRUCTION: OBSTETRICAL OPERATIVE AND THERAPEUTIC TERMS

Study the following:

Term	Meaning
OPERATIVE	
cesarean section (C-section) *se-zā′rē-ăn*	surgical delivery of a baby through an incision through the abdomen and into the uterus
episiotomy *e-piz-ē-ot′ō-mē*	incision of the perineum to facilitate delivery
THERAPEUTIC	
amnioinfusion *am′nē-ō-in-fyū′zhŭn*	introduction of a solution into the amniotic sac; an isotonic solution is most commonly used to relieve fetal distress
therapeutic abortion (TAB)	abortion induced by mechanical means or by drugs for medical reasons
version	manual method for reversing the position of the fetus, usually done to facilitate delivery
external version	abdominal manipulation
internal version	intravaginal manipulation

COMMON THERAPEUTIC DRUG CLASSIFICATIONS

abortifacient *ă-bōr-ti-fā′shent*	drug that causes abortion (e.g., mifepristone—formerly known as RU-486)
oxytocin *ok-sē-tō′sin*	hormone secreted by the pituitary gland that causes myometrial con traction, used to induce labor
Rh immune globulin *glob′yū-lin*	immunizing agent given to an Rh-negative mother within 72 hours after delivering an Rh-positive baby to suppress the Rh immune response
tocolytic agent *tō-kō-lit′ik*	drug used to stop labor contractions

PROGRAMMED REVIEW: OBSTETRICAL OPERATIVE AND THERAPEUTIC TERMS

Answers	Review
cesarean section	**15.143** The delivery of an infant through a surgical incision is named for a famous Roman emperor reputedly delivered in this manner: _____ _____ (C-section).
episi/o, -tomy episiotomy	**15.144** The two combining forms for vulva are *vulv/o* and _____. Recall that the suffix for incision is _____. Made with the latter combining form, the term for the surgical incision or the perineum to facilitate delivery is _____.
amnioinfusion	**15.145** To infuse means to introduce a fluid into a body area. The introduction of a solution into the amniotic sac is called _____.
abortion therapeutic abortion abortifacient	**15.146** Again, the expulsion of the products of conception is called an _____. When it is performed deliberately by mechanical or pharmacologic means, this is called a _____ _____ (TAB). A drug that causes abortion is an _____.
delivery external internal version	**15.147** Manual manipulation to change the position of the fetus to facilitate _____ is called version. This manipulation of the abdomen done from the outside is termed _____ version. Performed from within the vagina, it is called _____ _____.
oxytocin	**15.148** A hormone secreted by the pituitary gland causes uterine contractions. It is sometimes given to a pregnant woman to induce labor. This hormone is _____.
birth tocolytic	**15.149** Recall that the combining form *toc/o* means _____. The suffix *-lytic* can mean to stop something. A type of drug given to stop labor contractions is a _____.

immune, globulin

15.150 An Rh-negative mother who delivers an Rh-positive baby may have an immune response. This agent is given to the mother to suppress that response: Rh _____ _____ .

Practice Exercises

For the following terms, on the lines below the term, write out the indicated word parts: prefixes, combining forms, roots, and suffixes. Then define the word.

Example:

ectocervical

$$\underset{\text{P} \qquad \text{R} \qquad \text{S}}{\text{ecto/cervic/al}}$$

DEFINITION: outside/cervix or neck/pertaining to

1. vulvitis

_____ / _____
  R   S

DEFINITION: _____

2. polymastia

_____ / _____ / _____
    P   R   S

DEFINITION: _____

3. ovoid

_____ / _____
  R   S

DEFINITION: _____

4. tocolysis

_____ / _____
  CF   S

DEFINITION: _____

5. salpingotomy

_____ / _____
  CF   S

DEFINITION: _____

6. mammoplasty

_____ / _____
   CF   S

DEFINITION: _____

7. transvaginal

_____ / _____ / _____
   P   R   S

DEFINITION: _____

8. hysterorrhexis

_____ / _____
   CF   S

DEFINITION: _____

9. colposcopy

_____ / _____
   CF   S

DEFINITION: _____

10. mammography

_____ / _____
    CF   S

DEFINITION: _____

11. metrorrhagia

_____ / _____
    CF   S

DEFINITION: _____

12. ovariocentesis

_____ / _____
    CF   S

DEFINITION: _____

13. menarche

_____ / _____
    R   S

DEFINITION: _____

14. oophorectomy

_____ / _____
    R   S

DEFINITION: _____

15. oligomenorrhea

    ———— / ———— / ————
      P   CF   S

DEFINITION: _____

16. dystocia

    ———— / ———— / ————
      P   R   S

DEFINITION: _____

17. gynecologist

    ———— / ————
      CF   S

DEFINITION: _____

18. hysterosalpingogram

    ———— / ———— / ————
      CF   CF   S

DEFINITION: _____

19. episiotomy

    ———— / ————
      CF   S

DEFINITION: _____

20. colporrhaphy

    ———— / ————
      CF   S

DEFINITION: _____

21. hysterospasm

    ———— / ————
      CF   S

DEFINITION: _____

22. lactorrhea

    ———— / ————
      CF   S

DEFINITION: _____

23. ovigenesis

    ———— / ————
      CF   S

DEFINITION: _____

24. endocervical

_____ / _____ / _____
P   R   S

DEFINITION: _____

25. uterotomy

_____ / _____
CF   S

DEFINITION: _____

Define the following abbreviations:

26. IUD _____

27. HPV _____

28. CVS _____

29. D&C _____

30. HBV _____

31. EDC _____

32. HSV _____

33. STD _____

34. TAB _____

35. HRT _____

Match the following:

36. removal of a uterine tube and an ovary _____   a. PID

37. white vaginal discharge _____   b. chlamydia

38. condition when baby's head is too big _____ for birth canal   c. colporrhaphy

39. presence of more than one nipple on a breast _____   d. LEEP

40. implantation of a fertilized egg outside _____ the uterus   e. CPD

41. most common bacterial STD _____ in North America   f. leukorrhea

42. excisional biopsy _____   g. polythelia

43. painful intercourse _____   h. ectopic

44. surgical repair of cystocele _____   i. salpingo-oophorectomy

45. inflammation of entire female pelvic cavity_____   j. dyspareunia

Give the medical term for the following:

46. condition of benign lumps in breast that fluctuate with menstrual cycle

_____

47. abnormal opening between bladder and vagina _____

48. cutting and tying the uterine tubes _____

49. having more than two breasts _____

50. bacterial STD caused by a spirochete _____

51. x-ray of uterine tubes to determine patency _____

52. study of cervical cells to screen for cancer _____

53. condition of migration of endometrial tissue _____

54. abnormal opening between the rectum and vagina _____

55. surgical remedy for rectocele _____

Complete the following:

56. _____pause = cessation of menstruation

57. _____rrhea = painful menstruation

58. _____rrhea = absence of menstruation

59. _____rrhea = scanty menstruation

60. _____rrhagia = excessive bleeding at time of menstruation

61. _____rrhagia = bleeding from the uterus at any time other than the
normal period

62. _____mastia = development of mammary glands in a male

63. _____mastia = absence of a breast

64. _____mastia = unusually small breasts—a common surgical remedy
is _____ mammoplasty

65. _____mastia = unusually large breasts; a common surgical remedy is
_____mammoplasty

66. masto_____ = surgical fixation of a pendulous breast

67. _____ectomy = removal of a breast

68. _____ectomy = removal of a breast lump

Identify terms related to abortion:

69. _____ a naturally occurring miscarriage

70. _____ a miscarriage occurring in three or more consecutive pregnancies

71. _____ fetal expulsion with parts of placenta remaining with bleeding

72. _____ fetal death within the uterus

73. _____ one induced by mechanical means or by drugs

74. _____ bleeding with threat of miscarriage

Match the following:

75. retroflexion _____   a. forward bend of uterus

76. condylomata _____   b. toxemia of pregnancy

77. para 2 _____   c. backward bend of uterus

78. prolapse _____   d. a pregnant woman

79. cystocele _____   e. cervical cancer

80. gravida _____   f. genital warts

81. rectocele _____   g. woman who has given birth twice

82. eclampsia _____   h. first delivery

83. CIN-2 _____   i. protrusion of the rectum into the vagina

84. primipara _____   j. descent of uterus from normal position

85. anteflexion _____   k. cervical dysplasia

86. CIS _____   l. pouching of the bladder into the vagina

For each of the following, circle the combining form that corresponds to the meaning given:

87. **birth or labor**	tox/o	toc/o	troph/o
88. **vagina**	uter/o	metr/o	colp/o
89. **uterine tube**	vagin/o	oophor/o	salping/o
90. **menstruation**	men/o	mamm/o	mast/o
91. **cervix**	colp/o	cervic/o	salping/o
92. **egg**	oophor/o	ov/i	ovari/o
93. **vulva**	episi/o	vagin/o	metr/o

94. **uterus**	vagin/o	metr/o	oophor/o
95. **milk**	lact/o	leuk/o	lip/o
96. **ovary**	ov/o	oophor/o	salping/o
97. **breast**	men/o	metr/o	mast/o
98. **woman**	gen/o	gynec/o	hyster/o

Write in the missing words on lines in the following illustration of female reproductive anatomy:

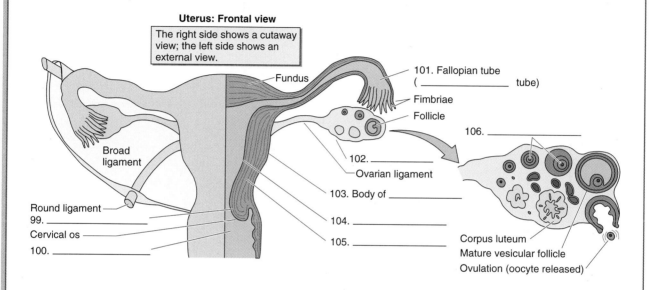

Uterus: Frontal view

The right side shows a cutaway view; the left side shows an external view.

Fundus

Fimbriae

Follicle

101. Fallopian tube (_____ tube)

106. _____

Broad ligament

102. _____
Ovarian ligament

103. Body of _____

Round ligament
99. _____

Cervical os

100. _____

104. _____

105. _____

Corpus luteum
Mature vesicular follicle
Ovulation (oocyte released)

For each of the following, circle the correct spelling of the term:

107.	gonorrhea	gonorhea	ghonarhea
108.	dispareunia	dyspareunia	dysparunia
109.	tokolytic	toecolytic	tocolytic
110.	polythelia	polythellia	polytelia
111.	meterorrhagia	metrorrhagia	metrorhagia
112.	dialation	dyelayshun	dilation
113.	salpingotomy	salpengotomy	salpigotomy
114.	nulligravida	nuligravida	nulligraveda
115.	meconeium	meconium	meconeum
116.	macrosomia	macrosomnia	macrasomia
117.	cureitage	curetage	curettage

118. eclampshea	eklampsia	eclampsia
119. amenorrhea	amennorhea	amenorhea
120. abortifacient	abortafacient	abortofacent

Give the noun that was used to form the following adjectives.

121. chlamydial   _____

122. areolar   _____

123. syphilitic   _____

124. cervical   _____

125. dysplastic   _____

126. endometrial   _____

Medical Record Analyses

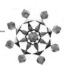

MEDICAL RECORD 15-1

GYN Chart Note

S: This 44 y.o. female, gravida 2, para 2, c/o extremely heavy periods for the past several years that have been getting worse for the past two months and have been accompanied by moderately severe cramps. PAP smears have been normal. She has no bladder or bowel complaints.

O: On pelvic exam, the uterus is found to be retroverted and irregularly enlarged with several large fibroids palpable. There are no adnexal masses.

A: Leiomyomata uteri with secondary menorrhagia

P: Schedule vaginal hysterectomy; donate one pint of blood for autologous transfusion, if necessary

1. What is the patient's OB history?
   a. never been pregnant
   b. been pregnant only once
   c. had two miscarriages
   d. has been pregnant four times
   e. has had two live births

2. Identify the patient's most significant symptom:
   a. amenorrhea
   b. dyspareunia
   c. leukorrhea
   d. menorrhagia
   e. metrorrhagia

3. Which of the following was one of the objective findings?
   a. tipped uterus
   b. forward bending uterus
   c. backward bending uterus
   d. presence of several ovarian tumors
   e. migration of portions of endometrial tissue

4. What was the condition of the patient's uterine tubes?
   a. not stated
   b. normal
   c. inflamed
   d. enlarged
   e. had been previously removed

5. What was the Dx?
   a. congenital tumor composed of displaced embryonic tissue
   b. cyst of the uterine tube
   c. inflammation of the organs of the pelvic cavity
   d. smooth muscle tumors in the uterus
   e. ovarian tumors

6. What surgical procedure is planned?
   a. incision into uterine tube to remove the cyst
   b. excision of uterus
   c. excision of ovaries
   d. dilation of cervix and scraping of endometrium
   e. excision of tubes and ovaries cavity

MEDICAL RECORD 15-2 FOR ADDITIONAL STUDY

CENTRAL MEDICAL CENTER

211 Medical Center Drive • Central City, US 90000-1234 • PHONE: (012) 125-6784 • FAX: (012) 125-9999

TO BE ADMITTED: 9/3/20xx

HISTORY

CHIEF COMPLAINT:
Right ovarian cyst.

HISTORY OF PRESENT ILLNESS:
This is a 32-year-old Caucasian female who had a routine examination on June 21, 20xx, at which time the examination revealed the right ovary to be approximately two to three times normal size. Otherwise, all was normal. The Papanicolaou smear revealed atypical cells of undetermined significance. The patient returned for a colposcopy, and this revealed what appeared to be squamous epithelial lesions CIN 1-2. Biopsies were performed which revealed chronic cervicitis and no evidence of CIN. The patient was placed on Lo-Ovral for two cycles and then was rechecked. The right ovary continued to enlarge and got to the point where it was approximately 4 x 5 cm, floating anteriorly in the pelvis, and was fairly firm to palpation. A pelvic sonogram corroborated the clinical findings in that superior to the right adnexa was a 4 x 5 cm mass, possibly with hemorrhage into either a paraovarian cyst or possibly a dermoid cyst. The patient is to be admitted now for an exploratory laparotomy.

PAST HISTORY:
There is no history of severe medical illnesses. The patient had the usual childhood diseases and has had good health as an adult.

PREVIOUS SURGERY: The patient had a hymenotomy and dilatation and curettage in 20xx

MENSTRUAL HISTORY: Menstrual cycle is 30 days, averaging a four to seven day flow.

OBSTETRICAL HISTORY: The patient is a Gravida 0.

FAMILY HISTORY:
Diabetes in the family. Mother and father are living and well

REVIEW OF SYSTEMS:
Noncontributory.

(continued)

P. Widetick, M.D.
P. Widetick, M.D.

PW:bst
D: 9/1/20xx T: 9/2/20xx

HISTORY AND PHYSICAL Page 1	PT. NAME: FOLEY, JANE J. ID NO: IP-751014 ROOM NO: 331 ATT. PHYS: P. WIDETICK, M.D.

MEDICAL RECORD 15-2 FOR ADDITIONAL STUDY CONTINUED

CENTRAL MEDICAL CENTER

211 Medical Center Drive • Central City, US 90000-1234 • PHONE: (012) 125-6784 • FAX: (012) 125-9999

PHYSICAL EXAMINATION

GENERAL:
The patient is a well-developed, well-nourished Caucasian female who is anxious but in no acute distress.

VITAL SIGNS:
HEIGHT: 5 feet 5 inches. WEIGHT: 154 pounds. BLOOD PRESSURE: 110/82.

HEENT:
Normal.

NECK:
Supple; the trachea is in the midline. The thyroid is not enlarged.

CHEST:
LUNGS: Clear to percussion and auscultation. HEART: Regular sinus rhythm with no murmur. BREASTS: Normal to palpation.

ABDOMEN:
Soft and flat. No scars or masses.

PELVIC:
The outlet and vagina are normal. The cervix is moderately eroded. The uterus is normal size and anterior. The left adnexa is negative. The right adnexa has a firm, irregular cystic ovary that is anterior and approximately 5 x 5 cm. This is mobile and nontender.

EXTREMITIES:
Normal. Reflexes are grossly intact.

DIAGNOSIS:
Right ovarian cyst.

PLAN:
The patient is to be admitted for exploratory laparotomy and ovarian cystectomy.

P. Widetick, M.D.
P. Widetick, M.D.

PW:bst
D: 9/1/20xx T: 9/2/20xx

HISTORY AND PHYSICAL PAGE 2	PT. NAME: FOLEY, JANE J. ID NO: IP-751014 ROOM NO: 331 ATT. PHYS: P. WIDETICK, M.D.

MEDICAL RECORD 15-2 FOR ADDITIONAL STUDY

Jane Foley has seen her gynecologist, Dr. Phyllis Widetick, yearly for a routine examination and Pap smear. Every year the results have been normal. Jane is generally a healthy, active woman. This year, however, Dr. Widetick's examination and Pap smear found a problem. When the test results were in, Jane returned for additional testing.

Read Medical Record 15-2 (page 670–671) for Ms. Foley, and answer the following questions. This record is the history and physical report dictated by Dr. Widetick after her examination. Write your answers in the spaces provided.

1. In your own words, not using medical terminology, briefly describe the patient's chief complaint.

_____

_____

_____

2. In your own words, not using medical terminology, briefly describe what a Pap smear is.

_____

_____

_____

3. Explain the result of Ms. Foley's Pap smear.

_____

_____

_____

4. Because of this result, Dr. Widetick used colposcopy for further testing. Translate into nonmedical language what she discovered with this diagnostic procedure.

_____

_____

_____

5. What was the positive finding from the biopsy? Define this in your own words.

_____

_____

_____

6. Ms. Foley underwent all the following procedures. Put these in correct sequence by numbering them 1 to 6 in the order they were performed.

_____ follow-up examination

_____ visualization with colposcope

_____ ultrasound

_____ Pap smear

_____ routine physical examination

_____ Bx

7. The sonogram _definitely_ showed what finding?

_____

What were the _possible_ findings?

_____

_____

8. In nonmedical language, define the two previous surgeries Ms. Foley has had.

_____

_____

_____

9. How many children has Ms. Foley had?

_____

10. Mark any of the following abnormal findings from the present physical examination:
    a. enlarged uterus
    b. gross reflexes
    c. eroded cervix
    d. hypertension
    e. enlarged thyroid
    f. mobile right ovarian cyst

11. Define Dr. Widetick's final diagnosis and explain what she will do next to treat Ms. Foley.

_____

_____

_____

Answers to Practice Exercises

1. vulv/itis
   R   S
   vulva (covering)/ inflammation
2. poly/mast/ia
   P   R   S
   many/breast/condition of
3. ov/oid
   R S
   egg/resembling
4. toco/lysis
   CF S
   birth or labor/breaking down or dissolution

5. salpingo/tomy
   CF   S
   uterine (fallopian) tube/ incision
6. mammo/plasty
   CF   S
   breast/surgical repair or reconstruction
7. trans/vagin/al
   P   R   S
   across or through/vagina/ pertaining to
8. hystero/rrhexis
   CF   S
   uterus/rupture

9. colpo/scopy
   CF   S
   vagina/process of examination
10. mammo/graphy
    CF   S
    breast/process of recording
11. metro/rrhagia
    CF   S
    uterus/to burst forth
12. ovario/centesis
    CF   S
    ovary/puncture for aspiration
13. men/arche
    R   S
    menstruation/beginning

14. oophor/ectomy
     R   S
    ovary/excision (removal)
15. oligo/meno/rrhea
     P   CF   S
    few or deficient/
       menstruation/discharge
16. dys/toc/ia
     P   R   S
    painful, difficult or faulty/
       labor or birth/condition of
17. gyneco/logist
       CF   S
    woman/one who specializes
       in the study or treatment of
18. hystero/salpingo/gram
       CF   CF   S
    uterus/uterine (fallopian)
       tube/record
19. episio/tomy
       CF   S
    vulva (covering)/incision
20. colpo/rrhaphy
       CF   S
    vagina/suture
21. hystero/spasm
       CF   S
    uterus/involuntary
       contraction
22. lacto/rrhea
       CF   S
    milk/discharge
23. ovi/genesis
       CF   S
    egg/origin or production
24. endo/cervic/al
       P   R   S
    within/cervix/pertaining to
25. utero/tomy
       CF   S
    uterus/incision
26. intrauterine device
27. human papilloma virus
28. chorionic villus sampling
29. dilation and curettage
30. hepatitis B virus
31. estimated date of
    confinement
32. herpes simplex virus
33. sexually transmitted disease
34. therapeutic abortion
35. hormone replacement
    therapy
36. l

37. f
38. e
39. g
40. h
41. b
42. d
43. j
44. c
45. a
46. fibrocystic breasts
47. vesicovaginal fistula
48. tubal ligation
49. polymastia
50. syphilis
51. hysterosalpingogram
52. Papanicolaou smear (Pap)
53. endometriosis
54. rectovaginal fistula
55. colporrhaphy—posterior
    repair
56. menopause
57. dysmenorrhea
58. amenorrhea
59. oligomenorrhea
60. menorrhagia
61. metrorrhagia
62. gynecomastia
63. amastia
64. hypomastia or micromastia;
    augmentation mammoplasty
65. hypermastia or macromastia;
    reduction mammoplasty
66. mastopexy
67. mastectomy
68. lumpectomy
69. spontaneous abortion
70. habitual abortion
71. incomplete abortion
72. missed abortion
73. therapeutic abortion
74. threatened abortion
75. c
76. f
77. g
78. j
79. l
80. d
81. i
82. b
83. k
84. h
85. a
86. e

87. toc/o
88. colp/o
89. salping/o
90. men/o
91. cervic/o
92. ov/i
93. episi/o
94. metr/o
95. lact/o
96. oophor/o
97. mast/o
98. gynec/o
99. cervix
100. vagina
101. uterine
102. ovary
103. uterus
104. endometrium
105. myometrium
106. eggs or ova
107. gonorrhea
108. dyspareunia
109. tocolytic
110. polythelia
111. metrorrhagia
112. dilation
113. salpingotomy
114. nulligravida
115. meconium
116. macrosomia
117. curettage
118. eclampsia
119. amenorrhea
120. abortifacient
121. chlamydia
122. areola
123. syphilis
124. cervix
125. dysplasia
126. endometrium

Answers to Medical Record Analyses

1. e
2. d
3. a
4. b
5. d
6. b

APPENDIX A

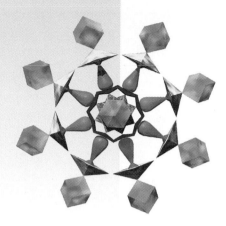

Glossary of Prefixes, Suffixes, and Combining Forms

TERM COMPONENT TO ENGLISH

a-	without	ambi-	both
ab-	away from	an-	without
abdomin/o	abdomen	an/o	anus
-ac	pertaining to	andr/o	male
acous/o	hearing	angi/o	vessel
acr/o	extremity or topmost	ankyl/o	crooked or stiff
-acusis	hearing condition	ante-	before
ad-	to, toward, or near	anti-	against or opposed to
aden/o	gland	aort/o	aorta
adip/o	fat	appendic/o	appendix
adren/o	adrenal gland	aque/o	water
adrenal/o	adrenal gland	-ar	pertaining to
aer/o	air or gas	-arche	beginning
-al	pertaining to	arteri/o	artery
albumin/o	protein	arthr/o	joint
-algia	pain	articul/o	joint
alveol/o	alveolus (air sac)	-ary	pertaining to

-ase	an enzyme	cephal/o	head
-asthenia	weakness	cerebell/o	cerebellum (little brain)
ather/o	fatty paste	cerebr/o	cerebrum (largest part of brain)
-ation	process	cerumin/o	wax
atri/o	atrium	cervic/o	neck or cervix
audi/o	hearing	cheil/o	lip
aur/i	ear	chol/e	bile
bacteri/o	bacteria	chondr/o	cartilage (gristle)
balan/o	glans penis	chrom/o	color
bi-	two or both	chromat/o	color
bil/i	bile	chyl/o	juice
-blast	germ or bud	circum-	around
blast/o	germ or bud	col/o	colon
blephar/o	eyelid	colon/o	colon
brachi/o	arm	colp/o	vagina (sheath)
brady-	slow	con-	together or with
bronch/o	bronchus (airway)	conjunctiv/o	conjunctiva (to join together)
bronchi/o	bronchus (airway)	contra-	against or opposed to
bronchiol/o	bronchiole (little airway)	corne/o	cornea
bucc/o	cheek	coron/o	circle or crown
capn/o	carbon dioxide	cost/o	rib
carb/o	carbon dioxide	crani/o	skull
carcin/o	cancer	crin/o	to secrete
cardi/o	heart	cutane/o	skin
cata-	down	cyan/o	blue
-cele	pouching or hernia	cyst/o	bladder or sac
celi/o	abdomen	cyt/o	cell
-centesis	puncture for aspiration	dacry/o	tear

dactyl/o	digit (finger or toe)	enter/o	small intestine
de-	from, down, or not	epi-	upon
dent/i	teeth	epididym/o	epididymis
derm/o	skin	episi/o	vulva (covering)
dermat/o	skin	erythr/o	red
-desis	binding	esophag/o	esophagus
dextr/o	right, or on the right side	esthesi/o	sensation
dia-	across or through	eu-	good or normal
diaphor/o	profuse sweating	ex-	out or away
dips/o	thirst	exo-	outside
dis-	separate from or apart	extra-	outside
doch/o	duct	fasci/o	fascia (a band)
duoden/o	duodenum	femor/o	femur
-dynia	pain	fibr/o	fiber
dys-	painful, difficult or faulty	gangli/o	ganglion (knot)
-e	noun marker	gastr/o	stomach
e-	out or away	-gen	origin or production
-eal	pertaining to	gen/o	origin or production
ec-	out or away	-genesis	origin or production
-ectasis	expansion or dilation	gingiv/o	gum
ecto-	outside	gli/o	glue
-ectomy	excision (removal)	glomerul/o	glomerulus (little ball)
-emesis	vomiting	gloss/o	tongue
-emia	blood condition	glott/o	opening
en-	within	gluc/o	sugar
encephal/o	entire brain	glyc/o	sugar
endo-	within	gnos/o	knowing

-gram	record
-graph	instrument for recording
-graphy	process of recording
gynec/o	woman
hem/o	blood
hemat/o	blood
hemi-	half
hepat/o	liver
hepatic/o	liver
herni/o	hernia
hidr/o	sweat
hist/o	tissue
histi/o	tissue
hormon/o	hormone (an urging on)
hydr/o	water
hyper-	above or excessive
hypo-	below or deficient
hypn/o	sleep
hyster/o	uterus
-ia	condition of
-iasis	formation of or presence of
-iatrics	treatment
-iatry	treatment
-ic	pertaining to
-icle	small
ile/o	ileum
immun/o	safe

infra-	below or under
inguin/o	groin
inter-	between
intra-	within
ir/o	iris (colored circle)
irid/o	iris (colored circle)
-ism	condition of
iso-	equal, like
-ist	one who specializes in
-itis	inflammation
-ium	structure or tissue
jejun/o	jejunum (empty)
kerat/o	hard or cornea
ket/o	ketone bodies
keton/o	ketone bodies
kinesi/o	movement
kyph/o	humped
lacrim/o	tear
lact/o	milk
lapar/o	abdomen
laryng/o	larynx (voice box)
lei/o	smooth
-lepsy	seizure
leuc/o	white
leuk/o	white
lex/o	word, phrase
lingu/o	tongue

lip/o	fat	-metry	process of measuring
lith/o	stone	micro-	small
lob/o	lobe (a portion)	mono-	one
-logist	one who specialized in the study or treatment of	morph/o	form
-logy	study of	multi-	many
lord/o	bent	muscul/o	muscle
lumb/o	loin (lower back)	my/o	muscle
lymph/o	clear fluid	myc/o	fungus
-lysis	breaking down or dissolution	myel/o	bone marrow or spinal cord
macr/o	large or long	myos/o	muscle
-malacia	softening	myring/o	eardrum
mamm/o	breast	narc/o	stupor, sleep
-mania	abnormal impulse (attraction) toward	nas/o	nose
mast/o	breast	nat/i	birth
meat/o	opening	necr/o	death
-megaly	enlargement	neo-	new
melan/o	black	nephr/o	kidney
men/o	menstruation	neur/o	nerve
mening/o	meninges (membrane)	ocul/o	eye
meningi/o	meninges (membrane)	-oid	resembling
meso-	middle	-ole	small
meta-	beyond, after, or change	olig/o	few or deficient
-meter	instrument for measuring	-oma	tumor
metr/o	uterus	onych/o	nail

oophor/o	ovary	pelv/i	hip bone
ophthalm/o	eye	pelv/o	hip bone
-opia	condition of vision	-penia	abnormal reduction
opt/o	eye	per-	through or by
orch/o	testis (testicle)	peri-	around
orchi/o	testis (testicle)	perine/o	perineum
orchid/o	testis (testicle)	peritone/o	peritoneum
or/o	mouth	-pexy	suspension or fixation
orth/o	straight, normal, or correct	phac/o	lens (lentil)
-osis	condition or increase	phag/o	eat or swallow
oste/o	bone	phak/o	lens (lentil)
ot/o	ear	pharyng/o	pharynx (throat)
-ous	pertaining to	phas/o	speech
ovari/o	ovary	-phil	attraction for
ov/i	egg	-philia	attraction for
ov/o	egg	phleb/o	vein
ox/o	oxygen	phob/o	exaggerated fear or sensitivity
pachy-	thick	phon/o	voice or sound
palat/o	palate	phor/o	to carry, bear
pan-	all	phot/o	light
pancreat/o	pancreas	phren/o	diaphragm; mind
para-	alongside of or abnormal	plas/o	formation
-paresis	slight paralysis	-plasia	formation
patell/o	patella (knee cap)	-plasty	surgical repair or reconstruction
path/o	disease	-plegia	paralysis
pector/o	chest	pleur/o	pleura
ped/o	child or foot	-pnea	breathing

pneum/o	air or lung	rhabd/o	rod shaped or striated (skeletal)
pneumon/o	air or lung	rhin/o	nose
pod/o	foot	-rrhage	to burst forth
-poiesis	formation	-rrhagia	to burst forth
poly-	many	-rrhaphy	suture
post-	after or behind	-rrhea	discharge
pre-	before	-rrhexis	rupture
presby/o	old age	salping/o	uterine (fallopian) tube; eustachian tube
pro-	before	sarc/o	flesh
proct/o	anus and rectum	schiz/o	split, division
prostat/o	prostate	scler/o	hard or sclera
psych/o	mind	scoli/o	twisted
-ptosis	falling or downward displacement	-scope	instrument for examination
pulmon/o	lung	-scopy	process of examination
purpur/o	purple	seb/o	sebum (oil)
py/o	pus	semi-	half
pyel/o	basin	sial/o	saliva
pylor/o	pylorus (gatekeeper)	sigmoid/o	sigmoid colon
quadr/i	four	sinistr/o	left, or on the left side
radi/o	radius; radiation (especially x-ray)	sinus/o	hollow (cavity)
re-	again or back	somat/o	body
rect/o	rectum	somn/o	sleep
ren/o	kidney	somn/i	sleep
reticul/o	a net	son/o	sound
retin/o	retina	-spasm	involuntary contraction
retro-	backward or behind	sperm/o	sperm (seed)

spermat/o	sperm (seed)	thromb/o	clot
sphygm/o	pulse	thym/o	thymus gland; mind
spin/o	spine (thorn)	thyr/o	thyroid gland (shield)
spir/o	breathing	thyroid/o	thyroid gland (shield)
splen/o	spleen	-tic	pertaining to
spondyl/o	vertebra	toc/o	labor
squam/o	scale	tom/o	to cut
-stasis	stop or stand	-tomy	incision
steat/o	fat	ton/o	tone or tension
sten/o	narrow	tonsill/o	tonsil
stere/o	three dimensional or solid	top/o	place
stern/o	sternum (breastbone)	tox/o	poison
steth/o	chest	toxic/o	poison
stomat/o	mouth	trache/o	trachea (windpipe)
-stomy	creation of an opening	trans-	across or through
sub-	below or under	tri-	three
super-	above or excessive	trich/o	hair
supra-	above or excessive	-tripsy	crushing
sym-	together or with	troph/o	nourishment or development
syn-	together or with	tympan/o	eardrum
tachy-	fast	-ula	small
tax/o	order or coordination	-ule	small
ten/o	tendon (to stretch)	uln/o	ulna
tend/o	tendon (to stretch)	ultra-	beyond or excessive
tendin/o	tendon (to stretch)	uni-	one
test/o	testis (testicle)	ur/o	urine
thalam/o	thalamus (a room)	ureter/o	ureter
thorac/o	chest	urethr/o	urethra

urin/o	urine	vertebr/o	vertebra
uter/o	uterus	vesic/o	bladder or sac
uvul/o	uvula	vesicul/o	bladder or sac
vagin/o	vagina (sheath)	vitre/o	glassy
varic/o	swollen or twisted vein	vulv/o	vulva (covering)
vas/o	vessel	xanth/o	yellow
vascul/o	vessel	xer/o	dry
ven/o	vein	-y	condition or process of
ventricul/o	ventricle (belly or pouch)		

ENGLISH TO TERM COMPONENT

abdomen	abdomin/o, celi/o, lapar/o	alveolus	alveol/o
abnormal	-para-	anus	an/o
abnormal reduction	-penia-	anus and rectum	proct/o
above	hyper-, super-, supra-	aorta	aort/o
across	dia-, trans-	apart	dis-
adrenal gland	adren/o, adrenal/o	appendix	appendic/o
after	post-, meta-	arm	brachi/o
again	re-	around	circum-, peri-
against	anti-, contra-	artery	arteri/o
air	aer/o, pneum/o, pneumon/o	atrium	atri/o
air sac	alveol/o	attraction for	-phil, -philia
airway	bronch/o, bronchi/o	away	e-, ec-, ex-
all	pan-	away from	ab-
alongside of	para-	back	re-

backward	retro-	bronchus	bronch/o, bronchi/o
bacteria	bacteri/o	bud	-blast, blast/o
basin	pyel/o	burst forth	-rrhage, -rrhagia
before	ante-, pre-, pro-	calculus	lith/o
beginning	-arche	cancer	carcin/o
behind	post-, retro-	carbon dioxide	capn/o, carb/o
below	hypo-, infra-, sub	carry	phor/o
bent	lord/o	cartilage	chondr/o
between	inter-	cavity (sinus)	atri/o, sin/o
beyond	meta-, ultra-	cell	cyt/o
bile	bil/i, chol/e	cerebellum	cerebell/o
bile duct	choledoch/o	cerebrum	cerebr/o
binding	-desis	cervix	cervic/o
birth	nat/i, toc/o	change	meta-
black	melan/o	cheek	bucc/o
bladder	cyst/o, vesic/o, vesicul/o	chest	pectoro, steth/o, thorac/o
blood	hem/o, hemat/o	child	ped/o
blood condition	-emia	circle	coron/o
blue	cyan/o	clear fluid	lymph/o
body	somat/o	clot	thromb/o
bone	oste/o	colon	col/o, colon/o
bone marrow	myel/o	colon, sigmoid	sigmoid/o
both	ambi-, bi-	color	chrom/o, chromat/o
brain	cerebr/o (largest part) encephal/o (entire brain)	colored circle	irid/o, ir/o
breaking down	-lysis	condition	-osis
breast	mamm/o, mast/o	condition of	-ia, -ism, -ium, -y
breathing	-pnea, spir/o	contraction, involuntary	-spasm

coordination	tax/o	egg	ov/i, ov/o
cornea	corne/o, kerat/o	enlargement	-megaly
correct	ortho-	enzyme	-ase
creation of an opening	-stomy	epididymis	epididym/o
crooked	ankyl/o	equal	iso-
crown	coron/o	esophagus	esophag/o
crushing	-tripsy	eustachian tube	salping/o
to cut	tom/o	examination	-scopy
death	necr/o	excessive	hyper-, super-, supra, ultra-
deficient	hypo-, olig/o	excision (removal)	-ectomy
development	troph/o	expansion or dilation	-ectasis
diaphragm	phren/o	extremity	acr/o
difficult	dys-	eye	ocul/o, ophthalm/o, opt/o
digit (finger or toe)	dactyl/o	eyelid	blephar/o
dilation or expansion	-ectasis	falling	-ptosis
discharge	-rrhea	fallopian tube	salping/o
disease	path/o	fascia	fasci/o
dissolution	-lysis	fast	tachy-
division	schiz/o	fat	adip/o, ather/o, lip/o, steat/o
down	de-	faulty	dys-
downward placement	-ptosis	fear, exaggerated	phob/o
dry	xer/o	femur	femor/o
duct	doch/o	few	olig/o
duodenum	duoden/o	fiber	fibr/o
ear	aur/i, ot/o	fixation	-pexy
eardrum	myring/o, tympan/o	flesh	sarc/o
eat, swallow	phag/o	foot	pod/o, ped/o

form	morph/o	humped	kyph/o
formation	-plasia, plas/o, -poiesis	ileum	ile/o
formation of	-lasis	incision	-tomy
four	quadri-	increase	-osis
from	de-	inflammation	-itis
fungus	myc/o	instrument for examination	-scope
ganglion	gangli/o	instrument for measuring	-meter
gas	aer/o	instrument for recording	-graph
germ or bud	-blast, blast/o	jejunum (empty)	jejun/o
gland	aden/o	joint	arthr/o, articul/o
glans penis	balan/o	juice	chyl/o
glassy	vitre/o	ketone bodies	ket/o, keton/o
glomerulus	glomerul/o	kidney	nephr/o, ren/o
glue	gli/o	kneecap	patell/o
good	eu-	knowing	gnos/o
groin	inguin/o	labor	toc/o
gums	gingiv/o	large	macr/o
hair	trich/o	larynx	laryng/o
half	hemi-, semi-	left or on left side	sinistr/o
hard	kerat/o, scler/o	lens	phac/o, phak/o
head	cephal/o	light	phot/o
hearing	acous/o, audi/o	like	iso-
hearing condition	-acusis	lip	cheil/o
heart	cardio/o	liver	hepat/o, hepatic/o
hernia	-cele, herni/o	lobe	lob/o
hip bone	pelvi/i, pelv/o	loin (lower back)	lumb/o
hormone	hormon/o	long	macr/o

lung	pneum/o, pneumon/o, pulmon/o	old age	presby-
male	andr/o	one	mono-
many	multi-, poly-	one who specializes in	-ist
measuring, instrument for	-meter	one who specializes in the study or treatment of	-logist
measuring process of	metry	opening	glott/o, meat/o
meninges	mening/o, meningi/o	opening, creation of	-stomy
menstruation	men/o	opposed to	anti-, contra-
milk	lact/o	order	tax/o
mind	psych/o, phren/o, thym/o	origin	-gen, -genesis, gen/o
mouth	or/o, stomat/o	out	e-, ec-, ex-
movement	kinesi/o	outside	ecto-, exo-, extra-
muscle	muscul/o, my/o, myos/o	ovary	oophor/o, ovari/o
nail	onych/o	oxygen	ox/o
narrow	sten/o	pain	-algia, -dynia
near	ad-	painful	dys-
neck	cervic/o	palate	palat/o
nerve	neur/o	pancreas	pancreat/o
net	reticul/o	paralysis	-plegia
new	neo-	paralysis, slight	-paresis
normal	eu-ortho-	perineum	perine/o
nose	nas/o, rhin/o	peritoneum	peritone/o
not	de-	pertaining to	-ac, -al, -ar, -ary, -eal, -ic, -ous, -tic
nourishment	troph/o	pharynx	pharyng/o
oil	seb/o	place	top/o

pleura	pleur/o	rupture	-rrhexis
poison	tox/o, toxic/o	sac	cyst/o, vesic/o, vesicul/o
portion	lob/o	safe	immun/o
pouching	-cele	saliva	sial/o
presence of	-iasis	scale	squam/o
process	-ation	sclera	scler/o
process of	-y	sebum	seb/o
production	-gen, gen/o, -genesis	secrete	crin/o
prostate	prostat/o	seizure	-lepsy
protein	albumin/o	sensation	esthesi/o
pulse	sphygm/o	sensitivity, exaggerated	phob/o
puncture for aspration	-centesis	separate from	dis-
purple	purpur/o	sigmoid colon	sigmoid/o
pus	py/o	sinus	sinus/o
pylorus	pylor/o	skeletal	rhabd/o
radius	radi/o	skin	cutane/o, derm/o, dermat/o
record	-gram	skull	crani/o
recording, process of	-graphy	sleep	hypn/o, somn/i, somn/o
rectum	proct/o, rect/o	slow	brady-
red	erythr/o	small	-icle, micro-, -ole, -ula, -ule
resembling	-oid	small intestine	enter/o
reticulum	reticul/o	smooth	lei/o
retina	retin/o	softening	-malacia
rib	cost/o	sound	phon/o, son/o
right or on the right side	dextr/o	sheath	vagin/o
rod shaped	rhabd/o	specializes, one who	-ist

speech	phas/o	tendon	ten/o, tend/o, tendin/o
sperm	sperm/o, spermat/o	tension	ton/o
spinal cord	myel/o	testis (testicle)	orch/o, orchi/o, orchid/o, test/o
spine	spin/o	thalamus	thalam/o
spleen	splen/o	thick	pachy-
split	schiz/o	thirst	dips/o
sternum	stern/o	three	tri-
stiff	ankyl/o	three dimensional or solid	stere/o
stomach	gastr/o	throat	pharyng/o
stone	lith/o	through	dia-, per-, trans-
stop or stand	-stasis	thymus gland	thym/o
straight	orth/o	thyroid gland	thyr/o, thyroid/o
striated	rhabd/o	tissue	hist/o, -ium
structure	-ium	to or toward	ad-
study of	-logy	together	con-, sym-, syn-
study of, one who specializes in	-logist	tone	ton/o
stupor	narc/o	tongue	gloss/o, lingu/o
sugar	gluc/o, glyc/o, glycos/o	tonsil	tonsill/o
surgical repair or reconstruction	-plasty	topmost	acr/o
suspension	-pexy	trachea	trache/o
suture	-rrhaphy	treatment	-iatrics, -iatry
swallow	phag/o	treatment, one who specializes in	-logist
sweat	hidr/o	tumor	-oma
sweat, profuse	diaphor/o	twisted	scoli/o
tear	dacry/o, lacrim/o	two	bi-
teeth	dent/i	ulna	uln/o

under	infra-, sub-	voice box	laryng/o
upon	epi-	vomiting	-emesis
ureter	ureter/o	vulva	vulv/o, episi/o
urethra	urethr/o	water	aque/o, hydr/o
urine	ur/o, urin/o	wax	cerumin/o
uterine tube	salping/o	weakness	-asthenia
uterus	hyster/o, metr/o, uter/o	white	leuc/o, leuk/o
vagina	colp/o, vagin/o	windpipe	trache/o
vein	phleb/o, ven/o	with	con-, sym-, syn-
vein, swollen or twisted	varic/o	within	en-, endo-, intra-
ventricle	ventricul/o	without	a-, an-
vertebra	vertebr/o, spondyl/o	woman	gynec/o
vessel	angi/o, vas/o, vascul/o	word, phrase	lex/o
vision, condition of	-opia	yellow	xanth/o
voice	phon/o		

APPENDIX B

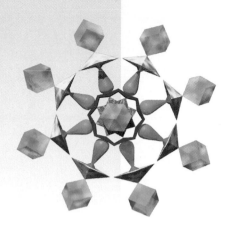

Abbreviations and Symbols

$\bar{a}$	before
A	anterior; assessment
A & P	auscultation and percussion
A&W	alive and well
AB	abortion
ABG	arterial blood gas
ac	before meals
ACE	angiotensin-converting enzyme
ACTH	adrenocorticotropic hormone
AD	right ear
ADH	antidiuretic hormone
ADHD	attention-deficit/hyperactivity disorder
ad lib	as desired
AIDS	acquired immunodeficiency syndrome
alb	albumin
am	morning
amt	amount
ANS	autonomic nervous system

AP	anterior posterior
aq	water
AS	left ear
ASD	atrial septal defect
ASHD	arteriosclerotic heart disease
AU	both ears
AV	atrioventricular
Ⓑ	bilateral
BD	bipolar disorder
bid	twice a day
BM	black male; bowel movement
BP	blood pressure
BPH	benign prostatic hypertrophy/hyperplasia
BRP	bathroom privileges
BS	blood sugar
BUN	blood urea nitrogen
Bx	biopsy
c̄	with
C	Celsius; centigrade
C&S	culture and sensitivity
CABG	coronary artery bypass graft
CAD	coronary artery disease
cap	capsule
CAT	computed axial tomography
CBC	complete blood count
cc	cubic centimeter
CC	chief complaint
CCU	coronary (cardiac) care unit
CHF	congestive heart failure

CIN	cervical intraepithelial neoplasia
CIS	carcinoma in situ
cm	centimeter
CNS	central nervous system
CO	cardiac output
c/o	complains of
COPD	chronic obstructive pulmonary disease
CP	cerebral palsy; chest pain
CPAP	continuous positive airway pressure
CPD	cephalopelvic disproportion
CPR	cardiopulmonary resuscitation
CSF	cerebrospinal fluid
CT	computed tomography
cu mm	cubic millimeter
CVA	cerebrovascular accident
CVS	chorionic villus sampling
CXR	chest x-ray
d	day
D&C	dilation and curettage
DC	discharge; discontinue; doctor of chiropractic
DDS	doctor of dental surgery
DJD	degenerative joint disease
DKA	diabetic ketoacidosis
DO	doctor of osteopathy
DPM	doctor of podiatric medicine
dr	dram
DRE	digital rectal examination
DTR	deep tendon reflex
DVT	deep vein thrombosis

Dx	diagnosis
ECG	electrocardiogram
ECHO	echocardiogram
ECT	electroconvulsive therapy
ECU	emergency care unit
EDC	estimated date of confinement
EDD	estimated date of delivery
EEG	electroencephalogram
EGD	esophagogastroduodenoscopy
EKG	electrocardiogram
EMG	electromyogram
ENT	ear, nose, throat
ER	emergency room
ERCP	endoscopic retrograde cholangiopancreatography
ESR	erythrocyte sedimentation rate
ESWL	extracorporeal shock wave lithotripsy
ETOH	ethyl alcohol
F	Fahrenheit
FBS	fasting blood sugar
FH	family history
fl oz	fluid ounce
FS	frozen section
FSH	follicle-stimulating hormone
Fx	fracture
g	gram
GAD	generalized anxiety disorder
GERD	gastroesophageal reflux disease
GH	growth hormone
GI	gastrointestinal

gm	gram
gr	grain
gt	drop
gtt	drops
GTT	glucose tolerance test
GYN	gynecology
h	hour
H & P	history and physical
HAV	hepatitis A virus
HBV	hepatitis B virus
HCT or Hct	hematocrit
HCV	hepatitis C virus
HD	Huntington disease
HEENT	head, eyes, ears, nose, throat
HGB or Hgb	hemoglobin
H & H	hemoglobin and hematocrit
HIV	human immunodeficiency virus
HPI	history of present illness
HPV	human papilloma virus
hs	hour of sleep
HSV-1	herpes simplex virus type 1
HSV-2	herpes simplex virus type 2
Ht	height
HTN	hypertension
Hx	history
I & D	incision and drainage
ICD	implantable cardioverter defibrillator
ICU	intensive care unit
ID	intradermal

IM	intramuscular
IMP	impression
IOL	intraocular lens implant
IP	inpatient
IUD	intrauterine device
IV	intravenous
IVP	intravenous pyelogram
kg	kilogram
KUB	kidney, ureter, bladder
L	left; liter
L&W	living and well
lb	pound
LEEP	loop electrosurgical excision procedure
LH	luteinizing hormone
LLETZ	large loop excision of transformation zone
LLQ	left lower quadrant
LP	lumbar puncture
LTB	laryngotracheobronchitis
LUQ	left upper quadrant
ⓜ	murmur
m	meter
MCH	mean corpuscular (cell) hemoglobin
MCHC	mean corpuscular (cell) hemoglobin concentration
MCV	mean corpuscular (cell) volume
MD	medical doctor; muscular dystrophy
mg	milligram
MI	myocardial infarction
ml, mL	milliliter
mm	millimeter

MPI	myocardial perfusion image
MRA	magnetic resonance angiography
MRI	magnetic resonance imaging
MS	multiple sclerosis; musculoskeletal
MSH	melanocyte-stimulating hormone
MVP	mitral valve prolapse
NAD	no acute distress
NCV	nerve conduction velocity
NG	nasogastric
NKA	no known allergy
NKDA	no known drug allergy
noc	night
NPO	nothing by mouth
NSAID	nonsteroidal anti-inflammatory drug
NSR	normal sinus rhythm
O	objective
OB	obstetrics
OCD	obsessive-compulsive disorder
OD	right eye; doctor of optometry
OH	occupational history
OP	outpatient
OR	operating room
ORIF	open reduction, internal fixation
OS	left eye
OU	both eyes
oz	ounce
$\bar{p}$	after
P	plan; posterior; pulse
PA	posterior anterior

$PaCO_2$	partial pressure of carbon dioxide
PaO_2	partial pressure of oxygen
PAP	Papanicolaou test (smear)
PAR	postanesthetic recovery
pc	after meals
PD	panic disorder
PDA	patent ductus arteriosus
PE	physical examination
PEFR	peak expiratory flow rate
per	by or through
PERRLA	pupils equal, round, and reactive to light and accommodation
PET	positron emission tomography
PF	peak flow
PFT	pulmonary function testing
PH	past history
PhD	doctor of philosophy
PI	present illness
PID	pelvic inflammatory disease
PIH	pregnancy induced hypertension
pm	after noon
PLT	platelet
PMH	past medical history
PNS	peripheral nervous system
po	by mouth
post op	postoperative
PPBS	post prandial blood sugar
PR	per rectum
pre op	preoperative
prn	as needed

PSA	prostate-specific antigen
PSG	polysomnography
pt	patient
PT	physical therapy; prothrombin time
PTCA	percutaneous transluminal coronary angioplasty
PTH	parathyroid hormone
PTSD	posttraumatic stress disorder
PTT	partial thromboplastin time
PUD	peptic ulcer disease
PV	per vagina
PVC	premature ventricular contraction
Px	physical examination
q	every
qd	every day
qh	every hour
q2h	every 2 hours
qid	four times a day
qns	quantity not sufficient
qod	every other day
qt	quart
R	right; respiration
RBC	red blood cell; red blood count
RLQ	right lower quadrant
R/O	rule out
ROM	range of motion
ROS	review of symptoms
RP	retrograde pyelogram
RRR	regular rate and rhythm
RTC	return to clinic

RTO	return to office
RUQ	right upper quadrant
Rx	recipe; take thou
s̄	without
S	subjective
SA	sinoatrial
SAB	spontaneous abortion
SAD	seasonal affective disorder
SC	subcutaneous
SH	social history
Sig:	instruction to patient
SLE	systemic lupus erythematosus
SOB	shortness of breath
SPECT	single photon emission computed tomography
SpGr	specific gravity
SQ	subcutaneous
SR	systems review
s̄s̄	one-half
STAT	immediately
STD	sexually transmitted disease
suppos	suppository
SV	stroke volume
Sx	symptom
T	temperature
T & A	tonsillectomy and adenoidectomy
tab	tablet
TAB	therapeutic abortion
TB	tuberculosis
TEDS	thrombo-embolic disease stockings

TEE	transesophageal echocardiogram
TIA	transient ischemic attack
tid	three times a day
TM	tympanic membrane
TMR	transmyocardial revascularization
Tr	treatment
TSH	thyroid-stimulating hormone
TURP	transurethral resection of the prostate
TV	tidal volume
Tx	treatment; traction
UA	urinalysis
UCHD	usual childhood diseases
URI	upper respiratory infection
US	ultrasound
UTI	urinary tract infection
VC	vital capacity
VCU	voiding cystourethrogram
VS	vital signs
VSD	ventricular septal defect
V_T	tidal volume
wa	while awake
WBC	white blood cell; white blood count
WDWN	well developed, well nourished
wk	week
WNL	within normal limits
Wt	weight
yo, y/o	year old
yr	year
♀	female

♂	male
#	number; pound
°	degree; hour
↑	increase; above
↓	decrease; below
Ø	none; negative
♀	standing
♀	sitting
○—	lying
×	times; for
>	greater than
<	less than
ī	one
īī	two
īīī	three
īv	four
I, II, III, IV, V, VI VII, VIII, IX, X	uppercase Roman numerals 1–10

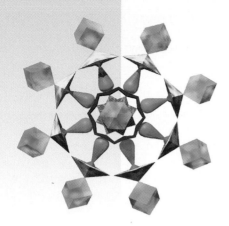

Commonly Prescribed Drugs and Their Applications

Compiled by Marjorie Canfield Willis, CMA-AC, and Michael J. Deimling, PhD, RPh

This alphabetical index of commonly prescribed drugs (trade and generic) is based on listings of new and refill prescriptions dispensed in the United States in 2000. The name of trade drugs are capitalized; their generic names accompany them in parentheses. All generic drug names are set in lower case.

Drug	Category/Application(s)
Accupril (quinapril hydro-chloride)	angiotensin-converting enzyme (ACE) inhibitor, antihypertensive, treats congestive heart failure
acetaminophen and codeine	analgesic/opiate combination
Accutane (isotretinoin)	retinoid, treats acne
Aciphex (rabeprazole)	proton pump inhibitor (PPI); treats peptic ulcer disease, gastroesophageal disease
Actos (pioglitazone)	oral hypoglycemic, antidiabetic
Adalat CC (nifedipine)	calcium channel blocker, antihypertensive, antianginal
Adderall (dextroamphetamine and amphetamine)	amphetamine combination, treats attention deficit/hyperactivity disorder
albuterol	β_2-adrenergic agonist, bronchodilator, antiasthmatic
Alesse-28 (ethinyl estradiol and levonorgestrel)	oral contraceptive
Allegra (fexofenadine)	second-generation antihistamine
Allegra-D (fexofenadine and pseudoephedrine)	antihistamine/decongestant combination
allopurinol	xanthine oxidase inhibitor, treats gout

Alphagan (brimonidine)	α_2-adrenergic agonist, treats glaucoma
alprazolam	benzodiazepine, anxiolytic (treats anxiety), sedative/hypnotic
Altase (ramipril)	angiotensin-converting enzyme (ACE) inhibitor, antihypertensive, treats congestive heart failure
Amaryl (glimepiride)	oral hypoglycemic, sulfonylurea
Ambien (zolpidem tartrate)	nonbenzodiazepine sedative/hypnotic
amitriptyline hydrochloride	tricyclic antidepressant
amoxicillin trihydrate	penicillin, antibiotic
Amoxil (amoxicillin trihydrate)	penicillin, antibiotic
Aricept (donepezil)	acetaylcholinesterase inhibitor (AchE), treats Alzheimer dementia
atenolol	β_1-adrenergic antagonist (blocker), cardioselective β-blocker, antihypertensive, antianginal, antiarrhythmic
Atrovent (ipratropium bromide)	anticholinergic, bronchodilator, antiasthmatic
Augmentin (amoxicillin/clavulanic acid)	penicillin/β-lactamase inhibitor combination
Avandia (rosiglitazone)	oral hypoglycemic, antidiabetic
Avapro (irbesartan)	angiotensin II receptor antagonist, antihypertensive
Azmacort (triamcinolone)	corticosteroid, anti-inflammatory
Bactroban (mupirocin)	topical antibacterial
Biaxin (chlarithromycin)	macrolide, antibiotic
BuSpar buspirone hydrochloride)	anxiolytic (treats anxiety)
Cardizem CD (diltiazem hydrochloride)	calcium channel blocker, antihypertensive, antianginal, antiarrhythmic
Cardura (doxazosin mesylate)	α_1-adrenergic antagonist, antihypertensive, vasodilator
Carisoprodol	skeletal muscle relaxant
Ceftin (cefuroxime)	second-generation cephalosporin, antibiotic
Cefzil (cefprozil)	second-generation cephalosporin, antibiotic
Celebrex (celecoxib)	cyclooxygenase-2 (COX-2) inhibitor, nonsteroidal anti-inflammatory drug (NSAID), analgesic, antipyretic

Celexa (citalopram)	antidepressant, selective serotonin reuptake inhibitor (SSR)
cephalexin	first-generation cephalosporin, antibiotic
Cipro (ciprofloxacin hydrochloride)	fluoroquinolone, antibacterial
Claritin (loratadine)	second-generation antihistamine
Claritin-D (loratadine and pseudoephedrine)	antihistamine/decongestant combination
Climara (estradiol) transdermal	estrogen, replacement therapy
Clonazepam	benzodiazepine, anticonvulsant, antiepileptic
clonidine hydrochloride	α_2-adrenergic agonist, central sympatholytic, antihypertensive
Combivent (ipratropium and albuterol)	anticholinergic/β_2-adrenergic agonist combination, bronchodilator, antiasthmatic
Contuss-XT (guaifenesin and phenylpropanolamine)	expectorant/decongestant
Coumadin (warfarin)	oral anticoagulant
Cozaar (losartan)	angiotensin II receptor antagonist, antihypertensive
cyclobenzaprine hydrochloride	skeletal muscle relaxant
Depakote (valproic acid and derivatives)	anticonvulsant, antiepileptic
Detrol (tolterodine)	anticholinergic, urinary antispasmodic
Dexedrine (dextroamphetamine)	amphetamine, central nervous system stimulant, treats attention deficit/hyperactivity disorder
diazepam	anxiolytic (treats anxiety), sedative, hypnotic, anticonvulsant, muscle relaxant
Diflucan (fluconazole)	antifungal
Dilantin (phenytoin)	hydantoin, anticonvulsant, antiepileptic
diltiazem hydrochloride	calcium channel blocker; antihypertensive, antianginal, antiarrhythmic
Diovan (valsartan)	angiotensin II receptor antagonist, antihypertensive
doxycycline hyclate	tracycline, antibiotic
Duragesic (fentanyl)	opioid, analgesic

Effexor XR (venlafaxine)	antidepressant, serotonin norepinephrine reuptake inhibitor (SNRI)
Elocon (mometasome furoate)	corticosteroid, anti-inflammatory
Ery-Tab (erythromycin)	macrolide, antibiotic
estradiol	estrogen, replacement therapy
Evista (raloxifene)	selective estrogen receptor modulator (SERM), treats osteoporosis
Flomax (tamsulosin)	α_1-adrenergic antagonist (blocker), treats benign prostatic hyperplasia
Flonase (fluticasone propionate)	corticosteroid, anti-inflammatory
Flovent (fluticasone)	corticosteroid, anti-inflammatory
folic acid	vitamin
Fosamax (alendronate)	bisphosphonate, treats Paget disease
furosemide	loop diuretic
gemfibrozil	antihyperlipidemic, fibric acid derivative
Glucophage (metfomin)	oral hypoglycemic, biguanide, antidiabetic
Glucotrol XL (glipizide)	oral hypoglycemic, sulfonylurea, antidiabetic
glyburide	oral hypoglycemic, sulfonylurea, antidiabetic
guaifenesin and phenyl-propanolamine	expectorant/decongestant combination
hydrochlorothiazide (HCTZ)	thiazide diuretic
hydrocodone and aceta-minophen	opiate/analgesic combination
hydroxyzine hydrochloride	first-generation antihistamine
Hyzaar (losartan and hydrochlorothiazide)	angiotensin II receptor antagonist/thiazide diuretic combination, antihypertensive
ibuprofen OTC	nonsteroidal anti-inflammatory drug (NSAID), analgesic, antipyretic
Imitrex (sumatriptan succinate)	serotonin (5-HT$_1$) agonist, treats migraine
isosorbide mononitrate	vasodilator, antianginal
K-Dur (potassium chloride)	potassium supplement

Klor-Con 10 (potassium chloride)	potassium supplement
Lanoxin (digoxin)	(+) inotropic, antiarrhythmic
Lescol (fluvastatin)	HGM-CoA reductase inhibitor, antihyperlipidemic agent
Levaquin (levofloxacin)	fluoroquinolone, antibacterial
Levothroid (levothyroxine)	thyroid hormone, replacement therapy
Levoxyl (levothyroxine)	thyroid hormone, replacement therapy
Lipitor (atorvastatin)	HMG-CoA reductase inhibitor, antihyperlipidemic agent
Lo/Ovral-28 (ethinyl estradiol)	oral contraceptive
lorazepam	benzodiazepine, anxiolytic (treats anxiety), anticonvulsant
Lotensin (benazepril hydrochloride)	angiotensin-converting enzyme (ACE) inhibitor, antihypertensive, treats congestive heart failure
Lotrel (amlodipine and benazepril)	calcium channel blocker/angiotensin converting enzyme (ACE) inhibitor combination, antihypertensive
Lotrisone (betamethasone dipropionate and clotrimazole)	corticosteroid/antifungal combination
Macrobid (nitrofurantoin)	antibacterial, urinary antiseptic
medroxyprogesterone	progestin, contraceptive
methylphenidate hydrochloride	central nervous system stimulant, treats attention deficit/hyperactivity disorder
methylprednisolone	corticosteroid, anti-inflammatory
metoprolol tartrate	β_1-adrenergic antagonist (blocker), cardioselective β-blocker, antihypertensive, antiarrhythmic
metronidazole	antimicrobial, antibacterial, antiprotazoal, amebicide, antiparasitic
Miacalcin (calcitonin)	parathyroid hormone, treats osteoporosis and Paget disease
Monopril (fosinopril)	angiotensin-converting enzyme (ACE) inhibitor, antihypertensive, treats congestive heart failure
Naproxen	nonsteroidal anti-inflammatory drug (NSAID), analgesic, antipyretic
Nasonex (mometasone furoate)	corticosteroid, anti-inflammatory

Necon 1/35/28 (norethin-drone and ethinyl estradiol)	oral contraceptive
neomycin, polymyxin b and hydrocortisone	antibiotic/corticosteroid combination
Neurontin (gabapentin)	anticonvulsant, antiepileptic
nitroglycerin	vasodilator, treats angina
Norvasc (amlodipine)	calcium channel blocker, antihypertensive, antianginal
Ortho-Cyclen-28 (ethinyl estradiol and norgestimate)	oral contraceptive
Ortho-Novum 7/7/7-28 (ethinyl estradiol and norethindrone)	oral contraceptive
Ortho-Tri-Cyclen 28 (ethinyl estradiol and norgestimate)	oral contraceptive
oxycodone and aceta-minophen	opiate/analgesic combination
OxyContin (oxycodone)	opiate, analgesic
Paxil (paroxetine)	antidepressant, selective serotonin reuptake inhibitor (SSRI)
Penicillin VK (penicillin v potassium)	penicillin; antibiotic
Pepcid (famotidine)	histamine H_2 receptor antagonist (H_2RA); treats peptic ulcer disease, gastroesophageal disease
Phenergan (promethazine hydrochloride)	antiemetic, antihistamine
Plavix (clopidogrel)	antiplatelet, antithrombotic
Plendil (felodipine)	calcium channel blocker, antihypertensive, antianginal
potassium chloride	potassium supplement
Pravachol (pravastatin sodium)	HMG-CoA reductase inhibitor, antihyperlipidemic
prednisone	corticosteroid, anti-inflammatory, immunosuppressant
Premarin (conjugated estrogens)	estrogen, conjugated estrogens
Prempro (estrogens and medroxy-progesterone)	estrogen/progestin combination, replacement therapy
Prevacid (lansoprazole)	proton pump inhibitor (PPI); treats peptic ulcer disease, gastroesophageal disease

Prilosec (omeprazole)	proton pump inhibitor (PPI); treats peptic ulcer disease, gastroesophageal disease
Prinivil (lisinopril)	angiotensin-converting enzyme (ACE) inhibitor, antihypertensive agent, treats congestive heart failure
Procardia XL (nifedipine)	calcium channel blocker; antihypertensive, antianginal
promethazine hydrochloride	antiemetic, antihistamine
promethazine hydrochloride and codeine	antihistamine/antitussive combination
propoxyphene napsylate and acetaminophen	opioid/analgesic combination
propanolol hydrochloride	β-adrenergic antagonist (blocker), antihypertensive, antiarrhythmic, antianginal
Proventil (albuterol)	β_2-selective adrenergic agonist, bronchodilator, antiasthmatic
Prozac (fluoxetine hydrochloride)	antidepressant, selective serotonin reuptake inhibitor (SSRI)
ranitidine hydrochloride	histamine H_2 receptor antagonist (H_2RA); treats peptic ulcer disease, gastroesophageal disease
Relafen (nabumetone)	nonsteroidal anti-inflammatory drug (NSAID), analgesic antipyretic
Remeron (mirtazapine)	atypical antidepressant
Risperdal (risperidone)	antipsychotic
Ritalin (methylphenidate hydrochloride)	central nervous system stimulant, treats attention deficit/hyperactivity disorder
Roxicet (oxycodone and acetaminophen)	opiate/analgesic combination
Serevent (salmeterol xinafoate)	β_2-selective adrenergic agonist, bronchodilator
Serzone (nefazodone)	atypical antidepressant
Skelaxin (metaxalone)	skeletal muscle relaxant
Singular (montelukast)	leukotriene D_4 (LTD_4) receptor antagonist, anti-inflammatory, antiasthmatic
Synthroid (levothyroxine sodium)	thyroid hormone
tamoxifen citrate	selective estrogen receptor modulator (SERM), antineoplastic

temazepam	benzodiazepine, anxiolytic (treats anxiety), sedative/hypnotic
Terazole (terconazole)	antifungal
terazosin	α_1 adrenergic antagonist (blocker), antihypertensive, vasodilator
tetracycline	tetracycline, antibiotic
Tiazac (diltiazem)	calcium channel blocker, antihypertensive antianginal antiarrhythmic
TobraDex (tobramycin and dexamethasone)	antibiotic/corticosteroid combination
Toprol-XL (metoprolol)	β_1-adrenergic antagonist (blocker), cardioselective β-blocker, antihypertensive, antiarrhythmic, antianginal
trazodone hydrochloride	atypical antidepressant
triamterene and hydrochlorothiazide (HCTZ)	potassium sparing diuretic/thiazide diuretic combination
trimethoprim-sulfamethoxazole (also known as co-trimoxazole)	antibacterial combination, sulfonamide
Trimox (amoxicillin trihydrate)	penicillin, antibiotic
Triphasil-28 (ethinyl estradiol and levonorgestrel)	oral contraceptive
Tussionex (hydrocodone and chlorpheniramine)	opiate/antihistamine combination, antitussive
Ultram (tramadol hydrochloride)	opioid, analgesic
Valtrex (valacyclovir)	antiviral
Vasotec (enalapril)	angiotensin-converting enzyme (ACE) inhibitor, antihypertensive, treats congestive heart failure
Veetids (penicillin V potassium)	penicillin, antibiotic
verapamil	calcium channel blocker, antihypertensive, antianginal, antiarrhythmic
Viagra (sildenafil)	phosphodiesterase type 5 (PDE5) inhibitor, treats erectile dysfunction
Vicoprofen (hydrocodone and ibuprofen)	opiate/analgesic combination
Vioxx (rofecoxib)	cyclooxygenase-2 (COX-2) inhibitor, nonsteroidal anti-inflammatory drug (NSAID), analgesic, antipyretic

warfarin	oral anticoagulant
Wellbutrin SR (bupropion)	atypical antidepressant
Xalantan (latanoprost)	prostaglandin, treats glaucoma
Zestoretic (lisinopril and hydrochlorothiazide)	angiotensin-converting enzyme (ACE) inhibitor/thiazide diuretic combination, antihypertensive
Zestril (lisinopril)	angiotensin-converting enzyme (ACE) inhibitor, antihypertensive, treats congestive heart failure
Ziac (bisoprolol and hydrochlorothiazide)	β_1-adrenergic antagonist/thiazide diuretic combination, antihypertensive
Zithromax (azithromycin dihydrate)	macrolide, antibiotic
Zocor (simvastatin)	HMG-CoA reductase inhibitor, antihyperlipidemic agent
Zoloft (sertraline hydrochloride)	antidepressant, selective serotonin reuptake inhibitor (SSRI)
Zyprexa (olanzapine)	antipsychotic
Zyrtec (cetirizine)	second-generation antihistamine

References

Lance LL, Lacy CF, Goldman MP, Armstrong LL, eds., Quick look drug book. Baltimore: Lippincott Williams & Wilkins, 2000.

Top 200 drugs of 1999. *Pharmacy Times,* www.pharmacytimes. com/top200.html.

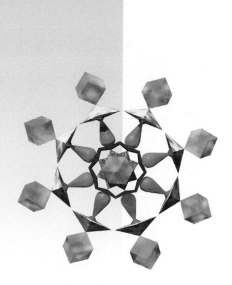

Figure Credit List

FIGURE 2-10. Courtesy of Deutsches Roentgen-Museum, Remscheid-Lennep, Germany.

FIGURE 2-11. B, Courtesy of GE Medical Systems. Inset, Courtesy of Orange Coast College.

FIGURE 2-12. Courtesy of ADAC Laboratories, a Philips Medical Systems Company, Bothell, WA.

FIGURE 2-13. B, Courtesy of Philips Medical Systems, Bothell, WA. Inset, Courtesy of Mission Regional Imaging, Mission Viejo, CA

FIGURE 2-14. B, Courtesy of Acuson Corporation, Mountain View, CA.

FIGURE 3-3. A–J, Courtesy of American Academy of Dermatology, Schaumburg, IL. S, Courtesy of LJ Underwood and RD Underwood, Mission Viejo, CA.

FIGURE 3-4. From Goodheart: A Photoguide of Common Skin Disorders: Diagnosis and Management (0.683.30257.4). Philadelphia: Lippincott Williams & Wilkins. 1999, pg 268 (**FIGURE** 21-17).

FIGURE 3-5. Reprinted with permission of Skin Cancer Foundation, New York, NY.

FIGURE 3-6. Reprinted with permission of Skin Cancer Foundation, New York, NY.

FIGURE 3-7. Courtesy of American Cancer Society, Atlanta, GA.

FIGURE 3-8. Courtesy of LJ Underwood and RD Underwood, Mission Viejo, CA.

FIGURE 3-9. Courtesy of LJ Underwood and RD Underwood, Mission Viejo, CA.

FIGURE 3-10. Courtesy of Ellman International, Hewlett, NY (Randolph Waldman, MD, photographer).

FIGURE 4-9. From Malone TR, ed. Hand and Wrist Injuries and Treatment. Baltimore: Williams & Wilkins, 1989:5.

FIGURE 4-11. From Harris JH Jr, Harris WH, Novelline RA. The Radiology of Emergency Medicine, 3rd ed. Baltimore: Williams & Wilkins, 1993:440, 467.

FIGURE 4-12. Courtesy of Orange Coast College Radiologic Technology Program

FIGURE 4-14. From Yochum TR, Rowe LJ. Essentials of skeletal radiology. Philadelphia: Lippincott Williams & Wilkins, 1987:xxvii.

FIGURE 4-15. Courtesy of West Coast Radiology Center, Santa Ana, CA.

FIGURE 4-16 . Courtesy of Coherent Medical, Inc., Palo Alto, CA.

FIGURE 4-18. Courtesy of Smith & Nephew Systems, Inc., Memphis, TN.

FIGURE 4-19. Courtesy of Camp International, Jackson, MI.

FIGURE 4-20. Courtesy of RGP Prosthetic Research Center, San Diego, CA.

FIGURE 5-6. Courtesy of Welch Allyn, Skaneateles Falls, NY.

FIGURE 5-12. C, From Weber J, Kelly J. Lippincott's Learning System: Health Assessment in Nursing. Philadelphia: Lippincott Williams & Wilkins, 1997: 699.

FIGURE 5-13. B, Courtesy of Burdick Corporation, Milton, WI.

FIGURE 5-15. A, Courtesy of Acuson Corporation, Mountain View, CA. B, Courtesy of Orange Coast College, Costa Mesa, CA.

FIGURE 5-16. Doppler color flow. Courtesy of Hoag Memorial Presbyterian Hospital, Newport Beach, CA.

FIGURE 5-19. PTCA. Courtesy of Medtronic Interventional Vascular, San Diego, CA.

FIGURE 5-20. A, Redrawn from About Your Pacemaker. Sylmar, CA: Siemens Pacesetter, p. 18. B, Courtesy of Philips Medical Systems, Shelton, CT.

FIGURE 6-3. White and red blood cells. Wintrobe's Clinical Hematology, 9th ed. Philadelphia: Lea & Febiger, 1993. Platelets. Courtesy of Mosby's Medical Nursing and Allied Health Dictionary, 4th ed. St. Louis: Mosby Yearbook, 1994:1230.

FIGURE 6-5. From Lee GR, et al. Wintrobe's Clinical Hematology, 10th ed. Philadelphia: Lippincott Williams & Wilkins, Fig 30.4A, pp. 910, 911.

FIGURE 6-6. From Lee GR, et al. Wintrobe's Clinical Hematology, 9th ed. Philadelphia: Lea & Febiger, 1993;1:758.

FIGURE 7-7. From Sheldon H. Boyd's Introduction to the Study of Disease, 11th ed. Philadelphia: Lea & Febiger, 1992:340.

FIGURE 7-9. Courtesy of Temple University Health Sciences Center, Philadelphia, PA.

FIGURE 7-10. Courtesy of Felix Wang, MD, University of California at Irvine, Irvine, CA.

FIGURE 7-11. Courtesy of SensorMedics, Yorba Linda, CA.

FIGURE 7-12. Courtesy of Felix Wang, MD, University of California at Irvine, Irvine, CA.

FIGURE 8-3. Inset. From Haines DL. Neuroanatomy: An Atlas of Structures, Sections, and Systems, 4th ed. Baltimore: Williams & Wilkins, 1995:29.

FIGURE 8-4. From Haines DL. Neuroanatomy: An Atlas of Structures, Sections, and Systems, 4th ed. Baltimore: Williams & Wilkins, 1995:131,237.

FIGURE 8-8. Courtesy of Saied Tohamy, MD.

FIGURE 8-9. Courtesy of Mission Regional Imaging, Mission Viejo, CA

FIGURE 8-10. From Pillitteri: Child Health Nursing: Care of the Child and Family. Philadelphia: Lippincott Williams & Wilkins 1999, Fig 18.13, p. 532.

FIGURE 8-11. From Haines DL. Neuroanatomy: An Atlas of Structures, Sections, and Systems, 4th ed. Baltimore: Williams & Wilkins, 1995:29.

FIGURE 8-12. Courtesy of SensorMedics, Yorba Linda, CA.

FIGURE 8-13. Courtesy of Newport Diagnostic Center, Newport Beach, CA.

FIGURE 8-16. Courtesy of Carl Zeiss, Inc.

FIGURE 8-18. Courtesy of Varian Medical Systems, Palo Alto, CA.

FIGURE 8-19. Courtesy of Radionics, Burlington, MA.

FIGURE 9-3. From Weber J, Kelly J. Lippincott's Learning System: Health Assessment in Nursing. Philadelphia: Lippincott Williams & Wilkins, 1997:188.

FIGURE 9-4. From Weber J, Kelly J. Lippincott's Learning System: Health Assessment in Nursing. Philadelphia: Lippincott Williams & Wilkins, 1997:188.

FIGURE 9-5. From Sheldon H. Boyd's Introduction to the Study of Disease, 11th ed. Philadelphia: Lea & Febiger, 1992:640.

FIGURE 9-6. From Weber J, Kelly J. Lippincott's Learning System: Health Assessment in Nursing. Philadelphia: Lippincott Williams & Wilkins, 1997:188.

FIGURE 9-7. Courtesy of Felix Wang MD, University of California, Irvine.

FIGURE 10-4. From Weber J, Kelly J. Lippincott's Learning System: Health Assessment in Nursing. Philadelphia: Lippincott Williams & Wilkins, 1997:254.

FIGURE 10-6. From Weber J, Kelly J. Lippincott's Learning System: Health Assessment in Nursing. Philadelphia: Lippincott Williams & Wilkins, 1997:254.

FIGURE 10-7. From Coles WH. Ophthalmology: A Diagnostic Text. Baltimore: Williams & Wilkins, 1989:203,205.

FIGURE 10-8. Courtesy of Welch Allyn, Skaneateles Falls, NY.

FIGURE 10-9. Courtesy of Nikon, Inc., Melville, NY.

FIGURE 11-2. Courtesy of Welch Allyn, Skaneateles Falls, NY.

FIGURE 12-5. From West J Med 1981;134:415.

FIGURE 12-6. Redrawn from poster created by Reed & Carnrick, Kenilworth, MJ. Endoscope and fiberoptics. Courtesy of Olympu America, Inc., Lake Success, NY. Photographs. Courtesy of Mission Hospital Regional Medical Center, Mission Viejo, CA.

FIGURE 12-12. From Am Fam Physician 1992;44:827.

FIGURE 12-13. Courtesy of William Brant, MD.

FIGURE 12-14. Courtesy of Acuson Corporation, Mountain View, CA.

FIGURE 13-3. From McClatchey KD, et al. Clinical Laboratory Medicine, 2nd ed. 2001.

FIGURE 13-4. From McClatchey KD, et al. Clinical Laboratory Medicine, 2nd ed. 2001.

FIGURE 13-5. From Sheldon H. Boyd's Introduction to the Study of Disease, 11th ed. Philadelphia: Lea & Febiger, 1992:436.

FIGURE 13-7. Courtesy of Mission Regional Imaging, Mission Viejo, CA.

FIGURE 13-9. Courtesy of Circon Corporation, Santa Barbara, CA.

FIGURE 13-10. Courtesy of Circon Corporation, Santa Barbara, CA.

FIGURE 14-5. Courtesy of LJ Underwood and RD Underwood, Mission Viejo, CA.

FIGURE 15-4. B, Courtesy of Medison American, Inc., Cypress, CA.

FIGURE 15-6. Courtesy of Cabbott Medical/Cryomedics, Langhorne, PA.

FIGURE 15-9. From Micha JP. Genital Warts: Treatable Warning of Cancer. Belle Mead, NJ: Excerpta Medica, p. 31.

FIGURE 15-12. Courtesy of Siemens Medical Systems, Inc., Danvers, MA.

FIGURE 15-17. From Georgiade GS, et al. Textbook of Plastic, Maxillofacial and Reconstructive Surgery, 2nd ed. Baltimore: Williams & Wilkins, 1992:853,863.

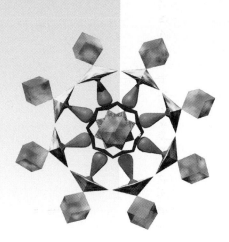

Index

Page numbers in *italics* denote figures.

Symbols
< (less than) symbol, 72, 702
> (greater than) symbol, 72, 702

A
-a, 12
A-, 14, 675
ā (before), 70
A (anterior, assessment), 691
A (assessment), 41
A & P (ausculation and percussion), 640, 691
A & W (alive and well), 41, 691
Ab-, 14, 675
AB (abortion), 653, 691
Abbreviations
    medical records, 64–66
    prescription, 70–72
    Roman numerals, symbols, 72, 702
    symbols, 65–66, 67, 701–702
    units of measure, 67–68
Abdomen
    anatomic divisions, 498, *499*
    diagnostic terms, 505–509, *506*, *507*, *509*
    diagnostic tests and procedures, 514–517
    medical record analysis, 536–541
    operative terms, 521–522, *522*
    practice exercises, 527–535, *534*, 542–543
    programmed review
        anatomic divisions, 499–500, *500*
        diagnostic terms, 510–514
        diagnostic tests and procedures, 517–520
        operative terms, 523–525
        symptomatic terms, 503–505
    symptomatic terms, *501*, 501–502

term component, 683
    therapeutic terms, 526–527
Abdominal aorta, *546*
Abdominal hysterectomy, 640
Abdominal sonogram, 517, *517*, 560
Abdomin/o, 22, 487, 675
Abdominocentesis, 521
Abduction, *147*, 148
ABGs (arterial blood gases), 298, 691
Abnormal, term component, 683
Abnormal reduction, term component, 683
Abortifacient, 659
Abortion (AB), 653
Above, term component, 683
Abruptio placentae, 654
Abscess, 105
Absence, 344
-ac, 9, 18, 675
ac (before meals), 70, 691
Accommodation, 434
ACE (angiotensin-converting enzyme) inhibitor, 223, 691
acetaminophen and codeine, 703
Acne, 104
Across, term component, 683
Acous/o, 459, 675
Acquired immunodeficiency syndrome (AIDS), 252, 691
Acr/o, 22, 675
Acromegaly, 403, *403*
ACTH (adrenocorticotrophic hormone), 395, 691
Actinic keratoses, 105
Active immunity, 248
-acusis (additional suffix), 460, 675
Acute, 62
Ad-, 14, 675
AD (right ear), 71, 691

P-1 a- an-	**P-6** bi-
P-2 ab-	**P-7** brady-
P-3 ad-	**P-8** circum- peri-
P-4 ante- pre- pro-	**P-9** con- syn- sym-
P-5 anti- contra-	**P-10** de-

two, or both

bilateral

without

aphagia
anesthesia

slow

bradycardia

away from

abnormal

around

circumcise
periosteal

to, toward, or near

adhesion

together or with

congenital
syndactylism
symbiosis

before

antepartum
premature
proactive

from, down, or not

degenerate

against or opposed to

antitoxic
contraindicated

P-11

dia-

trans-

P-16

epi-

P-12

dys-

P-17

eu-

P-13

e-

ec-

ex-

P-18

hemi-

semi-

P-14

ecto-

exo-

extra-

P-19

hyper-

P-15

en-

endo-

intra-

P-20

hypo-

upon

epidermal

across or through

diameter
transmission

good or normal

eugenic

painful, difficult, or faulty

dysfunction

half

hemicephalia

semilunar

out or away

evacuate
eccentric
excise

above or excessive

hyperlipemia

outside

ectomorphic
exocrine
extravasation

below or deficient

hypothermia

within

encapsulate
endoscope
intradermal

P-21

inter-

P-26

mono-
uni-

P-22

macro-

P-27

neo-

P-23

meso-

P-28

oligo-

P-24

meta-

P-29

pan-

P-25

micro-

P-30

para-

one

monocyte

unilateral

between

interaction

new

neoplasia

large or long

macrocyte

few or deficient

oligotrophia

middle

mesomorphic

all

panacea

beyond, after, or change

metastasis

metamorphosis

alongside of, or abnormal

paramedic

paranoia

small

microscope

P-31

poly-

multi-

P-36

sub-

infra-

P-32

post-

P-37

super-

supra-

P-33

quadri-

P-38

tachy-

P-34

re-

P-39

tri-

P-35

retro-

P-40

ultra-

below or under

<u>sub</u>cutaneous

<u>infra</u>umbilical

many

<u>poly</u>phobia

<u>multi</u>cellular

above or excessive

<u>super</u>numerary

<u>supra</u>renal

after, or behind

<u>post</u>operative

fast

<u>tachy</u>cardia

four

<u>quadri</u>plegia

three

<u>tri</u>angle

again or back

<u>re</u>activate

beyond or excessive

<u>ultra</u>sonic

backward or behind

<u>retro</u>grade

S-1 -ac -al -ar -ary	**S-5** -centesis
S-1 -eal -ous -ic -tic	**S-6** -desis
S-2 -algia -dynia	**S-7** -e
S-3 -ation	**S-8** -ectasis
S-4 -cele	**S-9** -ectomy

puncture for aspiration

abdomino<u>centesis</u>

pertaining to (adjective endings)

cardi<u>ac</u>
ped<u>al</u>
glandul<u>ar</u>
pulmon<u>ary</u>

binding

arthro<u>desis</u>

pertaining to (adjective endings)

esophag<u>eal</u>
fibr<u>ous</u>
tox<u>ic</u>
cyano<u>tic</u>

noun marker

erythrocyt<u>e</u>

pain

cephal<u>algia</u>
cephalo<u>dynia</u>

expansion or dilation

angi<u>ectasis</u>

process

extravas<u>ation</u>

excision (removal)

append<u>ectomy</u>

pouching or hernia

gastro<u>cele</u>

S-10

-emia

S-15

-iasis

S-11

-genesis

S-16

-icle
-ole
-ula

S-12

-gram
-graph
-graphy

S-17

-ule

-itis

S-13

-ia
-ism

S-18

-ium

S-14

-iatrics
-iatry

S-19

-logy
-logist
-ist

formation or presence of

lith<u>iasis</u>

blood condition

hyperlip<u>emia</u>

small

ventr<u>icle</u>
arteri<u>ole</u>
mac<u>ula</u>
pust<u>ule</u>

origin or production

patho<u>genesis</u>

inflammation

appendic<u>itis</u>

record
sono<u>gram</u>

instrument for recording
sono<u>graph</u>

process of recording
sono<u>graphy</u>

structure or tissue

epigastr<u>ium</u>
pericard<u>ium</u>

condition of

pneumon<u>ia</u>
perfection<u>ism</u>

study of
one who specializes in
histo<u>logy</u>

the study or treatment of
onco<u>logist</u>

one who specializes in
thera<u>pist</u>

treatment

ped<u>iatrics</u>
psych<u>iatry</u>

S-20 **-lysis**	S-25 **-oma**
S-21 **-malacia**	S-26 **-osis**
S-22 **-megaly**	S-27 **-penia**
S-23 **-meter** **-metry**	S-28 **-pexy**
S-24 **-oid**	S-29 **-phil** **-philia**

tumor

carcin<u>oma</u>

breaking down or dissolution

hemo<u>lysis</u>

condition or increase

scler<u>osis</u>
leukocyt<u>osis</u>

softening

osteo<u>malacia</u>

abnormal reduction

pancyto<u>penia</u>

enlargement

hepato<u>megaly</u>

suspension or fixation

nephro<u>pexy</u>

instrument for measuring

spiro<u>meter</u>

process of measuring

spiro<u>metry</u>

attraction for

neutro<u>phil</u>
pneumo<u>philia</u>

resembling

lip<u>oid</u>

S-30

-plasty

S-31

-poiesis

S-32

-ptosis

S-33

-rrhage
-rrhagia

S-34

-rrhaphy

S-35

-rrhea

S-36

-rrhexis

S-37

-scope

-scopy

S-38

-spasm

S-39

-stasis

discharge

ameno<u>rrhea</u>
rhino<u>rrhea</u>

**surgical repair
or reconstruction**

rhino<u>plasty</u>

rupture

cardio<u>rrhexis</u>

formation

hemo<u>poiesis</u>

instrument for examination

endo<u>scope</u>

process of examination

endo<u>scopy</u>

**falling or downward
displacement**

nephro<u>ptosis</u>

involuntary contraction

vaso<u>spasm</u>

to burst forth

hemo<u>rrhage</u>
meno<u>rrhagia</u>

stop or stand

hemo<u>stasis</u>

suture

osteo<u>rrhaphy</u>

-stomy

-tomy

-y

creation of an opening

colo<u>stomy</u>

incision

lapar<u>otomy</u>

condition or process of

adenopath<u>y</u>

CF-1 abdomin/o lapar/o	**CF-6** arthr/o
CF-2 acr/o	**CF-7** carcin/o
CF-3 aden/o	**CF-8** cardi/o
CF-4 aer/o	**CF-9** cephal/o
CF-5 angi/o vas/o vascul/o	**CF-10** col/o colon/o

joint

arthrodesis

abdomen

abdominal
laparoscopy

cancer

carcinogenic

extremity or topmost

acrodynia
acrophobia

heart

cardiologist

gland

adenoma

head

cephalic

air, gas

aerobic

colon (large intestine)

colostomy
colonoscopy

vessel

angioplasty
vasectomy
vascular

CF-11 crin/o	**CF-16** erythr/o
CF-12 cyan/o	**CF-17** esophag/o
CF-13 cyt/o	**CF-18** esthesi/o
CF-14 derm/o dermat/o cutane/o	**CF-19** fibr/o
CF-15 enter/o	**CF-20** gastr/o

red

erythrocyte

to secrete

endocrinology

esophagus

esophagitis

blue

cyanotic

sensation

anesthesia

cell

cytology

fiber

fibroma

skin

hypodermic
dermatologist
cutaneous

stomach

gastric

small intestine

enterospasm

CF-21	CF-26
gen/o	**hydr/o**
CF-22	CF-27
gynec/o	**leuk/o**
CF-23	CF-28
hem/o **hemat/o**	**lip/o**
CF-24	CF-29
hepat/o	**lith/o**
CF-25	CF-30
hist/o	**melan/o**

water hydrophobia	**origin or production** carcinogenic
white leukocyte	**woman** gynecology
fat lipoid	**blood** hemolysis hematoma
stone lithiasis	**liver** hepatomegaly
black melanoma	**tissue** histogenesis

CF-31	CF-36
morph/o	**onc/o**
CF-32	CF-37
nas/o **rhin/o**	**or/o**
CF-33	CF-38
necr/o	**orth/o**
CF-34	CF-39
nephr/o **ren/o**	**oste/o**
CF-35	CF-40
neur/o	**path/o**

tumor or mass oncology	**form** morphology
mouth oral	**nose** nasal rhinitis
straight, normal, correct orthopedic	**death** necrosis
bone osteogenic	**kidney** nephrectomy renal
disease pathology	**nerve** neuritis

CF-41

ped/o

CF-48

pneum/o
pneumon/o

CF-42

phag/o

CF-47

psych/o

CF-43

phas/o

CF-48

py/o

CF-44

phob/o

CF-49

scler/o

CF-45

plas/o

CF-50

son/o

air or lung

pneumogram
pneumonitis

child or foot

pediatrics
pedal

mind

psychiatry

eat or swallow

phagocyte

pus

pyorrhea

speech

dysphasia

hard

sclerosis

**exaggerated fear
or sensitivity**

hydrophobia
photophobia

sound

sonic

formation

dysplasia

sten/o

tox/o
toxic/o

troph/o

ur/o
urin/o

narrow

<u>steno</u>sis

poison

<u>tox</u>emia
<u>toxico</u>logy

nourishment or development

hyper<u>trophy</u>

urine

<u>uro</u>logy